PROFESSIONAL EDITION

2015
HCPCS Level II

INCLUDES NETTER'S ANATOMY ART

Carol J. Buck
MS, CPC, COC, CCS-P

Former Program Director
Medical Secretary Programs
Northwest Technical College
East Grand Forks, Minnesota

SAUNDERS

3251 Riverport Lane
St. Louis, Missouri 63043

2015 HCPCS LEVEL II, PROFESSIONAL EDITION

ISBN: 978-0-323-27986-4
ISSN: 2211-4985

Notices

Knowledge and best practice in this field are constantly changing. As new research and experience broaden our understanding, changes in research methods, professional practices, or medical treatment may become necessary.

Practitioners and researchers must always rely on their own experience and knowledge in evaluating and using any information, methods, compounds, or experiments described herein. In using such information or methods they should be mindful of their own safety and the safety of others, including parties for whom they have a professional responsibility.

With respect to any drug or pharmaceutical products identified, readers are advised to check the most current information provided (i) on procedures featured or (ii) by the manufacturer of each product to be administered, to verify the recommended dose or formula, the method and duration of administration, and contraindications. It is the responsibility of practitioners, relying on their own experience and knowledge of their patients, to make diagnoses, to determine dosages and the best treatment for each individual patient, and to take all appropriate safety precautions.

To the fullest extent of the law, neither the Publisher nor the authors, contributors, or editors, assume any liability for any injury and/or damage to persons or property as a matter of products liability, negligence or otherwise, or from any use or operation of any methods, products, instructions, or ideas contained in the material herein.

International Standard Book Number: 978-0-323-27986-4

Director, Private Sector Education & Professional/Reference: Jeanne Olson
Senior Content Development Specialist: Jenna Price
Publishing Services Manager: Pat Joiner
Senior Designer: Amy Buxton

Printed in Canada

Last digit is the print number: 9   8   7   6   5   4   3   2   1

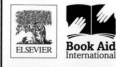

Working together
to grow libraries in
developing countries

www.elsevier.com • www.bookaid.org

TECHNICAL COLLABORATORS

Jacqueline Klitz Grass, MA, CPC
Coding and Reimbursement Specialist
Grand Forks, North Dakota

Nancy Maguire, ACS, CRT, PCS, FCS, HCS-D, APC, AFC
Physician Consultant for Auditing and Education
Winchester, Virginia

CONTENTS

Updates will be posted on codingupdates.com when available.

Check codingupdates.com for Practitioner and Facility Medically Unlikely Edits (MUEs) and Column 1 and Column 2 Edits.

Check the Centers for Medicare and Medicaid Services (www.cms.gov/Manuals/IOM/list.asp) website and codingupdates.com for full and select IOMs.

Notice: 2015 DMEPOS updates were unavailable at the time of printing. Check codingupdates.com for updates in January. Also available online are the 2015 PQRS Measures List and Specifications Manual.

GUIDE TO USING THE 2015 HCPCS LEVEL II CODES

Medical coding has long been a part of the health care profession. Through the years medical coding systems have become more complex and extensive. Today, medical coding is an intricate and immense process that is present in every health care setting. The increased use of electronic submissions for health care services only increases the need for coders who understand the coding process.

2015 HCPCS Level II was developed to help meet the needs of today's coder.

All material adheres to the latest government versions available at the time of printing.

Annotated

Throughout this text, revisions and additions are indicated by the following symbols:

◄ **New:** Additions to the previous edition are indicated by the color triangle.

↻ **Revised:** Revisions within the line or code from the previous edition are indicated by the color arrow.

✔ **Reinstated** indicates a code that was previously deleted and has now been reactivated.

✖ deleted words have been removed from this year's edition.

HCPCS Symbols

⊚ **Special coverage instructions** apply to these codes. Usually these special coverage instructions are included in the Internet Only Manuals (IOM). References to the IOM locations are given in the form of Medicare Pub. 100 reference numbers listed below the code. IOM select references are located at codingupdates.com.

⊘ **Not covered or valid by Medicare** is indicated by the "No" symbol. Usually the reason for the exclusion is included in the Internet Only Manuals (IOM) select references at codingupdates.com.

* **Carrier discretion** is an indication that you must contact the individual third-party payers to find out the coverage available for codes identified by this symbol.

NDC Drugs approved for Medicare Part B are listed as NDC (National Drug Code). All other FDA-approved drugs are listed as Other.

A2-Z3 **ASC Payment Indicators** identify the 2015 final payment for the code. A list of Payment Indicators is listed in the front material of this text.

A-Y **ASC Status Indicators** identify the 2015 final status assigned to the code. A list of Status Indicators is listed in the front material of this text.

Ⓑ Bill local carrier.

Ⓑ Bill DME MAC.

Coding Clinic Indicates the American Hospital Association *Coding Clinic for HCPCS* references by year, quarter, and page number.

♿ DMEPOS identifies durable medical equipment, prosthetics, orthotics, and supplies that may be eligible for payment from CMS.

♀ Indicates a code for female only.

♂ Indicates a code for male only.

Ⓐ Indicates a code with an indication of age

🅿 Indicates a code included in the 2014 PQRS Quality Measure Specifications Manual.

Qp Indicates there is a maximum allowable number of units of service, per day, per patient for physician/provider services (*see* codingupdates.com for Practitioner Medically Unlikely Edits).

Qh Indicates there is a maximum allowable number of units of service, per day, per patient in the outpatient hospital setting (*see* codingupdates.com for Hospital Medically Unlikely Edits).

Red, green, and blue typeface terms within the Table of Drugs and tabular section are terms added by the publisher and do not appear in the official code set. Information supplementing the official HCPCS Index produced by CMS is *italicized*.

SYMBOLS AND CONVENTIONS

HCPCS Symbols

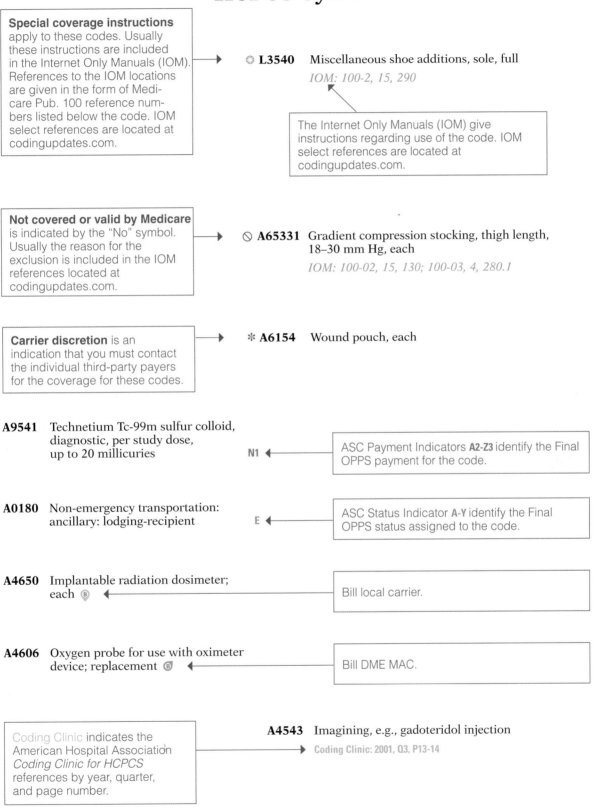

Special coverage instructions apply to these codes. Usually these instructions are included in the Internet Only Manuals (IOM). References to the IOM locations are given in the form of Medicare Pub. 100 reference numbers listed below the code. IOM select references are located at codingupdates.com.

⊛ **L3540**   Miscellaneous shoe additions, sole, full

IOM: 100-2, 15, 290

The Internet Only Manuals (IOM) give instructions regarding use of the code. IOM select references are located at codingupdates.com.

Not covered or valid by Medicare is indicated by the "No" symbol. Usually the reason for the exclusion is included in the IOM references located at codingupdates.com.

⊘ **A65331**   Gradient compression stocking, thigh length, 18–30 mm Hg, each

IOM: 100-02, 15, 130; 100-03, 4, 280.1

Carrier discretion is an indication that you must contact the individual third-party payers for the coverage for these codes.

✳ **A6154**   Wound pouch, each

A9541   Technetium Tc-99m sulfur colloid, diagnostic, per study dose, up to 20 millicuries

N1   ASC Payment Indicators **A2-Z3** identify the Final OPPS payment for the code.

A0180   Non-emergency transportation: ancillary: lodging-recipient

E   ASC Status Indicator **A-Y** identify the Final OPPS status assigned to the code.

A4650   Implantable radiation dosimeter; each ⓑ

Bill local carrier.

A4606   Oxygen probe for use with oximeter device; replacement ⓑ

Bill DME MAC.

Coding Clinic indicates the American Hospital Association *Coding Clinic for HCPCS* references by year, quarter, and page number.

A4543   Imagining, e.g., gadoteridol injection

Coding Clinic: 2001, Q3, P13-14

Codes shown are for illustration purposes only and may not be current codes.

DMEPOS symbol identifies durable medical equipment, prosthetics, orthotics, and supplies that may be eligible for payment from CMS.

→ **E2210**   Wheelchair accessory, bearings, any type, replacement only, each ♿

❋ **A4233**   Replacement battery, alkaline (other than J cell), for use with medically necessary home blood glucose monitor owned by patient, each ♿ ←

On DMEPOS Fee Schedule.

If "incident to" physician service, do not bill; otherwise bill DME MAC

DMEPOS Modifier(s): NU, KL ←

DMEPOS modifier(s).

✿ **B9000**   Enteral nutrition infusion pump - without alarm [Qp]   γ

Pump will be denied as not medically necessary if medical necessity of pump is not documented

IOM: 100-02, 15, 120; 100-03, 3, 180.2; 100-04, 20, 100.2.2

PEN: On Fee Schedule ←
PEN Modifier(s): NU, RR, UE

On the Parenteral and Enteral Nutrition Items or Services (PEN) with modifier(s) from current PEN Fee Schedule.

A4261   Cervical cap for contraceptive use ♀ ←

Indicates for female only.

A4267   Contraceptive supply, condom, male, each ♂ ←

Indicates for male only.

Indicates a **reinstated** code.

→ ✔ **D2970**   Temporary crown (fractured tooth)

Indicates **new** information or a new code.

→ ▶ **A4614**   Peak expiratory flow rate meter, hand-held

Indicates a **revision** within the line or code.

→ ↻ **J0270**   Injection alprostadil, per 1.25 mcg

Codes shown are for illustration purposes only and may not be current codes.

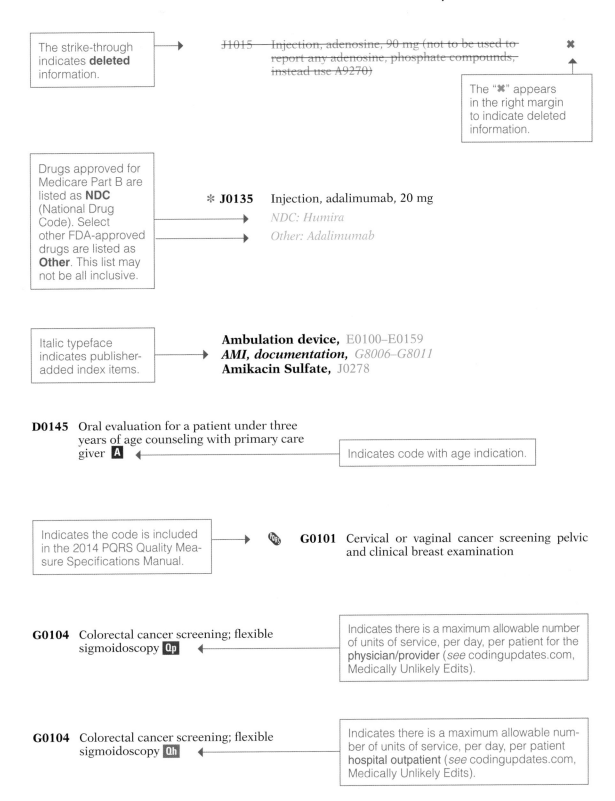

The strike-through indicates **deleted** information.

~~J1015   Injection, adenosine, 90 mg (not to be used to report any adenosine, phosphate compounds, instead use A9270)~~   ✖

The "✖" appears in the right margin to indicate deleted information.

Drugs approved for Medicare Part B are listed as **NDC** (National Drug Code). Select other FDA-approved drugs are listed as **Other**. This list may not be all inclusive.

✱ **J0135**   Injection, adalimumab, 20 mg
NDC: Humira
Other: Adalimumab

Italic typeface indicates publisher-added index items.

Ambulation device, *E0100–E0159*
AMI, documentation, *G8006–G8011*
Amikacin Sulfate, J0278

D0145   Oral evaluation for a patient under three years of age counseling with primary care giver **A**

Indicates code with age indication.

Indicates the code is included in the 2014 PQRS Quality Measure Specifications Manual.

G0101   Cervical or vaginal cancer screening pelvic and clinical breast examination

G0104   Colorectal cancer screening; flexible sigmoidoscopy **Qp**

Indicates there is a maximum allowable number of units of service, per day, per patient for the **physician/provider** (*see* codingupdates.com, Medically Unlikely Edits).

G0104   Colorectal cancer screening; flexible sigmoidoscopy **Qh**

Indicates there is a maximum allowable number of units of service, per day, per patient **hospital outpatient** (*see* codingupdates.com, Medically Unlikely Edits).

Codes shown are for illustration purposes only and may not be current codes.

2015 HCPCS UPDATES

2015 HCPCS New/Revised/Deleted Codes and Modifiers

HCPCS quarterly updates are posted on the companion website (www.codingupdates.com) when available.

NEW CODES/MODIFIERS

L1	C9740	G6011	G6038	G9365	G9396	G9421	G9448	J0153	K0901
PO	C9742	G6012	G6039	G9366	G9399	G9422	G9449	J0571	K0902
SZ	G0276	G6013	G6040	G9367	G9400	G9423	G9450	J0572	L3981
XE	G0277	G6014	G6041	G9368	G9401	G9424	G9451	J0573	L6026
XP	G0279	G6015	G6042	G9369	G9402	G9425	G9452	J0574	L7259
XS	G0464	G6016	G6043	G9370	G9403	G9426	G9453	J0575	L8696
XU	G0466	G6017	G6044	G9376	G9404	G9427	G9454	J0887	Q4150
A4459	G0467	G6018	G6045	G9377	G9405	G9428	G9455	J0888	Q4151
A4602	G0468	G6019	G6046	G9378	G9406	G9429	G9456	J1071	Q4152
A7048	G0469	G6020	G6047	G9379	G9407	G9430	G9457	J1322	Q4153
A9606	G0470	G6021	G6048	G9380	G9408	G9431	G9458	J1439	Q4154
C2624	G0471	G6022	G6049	G9381	G9409	G9432	G9459	J2274	Q4155
C2644	G0472	G6023	G6050	G9382	G9410	G9433	G9460	J2704	Q4156
C9025	G0473	G6024	G6051	G9383	G9411	G9434	G9463	J3121	Q4157
C9026	G6001	G6025	G6052	G9384	G9412	G9435	G9464	J3145	Q4158
C9027	G6002	G6027	G6053	G9385	G9413	G9436	G9465	J7181	Q4159
C9136	G6003	G6028	G6054	G9386	G9414	G9437	G9466	J7182	Q4160
C9349	G6004	G6030	G6055	G9389	G9415	G9438	G9467	J7200	S1034
C9442	G6005	G6031	G6056	G9390	G9416	G9439	G9468	J7201	S1035
C9443	G6006	G6032	G6057	G9391	G9417	G9440	G9469	J7327	S1036
C9444	G6007	G6034	G6058	G9392	G9418	G9441	G9470	J7336	S1037
C9446	G6008	G6035	G9362	G9393	G9419	G9442	G9471	J9267	S8032
C9447	G6009	G6036	G9363	G9394	G9420	G9443	G9472	J9301	S9901
C9739	G6010	G6037	G9364	G9395					

REVISED CODES/MODIFIERS

Change in description	G9296	L8680	A4740	E0764	E1600	E2504	J9218	Q4029
	G9297		A4750	E0849	E1610	E2506	J9219	Q4030
A4601	G9298	**Payment change**	A4755	E0855	E1615	E2508	J9300	Q4031
C9741	G9299		A4760	E0984	E1620	E2510	J9390	Q4032
E0856	G9303	A4248	A4765	E1002	E1625	E2599	K0607	Q4033
E0986	G9304	A4565	A4766	E1003	E1630	G0127	K0730	Q4034
G0204	G9329	A4639	A4770	E1004	E1632	G0247	Q0515	Q4035
G0206	G9340	A4651	A4771	E1005	E1634	G0364	Q4001	Q4036
G0416	G9341	A4652	A4772	E1006	E1635	G0448	Q4002	Q4037
G8461	G9342	A4653	A4773	E1007	E1636	J0120	Q4003	Q4038
G8474	G9343	A4657	A4774	E1008	E1637	J0200	Q4004	Q4039
G8476	G9344	A4660	A4802	E1010	E1639	J0205	Q4005	Q4040
G8477	G9345	A4663	A4860	E1014	E1699	J0395	Q4006	Q4041
G8483	G9346	A4671	A4870	E1029	E1700	J0725	Q4007	Q4042
G8484	G9347	A4672	A4890	E1030	E2227	J1364	Q4008	Q4043
G8571	J7195	A4673	A4911	E1161	E2310	J1435	Q4009	Q4044
G8572	J7301	A4674	A4913	E1232	E2311	J1455	Q4010	Q4045
G8720	L7367	A4680	A4918	E1233	E2312	J1460	Q4011	Q4046
G8840	Q4119	A4690	A4927	E1234	E2313	J1560	Q4012	Q4047
G8843	Q4147	A4706	A4928	E1235	E2321	J1562	Q4013	Q4048
G8861	S0183	A4707	A4929	E1236	E2322	J1570	Q4014	Q4049
G8876	V2799	A4708	A4930	E1237	E2325	J1600	Q4015	Q4121
G8924		A4709	A4931	E1238	E2326	J1930	Q4016	Q4131
G8936	**Change in administrative data field**	A4714	A7025	E1500	E2327	J2212	Q4017	Q4132
G8968		A4719	A9586	E1510	E2328	J2320	Q4018	Q4133
G9160		A4720	C9248	E1520	E2329	J2725	Q4019	Q9968
G9163		A4721	C9250	E1530	E2330	J2941	Q4020	V2630
G9166	A4466	A4722	C9290	E1540	E2351	J3070	Q4021	V2631
G9169	A9272	A4723	E0117	E1550	E2373	J3365	Q4022	V2632
G9172	A9274	A4724	E0144	E1560	E2374	J3485	Q4023	
G9175	A9279	A4725	E0198	E1570	E2376	J7178	Q4024	**Change in short description**
G9186	E1358	A4726	E0300	E1575	E2377	J7180	Q4025	
G9210	E2230	A4728	E0620	E1580	E2378	J7505	Q4026	
G9242	J1826	A4730	E0656	E1590	E2500	J9160	Q4027	J7302
G9277	J8565	A4736	E0657	E1592	E2502	J9215	Q4028	L3980
G9278	J9010	A4737	E0740	E1594				

DELETED CODES/MODIFIERS

A7042	G0456	G8492	G8594	G8705	G8772	G8888	G8943	G9224	J3130
A7043	G0457	G8493	G8595	G8706	G8773	G8889	G8949	G9248	J3140
C1300	G0461	G8501	G8597	G8707	G8774	G8890	G8957	G9249	J3150
C9021	G0462	G8502	G8629	G8736	G8775	G8891	G9193	G9252	J7335
C9022	G0908	G8547	G8630	G8737	G8776	G8892	G9194	G9253	J9265
C9023	G0909	G8552	G8631	G8738	G8777	G8893	G9195	G9271	L6025
C9133	G0910	G8579	G8632	G8739	G8778	G8894	G9199	G9272	L7260
C9134	G0919	G8580	G8682	G8740	G8779	G8895	G9200	J0150	L7261
C9135	G0920	G8581	G8683	G8751	G8780	G8896	G9201	J0151	M0064
C9441	G0921	G8582	G8685	G8763	G8781	G8897	G9202	J0900	Q9970
C9735	G0922	G8583	G8699	G8764	G8782	G8904	G9214	J1060	Q9972
G0173	G8126	G8584	G8700	G8767	G8859	G8905	G9215	J1070	Q9973
G0251	G8127	G8585	G8701	G8768	G8860	G8930	G9216	J1080	Q9974
G0417	G8128	G8586	G8702	G8769	G8862	G8931	G9218	J2271	S0144
G0418	G8406	G8587	G8703	G8770	G8886	G8932	G9220	J2275	S3855
G0419	G8464	G8593	G8704	G8771	G8887	G8933	G9221	J3120	

ADDED AND DELETED DURING 2014

C9021	C9022	C9023	C9134	C9135	Q9970	Q9972	Q9973	Q9974	S0144

NEW, REVISED, AND DELETED DENTAL CODES

New	D6114	D9987	D2915	D6059	D6067	D6075	D6103	D8660	**Deleted**
D0171	D6115		D2920	D6060	D6068	D6076	D6194	D8670	D6053
D0351	D6116	**Revised**	D2975	D6061	D6069	D6077	D6930	D8693	D6054
D1353	D6117	D0350	D3351	D6062	D6070	D6092	D7285	D9221	D6078
D6110	D6549	D0481	D4249	D6063	D6071	D6093	D7286	D9241	D6079
D6111	D9219	D1208	D4260	D6064	D6072	D6094	D7292	D9242	D6975
D6112	D9931	D1550	D4261	D6065	D6073	D6101	D7293	D9248	
D6113	D9986	D2910	D6058	D6066	D6074	D6102	D7294		

A2-Z3 ASC Payment Indicators

Final ASC Payment Indicators for CY 2015	
Payment Indicator	**Payment Indicator Definition**
A2	Surgical procedure on ASC list in CY 2007; payment based on OPPS relative payment weight.
D5	Deleted/discontinued code; no payment made.
F4	Corneal tissue acquisition, hepatitis B vaccine; paid at reasonable cost.
G2	Non office-based surgical procedure added in CY 2008 or later; payment based on OPPS relative payment weight.
H2	Brachytherapy source paid separately when provided integral to a surgical procedure on ASC list; payment OPPS rate.
J7	OPPS pass-through device paid separately when provided integral to a surgical procedure on ASC list; payment contractor-priced.
J8	Device-intensive procedure; paid at adjusted rate.
K2	Drugs and biologicals paid separately when provided integral to a surgical procedure on ASC list; payment based on OPPS rate.
K7	Unclassified drugs and biologicals; payment contractor-priced.
L1	Influenza vaccine; pneumococcal vaccine. Packaged item/service; no separate payment made.
L6	New Technology Intraocular Lens (NTIOL); special payment.
N1	Packaged service/item; no separate payment made.
P2	Office-based surgical procedure added to ASC list in CY 2008 or later with MPFS nonfacility PE RVUs; payment based on OPPS relative payment weight.
P3	Office-based surgical procedure added to ASC list in CY 2008 or later with MPFS nonfacility PE RVUs; payment based on MPFS nonfacility PE RVUs.
R2	Office-based surgical procedure added to ASC list in CY 2008 or later without MPFS nonfacility PE RVUs; payment based on OPPS relative payment weight.
Z2	Radiology or diagnostic service paid separately when provided integral to a surgical procedure on ASC list; payment based on OPPS relative payment weight.
Z3	Radiology or diagnostic service paid separately when provided integral to a surgical procedure on ASC list; payment based on MPFS nonfacility PE RVUs.

CMS-1613-FC, Final Changes to the ASC Payment System and CY 2015 Payment Rates, http://www.cms.gov/Medicare/Medicare-Fee-for-Service-Payment/ASCPayment/ASC-Regulations-and-Notices.

A-Y ASC Status Indicators

	Final OPPS Payment Status Indicators for CY 2015	
Indicator	**Item/Code/Service**	**OPPS Payment Status**
A	Services furnished to a hospital outpatient that are paid under a fee schedule or payment system other than OPPS, for example:	Not paid under OPPS. Paid by MACs under a fee schedule or payment system other than OPPS. Services are subject to deductible or coinsurance unless indicated otherwise.
	• Ambulance Services	
	• Separately Payable Clinical Diagnostic Laboratory Services	Not subject to deductible or coinsurance.
	• Separately Payable Non-Implantable Prosthetics and Orthotics	
	• Physical, Occupational, and Speech Therapy	
	• Diagnostic Mammography	
	• Screening Mammography	Not subject to deductible or coinsurance.
B	Codes that are not recognized by OPPS when submitted on an outpatient hospital Part B bill type (12x and 13x)	Not paid under OPPS. • May be paid by MACs when submitted on a different bill type, for example, 75x (CORF), but not paid under OPPS. • An alternate code that is recognized by OPPS when submitted on an outpatient hospital Part B bill type (12x and 13x) may be available.
C	Inpatient Procedures	Not paid under OPPS. Admit patient. Bill as inpatient.
D	Discontinued Codes	Not paid under OPPS or any other Medicare payment system.
E	Items, Codes, and Services:	Not paid by Medicare when submitted on outpatient claims (any outpatient bill type).
	• For which pricing information is not available	
	• Not covered by any Medicare outpatient benefit category	
	• Statutorily excluded by Medicare	
	• Not reasonable and necessary	
F	Corneal Tissue Acquisition; Certain CRNA Services and Hepatitis B Vaccines	Not paid under OPPS. Paid at reasonable cost.
G	Pass-Through Drugs and Biologicals	Paid under OPPS; separate APC payment.
H	Pass-Through Device Categories	Separate cost-based pass-through payment; not subject to copayment.
J1	Hospital Part B services paid through a comprehensive APC	Paid under OPPS; all covered Part B services on the claim are packaged with the primary "J1" service for the claim, except services with OPPS SI=F, G, H, L and U; ambulance services; diagnostic and screening mammography; all preventive services; and certain Part B inpatient services.
K	Nonpass-Through Drugs and Nonimplantable Biologicals, including Therapeutic Radiopharmaceuticals	Paid under OPPS: separate APC payment.
L	Influenza Vaccine; Pneumococcal Pneumonia Vaccine	Not paid under OPPS. Paid at reasonable cost; not subject to deductible or coinsurance.
M	Items and Services Not Billable to the MAC	Not paid under OPPS.
N	Items and Services Packaged into APC Rates	Paid under OPPS; payment is packaged into payment for other services. Therefore, there is no separate APC payment.
P	Partial Hospitalization	Paid under OPPS; per diem APC payment.

A-Y ASC Status Indicators—cont'd

	Final OPPS Payment Status Indicators for CY 2015	
Indicator	**Item/Code/Service**	**OPPS Payment Status**
Q1	STV-Packaged Codes	Paid under OPPS; Addendum B displays APC assignments when services are separately payable. (1) Packaged APC payment if billed on the same date of service as a HCPCS code assigned status indicator "S," "T," or "V." (2) In other circumstances, payment is made through a separate APC payment.
Q2	T-Packaged Codes	Paid under OPPS; Addendum B displays APC assignments when services are separately payable. (1) Packaged APC payment if billed on the same date of service as a HCPCS code assigned status indicator "T." (2) In other circumstances, payment is made through a separate APC payment.
Q3	Codes That May Be Paid Through a Composite APC	Paid under OPPS; Addendum B displays APC assignments when services are separately payable. Addendum M displays composite APC assignments when codes are paid through a composite APC. (1) Composite APC payment based on OPPS composite-specific payment criteria. Payment is packaged into a single payment for specific combinations of service. (2) In other circumstances, payment is made through a separate APC payment or packaged into payment for other services.
R	Blood and Blood Products	Paid under OPPS; separate APC payment.
S	Procedure or Service, Not Discounted when Multiple	Paid under OPPS; separate APC payment.
T	Procedure or Service, Multiple Procedure Reduction Applies	Paid under OPPS; separate APC payment.
U	Brachytherapy Sources	Paid under OPPS; separate APC payment.
V	Clinic or Emergency Department Visit	Paid under OPPS; separate APC payment.
Y	Non-Implantable Durable Medical Equipment	Not paid under OPPS. All institutional providers other than home health agencies bill to DMERC.

CMS-1613-FC, Final Changes to the ASC Payment System and CY 2015 Payment Rates, http://www.cms.gov/Medicare/Medicare-Fee-for-Service-Payment/HospitalOutpatientPPS/Hospital-Outpatient-Regulations-and-Notices.html.

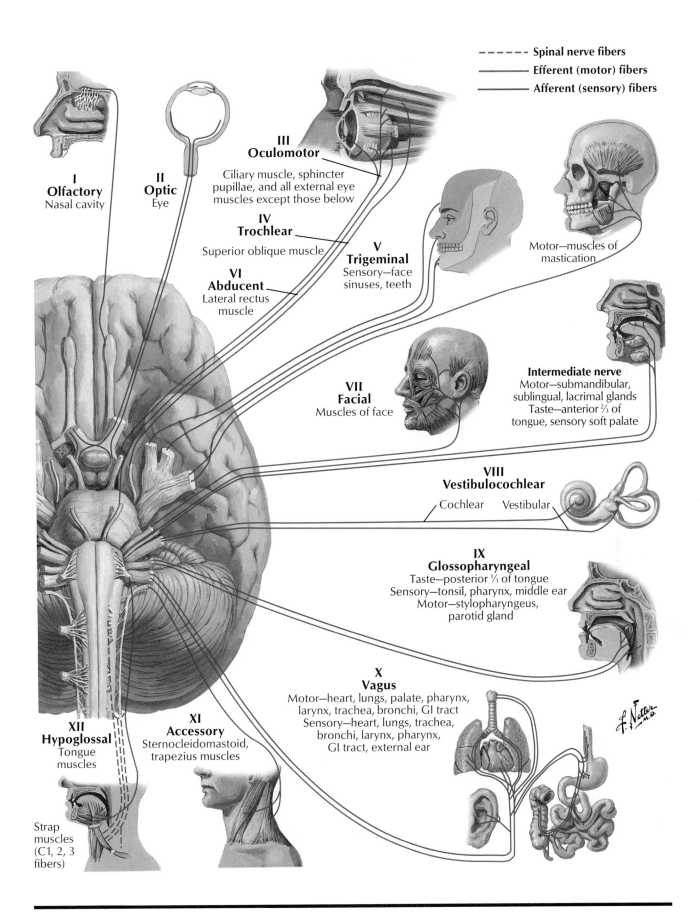

- - - - - Spinal nerve fibers
——— Efferent (motor) fibers
——— Afferent (sensory) fibers

I Olfactory
Nasal cavity

II Optic
Eye

III Oculomotor
Ciliary muscle, sphincter pupillae, and all external eye muscles except those below

IV Trochlear
Superior oblique muscle

V Trigeminal
Sensory—face sinuses, teeth

VI Abducent
Lateral rectus muscle

Motor—muscles of mastication

VII Facial
Muscles of face

Intermediate nerve
Motor—submandibular, sublingual, lacrimal glands
Taste—anterior ⅔ of tongue, sensory soft palate

VIII Vestibulocochlear
Cochlear   Vestibular

IX Glossopharyngeal
Taste—posterior ⅓ of tongue
Sensory—tonsil, pharynx, middle ear
Motor—stylopharyngeus, parotid gland

X Vagus
Motor—heart, lungs, palate, pharynx, larynx, trachea, bronchi, GI tract
Sensory—heart, lungs, trachea, bronchi, larynx, pharynx, GI tract, external ear

XII Hypoglossal
Tongue muscles

XI Accessory
Sternocleidomastoid, trapezius muscles

Strap muscles (C1, 2, 3 fibers)

Plate 118 Cranial Nerves (Motor and Sensory Distribution): Schema. (Netter: Atlas of Human Anatomy, 4 ed, 2006, Saunders.)

Superior view

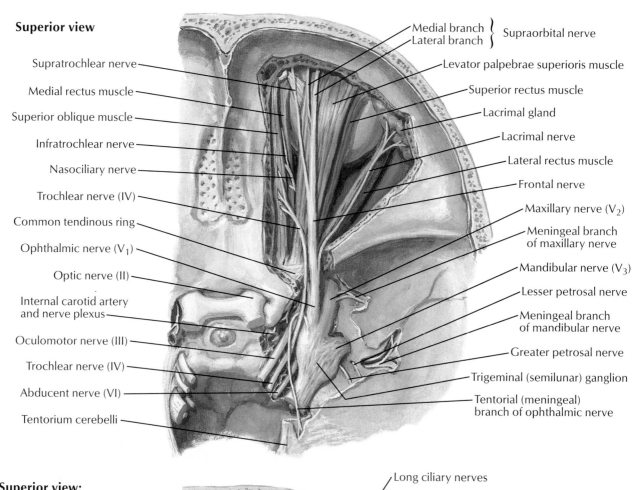

Supratrochlear nerve

Medial rectus muscle

Superior oblique muscle

Infratrochlear nerve

Nasociliary nerve

Trochlear nerve (IV)

Common tendinous ring

Ophthalmic nerve (V₁)

Optic nerve (II)

Internal carotid artery and nerve plexus

Oculomotor nerve (III)

Trochlear nerve (IV)

Abducent nerve (VI)

Tentorium cerebelli

Medial branch
Lateral branch } Supraorbital nerve

Levator palpebrae superioris muscle

Superior rectus muscle

Lacrimal gland

Lacrimal nerve

Lateral rectus muscle

Frontal nerve

Maxillary nerve (V₂)

Meningeal branch of maxillary nerve

Mandibular nerve (V₃)

Lesser petrosal nerve

Meningeal branch of mandibular nerve

Greater petrosal nerve

Trigeminal (semilunar) ganglion

Tentorial (meningeal) branch of ophthalmic nerve

Superior view:
levator palpebrae superioris, superior rectus, and superior oblique muscles partially cut away

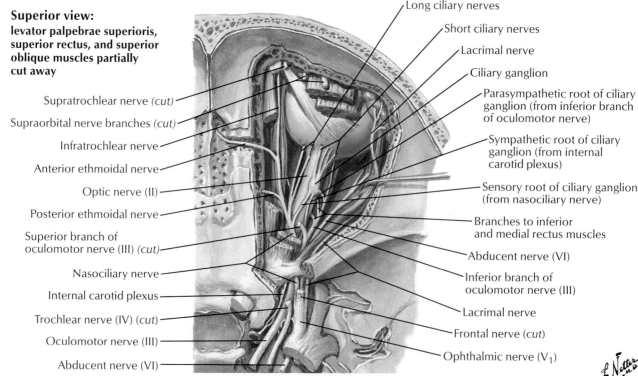

Supratrochlear nerve *(cut)*

Supraorbital nerve branches *(cut)*

Infratrochlear nerve

Anterior ethmoidal nerve

Optic nerve (II)

Posterior ethmoidal nerve

Superior branch of oculomotor nerve (III) *(cut)*

Nasociliary nerve

Internal carotid plexus

Trochlear nerve (IV) *(cut)*

Oculomotor nerve (III)

Abducent nerve (VI)

Long ciliary nerves

Short ciliary nerves

Lacrimal nerve

Ciliary ganglion

Parasympathetic root of ciliary ganglion (from inferior branch of oculomotor nerve)

Sympathetic root of ciliary ganglion (from internal carotid plexus)

Sensory root of ciliary ganglion (from nasociliary nerve)

Branches to inferior and medial rectus muscles

Abducent nerve (VI)

Inferior branch of oculomotor nerve (III)

Lacrimal nerve

Frontal nerve *(cut)*

Ophthalmic nerve (V₁)

Plate 86 Nerves of Orbit. (Netter: Atlas of Human Anatomy, 4 ed, 2006, Saunders.)

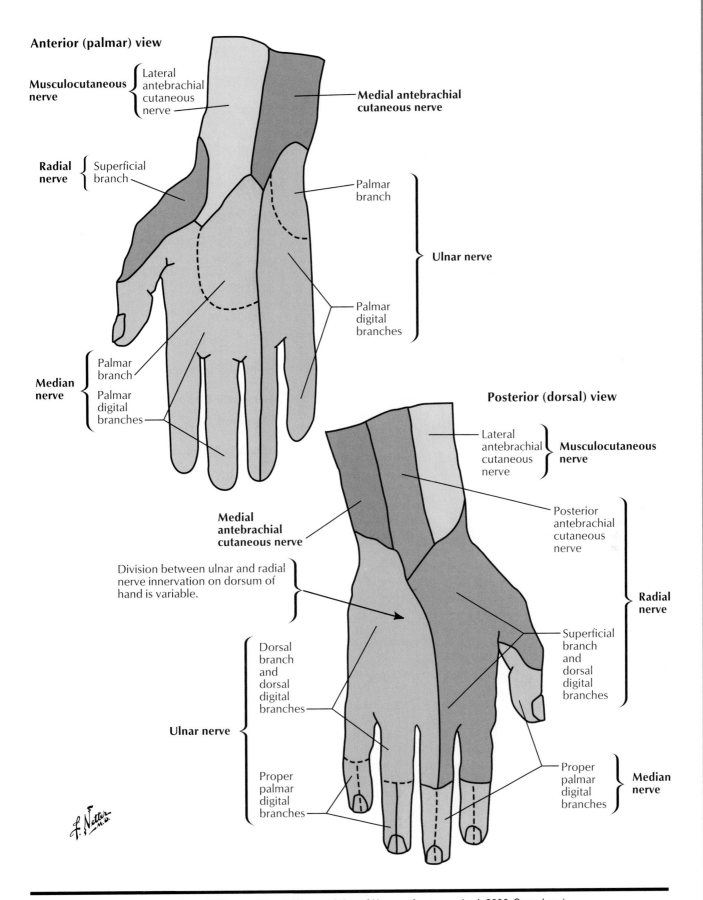

Anterior (palmar) view

Musculocutaneous nerve { Lateral antebrachial cutaneous nerve

Medial antebrachial cutaneous nerve

Radial nerve { Superficial branch

Palmar branch

Ulnar nerve

Palmar digital branches

Median nerve { Palmar branch — Palmar digital branches

Posterior (dorsal) view

Lateral antebrachial cutaneous nerve } **Musculocutaneous nerve**

Medial antebrachial cutaneous nerve

Posterior antebrachial cutaneous nerve

Division between ulnar and radial nerve innervation on dorsum of hand is variable.

Radial nerve

Dorsal branch and dorsal digital branches

Superficial branch and dorsal digital branches

Ulnar nerve

Proper palmar digital branches

Proper palmar digital branches } **Median nerve**

Plate 472 Cutaneous Innervation of Wrist and Hand. (Netter: Atlas of Human Anatomy, 4 ed, 2006, Saunders.)

Anterior view

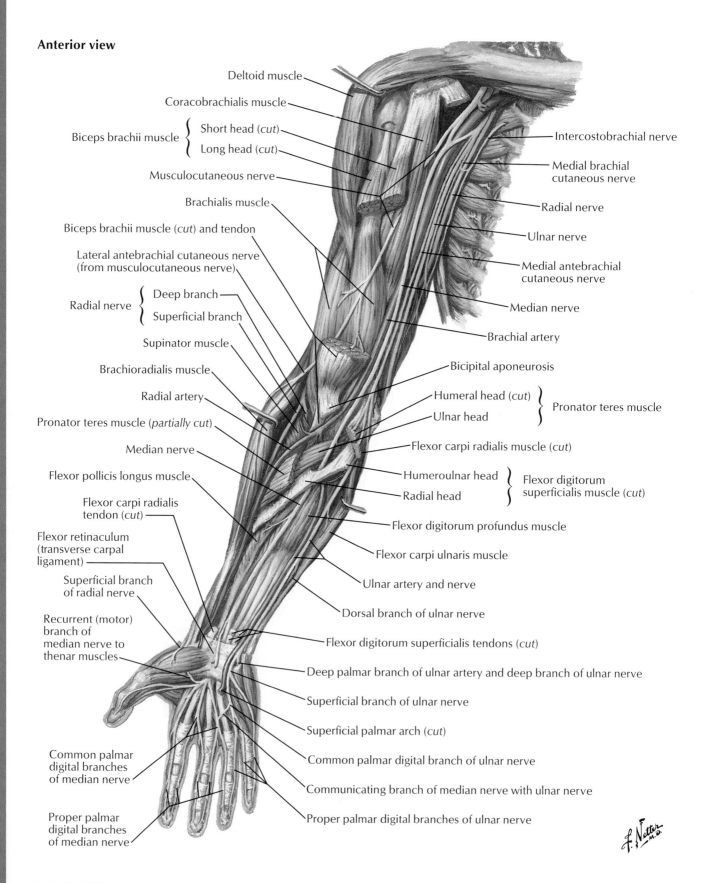

Deltoid muscle

Coracobrachialis muscle

Biceps brachii muscle
- Short head (*cut*)
- Long head (*cut*)

Musculocutaneous nerve

Brachialis muscle

Biceps brachii muscle (*cut*) and tendon

Lateral antebrachial cutaneous nerve (from musculocutaneous nerve)

Radial nerve
- Deep branch
- Superficial branch

Supinator muscle

Brachioradialis muscle

Radial artery

Pronator teres muscle (*partially cut*)

Median nerve

Flexor pollicis longus muscle

Flexor carpi radialis tendon (*cut*)

Flexor retinaculum (transverse carpal ligament)

Superficial branch of radial nerve

Recurrent (motor) branch of median nerve to thenar muscles

Common palmar digital branches of median nerve

Proper palmar digital branches of median nerve

Intercostobrachial nerve

Medial brachial cutaneous nerve

Radial nerve

Ulnar nerve

Medial antebrachial cutaneous nerve

Median nerve

Brachial artery

Bicipital aponeurosis

Humeral head (*cut*)
Ulnar head
} Pronator teres muscle

Flexor carpi radialis muscle (*cut*)

Humeroulnar head
Radial head
} Flexor digitorum superficialis muscle (*cut*)

Flexor digitorum profundus muscle

Flexor carpi ulnaris muscle

Ulnar artery and nerve

Dorsal branch of ulnar nerve

Flexor digitorum superficialis tendons (*cut*)

Deep palmar branch of ulnar artery and deep branch of ulnar nerve

Superficial branch of ulnar nerve

Superficial palmar arch (*cut*)

Common palmar digital branch of ulnar nerve

Communicating branch of median nerve with ulnar nerve

Proper palmar digital branches of ulnar nerve

Plate 473 Arteries and Nerves of Upper Limb. (Netter: Atlas of Human Anatomy, 4 ed, 2006, Saunders.)

NETTER'S ANATOMY ILLUSTRATIONS

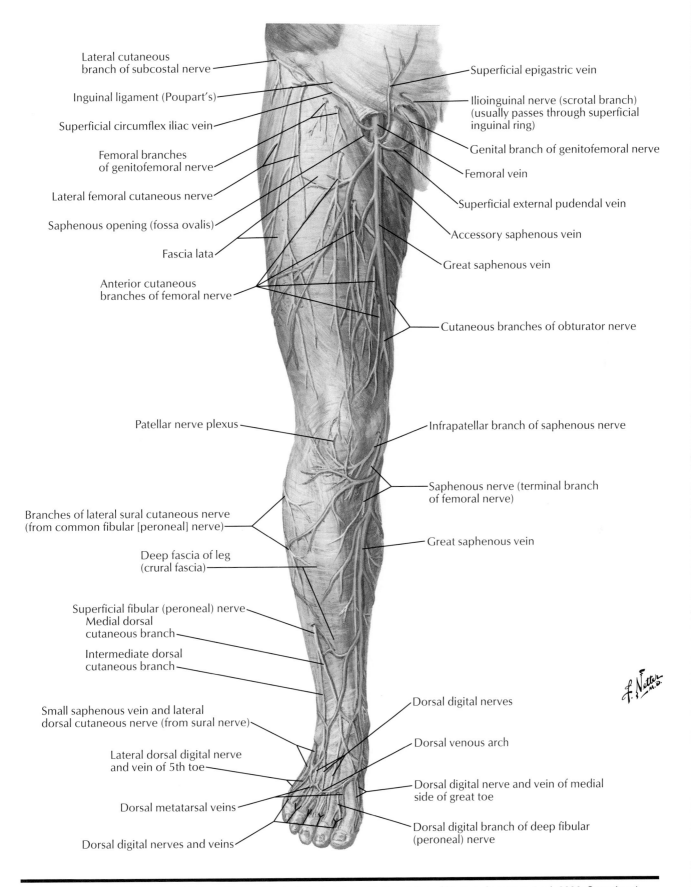

Lateral cutaneous branch of subcostal nerve

Inguinal ligament (Poupart's)

Superficial circumflex iliac vein

Femoral branches of genitofemoral nerve

Lateral femoral cutaneous nerve

Saphenous opening (fossa ovalis)

Fascia lata

Anterior cutaneous branches of femoral nerve

Patellar nerve plexus

Branches of lateral sural cutaneous nerve (from common fibular [peroneal] nerve)

Deep fascia of leg (crural fascia)

Superficial fibular (peroneal) nerve
Medial dorsal cutaneous branch

Intermediate dorsal cutaneous branch

Small saphenous vein and lateral dorsal cutaneous nerve (from sural nerve)

Lateral dorsal digital nerve and vein of 5th toe

Dorsal metatarsal veins

Dorsal digital nerves and veins

Superficial epigastric vein

Ilioinguinal nerve (scrotal branch) (usually passes through superficial inguinal ring)

Genital branch of genitofemoral nerve

Femoral vein

Superficial external pudendal vein

Accessory saphenous vein

Great saphenous vein

Cutaneous branches of obturator nerve

Infrapatellar branch of saphenous nerve

Saphenous nerve (terminal branch of femoral nerve)

Great saphenous vein

Dorsal digital nerves

Dorsal venous arch

Dorsal digital nerve and vein of medial side of great toe

Dorsal digital branch of deep fibular (peroneal) nerve

Plate 544   Superficial Nerves and Veins of Lower Limb: Anterior View. (Netter: Atlas of Human Anatomy, 4 ed, 2006, Saunders.)

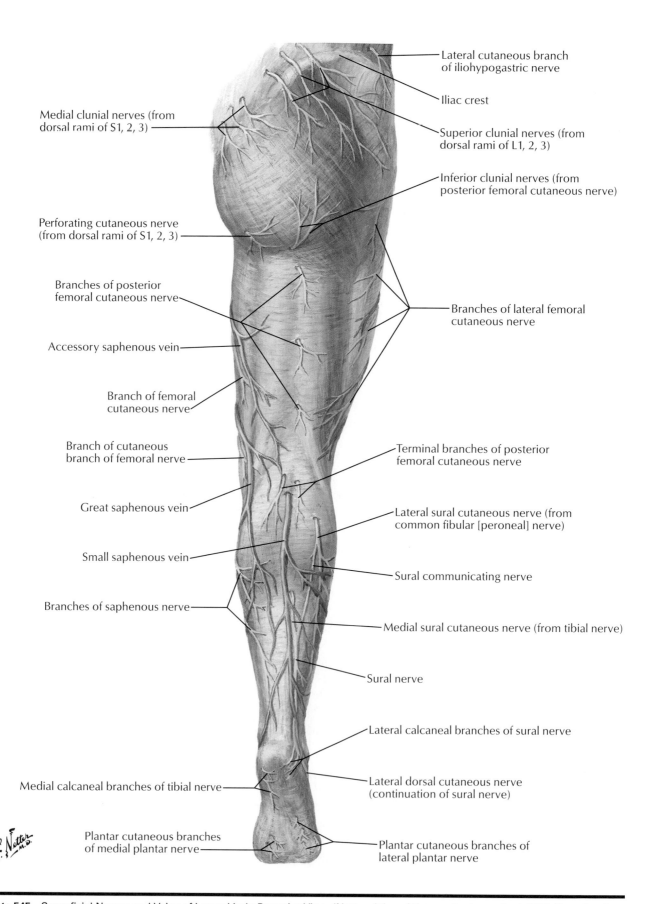

Lateral cutaneous branch of iliohypogastric nerve

Iliac crest

Medial clunial nerves (from dorsal rami of S1, 2, 3)

Superior clunial nerves (from dorsal rami of L1, 2, 3)

Inferior clunial nerves (from posterior femoral cutaneous nerve)

Perforating cutaneous nerve (from dorsal rami of S1, 2, 3)

Branches of posterior femoral cutaneous nerve

Branches of lateral femoral cutaneous nerve

Accessory saphenous vein

Branch of femoral cutaneous nerve

Branch of cutaneous branch of femoral nerve

Terminal branches of posterior femoral cutaneous nerve

Great saphenous vein

Lateral sural cutaneous nerve (from common fibular [peroneal] nerve)

Small saphenous vein

Sural communicating nerve

Branches of saphenous nerve

Medial sural cutaneous nerve (from tibial nerve)

Sural nerve

Lateral calcaneal branches of sural nerve

Medial calcaneal branches of tibial nerve

Lateral dorsal cutaneous nerve (continuation of sural nerve)

Plantar cutaneous branches of medial plantar nerve

Plantar cutaneous branches of lateral plantar nerve

Plate 545 Superficial Nerves and Veins of Lower Limb: Posterior View. (Netter: Atlas of Human Anatomy, 4 ed, 2006, Saunders.)

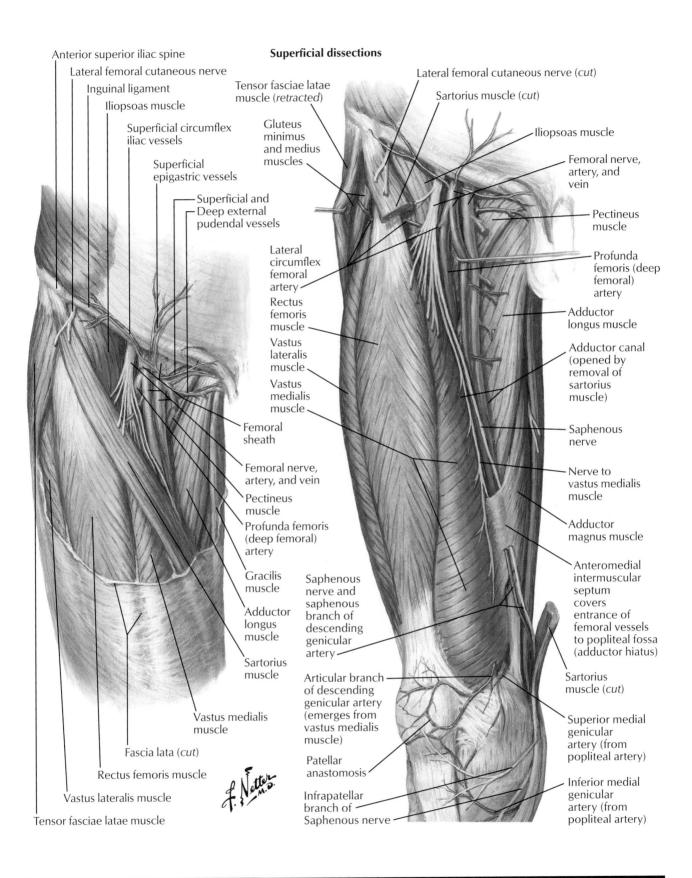

Anterior superior iliac spine

Lateral femoral cutaneous nerve

Inguinal ligament

Iliopsoas muscle

Superficial circumflex iliac vessels

Superficial epigastric vessels

Superficial and Deep external pudendal vessels

Superficial dissections

Tensor fasciae latae muscle (*retracted*)

Gluteus minimus and medius muscles

Lateral circumflex femoral artery

Rectus femoris muscle

Vastus lateralis muscle

Vastus medialis muscle

Femoral sheath

Femoral nerve, artery, and vein

Pectineus muscle

Profunda femoris (deep femoral) artery

Gracilis muscle

Adductor longus muscle

Saphenous nerve and saphenous branch of descending genicular artery

Sartorius muscle

Vastus medialis muscle

Fascia lata (*cut*)

Rectus femoris muscle

Vastus lateralis muscle

Tensor fasciae latae muscle

Articular branch of descending genicular artery (emerges from vastus medialis muscle)

Patellar anastomosis

Infrapatellar branch of Saphenous nerve

Lateral femoral cutaneous nerve (*cut*)

Sartorius muscle (*cut*)

Iliopsoas muscle

Femoral nerve, artery, and vein

Pectineus muscle

Profunda femoris (deep femoral) artery

Adductor longus muscle

Adductor canal (opened by removal of sartorius muscle)

Saphenous nerve

Nerve to vastus medialis muscle

Adductor magnus muscle

Anteromedial intermuscular septum covers entrance of femoral vessels to popliteal fossa (adductor hiatus)

Sartorius muscle (*cut*)

Superior medial genicular artery (from popliteal artery)

Inferior medial genicular artery (from popliteal artery)

Plate 500   Arteries and Nerves of Thigh: Anterior View. (Netter: Atlas of Human Anatomy, 4 ed, 2006, Saunders.)

Deep dissection

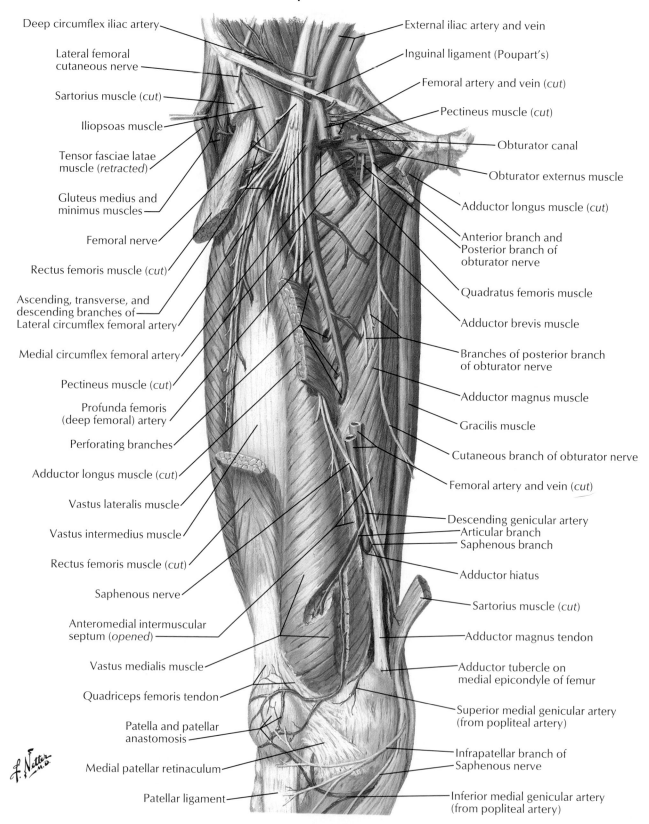

Deep circumflex iliac artery

Lateral femoral cutaneous nerve

Sartorius muscle (*cut*)

Iliopsoas muscle

Tensor fasciae latae muscle (*retracted*)

Gluteus medius and minimus muscles

Femoral nerve

Rectus femoris muscle (*cut*)

Ascending, transverse, and descending branches of Lateral circumflex femoral artery

Medial circumflex femoral artery

Pectineus muscle (*cut*)

Profunda femoris (deep femoral) artery

Perforating branches

Adductor longus muscle (*cut*)

Vastus lateralis muscle

Vastus intermedius muscle

Rectus femoris muscle (*cut*)

Saphenous nerve

Anteromedial intermuscular septum (*opened*)

Vastus medialis muscle

Quadriceps femoris tendon

Patella and patellar anastomosis

Medial patellar retinaculum

Patellar ligament

External iliac artery and vein

Inguinal ligament (Poupart's)

Femoral artery and vein (*cut*)

Pectineus muscle (*cut*)

Obturator canal

Obturator externus muscle

Adductor longus muscle (*cut*)

Anterior branch and Posterior branch of obturator nerve

Quadratus femoris muscle

Adductor brevis muscle

Branches of posterior branch of obturator nerve

Adductor magnus muscle

Gracilis muscle

Cutaneous branch of obturator nerve

Femoral artery and vein (*cut*)

Descending genicular artery
Articular branch
Saphenous branch

Adductor hiatus

Sartorius muscle (*cut*)

Adductor magnus tendon

Adductor tubercle on medial epicondyle of femur

Superior medial genicular artery (from popliteal artery)

Infrapatellar branch of Saphenous nerve

Inferior medial genicular artery (from popliteal artery)

Plate 501 Arteries and Nerves of Thigh: Anterior View. (Netter: Atlas of Human Anatomy, 4 ed, 2006, Saunders.)

Deep dissection

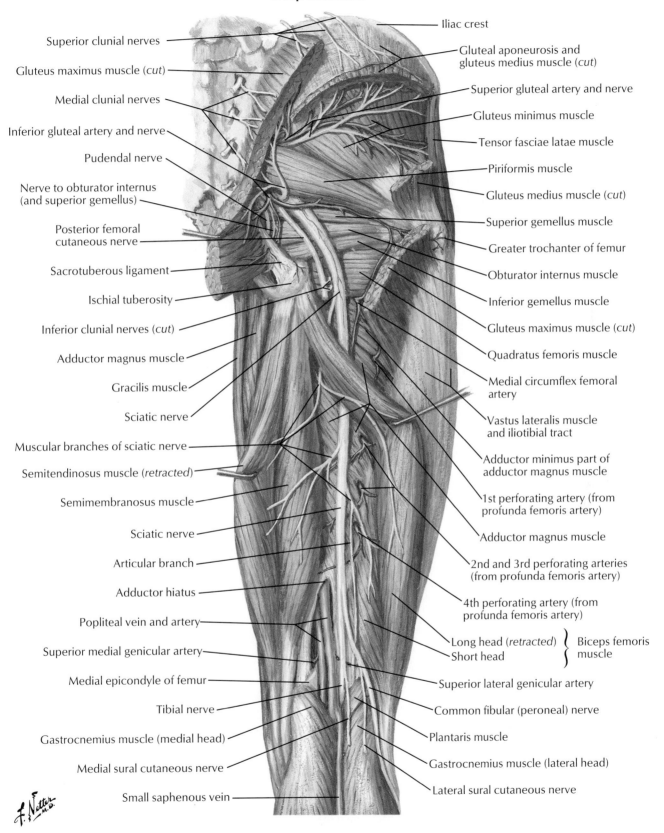

Superior clunial nerves

Gluteus maximus muscle (*cut*)

Medial clunial nerves

Inferior gluteal artery and nerve

Pudendal nerve

Nerve to obturator internus
(and superior gemellus)

Posterior femoral
cutaneous nerve

Sacrotuberous ligament

Ischial tuberosity

Inferior clunial nerves (*cut*)

Adductor magnus muscle

Gracilis muscle

Sciatic nerve

Muscular branches of sciatic nerve

Semitendinosus muscle (*retracted*)

Semimembranosus muscle

Sciatic nerve

Articular branch

Adductor hiatus

Popliteal vein and artery

Superior medial genicular artery

Medial epicondyle of femur

Tibial nerve

Gastrocnemius muscle (medial head)

Medial sural cutaneous nerve

Small saphenous vein

Iliac crest

Gluteal aponeurosis and
gluteus medius muscle (*cut*)

Superior gluteal artery and nerve

Gluteus minimus muscle

Tensor fasciae latae muscle

Piriformis muscle

Gluteus medius muscle (*cut*)

Superior gemellus muscle

Greater trochanter of femur

Obturator internus muscle

Inferior gemellus muscle

Gluteus maximus muscle (*cut*)

Quadratus femoris muscle

Medial circumflex femoral
artery

Vastus lateralis muscle
and iliotibial tract

Adductor minimus part of
adductor magnus muscle

1st perforating artery (from
profunda femoris artery)

Adductor magnus muscle

2nd and 3rd perforating arteries
(from profunda femoris artery)

4th perforating artery (from
profunda femoris artery)

Long head (*retracted*) ⎫ Biceps femoris
Short head   ⎭ muscle

Superior lateral genicular artery

Common fibular (peroneal) nerve

Plantaris muscle

Gastrocnemius muscle (lateral head)

Lateral sural cutaneous nerve

Plate 502 Arteries and Nerves of Thigh: Posterior View. (Netter: Atlas of Human Anatomy, 4 ed, 2006, Saunders.)

NETTER'S ANATOMY ILLUSTRATIONS

Horizontal section

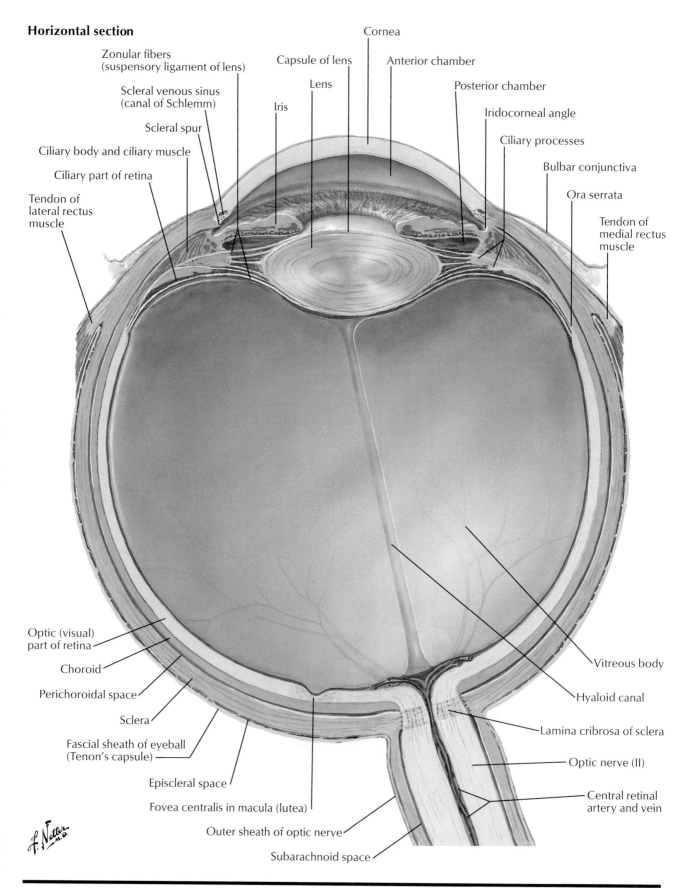

Zonular fibers (suspensory ligament of lens)

Scleral venous sinus (canal of Schlemm)

Scleral spur

Ciliary body and ciliary muscle

Ciliary part of retina

Tendon of lateral rectus muscle

Iris

Capsule of lens

Lens

Cornea

Anterior chamber

Posterior chamber

Iridocorneal angle

Ciliary processes

Bulbar conjunctiva

Ora serrata

Tendon of medial rectus muscle

Optic (visual) part of retina

Choroid

Perichoroidal space

Sclera

Fascial sheath of eyeball (Tenon's capsule)

Episcleral space

Fovea centralis in macula (lutea)

Outer sheath of optic nerve

Subarachnoid space

Vitreous body

Hyaloid canal

Lamina cribrosa of sclera

Optic nerve (II)

Central retinal artery and vein

Plate 87 Eyeball. (Netter: Atlas of Human Anatomy, 4 ed, 2006, Saunders.)

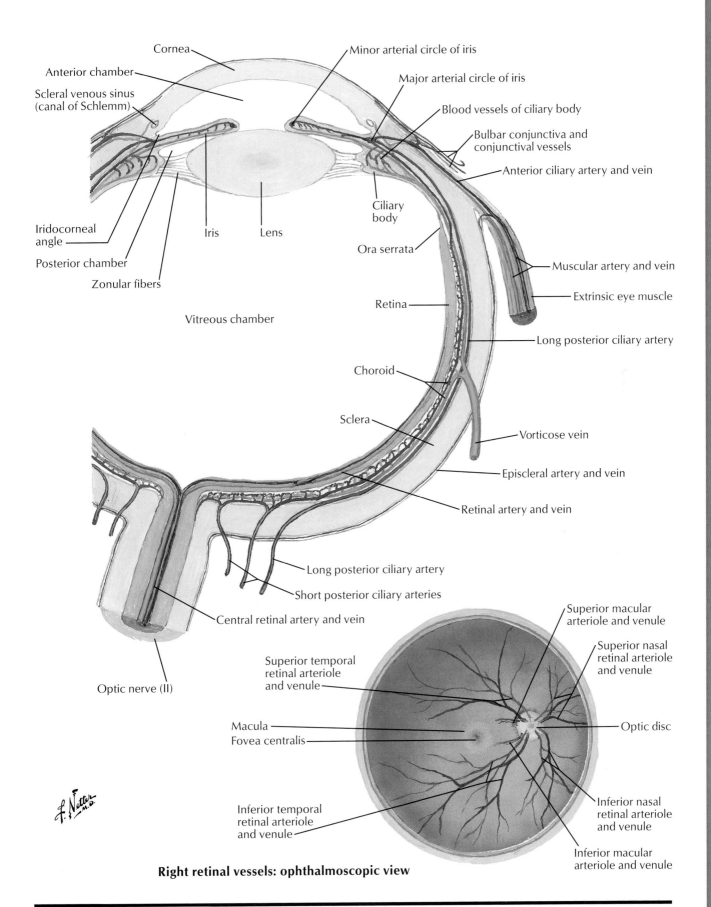

Cornea

Minor arterial circle of iris

Anterior chamber

Major arterial circle of iris

Scleral venous sinus (canal of Schlemm)

Blood vessels of ciliary body

Bulbar conjunctiva and conjunctival vessels

Anterior ciliary artery and vein

Ciliary body

Iridocorneal angle

Iris   Lens

Ora serrata

Muscular artery and vein

Posterior chamber

Extrinsic eye muscle

Zonular fibers

Retina

Long posterior ciliary artery

Vitreous chamber

Choroid

Sclera

Vorticose vein

Episcleral artery and vein

Retinal artery and vein

Long posterior ciliary artery

Short posterior ciliary arteries

Central retinal artery and vein

Optic nerve (II)

Superior macular arteriole and venule

Superior nasal retinal arteriole and venule

Superior temporal retinal arteriole and venule

Macula

Fovea centralis

Optic disc

Inferior nasal retinal arteriole and venule

Inferior temporal retinal arteriole and venule

Inferior macular arteriole and venule

Right retinal vessels: ophthalmoscopic view

Plate 90   Intrinsic Arteries and Veins of Eye. (Netter: Atlas of Human Anatomy, 4 ed, 2006, Saunders.)

NETTER'S ANATOMY ILLUSTRATIONS

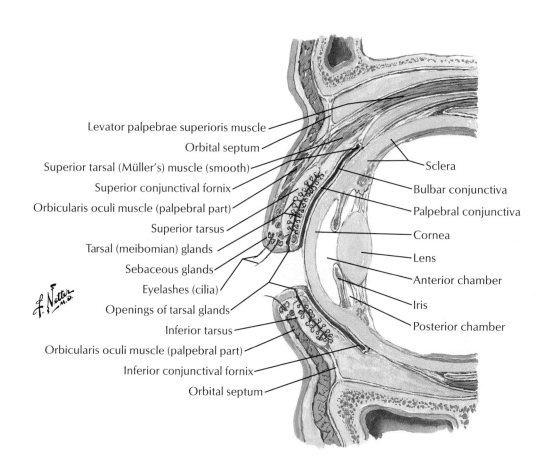

Levator palpebrae superioris muscle

Orbital septum

Superior tarsal (Müller's) muscle (smooth)

Superior conjunctival fornix

Orbicularis oculi muscle (palpebral part)

Superior tarsus

Tarsal (meibomian) glands

Sebaceous glands

Eyelashes (cilia)

Openings of tarsal glands

Inferior tarsus

Orbicularis oculi muscle (palpebral part)

Inferior conjunctival fornix

Orbital septum

Sclera

Bulbar conjunctiva

Palpebral conjunctiva

Cornea

Lens

Anterior chamber

Iris

Posterior chamber

Plate 81, Middle   Eyelid. (Netter: Atlas of Human Anatomy, 4 ed, 2006, Saunders.)

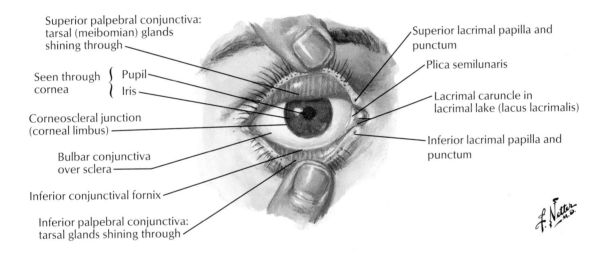

Superior palpebral conjunctiva: tarsal (meibomian) glands shining through

Seen through cornea { Pupil
Iris

Corneoscleral junction (corneal limbus)

Bulbar conjunctiva over sclera

Inferior conjunctival fornix

Inferior palpebral conjunctiva: tarsal glands shining through

Superior lacrimal papilla and punctum

Plica semilunaris

Lacrimal caruncle in lacrimal lake (lacus lacrimalis)

Inferior lacrimal papilla and punctum

Plate 81, Upper   Eyelid. (Netter: Atlas of Human Anatomy, 4 ed, 2006, Saunders.)

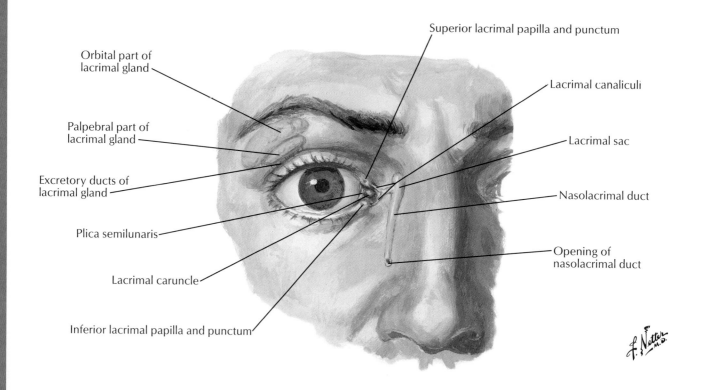

Orbital part of lacrimal gland

Palpebral part of lacrimal gland

Excretory ducts of lacrimal gland

Plica semilunaris

Lacrimal caruncle

Inferior lacrimal papilla and punctum

Superior lacrimal papilla and punctum

Lacrimal canaliculi

Lacrimal sac

Nasolacrimal duct

Opening of nasolacrimal duct

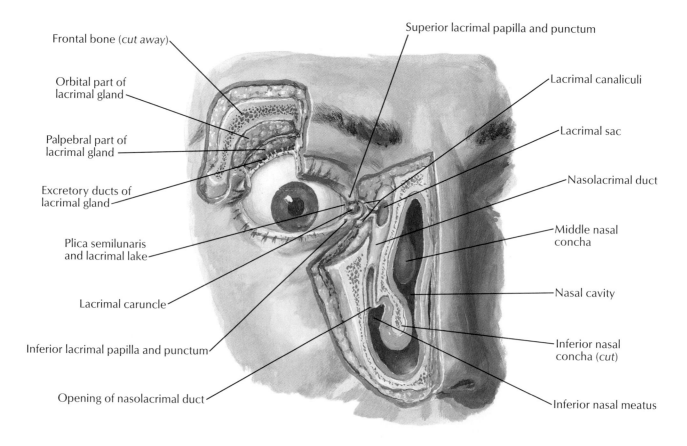

Frontal bone (*cut away*)

Orbital part of lacrimal gland

Palpebral part of lacrimal gland

Excretory ducts of lacrimal gland

Plica semilunaris and lacrimal lake

Lacrimal caruncle

Inferior lacrimal papilla and punctum

Opening of nasolacrimal duct

Superior lacrimal papilla and punctum

Lacrimal canaliculi

Lacrimal sac

Nasolacrimal duct

Middle nasal concha

Nasal cavity

Inferior nasal concha (*cut*)

Inferior nasal meatus

Plate 82   Lacrimal Apparatus. (Netter: Atlas of Human Anatomy, 4 ed, 2006, Saunders.)

Frontal section

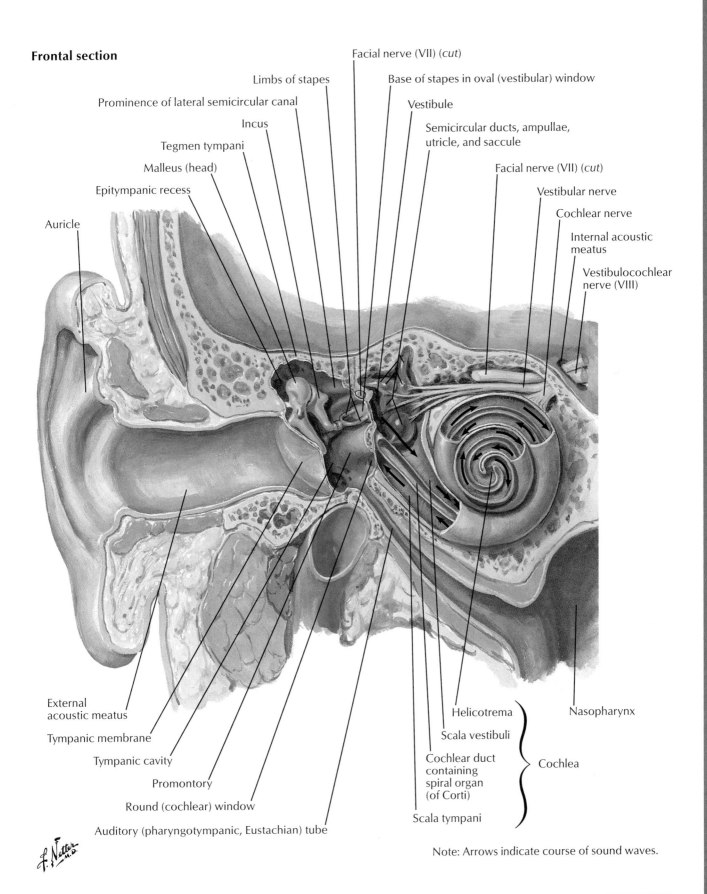

Facial nerve (VII) (*cut*)

Base of stapes in oval (vestibular) window

Limbs of stapes

Vestibule

Prominence of lateral semicircular canal

Semicircular ducts, ampullae, utricle, and saccule

Incus

Facial nerve (VII) (*cut*)

Tegmen tympani

Vestibular nerve

Malleus (head)

Cochlear nerve

Epitympanic recess

Internal acoustic meatus

Auricle

Vestibulocochlear nerve (VIII)

External acoustic meatus

Tympanic membrane

Helicotrema

Nasopharynx

Tympanic cavity

Scala vestibuli

Promontory

Cochlear duct containing spiral organ (of Corti)

Round (cochlear) window

Cochlea

Auditory (pharyngotympanic, Eustachian) tube

Scala tympani

Note: Arrows indicate course of sound waves.

Plate 92   Pathway of Sound Reception. (Netter: Atlas of Human Anatomy, 4 ed, 2006, Saunders.)

NETTER'S ANATOMY ILLUSTRATIONS

Medial wall of tympanic cavity: lateral view

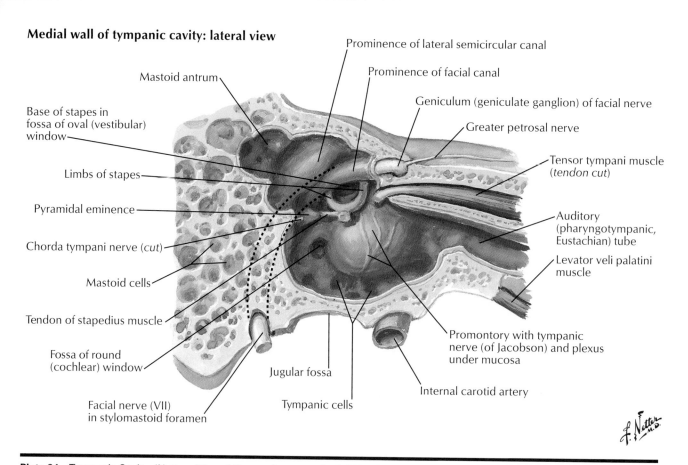

Mastoid antrum

Base of stapes in fossa of oval (vestibular) window

Limbs of stapes

Pyramidal eminence

Chorda tympani nerve (*cut*)

Mastoid cells

Tendon of stapedius muscle

Fossa of round (cochlear) window

Facial nerve (VII) in stylomastoid foramen

Jugular fossa

Tympanic cells

Prominence of lateral semicircular canal

Prominence of facial canal

Geniculum (geniculate ganglion) of facial nerve

Greater petrosal nerve

Tensor tympani muscle (*tendon cut*)

Auditory (pharyngotympanic, Eustachian) tube

Levator veli palatini muscle

Promontory with tympanic nerve (of Jacobson) and plexus under mucosa

Internal carotid artery

Plate 94 Tympanic Cavity. (Netter: Atlas of Human Anatomy, 4 ed, 2006, Saunders.)

Otoscopic view of right tympanic membrane

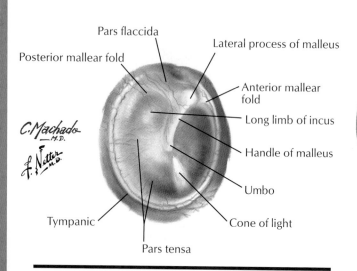

Pars flaccida

Posterior mallear fold

Lateral process of malleus

Anterior mallear fold

Long limb of incus

Handle of malleus

Umbo

Cone of light

Tympanic

Pars tensa

Plate 93 Tympanic Cavity. (Netter: Atlas of Human Anatomy, 4 ed, 2006, Saunders.)

Dissected right bony labyrinth (otic capsule): membranous labyrinth removed

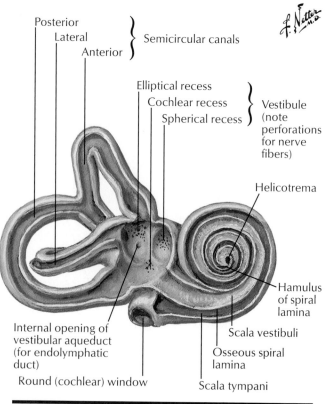

Posterior
Lateral
Anterior } Semicircular canals

Elliptical recess
Cochlear recess
Spherical recess } Vestibule (note perforations for nerve fibers)

Helicotrema

Hamulus of spiral lamina

Scala vestibuli

Osseous spiral lamina

Scala tympani

Internal opening of vestibular aqueduct (for endolymphatic duct)

Round (cochlear) window

Plate 95 Bony Membranous Labyrinth. (Netter: Atlas of Human Anatomy, 4 ed, 2006, Saunders.)

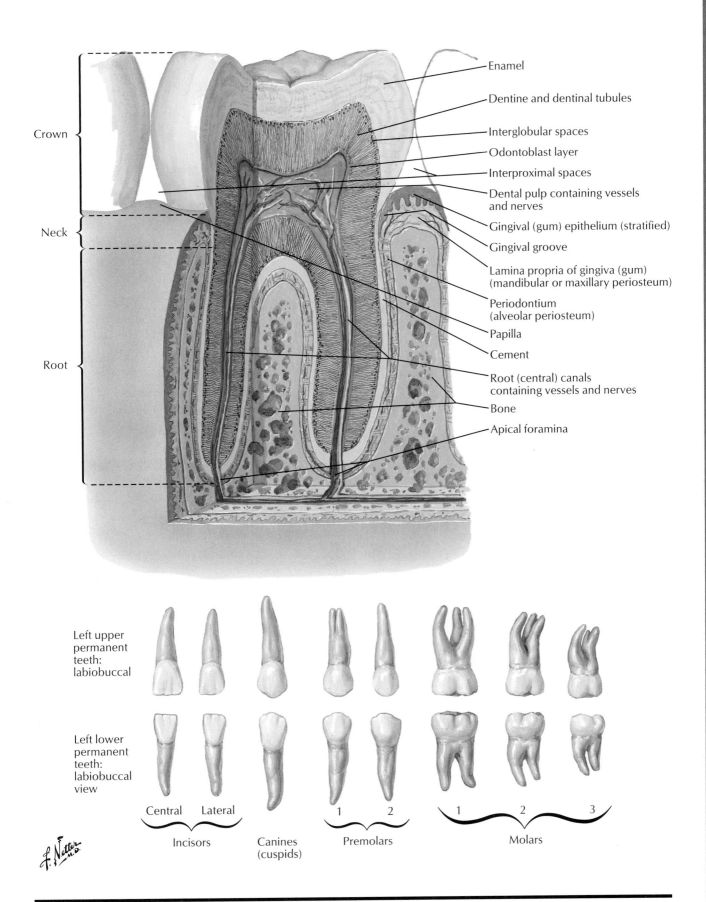

Crown

Neck

Root

Enamel

Dentine and dentinal tubules

Interglobular spaces

Odontoblast layer

Interproximal spaces

Dental pulp containing vessels and nerves

Gingival (gum) epithelium (stratified)

Gingival groove

Lamina propria of gingiva (gum) (mandibular or maxillary periosteum)

Periodontium (alveolar periosteum)

Papilla

Cement

Root (central) canals containing vessels and nerves

Bone

Apical foramina

Left upper permanent teeth: labiobuccal

Left lower permanent teeth: labiobuccal view

Central   Lateral

Incisors

Canines (cuspids)

1   2

Premolars

1   2   3

Molars

Plate 57   Teeth. (Netter: Atlas of Human Anatomy, 4 ed, 2006, Saunders.)

Tongue

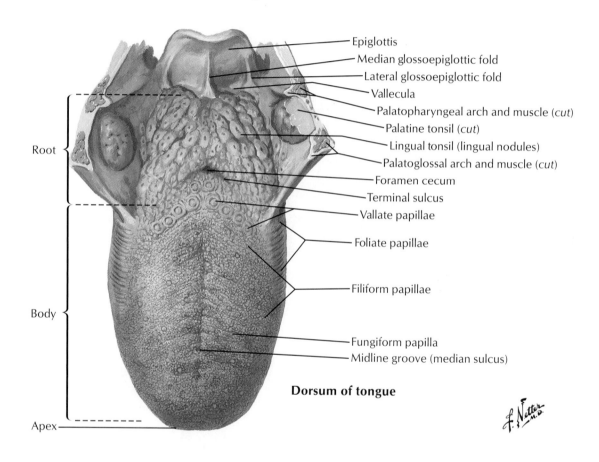

Root

Body

Apex

Epiglottis
Median glossoepiglottic fold
Lateral glossoepiglottic fold
Vallecula
Palatopharyngeal arch and muscle (*cut*)
Palatine tonsil (*cut*)
Lingual tonsil (lingual nodules)
Palatoglossal arch and muscle (*cut*)
Foramen cecum
Terminal sulcus
Vallate papillae
Foliate papillae
Filiform papillae
Fungiform papilla
Midline groove (median sulcus)

Dorsum of tongue

Plate 58   Tongue. (Netter: Atlas of Human Anatomy, 4 ed, 2006, Saunders.)

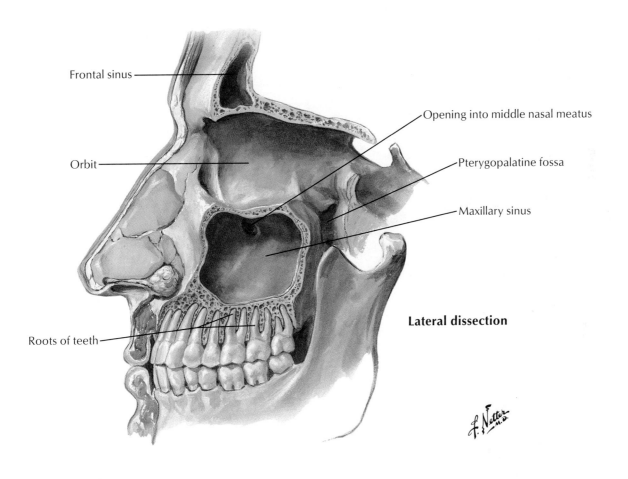

Frontal sinus

Orbit

Roots of teeth

Opening into middle nasal meatus

Pterygopalatine fossa

Maxillary sinus

Lateral dissection

Plate 49   Paranasal Sinuses. (Netter: Atlas of Human Anatomy, 4 ed, 2006, Saunders.)

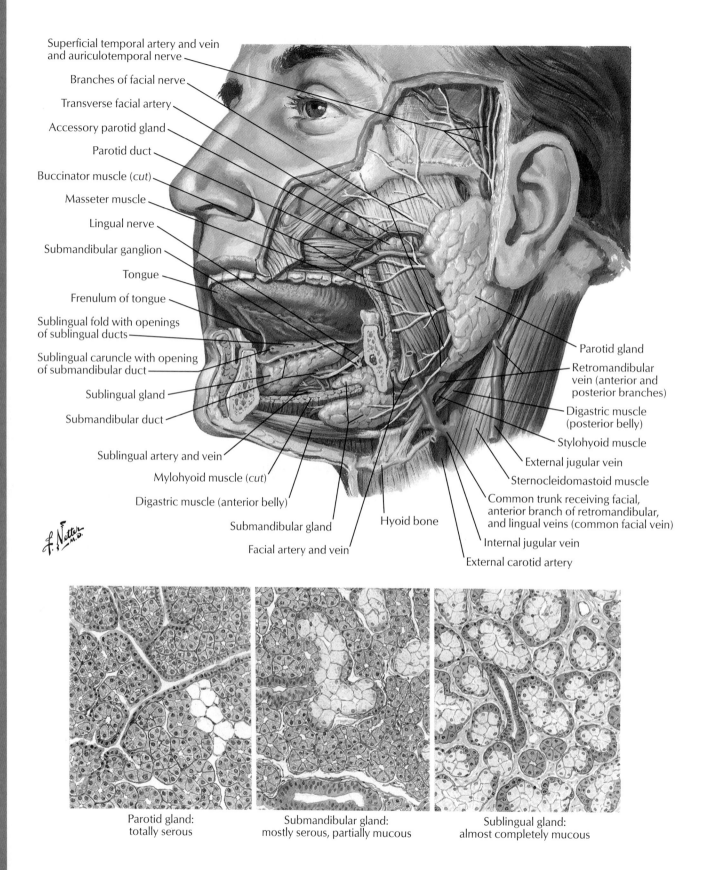

Superficial temporal artery and vein and auriculotemporal nerve

Branches of facial nerve

Transverse facial artery

Accessory parotid gland

Parotid duct

Buccinator muscle (*cut*)

Masseter muscle

Lingual nerve

Submandibular ganglion

Tongue

Frenulum of tongue

Sublingual fold with openings of sublingual ducts

Sublingual caruncle with opening of submandibular duct

Sublingual gland

Submandibular duct

Sublingual artery and vein

Mylohyoid muscle (*cut*)

Digastric muscle (anterior belly)

Submandibular gland

Facial artery and vein

Hyoid bone

Parotid gland

Retromandibular vein (anterior and posterior branches)

Digastric muscle (posterior belly)

Stylohyoid muscle

External jugular vein

Sternocleidomastoid muscle

Common trunk receiving facial, anterior branch of retromandibular, and lingual veins (common facial vein)

Internal jugular vein

External carotid artery

Parotid gland: totally serous

Submandibular gland: mostly serous, partially mucous

Sublingual gland: almost completely mucous

Plate 61 Salivary Glands. (Netter: Atlas of Human Anatomy, 4 ed, 2006, Saunders.)

Right coronary artery: left anterior oblique view

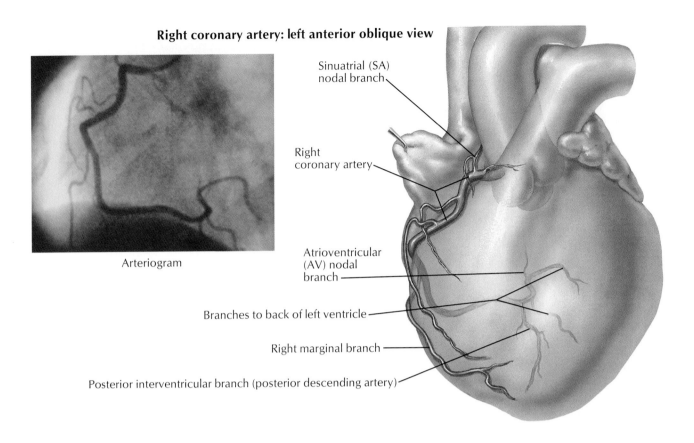

Arteriogram

Sinuatrial (SA) nodal branch

Right coronary artery

Atrioventricular (AV) nodal branch

Branches to back of left ventricle

Right marginal branch

Posterior interventricular branch (posterior descending artery)

Right coronary artery: right anterior oblique view

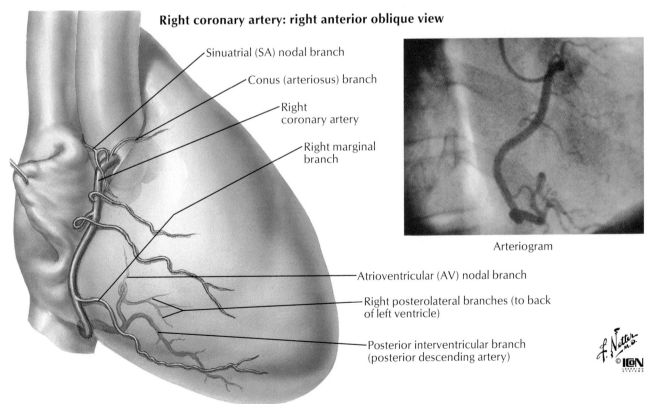

Sinuatrial (SA) nodal branch

Conus (arteriosus) branch

Right coronary artery

Right marginal branch

Arteriogram

Atrioventricular (AV) nodal branch

Right posterolateral branches (to back of left ventricle)

Posterior interventricular branch (posterior descending artery)

Plate 218   Coronary Arteries: Arteriographic Views. (Netter: Atlas of Human Anatomy, 4 ed, 2006, Saunders.)

Left coronary artery: left anterior oblique view

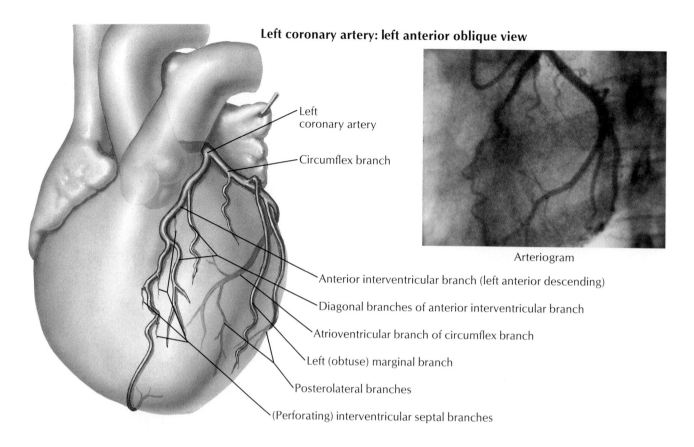

Left coronary artery

Circumflex branch

Arteriogram

Anterior interventricular branch (left anterior descending)

Diagonal branches of anterior interventricular branch

Atrioventricular branch of circumflex branch

Left (obtuse) marginal branch

Posterolateral branches

(Perforating) interventricular septal branches

Left coronary artery: right anterior oblique view

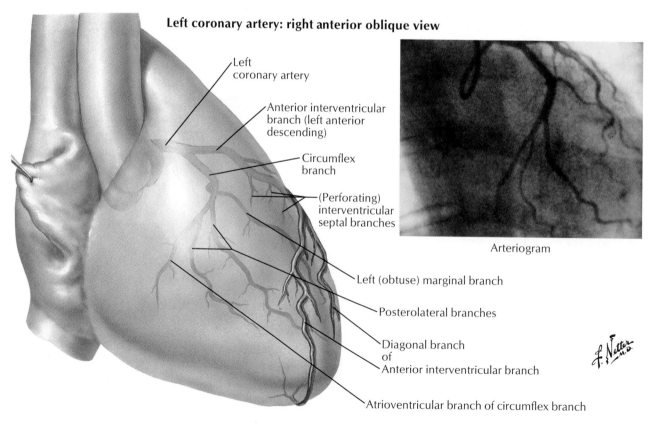

Left coronary artery

Anterior interventricular branch (left anterior descending)

Circumflex branch

(Perforating) interventricular septal branches

Arteriogram

Left (obtuse) marginal branch

Posterolateral branches

Diagonal branch of Anterior interventricular branch

Atrioventricular branch of circumflex branch

Plate 219 Coronary Arteries: Arteriographic Views. (Netter: Atlas of Human Anatomy, 4 ed, 2006, Saunders.)

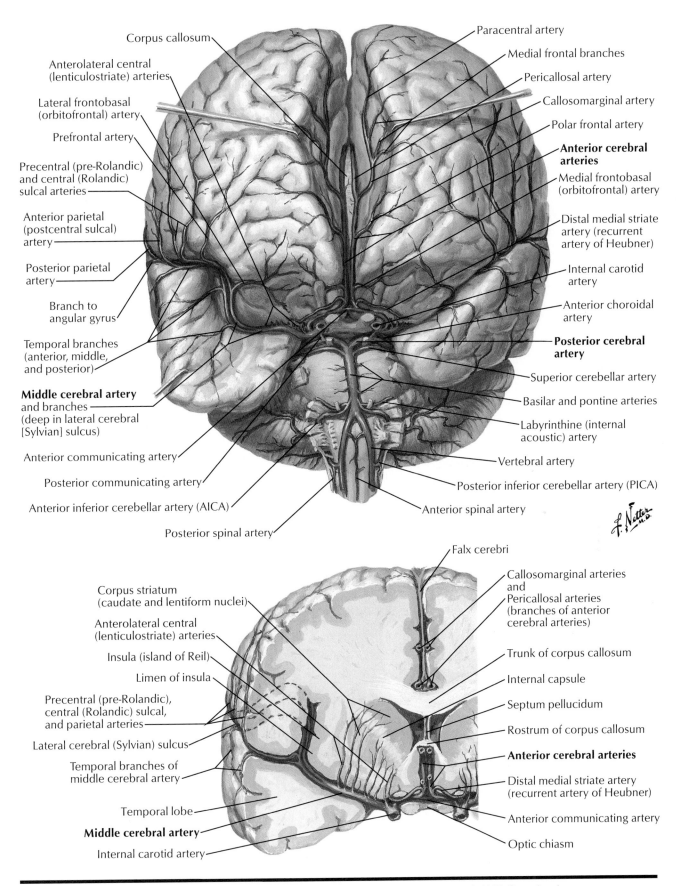

Corpus callosum

Anterolateral central (lenticulostriate) arteries

Lateral frontobasal (orbitofrontal) artery

Prefrontal artery

Precentral (pre-Rolandic) and central (Rolandic) sulcal arteries

Anterior parietal (postcentral sulcal) artery

Posterior parietal artery

Branch to angular gyrus

Temporal branches (anterior, middle, and posterior)

Middle cerebral artery and branches (deep in lateral cerebral [Sylvian] sulcus)

Anterior communicating artery

Posterior communicating artery

Anterior inferior cerebellar artery (AICA)

Posterior spinal artery

Paracentral artery

Medial frontal branches

Pericallosal artery

Callosomarginal artery

Polar frontal artery

Anterior cerebral arteries

Medial frontobasal (orbitofrontal) artery

Distal medial striate artery (recurrent artery of Heubner)

Internal carotid artery

Anterior choroidal artery

Posterior cerebral artery

Superior cerebellar artery

Basilar and pontine arteries

Labyrinthine (internal acoustic) artery

Vertebral artery

Posterior inferior cerebellar artery (PICA)

Anterior spinal artery

Corpus striatum (caudate and lentiform nuclei)

Anterolateral central (lenticulostriate) arteries

Insula (island of Reil)

Limen of insula

Precentral (pre-Rolandic), central (Rolandic) sulcal, and parietal arteries

Lateral cerebral (Sylvian) sulcus

Temporal branches of middle cerebral artery

Temporal lobe

Middle cerebral artery

Internal carotid artery

Falx cerebri

Callosomarginal arteries and Pericallosal arteries (branches of anterior cerebral arteries)

Trunk of corpus callosum

Internal capsule

Septum pellucidum

Rostrum of corpus callosum

Anterior cerebral arteries

Distal medial striate artery (recurrent artery of Heubner)

Anterior communicating artery

Optic chiasm

Plate 141 Arteries of Brain: Frontal View and Section. (Netter: Atlas of Human Anatomy, 4 ed, 2006, Saunders.)

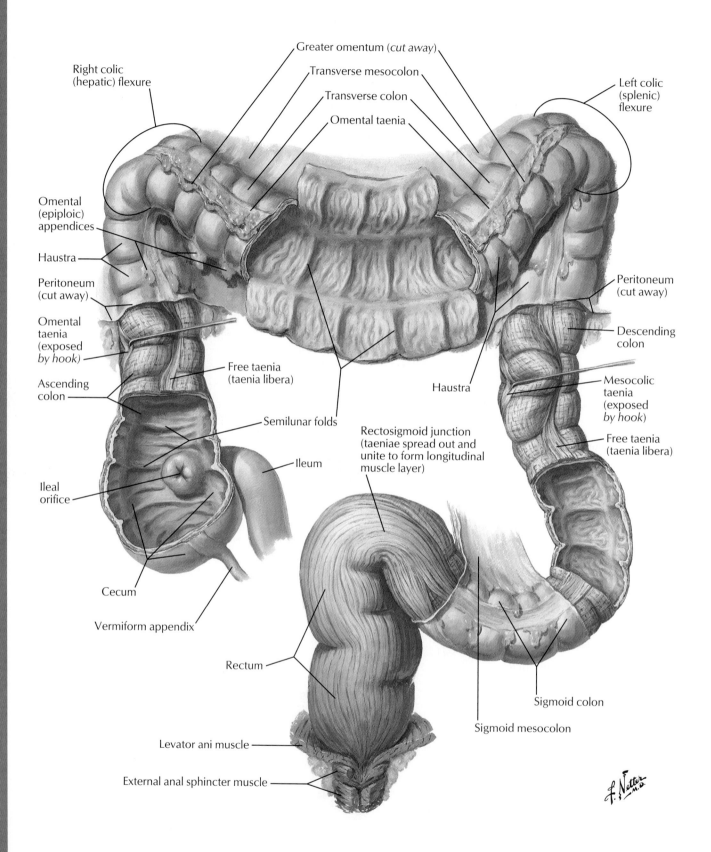

Right colic
(hepatic) flexure

Greater omentum (*cut away*)

Transverse mesocolon

Transverse colon

Omental taenia

Left colic
(splenic)
flexure

Omental
(epiploic)
appendices

Haustra

Peritoneum
(cut away)

Omental
taenia
(exposed
by hook)

Ascending
colon

Ileal
orifice

Cecum

Vermiform appendix

Free taenia
(taenia libera)

Semilunar folds

Ileum

Rectosigmoid junction
(taeniae spread out and
unite to form longitudinal
muscle layer)

Haustra

Peritoneum
(cut away)

Descending
colon

Mesocolic
taenia
(exposed
by hook)

Free taenia
(taenia libera)

Rectum

Levator ani muscle

External anal sphincter muscle

Sigmoid colon

Sigmoid mesocolon

Plate 284   Mucosa and Musculature of Large Intestine. (Netter: Atlas of Human Anatomy, 4 ed, 2006, Saunders.)

Transverse Section: T3–4 Intervertebral Disc, Manubrium

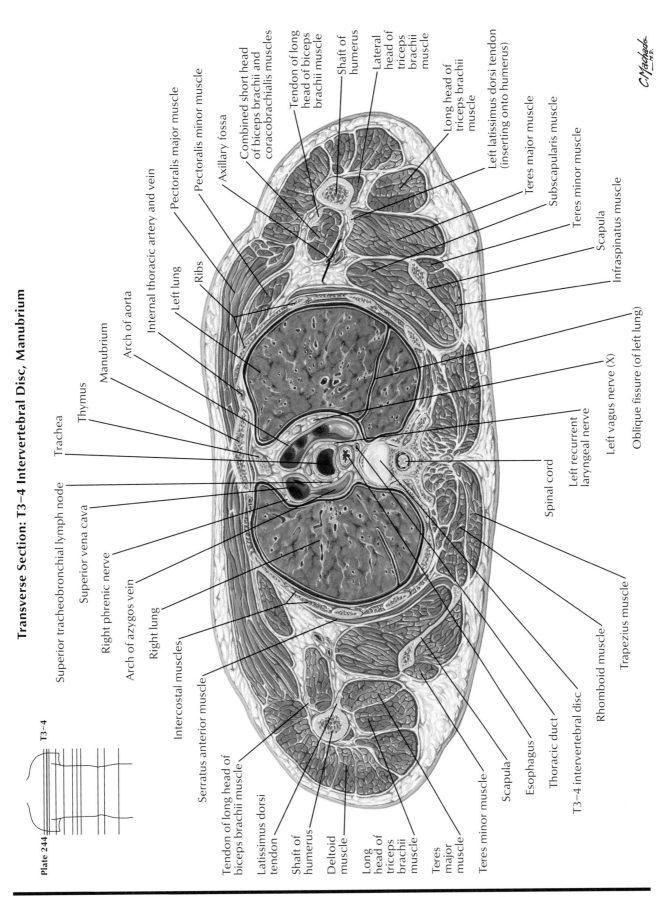

Superior tracheobronchial lymph node

Trachea

Thymus

Manubrium

Right phrenic nerve

Superior vena cava

Arch of aorta

Arch of azygos vein

Right lung

Internal thoracic artery and vein

Left lung

Pectoralis major muscle

Pectoralis minor muscle

Axillary fossa

Ribs

Combined short head of biceps brachii and coracobrachialis muscles

Tendon of long head of biceps brachii muscle

Shaft of humerus

Lateral head of triceps brachii muscle

Long head of triceps brachii muscle

Left latissimus dorsi tendon (inserting onto humerus)

Teres major muscle

Subscapularis muscle

Teres minor muscle

Scapula

Infraspinatus muscle

Oblique fissure (of left lung)

Left vagus nerve (X)

Left recurrent laryngeal nerve

Spinal cord

Trapezius muscle

Rhomboid muscle

T3–4 intervertebral disc

Thoracic duct

Esophagus

Scapula

Teres minor muscle

Teres major muscle

Long head of triceps brachii muscle

Deltoid muscle

Shaft of humerus

Latissimus dorsi tendon

Tendon of long head of biceps brachii muscle

Serratus anterior muscle

Intercostal muscles

Plate 244

T3–4

C.Machado
_M.D.

Plate 244   Cross Section of Thorax at T3-4 Disc Level. (Netter: Atlas of Human Anatomy, 4 ed, 2006, Saunders.)

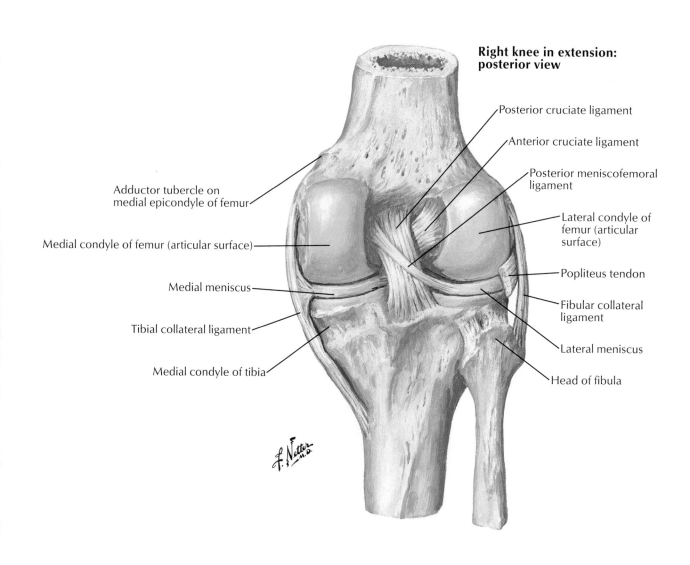

Right knee in extension: posterior view

Posterior cruciate ligament

Anterior cruciate ligament

Posterior meniscofemoral ligament

Lateral condyle of femur (articular surface)

Popliteus tendon

Fibular collateral ligament

Lateral meniscus

Head of fibula

Adductor tubercle on medial epicondyle of femur

Medial condyle of femur (articular surface)

Medial meniscus

Tibial collateral ligament

Medial condyle of tibia

Plate 509 Knee: Cruciate and Collateral Ligaments. (Netter: Atlas of Human Anatomy, 4 ed, 2006, Saunders.)

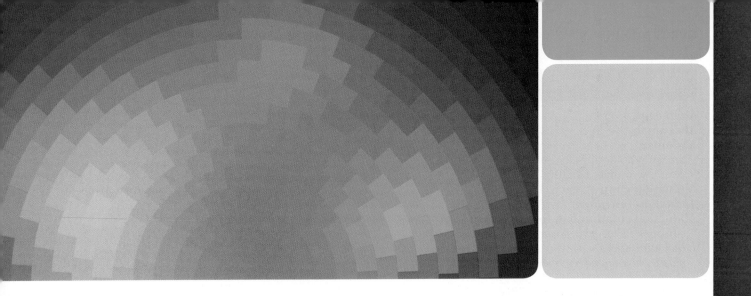

HCPCS 2015 INDEX

A

Abatacept, J0129

Abciximab, J0130

Abdomen

  dressing holder/binder, A4462

  pad, low profile, L1270

Abduction control, each, L2624

Abduction restrainer, A4566

Abduction rotation bar, foot, L3140–L3170

  adjustable shoe style positioning device, L3160

  including shoes, L3140

  plastic, heel-stabilizer, off-shelf, L3170

  without shoes, L3150

AbobotulinumtypeA, J0586

Absorption dressing, A6251–A6256

Access, site, occlusive, device, G0269

Access system, A4301

Accessories

  ambulation devices, E0153–E0159

    crutch attachment, walker, E0157

    forearm crutch, platform attachment, E0153

    leg extension, walker, E0158

    replacement, brake attachment, walker, E0159

    seat attachment, walker, E0156

    walker, platform attachment, E0154

    wheel attachment, walker, per pair, E0155

  artificial kidney and machine (see also **ESRD**), E1510–E1699

    adjustable chair, ESRD patients, E1570

    automatic peritoneal dialysis system, intermittent, E1592

    bath conductivity meter, hemodialysis, E1550

    blood leak detector, hemodialysis, replacement, E1560

    blood pump, hemodialysis, replacement, E1620

    cycler dialysis machine, peritoneal, E1594

    deionizer water system, hemodialysis, E1615

    delivery/instillation charges, hemodialysis equipment, E1600

    hemodialysis machine E1590

    hemostats, E1637

    heparin infusion pump, hemodialysis, E1520

    kidney machine, dialysate delivery system, E1510

    peritoneal dialysis clamps, E1634

    portable travel hemodialyzer, E1635

    reciprocating peritoneal dialysis system, E1630

    replacement, air bubble detector, hemodialysis, E1530

    replacement, pressure alarm, hemodialysis, E1540

    reverse osmosis water system, hemodialysis, E1610

    scale, E1639

    sorbent cartridges, hemodialysis, E1636

    transducer protectors, E1575

    unipuncture control system, E1580

    water softening system, hemodialysis, E1625

    wearable artificial kidney, E1632

Accessories *(Continued)*

  beds, E0271–E0280, *E0300–E0316, E0328–E0329*

    bed board, E0273

    bed cradle, E0280

    bed pan, standard, E0275

    bed side rails, E0305, E0310

    bed, board/table, E0315

    bed-pan fracture, E0276

    hospital bed, extra heavy duty, E0302, E0304

    hospital bed, heavy duty, E0301, E0303

    hospital bed, pediatric, electric, E0329

    hospital bed, safety enclosure frame, E0316

    mattress, foam rubber, E0272

    mattress, interspring, E0271

    over-bed table, E0274

    pediatric crib, E0300

    powered pressure-reducing air mattress, E0277

  wheelchairs, E0950–E1030, E1050–E1298, *E2201–E2295, E2300–E2399, K0001–K0109*

    accessory tray, E0950

    arm rest, E0994

    back upholstery replacement, E0982

    calf rest/pad, E0995

    commode seat, E0968

    detachable armrest, E0973

    elevating leg rest, E0990

    headrest cushion, E0955

    lateral trunk/hip support, E0956

    loop-holder, E0951–E0952

    manual swingaway, E1028

    manual wheelchair, adapter, amputee, E0959

    manual wheelchair, anti-rollback device, E0974

    manual wheelchair, anti-tipping device, E0971

    manual wheelchair, hand rim with projections, E0967

    manual wheelchair, headrest extension, E0966

    manual wheelchair, lever-activated, wheel drive, E0988

    manual wheelchair, one-arm drive attachment, E0958

    manual wheelchair, power add-on, E0983–E0984

    manual wheelchair, push activated power assist, E0986

    manual wheelchair, solid seat insert, E0992

    medial thigh support, E0957

    modification, pediatric size, E1011

    narrowing device, E0969

    No. 2 footplates, E0970

    oxygen related accessories, E1352–E1406

    positioning belt/safety belt/pelvic strap, E0978

    power-seating system, E1002–E1010

    reclining back addition, pediatric size wheelchair E1014

    residual limb support system, E1020

    safety vest, E0980

    seat lift mechanism, E0985

    seat upholstery replacement, E0981

    shock absorber, E1015–E1018

◀ **New**   ⟳ **Revised**   ✔ **Reinstated**   ~~deleted~~ **Deleted**

Accessories *(Continued)*
    shoulder harness strap, E0960
    ventilator tray, E1029–E1030
    wheel lock brake extension, manual, E0961
    wheelchair, amputee, accessories, E1170–E1200
    wheelchair, fully inclining, accessories,
    E1050–E1093
    wheelchair, heavy duty, accessories, E1280–E1298
    wheelchair, lightweight, accessories, E1240–E1270
    wheelchair, semi-reclining, accessories,
    E1100–E1110
    wheelchair, special size, E1220–E1239
    wheelchair, standard, accessories, E1130–E1161
   whirlpool equipment, E1300–E1310
Ace type, elastic bandage, A6448–A6450
Acetaminophen, J0131
Acetazolamide sodium, J1120
Acetylcysteine
   inhalation solution, J7604, J7608
   injection, J0132
Activity, therapy, G0176
Acyclovir, J0133
Adalimumab, J0135
Additions to
   fracture orthosis, L2180–L2192
    abduction bar, L2300–L2310
    adjustable motion knee joint, L2186
    anterior swing band, L2335
    BK socket, PTB and AFO, L2350
    disk or dial lock, knee flexion, L2425
    dorsiflexion and plantar flexion, L2220
    dorsiflexion assist, L2210
    drop lock knee joint, L2182
    drop lock, L2405
    extended steel shank, L2360
    foot plate, stirrup attachment, L2250
    hip joint, pelvic band, thigh flange, pelvic
    belt, E2192
    integrated release mechanism, L2515
    lacer custom-fabricated, L2320–L2330
    lift loop, drop lock ring, L2492
    limited ankle motion, L2200
    limited motion knee joint, L2184
    long tongue stirrup, L2265
    lower extremity orthrosis, L2200–L2397
    molded inner boot, L2280
    offset knee joint, heavy duty, L2395
    offset knee joint, L2390
    Patten bottom, L2370
    pelvic and thoracic control, L2570–L2680
    plastic shoe insert with ankle joints, L2180
    polycentric knee joint, L2387
    pre-tibial shell, L2340
    quadrilateral, L2188
    ratchet lock knee extension, L2430
    reinforced solid stirrup, L2260
    rocker bottom, custom fabricated, L2232
    round caliper/plate attachment, L2240

Additions to *(Continued)*
    split flat caliper stirrups, L2230
    straight knee joint, heavy duty, L2385
    straight knee, or offset knee joints, L2405–L2492
    suspension sleeve, L2397
    thigh/weight bearing, L2500–L2550
    torsion control, ankle joint, L2375
    torsion control, straight knee joint, L2380
    varus/valgus correction, L2270–L2275
    waist belt, L2190
   general additions, orthosis, L2750–L2999
    lower extremity orthrosis, non-corrosive finish, per
    bar, L2780
    lower extremity orthrosis, NOS, L2999
    lower extremity, above knee section, soft
    interface, L2830
    lower extremity, concentric adjustable torsion style
    mechanism, L2861
    lower extremity, drop lock retainer, L2785
    lower extremity, extension, per extension, per
    bar, L2760
    lower extremity, femoral length sock, L2850
    lower extremity, full kneecap, L2795
    lower extremity, high strength, lightweight material,
    hybrid lamination, L2755
    lower extremity, knee control, condylar pad, L2810
    lower extremity, knee control, knee cap, medial or
    lateral, L2800
    lower extremity, plating chrome or nickel, per
    bar, L2750
    lower extremity, soft interface, below knee, L2820
    lower extremity, tibial length sock, L2840
    orthotic side bar, disconnect device, L2768
Adenosine, J0151, J0153↻
Adhesive, A4364
   bandage, A6413
   disc or foam pad, A5126
   remover, A4455, A4456
   support, breast prosthesis, A4280
   wound, closure, G0168
Adjunctive, dental, D9110–D9999
Administration, chemotherapy, Q0083–Q0085
   both infusion and other technique, Q0085
   infusion technique only, Q0084
   other than infusion technique, Q0083
Administration, Part D
   supply, tositumomab, G3001
   vaccine, hepatitis B, G0010
   vaccine, influenza, G0008
   vaccine, pneumococcal, G0009
Admission, observation, G0379
Administrative, Miscellaneous and Investigational,
   A9000–A9999
   alert or alarm device, A9280
   artificial saliva, A9155
   DME delivery set-up, A9901
   eaching grabbing device, A9281
   exercise equipment, A9300

◀ **New**   ↻ **Revised**   ✔ **Reinstated**   ~~deleted~~ **Deleted**

Administrative, Miscellaneous and Investigational
(Continued)
external ambulatory insulin delivery system, *A9274*
foot pressure off loading/supportive device, *A9283*
helmets, *A8000–A8004*
home glucose disposable monitor, *A9275*
hot-water bottle, ice cap, heat wrap, *A9273*
miscellaneous DME, NOS, *A9999*
miscellaneous DME supply, *A9900*
monitoring feature/device, stand-alone or integrated, *A9279*
multiple vitamins, oral, per dose, *A9153*
non-covered item, *A9270*
non-prescription drugs, *A9150*
pediculosis treatment, topical, *A9180*
radiopharmaceuticals, *A9500–A9700*
receiver, external, interstitial glucose monitoring system, *A9278*
sensor, invasive, interstitial continuous glucose monitoring, *A9276*
single vitamin/mineral trace element, *A9152*
spirometer, non-electronic, *A9284*
transmitter, interstitial continuous glucose monitoring system, *A9277*
wig, any type, *A9282*
wound suction, disposable, *A9272*
Ado-trastuzumab, J9354
Adrenalin, J0171
Advanced life support, *A0390, A0426, A0427, A0433*
ALS emergency transport, *A0427*
ALS mileage, *A0390*
ALS, non-emergency transport, *A0426*
ALS2, *A0433*
Aerosol
compressor, E0571–E0572
compressor filter, K0178–K0179
mask, K0180
Aflibercept, J0178
AFO, E1815, E1830, L1900–L1990, L4392, L4396
Agalsidase beta, J0180
Aggrastat, J3245
A-hydroCort, J1710
Aid, hearing, V5030–V5263
Aide, home, health, G0156, S9122, T1021
home health aide/certified nurse assistant, in home, *S9122*
home health aide/certified nurse assistant, per visit, *T1021*
home health or hospital setting, *G0156*
Air bubble detector, dialysis, E1530
Air fluidized bed, E0194
Air pressure pad/mattress, E0186, E0197
Air travel and nonemergency transportation, A0140
Alarm
not otherwise classified, *A9280*
pressure, dialysis, E1540
Alatrofloxacin mesylate, J0200

Albumin, human, P9041, P9042
Albuterol
all formulations, inhalation solution, concentrated, J7610, J7611
all formulations, inhalation solution, unit dose, J7609, J7613
all formulations, inhalation solution, J7620
Alcohol/substance, assessment, G0396, G0397, H0001, H0003, H0049
alcohol abuse structured assessment, 15–30 min. *G0396*
alcohol abuse structured assessment, greater than 30 min. *G0397*
alcohol and/or drug assessment, Medicaid, *H0001*
alcohol and/or drug screening, Medicaid, *H0049*
alcohol and/or drug screening; laboratory analysis, Medicaid, *H0003*
Alcohol, A4244
Alcohol wipes, A4245
Aldesleukin (IL2), J9015
Alefacept, J0215
Alemtuzumab, J9010
Alert device, A9280
Alginate dressing, A6196–A6199
alginate, wound filler, sterile, *A6199*
alginate, pad more than 48 sq. cm, *A6198*
alginate, pad size 16 sq. cm, *A6196*
alginate, pad size more than 16 sq. cm, *A6197*
Alglucerase, J0205
Alglucosidase, J0220
Alglucosidase alfa, J0221
Alphanate, J7186
Alpha-1–proteinase inhibitor, human, J0256, J0257
Alprostadil
injection, J0270
urethral suppository, J0275
ALS mileage, A0390
Alteplase recombinant, J2997
Alternating pressure mattress/pad, A4640, E0181, E0277
overlay/pad, alternating, pump, heavy duty, *E0181*
powered pressure-reducing air mattress, *E0277*
replacement pad, owned by patient, *A4640*
Alveoloplasty, D7310–D7321
in conjunction with extractions, four or more teeth, *D7310*
in conjunction with extractions, one to three teeth, *D7311*
not in conjunction with extractions, four or more teeth, *D7320*
not in conjunction with extractions, one to three teeth, *D7321*
Amalgam dental restoration, D2140–D2161
four or more surfaces, primary or permanent, *D2161*
one surface, primary or permanent, *D2140*
three surfaces, primary or permanent, *D2160*
two surfaces, primary or permanent, *D2150*

◄ **New**   ↻ **Revised**   ✓ **Reinstated**   ~~deleted~~ **Deleted**

Ambulance, A0021–A0999
 air, A0430, A0431, A0435, A0436
  conventional, transport, one way, fixed wing, A0430
  conventional, transport, one way, rotary wing, A0431
  fixed wing air mileage, A0435
  rotary wing air mileage, A0436
 disposable supplies, A0382–A0398
  ALS routine disposable supplies, A0398
  ALS specialized service disposable supplies, A0394
  *ALS specialized service, esophageal
  intubation, A0396*
  BLS routine disposable, A0832
  *BLS specialized service disposable supplies, defibril-
  lation, A0384, A0392*
 non-emergency transport, fixed wing, S9960
 non-emergency transport, rotary wing, S9961
 oxygen, A0422
Ambulation device, E0100–E0159
 *brake attachment, wheeled walker
  replacement, E0159*
 cane, adjustable or fixed, with tip, E0100
 *cane, quad or three prong, adjustable or fixed, with
  tip, E0105*
 crutch attachment, walker, E0157
 crutch forearm, each, with tips and handgrips, E0111
 *crutch substitute, lower leg platform, with or without
  wheels, each, E0118*
 *crutch, underarm, articulating, spring assisted,
  each, E0117*
 crutches forearm, pair, tips and handgrips, E0110
 *crutches, underarm, other than wood, pair, with
  pads, tips and handgrips, E0114*
 *crutches, underarm, other than wood, with pad, tip,
  handgrip, with or without shock absorber,
  each, E0116*
 *crutches, underarm, wood, each, with pad, tip and
  handgrip, E0113*
 leg extensions, walker, set (4), E0158
 platform attachment, forearm crutch, each, E0153
 platform attachment, walker, E0154
 seat attachment, walker, E0156
 *walker, enclosed, four-sided frame, wheeled, posterior
  seat, E0144*
 walker, folding, adjustable or fixed height, E0135
 *walker, folding, wheeled, adjustable or fixed
  height, E0143*
 *walker, heavy duty, multiple braking system, variable
  wheel resistance, E0147*
 walker, heavy duty, wheeled, rigid or folding, E0149
 *walker, heavy duty, without wheels, rigid or
  folding, E0148*
 walker, rigid, adjustable or fixed height, E0130
 *walker, rigid, wheeled, adjustable or fixed
  height, E0141*
 *walker, with trunk support, adjystable or fixed height,
  any, E0140*
 *wheel attachment, rigid, pick up walker, per
  pair, E0155*

Amikacin Sulfate, J0278
Aminolevulinate, J7309
Aminolevulinic acid HCl, J7308
Aminophylline, J0280
Amiodarone HCl, J0282
Amitriptyline HCl, J1320
Ammonia N-13, A9526
Ammonia test paper, A4774
Amniotic membrane, V2790
Amobarbital, J0300
Amphotericin B, J0285
 Lipid Complex, J0287–J0289
Ampicillin
 sodium, J0290
 sodium/sulbactam sodium, J0295
Amputee
 adapter, wheelchair, E0959
 prosthesis, L5000–L7510, L7520, L7900,
  L8400–L8465
  above knee, L5200–L5230
  *additions to exoskeletal knee-shin systems,
  L5710–L5782*
  additions to lower extremity, L5610–L5617
  *additions to socket insert and suspension,
  L5654–L5699*
  additions to socket variations, L5630–L5653
  additions to test sockets, L5618–L5629
  *additions/replacements feet-ankle units,
  L5700–L5707*
  ankle, L5050–L5060
  below knee, L5100–L5105
  component modification, L5785–L5795
  endoskeletal, L5810–L5999
  endoskeleton, below knee, L5301–L5312
  endoskeleton, hip disarticulation, L5331–L5341
  fitting endoskeleton, above knee, L5321
  fitting procedures, L5400–L5460
  hemipelvectomy, L5280
  hip disarticulation, L520–L5270
  initial prosthesis, L5500–L5505
  knee disarticulation, L5150–L5160
  male vacuum erection system, L7900
  partial foot, L5000–L5020
  preparatory prosthesis, L5510–L5600
  prosthetic socks, L8400–L8485
  repair, prosthetic device, L7520
  tension ring, vacuum erection device, L7902
  upper extremity, battery components, L7360–L7368
  upper extremity, other/repair, L7400–L7510
  upper extremity, preparatory, elbow, L6584–L6586
  upper limb, above elbow, L6250
  upper limb, additions, L6600–L6698
  upper limb, below elbow, L6100–L6130
  upper limb, elbow disarticulation, L6200–L6205
  upper limb, endoskeletal, above elbow, L6500
  upper limb, endoskeletal, below elbow, L6400
  *upper limb, endoskeletal, elbow
  disarticulation, L6450*

◀ **New** ↺ **Revised** ✔ **Reinstated** ~~deleted~~ **Deleted**

Amputee *(Continued)*
  upper limb, endoskeletal, interscapular thoracic, L6570
  upper limb, endoskeletal, shoulder disarticulation, L6550
  upper limb, external power, device, L6920–L6975
  upper limb, interscapular thoracic, L6350–L6370
  upper limb, partial hand, L6000–L6025
  upper limb, postsurgical procedures, L6380–L6388
  upper limb, preparatory, shoulder, interscapular, L6588–L6590
  upper limb, preparatory, wrist, L6580–L6582
  upper limb, shoulder disarticulation, L6300–L6320
  upper limb, terminal devices, L6703–L6915
  upper limb, terminal devices, L7007–L7261
  upper limb, wrist disarticulation, L6050–L6055
  stump sock, L8470–L8485
  single ply, fitting above knee, L8480
  single ply, fitting, below knee, L8470
  single ply, fitting, upper limb, L8485
  wheelchair, E1170–E1190, E1200, K0100
  detachable arms, swing away detachable elevating footrests, E1190
  detachable arms, swing away detachable footrests, E1180
  detachable arms, without footrests or legrest, E1172
  detachable elevating legrest, fixed full length arms, E1170
  fixed full length arms, swing away detachable footrest, E1200
  heavy duty wheelchair, swing away detachable elevating legrests, E1195
  without footrests or legrest, fixed full length arms, E1171
Amygdalin, J3570
Anadulafungin, J0348
Analgesia, dental, D9230
Analysis
  saliva, D0418
  semen, G0027
Angiography, iliac, artery, G0278
Angiography, renal, non-selective, G0275
  non-ophthalmic fluorescent vascular, C9733
  reconstruction, G0288
Anistreplase, J0350
Ankle splint, recumbent, K0126–K0130
Ankle-foot orthosis (AFO), L1900–L1990, L2106–L2116, L4361, L4392, L4396
  ankle gauntlet, custom fabricated, L1904
  ankle gauntlet, prefabricated, off-shelf, L1902
  double upright free plantar dorsiflexion, olid stirrup, calf-band/cuff , custom, L1990
  fracture orthrosis, tibial fracture, thermoplastic cast material, custom, L2106
  multiligamentus ankle support, prefabricated, off-shelf, L1906
  plastic or other material, custom fabricated, L1940

Ankle-foot orthosis (AFO) *(Continued)*
  plastic or other material, prefabricated, fitting and adjustment, L1932
  plastic or other material, prefabricated, fitting and adjustment, L1951
  plastic or other material, with ankle joint, prefabricated, fitting and adjustment, L1971
  plastic, rigid anterior tibial section, custom fabricated, L1945
  plastic, with ankle joint, custom, L1970
  posterior, single bar, clasp attachment to shoe, L1910
  posterior, solid ankle, plastic, custom, L1960
  replacement, soft interface material, static AFO, L4392
  single upright free plantar dorsiflection, solid stirrup, calf-band/cuff, custom, L1980
  single upright with static or adjustable stop, custom, L1920
  spiral, plastic, custom fabricated, L1950
  spring wire, dorsiflexion assist calf band, L1900
  static or dynamic AFO, adjustable for fit, minimal ambulation, L4396
  supramalleolar with straps, custom fabricated, L1907
  tibial fracture cast orthrosis, custom, L2108
  tibial fracture orthrosis, rigid, prefabricated, fitting and adjustment, L2116
  tibial fracture orthrosis, semi-rigid, prefabricated, fitting and adjustment, L2114
  tibial fracture orthrosis, soft prefabricated, fitting and adjustment, L2112
  walking boot, prefabricated, off-the-shelf, L4361
Anterior-posterior-lateral orthosis, L0700, L0710
Antibiotic, G8708–G8712
  antibiotic not prescribed or dispensed, G8712
  patient not prescribed or dispensed antibiotic, G8708
  patient prescribed antibiotic, documented condition, G8709
  patient prescribed or dispensed antibiotic, G8710
  prescribed or dispensed antibiotic, G8711
Antidepressant, documentation, G8126–G8128
Anti-emetic, oral, Q0163–Q0181, J8498, J8597
  antiemetic drug, oral NOS, J8597
  antiemetic drug, rectal suppository, NOS, J8498
  diphenhydramine hydrochloride, 50 mg, oral, Q0163
  dolasetron mesylate, 100 mg, oral, Q0180
  dronabinol, 2.5 mg, Q0167
  granisetron hydrochloride, 1 mg, oral, Q0166
  hydroxyzine pomoate, 25 mg, oral, Q0177
  perphenazine, 4 mg, oral, Q0175
  prochlorperazine maleate,mg, oral, Q0164
  promethazine hydrochloride, 12.5 mg, oral, Q0169
  thiethylperazine maleate, 10 mg, oral, Q0174
  trimethobenzamide hydrochloride, 250 mg, oral, Q0173
  unspecified oral dose, Q0181
Anti-hemophilic factor (Factor VIII), J7190–J7192
Anti-inhibitors, per I.U., J7198

◄ **New**   ⊃ **Revised**   ✓ **Reinstated**   ~~deleted~~ **Deleted**

Antimicrobial, prophylaxis, documentation, G8201, D4281

Anti-neoplastic drug, NOC, J9999

Antithrombin III, J7197

Antithrombin recombinant, J7196

Antral fistula closure, oral, D7260

Apexification, dental, D3351–D3353

Apicoectomy, D3410–D3426
  (each additional root), D3426
  anterior, periradicular surgery, D3410
  biscuspid (first root), D3421
  molar (first root), D3425

Apomorphine, J0364

Appliance
  cleaner, A5131
  pneumatic, E0655–E0673
    non-segmental pneumatic appliance, E0655, E0660, E0665, E0666
    segmental gradient pressure, pneumatic appliance, E0671–E0673
    segmental pneumatic appliance, E0656, E0657, E0667, E0668, E0669, E0670

Application, heat, cold, E0200–E0239
  electric heat pad, moist, E0215
  electric heat pad, standard, E0210
  heat lamp with stand, E0205
  heat lamp without stand, E0200
  hydrocollator unit, pads, E0225
  hydrocollator unit, portable, E0239
  infrared heating pad system, E0221
  non-contact wound warming device, E0231
  paraffin bath unit, E0235
  phototherapy (bilirubin), E0202
  pump for water circulating pad, E0236
  therapeutic lightbox, E0203
  warming card, E0232
  water circulating cold pad with pump, E0218
  water circulating heat pad with pump, E0217

Aprotinin, J0365

Aqueous
  shunt, L8612
  sterile, J7051

ARB/ACE therapy, G8473–G8475

Arbutamine HCl, J0395

Arch support, L3040–L3100
  hallus-valgus night dynamic splint, off-shelf, L3100
  intralesional, J3302
  non-removable, attached to shoe, longitudinal, L3070
  non-removable, attached to shoe, longitudinal/ metatarsal, each, L3090
  non-removable, attached to shoe, metatarsal, L3080
  removable, premolded, longitudinal, L3040
  removable, premolded, longitudinal/metatarsal, each, L3060
  removable, premolded, metatarsal, L3050

Arformoterol, J7605

Aripiprazole, J0400, J0401

Arm, wheelchair, E0973

Arsenic trioxide, J9017

Artificial
  Cornea, L8609
  kidney machines and accessories (*see also* Dialysis), E1510–E1699
  larynx, L8500
  saliva, A9155

Arthrography, injection, sacroiliac, joint, G0259, G0260

Arthroscopy, knee, surgical, G0289, S2112
  chondroplasty, different compartment, knee, G0289
  harvesting of cartilage, knee, S2112

Asparaginase, J9019–J9020

Aspiration, bone marrow, G0364

Aspirator, VABRA, A4480

Assessment
  alcohol/substance, G0396, G0397, H0001, H0003, H0049 (*see also* Alcohol/substance, assessment)
  audiologic, V5008–V5020
  assessment for hearing, V5010
  conformity evaluation, V5020
  fitting/orientation, hearing aid, V5014
  hearing screening, V5008
  repair/modification hearing aid, V5014
  cardiac output, M0302
  speech, V5362–V5364

Assistive listening devices and accessories, V5281–V5290
  FMlDM system, monaural, V5281

Astramorph, J2275

Atherectomy, PTCA C9602, C9603

Atropine
  inhalation solution, concentrated, J7635
  inhalation solution, unit dose, J7636

Atropine sulfate, J0461

Attachment, walker, E0154–E0159
  brake attachment, wheeled walker, replacement, E0159
  crutch attachment, walker, E0157
  leg extension, walker, E0158
  platform attachment, walker, E0154
  seat attachment, walker, E0156
  wheel attachment, rigid pick up walker, E0155

Audiologic assessment, V5008–V5020

Auditory osseointegrated device, L8690–L8693

Auricular prosthesis, D5914, D5927

Aurothioglucose, J2910

Azacitidine, J9025

Azathioprine, J7500, J7501

Azithromycin injection, J0456

B

Back supports, L0621–L0861, L0960
  lumbar orthosis, L0625–L0627
  lumbar orthosis, sagittal control, L0641–L0648
  lumbar-sacral orthrosis, L628–L0640

◀ **New**   ⊃ **Revised**   ✔ **Reinstated**   ~~deleted~~ **Deleted**

Back supports *(Continued)*
  lumbar-sacral orthrosis, sagittal-coronal control,
    L0640, L0649–L0651
  sacroiliac orthrosis, L0621–L0624
Baclofen, J0475, J0476
Bacterial sensitivity study, P7001
Bag
  drainage, A4357
  enema, A4458
  irrigation supply, A4398
  urinary, A4358, A5112
Bandage, conforming
  elastic, <3", A6448
  elastic, >5", A6450
  elastic, >3", <5", A6449
  elastic, load resistance <1.35 foot pounds, >3", <5",
    A6452
  elastic, load resistance 1.25 to 1.34 foot pounds, >3",
    <5", A6451
  non-elastic, non-sterile, >5", A6444
  non-elastic, non-sterile, width greater than or equal
    to 3 inches, <5 inches, A6443
  non-elastic, non-sterile, width <3 inches, A6442
  non-elastic, sterile, >3" and <5", A6446
  non-elastic, sterile, >5", A6447
Basiliximab, J0480
Bath, aid, E0160–E0162, E0235, E0240–E0249
  bath tub rail, floor base, E0242
  bath tub wall rail, E0241
  bath/shower chair, with/without wheels, E0240
  pad for water circulating heat unit, replacement,
    E0249
  paraffin bath unit, portable, E0235
  raised toilet seat, E0244
  sitz bath chair, E0162
  sitz type bath, portable, with faucet
    attachment, E0161
  sitz type bath, portable, with/without
    commode, E0160
  toilet rail, E0243
  transfer bench, tub or toilet, E0248
  transfer tub rail attachment, E0246
  tub stool or bench, E0245
Bathtub
  chair, E0240
  stool or bench, E0245, E0247–E0248
  transfer rail, E0246
  wall rail, E0241, E0242
Battery, L7360, L7364–L7368
  charger, E1066, L7362, L7366
  replacement for blood glucose monitor,
    A4233–A4234
  replacement for cochlear implant device,
    L8623–L8624
  replacement for TENS, A4630
  ventilator, A4611–A4613
BCG live, intravesical, J9031
Beclomethasone inhalation solution, J7622

Bed
  accessories, E0271–E0280, E0300–E0326
    bed board, E0273
    bed cradle, E0280
    bed pan, fracture, metal, E0276
    bed pan, standard, metal, E0275
    mattress innerspring, E0271
    mattress, foam rubber, E0272
    over-bed table, E0274
    power pressure-reducing air mattress, E0277
  air fluidized, E0194
  cradle, any type, E0280
  drainage bag, bottle, A4357, A5102
  hospital, E0250–E0270, E0300–E0329
  pan, E0275, E0276
  rail, E0305, E0310
  safety enclosure frame/canopy, E0316
Behavioral therapy, cardiovascular
    disease, G0446
Behavioral, health, treatment services,
    H0002–H2037 (Medicaid)
  activity therapy, H2032
  alcohol/drug services, H0001, H0003, H0005–H0016,
    H0020–H0022, H0026–H0029, H0049–H0050,
    H2034–H2036
  assertive community treatment, H0040
  community based wrap-around services,
    H2021–H2022
  comprehensive community
    support, H2015–H2016
  comprehensive medication services, H2010
  comprehensive multidisciplinary
    evaluation, H2000
  crisis intervention, H2011
  day treatment, per diem, H2013
  day treatment, per hour, H2012
  developmental delay prevention activities, dependent
    child of client, H2037
  family assessment, H1011
  foster care, child, H0041–H0042
  health screening, H0002
  hotline service, H0030
  medication training, H0034
  mental health clubhouse services, H2030–H2031
  multisystemic therapy, juveniles, H2033
  non-medical family planning, H1010
  outreach service, H0023
  partial hospitalization, H0035
  plan development, non-physician, H0033
  prenatal care, at risk, H1000–H1005
  prevention, H0024–H0025
  psychiatric supportive treatment, community,
    H0036–H0037
  psychoeducational service, H2027
  psychoscial rehabilitation, H2017–H2018
  rehabilitation program, H2010
  residential treatment program, H0017–H0019
  respite care, not home, H0045

◄ **New**   ↻ **Revised**   ✓ **Reinstated**   ~~deleted~~ **Deleted**

Behavioral, health, treatment services *(Continued)*
  self-help/peer services, H0039
  sexual offender treatment, H2028–H2029
  skill training, H2014
  supported employment, H2024–H2026
  supported housing, H0043–H0044
  therapeutic behavioral services, H2019–H2020
Belatacept, J0485
Belimumab, J0490
Belt
  extremity, E0945
  ostomy, A4367
  pelvic, E0944
  safety, K0031
  wheelchair, E0978, E0979
Bench, bathtub *(see also* **Bathtub),** E0245
Bendamustine HCl, J9033
Benesch boot, L3212–L3214
Benztropine, J0515
Beta-blocker therapy, G9188–G9192
Betadine, A4246, A4247
Betameth, J0704
Betamethasone
  acetate and betamethasone sodium
    phosphate, J0702
  inhalation solution, J7624
Bethanechol chloride, J0520
Bevacizumab, J9035, Q2024
Bicuspid (excluding final restoration), D3320
  retreatment, by report, D3347
  surgery, first root, D3421
Bifocal, glass or plastic, V2200–V2299
  aniseikonic, bifocal, V2218
  bifocal add-over 3.25 d, V2220
  bifocal seg width over 28 mm, V2219
  lenticular lens, V2221
  lenticular, bifocal, myodisc, V2215
  specialty bifocal, by report, V2200
  sphere, bifocal, V2200–V2202
  spherocylinder, bifocal, V2203–V2214
Bilirubin (phototherapy) light, E0202
Binder, A4465
Biofeedback device, E0746
Bioimpedance, electrical, cardiac output, M0302
Biperiden lactate, J0190
Bitewing, D0270–D0277
  four radiographic images, D0274
  single radiographic image, D0270
  three radiographic images, D0273
  two radiographic images, D0272
  vertical bitewings, 7–8 radiographic images, D0277
Bitolterol mesylate, inhalation solution
  concentrated, J7628
  unit dose, J7629
Bivalirudin, J0583
Bivigam, 500 mg, J1556
Bladder calculi irrigation solution, Q2004
Bleomycin sulfate, J9040

Blood
  count, G0306, G0307, S3630
    complete CBC, automated without platelet count,
    automated WBC differential, G0306
    complete CBC, automated, without platelet count,
    G0307
    eosinophil count, blood, direct, S3630
  fresh frozen plasma, P9017
  glucose monitor, E0607, E2100, E2101,
    S1030, S1031, S1034
    blood glucose monitor with integrated lancing/
    blood sample, E2101
    blood glucose monitor, integrated voice
    synthesizer, E2100
    continuous noninvasive device, purchase, S1030
    continuous noninvasive device, rental, S1031
    home blood glucose monitor, E0607
  glucose test, A4253
  glucose, test strips, dialysis, A4772
  granulocytes, pheresis, P9050
  ketone test, A4252
  leak detector, dialysis, E1560
  leukocyte poor, P9016
  mucoprotein, P2038
  platelets, P9019
  platelets, irradiated, P9032
  platelets, leukocytes reduced, P9031
  platelets, leukocytes reduced, irradiated, P9033
  platelets, pheresis, P9034
  platelets, pheresis, irradiated, P9036
  platelets, pheresis, leukocytes reduced, P9035
  platelets, pheresis, leukocytes reduced,
    irradiated, P9037
  pressure monitor, A4660, A4663, A4670
  pump, dialysis, E1620
  red blood cells, deglycerolized, P9039
  red blood cells, irradiated, P9038
  red blood cells, leukocytes reduced, P9016
  red blood cells, leukocytes reduced,
    irradiated, P9040
  red blood cells, washed, P9022
  strips, A4253
  supply, P9010 P9022
  testing supplies, A4770
  tubing, A4750, A4755
Blood collection devices accessory, A4257, E0620
BMI, G8417–G8422
Body jacket
  scoliosis, L1300, L1310
Body sock, L0984
Body, mass, index, G8417–G8422
Bond or cement, ostomy skin, A4364
Bone
  density, study, G0130
  marrow, aspiration, G0364
Boot
  pelvic, E0944
  surgical, ambulatory, L3260

◄ **New**   ⟳ **Revised**   ✔ **Reinstated**   ~~deleted~~ **Deleted**

Bortezomib, J9041
Brachytherapy radioelements, Q3001
  brachytherapy, LDR, prostate, G0458
  brachytherapy, source, hospital outpatient,
    C1716–C1717, C1719
Breast prosthesis, L8000–L8035, L8600
  adhesive skin support, A4280
  custom breast prosthesis, post mastectomy, L8035
  garment with mastectomy form, post
    mastectomy, L8015
  implantable, silicone or equal, L8600
  mastectomy bra, with integrated breast prosthesis
    form, unilateral, L8001
  mastectomy bra, with prosthesis form,
    bilateral, L8002
  mastectomy bra, without integrated breast prosthesis
    form, L8000
  mastectomy form, L8020
  mastectomy sleeve, L8010
  nipple prosthesis, L8032
  silicone or equal with integral adhesive, L8031
  silicone or equal, without integral adhesive, L8030
Breast pump
  accessories, A4281–A4286
    adapter, replacement, A4282
    cap, breast pump bottle, replacement, A4283
    locking ring, replacement, A4286
    polycarbonate bottle, replacement, A4285
    shield and splash protector, replacement, A4284
    tubing, replacement, A4281
  electric, any type, E0603
  heavy duty, hospital grade, E0604
  manual, any type, E0602
Breathing circuit, A4618
Brentuximab Vedotin, J9042
Bridge
  replacement, D6930
  repair, by report, D6980
Brompheniramine maleate, J0945
Budesonide inhalation solution, J7626, J7627,
  J7633, J7634
Bulking agent, L8604
Buprenorphine hydrochloride, J0592
Buprenorphine/Naloxone, J0571–J0575◄
Burn, compression garment, A6501–A6513
  bodysuit, head-foot, A6501
  burn mask, face and/or neck, A6513
  chin strap, A6502
  facial hood, A6503
  foot to knee length, A6507
  foot to thigh length, A6508
  glove to axilla, A6506
  glove to elbow, A6505
  glove to wrist, A6504
  lower trunk, including leg openings, A6511
  trunk, including arms, down to leg openings, A6510
  upper trunk to waist, including arm
    openings, A6509

Bus, nonemergency transportation, A0110
Busulfan, J0594, J8510
Butorphanol tartrate, J0595
Bypass, graft, coronary, artery
  documentation, G8160–G8163
  surgery, S2205–S2209

C

C-1 Esterase Inhibitor, J0597–J0598
Cabazitaxel, J9043
Cabergoline, oral, J8515
Caffeine citrate, J0706
CABG, documentation, G8160–G8163
Cabinet/System, ultraviolet, E0691–E0694
  multidirectional light system, 6 ft. cabinet, E0694
  timer and eye protection, 4 foot, E0692
  timer and eye protection, 6 foot, E0693
  ultraviolet light therapy system, treatment area
    2 sq ft., E0691
CAD documentation, G8160–G8163
Calcitriol, J0636
Calcitonin-salmon, J0630
Calcitrol, S0169
Calcium
  disodium edetate, J0600
  gluconate, J0610
  glycerophosphate and calcium lactate, J0620
  lactate and calcium glycerophosphate, J0620
  leucovorin, J0640
Calibrator solution, A4256
Canakinumab, J0638
Cancer, screening
  cervical or vaginal, G0101
  colorectal, G0104–G0106, G0120–G0122,
    G0328, S3890
    alternative to screening colonoscopy, barium
    enema, G0120
    alternative to screening sigmoidoscopy, barium
    enema, G0106
    barium enema, G0122
    colonoscopy, high risk, G0105
    colonoscopy, not at high-risk, G0121
    DNA analysis, fecal, colorectal cancer
    screening, S3890
    fecal occult blood test-1–3 simultaneous, G0328
    flexible sigmoidoscopy, G0104
    prostate, G0102, G0103
Cane, E0100, E0105
  accessory, A4636, A4637
Canister
  disposable, used with suction pump, A7000
  non-disposable, used with suction pump, A7001
Cannula, nasal, A4615
Capecitabine, oral, J8520, J8521
Capsaicin patch, J7336↺
Carbon filter, A4680

◄ New   ↺ Revised   ✓ Reinstated   ~~deleted~~ Deleted

Carboplatin, J9045
Cardia Event, recorder, implantable, E0616
Cardiokymography, Q0035
Cardiovascular services, M0300–M0301
  Fabric wrapping abdominal aneurysm, M0301
  IV chelation therapy, M0300
Cardioverter-defibrillator, G0448
Carfilzomib, J9047
Carmustine, J9050
Caries susceptibility test, D0425
Care, coordinated, G9001–G9011, H1002
  coordinated care fee, maintenance rate, G9002
  coordinated care fee, home monitoring, G9006
  coordinated care fee, initial rate, G9001
  coordinated care fee, physician coordinated care over-
    sight, G9008
  coordinated care fee, risk adjusted high,
    initial, G9003
  coordinated care fee, risk adjusted low,
    initial, G9004
  coordinated care fee, risk adjusted maintenance,
    G9005
  coordinated care fee, risk adjusted maintenance,
    level 3, G9009
  coordinated care fee, risk adjusted maintenance,
    level 4, G9010
  coordinated care fee, risk adjusted maintenance,
    level 5, G9011
  coordinated care fee, scheduled team
    conference, G9007
  prenatal care, at-risk, enhanced service, care coordi-
    nation, H1002
Case management, T1016, T1017
Care plan, G0162
Caspofungin acetate, J0637
Cast
  diagnostic, dental, D0470
  hand restoration, L6900–L6915
  materials, special, A4590
  supplies, A4580, A4590, Q4001–Q4051
    body cast, adult, Q4001–Q4002
    cast supplies, (e.g. plaster), A4580
    cast supplies, unlisted types, Q4050
    finger splint, static, Q4049
    gauntlet cast, adult, Q4013–Q4014
    gauntlet cast, pediatric, Q4015–Q4016
    hip spica, adult, Q4025–Q4026
    hip spica, pediatric, Q4027–Q4028
    long arm cast, adult, Q4005–Q4006
    long arm cast, pediatric, Q4007–Q4008
    long arm splint, adult, Q4017–Q4018
    long arm splint, pediatric, Q4019–Q4020
    long leg cast, adult, Q4029–Q4030
    long leg cast, pediatric, Q4031–Q4032
    long leg cylinder cast, adult, Q4033–Q4034
    long leg cylinder cast, pediatric, Q4035–Q4036
    long leg splint, adult, Q4041–Q4042
    long leg splint, pediatric, Q4043–Q4044

Cast *(Continued)*
    short arm cast, adult, Q4009–Q4010
    short arm cast, pediatric, Q4011–Q4012
    short arm splint, adult, Q4021–Q4022
    short arm splint, pediatric, Q4023–Q4024
    short leg cast, adult, Q4037–Q4038
    short leg cast, pediatric, Q4039–Q4040
    short leg splint, adult, Q4045–Q4046
    short leg splint, pediatric, Q4047–Q4048
    shoulder cast, adult, Q4003–Q4004
    special casting material (fiberglass), A4590
    splint supplies, miscellaneous, Q4051
  thermoplastic, L2106, L2126
Caster
  front, for power wheelchair, K0099
  wheelchair, E0997, E0998
Catheter, A4300–A4355
  anchoring device, A5200, A4333, A4334
  cap, disposable (dialysis), A4860
  external collection device, A4327–A4330, A4347,
    A7048↵
  implanted, A7042, A7043✗
  indwelling, A4338–A4346
  insertion tray, A4354
  intermittent with insertion supplies, A4353
  irrigation supplies, A4355
  male external, A4324, A4325, A4348
  oropharyngeal suction, A4628
  starter set, A4329
  trachea (suction), A4609, A4610, A4624
  transtracheal oxygen, A4608
  vascular, A4300, A4301
Catheterization, specimen collection, P9612, P9615
CBC, G0306, G0307
Cefazolin sodium, J0690
Cefepime HCl, J0692
Cefotaxime sodium, J0698
Ceftaroline fosamil, J0712
Ceftazidime, J0713
Ceftizoxime sodium, J0715
Ceftriaxone sodium, J0696
Cefuroxime sodium, J0697
CellCept, K0412
Cellular therapy, M0075
Cement, ostomy, A4364
Centrifuge, A4650
Centruroides Immune F(ab), J0716
Cephalin Floculation, blood, P2028
Cephalothin sodium, J1890
Cephapirin sodium, J0710
Certification, physician, home, health (per calendar
    month), G0179–G0182
  Physician certification, home health, G0180
  Physician recertification, home health, G0179
  Physician supervision, home health, complex care,
    30 min or more, G0181
  Physician supervision, hospice 30 min
    or more, G0102

◄ **New**   ↵ **Revised**   ✔ **Reinstated**   ~~deleted~~ **Deleted**

11

Certolizumab pegol, J0717
Cerumen, removal, G0268
Cervical
cancer, screening, G0101
cytopathology, G0123, G0124, G0141–G0148
  screening smears, automated system, manual re-screening, G0148
  screening smears, automated system, physician supervision, G0147
  screening, automated thin layer preparation, cyto-technologist, physician interpretation, G0143
  screening, automated thin layer preparation, physi-cian supervision, G0144
  screening, automated thin layer, manual rescreen-ing, physician supervision, G0145
  screening, by cytotechnologist, physician supervi-sion, G0123
  screening, cytopathology smears, automated sys-tem, physician interpretation, G0141
  screening, interpretation by physician, G0124
halo, L0810–L0830
head harness/halter, E0942
orthosis, L0100–L0200
  cervical collar molded to patient, L0170
  cervical, flexible collar, L0120–L0130
  cervical, multiple post collar, supports, L0180–L0200
  cervical, semi-rigid collar, L0150–L0160, L0172, L0174
  cranial cervical, L0112–L0113
traction, E0855, E0856
Cervical cap contraceptive, A4261
Cervical-thoracic-lumbar-sacral orthosis (CTLSO), L0700, L0710
Cetuximab, J9055
Chair
adjustable, dialysis, E1570
lift, E0627
rollabout, E1031
sitz bath, E0160–E0162
transport, E1035–E1039
  chair, adult size, heavy duty, greater than 300 pounds, E1039
  chair, adult size, up to 300 pounds, E1038
  chair, pediatric, E1037
  multi-positional patient transfer system, extra-wide, greater than 300 pounds, E1036
  multi-positional patient transfer system, up to 300 pounds, E1035
Chelation therapy, M0300
Chemical endarterectomy, M0300
Chemistry and toxicology tests, P2028–P3001
Chemotherapy
administration (hospital reporting only), Q0083–Q0085
drug, oral, not otherwise classified, J8999
drugs (see also drug by name), J9000–J9999
Chest shell (cuirass), E0457

Chest Wall Oscillation System, E0483
hose, replacement, A7026
vest, replacement, A7025
Chest wrap, E0459
Chin cup, cervical, L0150
Chloramphenicol sodium succinate, J0720
Chlordiazepoxide HCl, J1990
Chloromycetin sodium succinate, J0720
Chloroprocaine HCl, J2400
Chloroquine HCl, J0390
Chlorothiazide sodium, J1205
Chlorpromazine HCl, J3230
Chlorpromazine HCL, 5 mg, oral, Q0161
Choroid, lesion, destruction, G0186
Chorionic gonadotropin, J0725
Chromic phosphate P32 suspension, A9564
Chromium CR-51 sodium chromate, A9553
Cidofovir, J0740
Cilastatin sodium, imipenem, J0743
Ciprofloxacin, for intravenous infusion, J0744
Cisplatin, J9060
Cladribine, J9065
Clamp
dialysis, A4910, A4918, A4920
external urethral, A4356
Cleanser, wound, A6260
Cleansing agent, dialysis equipment, A4790
Clofarabine, J9027
Clonidine, J0735
Closure, wound, adhesive, tissue, G0168
Clotting time tube, A4771
Clubfoot wedge, L3380
Cochlear prosthetic implant, L8614
accessories, L8615–L8617
batteries, L8621–L8624
replacement, L8619, L8627–L8629
  external controller component, L8628
  external speech processor and controller, integrated system, L8619
  external speech processor, component, L8627
  transmitting coil and cable, integrated, L8629
Codeine phosphate, J0745
Colchicine, J0760
Cold/Heat, application, E0200–E0239
  bilirubin light, E0202
  electric heat pad, standard, E0210
  electric heat pad, moist, E0215
  heat lamp with stand, E0205
  heat lamp, without stand, E0200
  hydrocollator unit, E0225
  hydrocollator unit, portable, E0239
  infrared heating pad system, E0221
  non-contact wound warming device, E0231
  paraffin bath unit, E0235
  pump for water circulating pad, E0236
  therapeutic lightbox, E0203
  warming card, non-contact wound warming device, E0232

◄ **New**   ↺ **Revised**   ✔ **Reinstated**   ~~deleted~~ **Deleted**

◄ New ↻ Revised ✔ Reinstated ~~deleted~~ Deleted

Corset, spinal orthosis, L0970–L0976
  LSO full corset, L0976
  LSO, corset front, L0972
  TLSO, corset front, L0970
  TLSO, full corset, L0974
Corticorelin ovine triflutate, J0795
Corticotropin, J0800
Corvert, *see* **Ibutilide fumarate**
Cosyntropin, J0833, J0834
Cough stimulating device, A7020, E0482
Counseling
  alcohol misuse, G0443
  cardiovascular disease, G0448
  control of dental disease, D1310, D1320
  obesity, G0447
  sexually transmitted infection, G0445
  smoking and tobacco cessation, G0436, G0437
Count, blood, *G0306, G0307, S3636*
Counterpulsation, external, *G0166*
Cover, wound
  alginate dressing, A6196–A6198
  foam dressing, A6209–A6214
  hydrogel dressing, A6242–A6248
  non-contact wound warming cover, and accessory, A6000, E0231, E0232
  specialty absorptive dressing, A6251–A6256
CPAP (continuous positive airway pressure) device, E0601
  headgear, K0185
  humidifier, A7046
  intermittent assist, E0452
Cradle, bed, E0280
Crib, E0300
Cromolyn sodium, inhalation solution, unit dose, J7631, J7632
Crotalidae polyvalent immune fab, J0840
Crowns, *D2710–D2983, D4249, D6720–D6794*
  clinical crown lengthening-hard tissue, D4249
  fixed partial denture retainers, crowns, D6710–D6794
  single restoration, D2710–D2983
Crutches, E0110–E0118
  accessories, A4635–A4637, K0102
  crutch substitute, lower leg, E0118
  forearm, E0110–E0111
  underarm, E0112–E0117
Cryoprecipitate, each unit, P9012
CTLSO, L1000–L1120, L0700, L0710
  addition, axilla sling, L1010
  addition, cover for upright, each, L1120
  addition, kyphosis pad, floating, L1025
  addition, kyphosis pad, L1020
  addition, lumbar bolster pad, L1030
  addition, lumbar rib pad, L1040
  addition, lumbar sling, L1090
  addition, outrigger bilateral, vertical extensions, L1085
  addition, outrigger, L1080
  addition, ring flange, L1100

CTLSO *(Continued)*
  addition, ring flange, molded to patient model, L1110
  addition, sternal pad, L1050
  addition, thoracic pad, L1060
  addition, trapezius sling, L1070
  anterior-posterior-lateral control, molded to patient model (CTLSO), L0710
  cervical, thoracic, lumbar, sacral orthrosis (CTLSO), L0700
  furnishing initial orthosis, L1000
  immobilizer, infant size, L1001
  tension based scoliosis orthosis, fitting, L1005
Cuirass, E0457
Culture sensitivity study, P7001
Cushion, wheelchair, E0977
Cyanocobalamin Cobalt C057, A9559
Cycler dialysis machine, E1594
Cyclophosphamide, J9070
  oral, J8530
Cyclosporine, J7502, J7515, J7516
Cytarabine, J9100
  liposome, J9098
Cytomegalovirus immune globulin (human), J0850
Cytopathology, cervical or vaginal, G0123, G0124, G0141–G0148

D

Dacarbazine, J9130
Daclizumab, J7513
Dactinomycin, J9120
Dalalone, J1100
Dalteparin sodium, J1645
Daptomycin, J0878
Darbepoetin Alfa, J0881–J0882
Daunorubicin
  Citrate, J9151
  HCl, J9150
DaunoXome, *see* **Daunorubicin citrate**
Decitabine, J0894
Decubitus care equipment, E0181–E0199
  air fluidized bed, E0194
  air pressure mattress, E0186
  air pressure pad, standard mattress, E0197
  dry pressure mattress, E0184
  dry pressure pad, standard mattress, E0199
  gel or gel-like pressure pad mattress, standard, E0185
  gel pressure mattress, E0196
  heel or elbow protector, E0191
  positioning cushion, E0190
  power pressure reducing mattress overlay, with pump, E0181
  powered air flotation bed, E0193
  pump, alternating pressure pad, replacement, E0182
  synthetic sheepskin pad, E0189
  water pressure mattress, E0187
  water pressure pad, standard mattress, E0198

◄ New   ↻ Revised   ✔ Reinstated   ~~deleted~~ Deleted

Deferoxamine mesylate, J0895
Defibrillator, external, E0617, K0606
  battery, K0607
  electrode, K0609
  garment, K0608
Degarelix, J9155
Deionizer, water purification system, E1615
Delivery/set-up/dispensing, A9901
Denileukin diftitox, J9160
Denosumab, J0897
Density, bone, study, G0130
Dental procedures
  adjunctive general services, D9000–D9999
  alveoloplasty, D7310–D7320
  analgesia, D9230
  diagnostic, D0100–D0999
  endodontics, D3000–D3999
  evaluations, D0120–D0180
  implant services, D6000–D6199
  implants, D3460, D5925, D6010–D6067,
    D6075–D6199
  laboratory, D0415–D0999
  maxillofacial, D5900–D5999
  orthodontics, D8000–D8999
  periodontics, D4000–D4999
  preventive, D1000–D1999
  prosthetics, D5911–D5960, D5999
  prosthodontics, fixed, D6200–D6999
  prosthodontics, removable, D5000–D5999
  restorative, D2000–D2999
Dentures, D5110–D5899
Depo-estradiol cypionate, J1000
Dermal filler injection, G0429
Desmopressin acetate, J2597
Destruction, lesion, choroid, G0186
Detector, blood leak, dialysis, E1560
Developmental testing, G0451
Devices, other orthopedic, E1800–E1841
  assistive listening device, V5267–V5290
Dexamethasone
  acetate, J1094
  inhalation solution, concentrated, J7637
  inhalation solution, unit dose, J7638
  intravitreal implant, J7312
  oral, J8540
  sodium phosphate, J1100
Dextran, J7100
Dextrose
  saline (normal), J7042
  water, J7060, J7070
Dextrostick, A4772
Diabetes
  evaluation, G0245, G0246
  shoes, A5500–A5508 (fitting/modifications)
    deluxe feature, depth-inlay shoe, A5508
    depth inlay shoe, A5500
    molded from cast patient's foot, A5501
    shoe with metatarsal bar, A5505

Diabetes (Continued)
  shoe with off-set heel(s), A5506
  shoe with rocker or rigid-bottom rocker, A5503
  shoe with wedge(s), A5504
  specified modification NOS, depth-inlay
    shoe, A5507
  training, outpatient, G0108, G0109
Diagnostic
  dental services, D0100–D0999
  mammography, digital image, bilateral,
    G0204, G0206
  radiology services, R0070–R0076
Dialysate
  concentrate additives, *peritoneal dialysis,* A4765
  solution, *A4720–A4728*
  testing solution, *test kit, peritoneal,* A4760
Dialysis
  air bubble detector, E1530
  bath conductivity, meter, E1550
  chemicals/antiseptics solution, A4674
  disposable cycler set, A4671
  emergency, G0257
  equipment, E1510–E1702
  extension line, A4672–A4673
  filter, A4680
  fluid barrier, E1575
  forceps, A4910
  home, S9335, S9339
  kit, A4820
  pressure alarm, E1540
  shunt, A4740
  supplies, A4650–A4927
  thermometer, A4910
  tourniquet, A4910
  unipuncture control system, E1580
  unscheduled, G0257
  venous pressure clamp, A4918
Dialyzer, A4690
Diaper, T1500, T4521–T4540, T4543, T4544
  adult incontinence garment, A4520
Diazepam, J3360
Diazoxide, J1730
Dicyclomine HCl, J0500
Diethylstilbestrol diphosphate, J9165
Digoxin, J1160
Digoxin immune fab (ovine), J1162
Dihydroergotamine mesylate, J1110
Dimenhydrinate, J1240
Dimercaprol, J0470
Dimethyl sulfoxide (DMSO), J1212
Diphenhydramine HCl, J1200
Dipyridamole, J1245
Disarticulation
  lower extremities, prosthesis, L5000–L5999
    above knee, L5200–L5230
    additions exoskeletal-knee-shin system,
      L5710–L5782
    additions to lower extremities, L5610–L5617

◀ **New**   ↻ **Revised**   ✔ **Reinstated**   ~~deleted~~ **Deleted**

◄ **New**   ⊋ **Revised**   ✓ **Reinstated**   ~~deleted~~ **Deleted**

Drugs *(Continued)*
  disposable delivery system, 50 ml or greater
    per hour, A4305
  immunosuppressive, J7500–J7599
  infusion supplies, A4230–A4232, A4221, A4222
  inhalation solutions, J7608–J7699
  non-prescription, A9150
  not otherwise classified, J3490, J7599, J7699, J7799,
    J8499, J8999, J9999
  oral, NOS, J8499
  prescription, oral, J8499, J8999
Dry pressure pad/mattress, E0179, E0184, E0199
Durable medical equipment (DME),
    E0100–E1830, K Codes
  additional oxygen related equipment, E1352–E1406
  arm support, wheelchair, E2626–E2633
  artificial kidney machines/accessories, E1500–E1699
  attachments, E0156–E0159
  bath and toilet aides, E0240–E0249
  canes, E0100–E0105
  commodes, E0160–E0175
  crutches, E0110–E0118
  decubitus care equipment, E0181–E0199
  DME, respiratory, inexpensive, purchased,
    A7000–A7509
  gait trainer, E8000–E8002
  heat/cold application, E0200–E0239
  hospital beds and accessories, E0250–E0373
  humidifiers/nebulizers/compressors, oxygen IPPB,
    E0550–E0585
  infusion supplies, E0776–E0791
  IPPB machines, E0500
  jaw motion rehabilitation system, E1700–E1702
  miscellaneous, E1902–E2120)
  monitoring equipment, home glucose, E0607
  negative pressure, E2402
  other orthopedic devices, E1800–E1841
  oxygen/respiratory equipment, E0424–E0487
  pacemaker monitor, E0610–E0620
  patient lifts, E0621–E0642
  pneumatic compressor, E0650–E0676
  rollout chair/transfer system, E1031–E1039
  safety equipment, E0700–E0705
  speech device, E2500–E2599
  suction pump/room vaporizers, E0600–E0606
  temporary DME codes, regional carriers,
    K0000–K9999
  TENS/stimulation device(s), E0720–E0770
  traction equipment, E0830–E0900
  trapeze equipment, fracture frame, E0910–E0948
  walkers, E0130–E0155
  wheelchair accessories, E2201–E2397
  wheelchair cusion/protection, E2601–E2621
  wheelchair, accessories, E0950–E1030
  wheelchair, amputee, E1170–E1200
  wheelchair, fully reclining, E1050–E1093
  wheelchair, heavy duty, E1280–E1298
  wheelchair, lightweight, E1240–E1270

Durable medical equipment (DME) *(Continued)*
  wheelchair, semi-reclining, E1100–E1110
  wheelchair, skin protection, E2622–E2625
  wheelchair, special size, E1220–E1239
  wheelchair, standard, E1130–E1161
  whirlpool equipment, E1300–E1310
Duraclon, *see* **Clonidine**
Dyphylline, J1180
Dysphagia, screening, documentation, G8232,
    V5364
Dystrophic, nails, trimming, G0127

E

Ear mold, V5264
Ecallantide, J1290
Echocardiography injectable contrast
    material, A9700
  ECG, 12–lead, G8704
Eculizumab, J1300
ED, visit, G0380–G0384
Edetate
  calcium disodium, J0600
  disodium, J3520
Educational Services
  chronic kidney disease, G0420, G0421
Eggcrate dry pressure pad/mattress, E0184, E0199
EKG, G0403–G0405
Elastic garments, A4466
Elbow
  disarticulation, endoskeletal, L6450
  orthosis (EO), E1800, L3702–L3740, L3760
    dynamic adjustable elbow flexion device, E1800
    elbow arthrosis, L3702–L3766
  protector, E0191
Electric hand, L7007–L7008
Electric, nerve, stimulator, transcutaneous, A4595,
    E0720–E0749
  conductive garment, E0731
  electric joint stimulation device, E0762
  electrical stimulator supplies, A4595
  electromagnetic wound treatment device, E0769
  electronic salivary reflex stimulator, E0755
  EMG, biofeedback device, E0746
  functional electrical stimulator, nerve and/or muscle
    groups, E0770
  functional stimulator sequential muscle groups, E0764
  incontinence treatment system, E0740
  nerve stimulator (FDA), treatment nausea and vomit-
    ing, E0765
  osteogenesis stimulator, electrical, surgically
    implanted, E0749
  osteogenesis stimulator, low-intensity
    ultrasound, E0760
  osteogenesis stimulator, non-invasive, not
    spinal, E0747
  osteogenesis stimulator, non-invasive, spinal, E0748

◀ **New**   ⟳ **Revised**   ✔ **Reinstated**   ~~deleted~~ **Deleted**

Electric, nerve, stimulator, transcutaneous
(Continued)
radiowaves, non-thermal, high frequency, E0761
stimulator, electrical shock unit, E0745
stimulator for scoliosis, E0744
TENS, 2 lead, E0720
TENS, four or more leads, E0730
Electrical work, dialysis equipment, A4870
Electrical stimulation device used for cancer treatment, E0766
Electromagnetic, therapy, G0295, G0329
Electronic medication compliance, T1505
Electrodes, per pair, A4555, A4556
Elevating leg rest, K0195
Elliotts b solution, J9175
Emergency department, visit, G0380–G0384
EMG, E0746
Eminase, J0350
Endarterectomy, chemical, M0300
Endodontic procedures, D3000–D3999
periapical services, D3410–D3470
pulp capping, D3110, D3120
root canal therapy, D3310–D3353
therapy, D3310–D3330
Endoscope sheath, A4270
Endoskeletal system, addition, L5848,
L5856–L5857, L5925, L5961, L5969
Endodontics, dental, D3000–D3999
Enfuvirtide, J1324
Enoxaparin sodium, J1650
Enema, bag, A4458
Enteral
feeding supply kit (syringe) (pump) (gravity),
B4034–B4036
formulae, B4149–B4156
nutrition infusion pump (with alarm) (without),
B9000, B9002
therapy, supplies, B4000–B9999
enteral and parenteral pumps, B9000–B9999
enteral formula/medical supplies, B0434–B4162
parenteral solutions/supplies, B4164–B5200
Epinephrine, J0171
Epirubicin HCl, J9178
Epoetin alpha, J0885–J0886, Q4081
Epoetin beta, J0887–J0888◀
Epoprostenol, J1325
Equipment
decubitus, E0181–E0199
exercise, A9300, E0935, E0936
orthopedic, E0910–E0948, E1800–E8002
oxygen, E0424–E0486, E1353–E1406
pump, E0781, E0784, E0791
respiratory, E0424–E0601
safety, E0700, E0705
traction, E0830–E0900
transfer, E0705
trapeze, E0910–E0912, E0940
whirlpool, E1300, E1310

Erection device, tension ring, L7902
Ergonovine maleate, J1330
Eribulin mesylate, J9179
Ertapenem sodium, J1335
Erythromycin lactobionate, J1364
ESRD (End-Stage Renal Disease; see also Dialysis)
machines and accessories, E1500–E1699
adjustable chair, ESRD, E1570
centrifuge, dialysis, E1500
dialysis equipment, NOS, E1699
hemodialysis equipment, delivery/instillation
charges, E1600
hemodialysis machine, E1590
hemodialysis, air bubble detector,
replacement, E1530
hemodialysis, bath conductivity meter, E1550
hemodialysis, blood leak detector,
replacement, E1560
hemodialysis, blood pump, replacement, E1620
hemodialysis, heparin infusion pump, E1520
hemodialysis, portable travel hemodialyzer
system, E1635
hemodialysis, pressure alarm, E1540
hemodialysis, reverse osmosis water system, E1615
hemodialysis, sorbent cartridges, E1636
hemodialysis, transducer protectors, E1575
hemodialysis, unipuncture control system, E1580
hemodialysis, water softening system, E1625
hemostats, E1637
peritoneal dialysis clamps, E1634
peritoneal dialysis, automatic intermittent
system, E1592
peritoneal dialysis, cycler dialysis machine, E1594
peritoneal dialysis, reciprocating system, E1630
scale, E1639
wearable artificial kidney, E1632
plumbing, A4870
supplies, A4653–A4932
acetate concentrate solution, hemodialysis, A4708
acid concentrate solution, hemodialysis, A4709
activated carbon filters, hemodialysis, A4680
ammonia test strip, dialysis, A4774
automatic blood pressure monitor, A4670
bicarbonate concentrate, powder,
hemodialysis, A4707
bicarbonate concentrate, solution, A4706
blood collection tube, vaccum, dialysis, A4770
blood glucose test strip, dialysis, A4772
blood pressure cuff only, A4663
blood tubing, arterial and venous,
hemodialysis, A4755
blood tubing, arterial or venous,
hemodialysis, A4750
chemicals/antiseptics solution, clean dialysis
equipment, A4674
dialysate solution, non-dextrose, A4728
dialysate solution, peritoneal dialysis,
A4720–A4726, A4760–A4766

◀ New   ⊋ Revised   ✔ Reinstated   ~~deleted~~ Deleted

ESRD *(Continued)*
  dialyzers, hemodialysis, A4690
  disposable catheter tips, peritoneal dialysis, A4860
  disposable cycler set, dialysis machine, A4671
  drainage extension line, dialysis, sterile, A4672
  extension line easy lock connectors, dialysis, A4673
  fistula cannulation set, hemodialysis, A4730
  injectable anesthetic, dialysis, A4737
  occult blood test strips, dialysis, A4773
  peritoneal dialysis, catheter anchoring device, A4653
  protamine sulfate, hemodialysis, A4802
  serum clotting timetube, dialysis, A771
  shunt accessory, hemodialysis, A4740
  sphygmomanometer, cuff and stethoscope, A4660
  syringes, A4657
  topical anesthetic, dialysis, A4736
  treated water, peritoneal dialysis, A4714
  "Y set" tubing, peritoneal dialysis, A4719
Estrogen conjugated, J1410
Estrone (5, Aqueous), J1435
Ethanolamine oleate, J1430
Etidronate disodium, J1436
Etonogestrel implant system, J7307
Etoposide, J9181
  oral, J8560
Euflexxa, J7323
Evaluation
  conformity, V5020
  contact lens, S0592
  dental, D0120–D0180
  diabetic, G0245, G0246
  footwear, G8410–G8416
  fundus, G8325–G8328
  hearing, S0618, V5008, V5010
  hospice, G0337
  multidisciplinary, H2000
  nursing, T1001
  ocularist, S9150
  performance measurement, S3005
  resident, T2011
  speech, S9152
  team, T1024
  treatment response, G0254
Everolimus, J7527
Examination
  gynecological, S0610–S0613
  ophthalmological, S0620, S0621
  oral, D0120–D0160
  pinworm, Q0113
  ringworm, S0605
Exercise
  class, S9451
  equipment, A9300, E0935, E0936
External
  ambulatory infusion pump, E0781, E0784
  ambulatory insulin delivery system, A9274
  power, battery components, L7360–L7368

External *(Continued)*
  power, elbow, L7160–L7191
  urinary supplies, A4356–A4359
Extractions (see also Dental procedures), D7110–D7130, D7250
Extraoral films, D0250, D0260
Extremity
  belt/harness, E0945
  traction, E0870–E0880
Eye
  case, V2756
  functions, documentation, G8315–G8333
  lens (contact) (spectacle), V2100–V2615
  pad, patch, A6410–A6412
  prosthetic, V2623, V2629
  service (miscellaneous), V2700–V2799

F

Faceplate, ostomy, A4361
Face tent, oxygen, A4619
Factor VIIA coagulation factor, recombinant, J7189
Factor VIII, anti-hemophilic factor, J7182, J7185, J7190–J7192↻
Factor IX, J7193, J7194, J7195, J7200, J7201↻
Factor XIII, anti-hemophilic factor, J7180
Factor XIII, A-subunit, J7181◄
Family Planning Education, H1010
Fee
  coordinated care, G9001–G9011
  dispensing, pharmacy, G0333, Q0510–Q0514, S9430
Fentanyl citrate, J3010
  and droperidol, J1810
Fern test, Q0114
Ferumoxytol, Q0138, Q0139
Filgrastim (G-CSF & TBO), J1442, J1446
Filler, wound
  alginate dressing, A6199
  foam dressing, A6215
  hydrocolloid dressing, A6240, A6241
  hydrogel dressing, A6248
  not elsewhere classified, A6261, A6262
Film, transparent (for dressing), A6257–A6259
Filter
  aerosol compressor, A7014
  dialysis carbon, A4680
  ostomy, A4368
  tracheostoma, A4481
  ultrasonic generator, A7014
Fistula cannulation set, A4730
Flebogamma, J1572
Florbetapir F18, A9586
Flowmeter, E0440, E0555, E0580
Floxuridine, J9200
Fluconazole, injection, J1450
Fludarabine phosphate, J8562, J9185

◄ New　　↻ Revised　　✔ Reinstated　　~~deleted~~ Deleted

Fluid barrier, dialysis, E1575
Flunisolide inhalation solution, J7641
Fluocinolone, J7311
Fluoride treatment, D1201–D1205
Fluorodeoxyglucose F-18 FDG, A9552
Fluorouracil, J9190
Fluphenazine decanoate, J2680
Foam
   dressing, A6209–A6215
   pad adhesive, A5126
Folding walker, E0135, E0143
Foley catheter, A4312–A4316, A4338–A4346
   indwelling catheter, specialty type, A4340
   indwelling catheter, three-way, continuous irrigation, A4346
   indwelling catheter, two-way latex, A4338
   indwelling catheter, two-way, all silicone, A4344
   insertion tray with drainage bag, A4312
   insertion tray with drainage bag, three-way, continuous irrigation, A4316
   insertion tray with drainage bag, two-way latex, A4314
   insertion tray with drainage bag, two-way, silicone, A4315
   insertion tray without drainage bag, A4313
Fomepizole, J1451
Fomivirsen sodium intraocular, J1452
Fondaparinux sodium, J1652
Foot care, G0247
Footdrop splint, L4398
Footplate, E0175, E0970, L3031
Footwear, orthopedic, L3201–L3265
   additional charge for split size, L3257
   Benesch boot, pair, child, L3213
   Benesch boot, pair, infant, L3212
   Benesch boot, pair, junior, L3214
   custom molded shoe, prosthetic shoe, L3250
   custom shoe, depth inlay, L3230
   ladies shoe, hightop, L3217
   ladies shoe, oxford, L3216
   ladies shoe, oxford/brace, L3224
   mens shoe, depth inlay, L3221
   mens shoe, hightop, L3222
   mens shoe, oxford, L3219
   mens shoe, oxford/brace, L3225
   molded shoe, custom fitted, Plastazote, L3253
   non-standard size or length, L3255
   non-standard size or width, L3254
   Plastazote sandal, L3265
   shoe molded/patient model, Plastazote, L3252
   shoe, hightop, child, L3206
   shoe, hightop, infant, L3204
   shoe, hightop, junior, L3207
   shoe, molded/patient model, silicone, L3251
   shoe, oxford, child, L3202
   shoe, oxford, infant, L3201
   shoe, oxford, junior, L3203
   surgical boot, child, L3209

Footwear, orthopedic *(Continued)*
   surgical boot, infant, L3208
   surgical boot, junior, L3211
   surgical boot/shoe, L3260
Forearm crutches, E0110, E0111
Formoterol, J7640
   fumarate, J7606
Fosaprepitant, J1453
Foscarnet sodium, J1455
Fosphenytoin, Q2009
Fracture
   bedpan, E0276
   frame, E0920, E0930, E0946–E0948
     attached to bed/weights, E0920
     attachments for complex cervical traction, E0948
     attachments for complex pelvic traction, E0947
     dual, cross bars, attached to bed, E0946
     free standing/weights, E0930
   orthosis, L2106–L2136, L3980–L3984
     ankle/foot orthosis, fracture, L2106–L2128
     KAFO, fracture orthosis, L2132–L2136
     Upper extremity, fracture orthosis, L3980–L3984
   orthotic additions, L2180–L2192, L3995
     addition to upper extremity orthosis, sock, fracture, L3995
     additions lower extremity fracture, L2180–L2192
Fragmin, *see* **Dalteparin sodium**
Frames (spectacles), V2020, V2025
   Deluxe frame, V2025
   Purchases, V2020
Fulvestrant, J9395
Furosemide, J1940

G

Gadobutrol, A9585
Gadofosveset trisodium, A9583
Gadoxetate disodium, A9581
Gait trainer, E8000–E8002
Gallium Ga67, A9556
Gallium nitrate, J1457
Galsulfase, J1458
Gammagard liquid, J1569
Gamma globulin, J1460, J1560
   injection, gamma globulin (IM), 1cc, J1460
   injection, gamma globulin, (IM), over 10cc, J1560
Gammaplex, J1557
Gamunex, J1561
Ganciclovir
   implant, J7310
   sodium, J1570
Garamycin, J1580
Gas system
   compressed, E0424, E0425
   gaseous, E0430, E0431, E0441, E0443
   liquid, E0434–E0440, E0442, E0444
Gastric freezing, hypothermia, M0100

◄ New   ⮌ Revised   ✔ Reinstated   ~~deleted~~ Deleted

Gatifloxacin, J1590
Gauze (*see also* Bandage)
    impregnated, A6222–A6233, A6266
    non-impregnated, A6402–A6404
Gefitinib, J8565
Gel
    conductive, A4558
    pressure pad, E0185, E0196
Gemcitabine HCl, J9201
Gemtuzumab ozogamicin, J9300
Generator
    ultrasonic with nebulizer, E0574
Gentamicin (Sulfate), J1580
Gingival procedures, *D4210–D4240*
    gingival flap procedure, D4240–D4241
    gingivectomy or gingivoplasty, D4210–D4212
Glasses
    air conduction, V5070
    binaural, V5120–V5150
        behind the ear, V5140
        body, V5120
        glasses, V5150
        in the ear, V5130
    bone conduction, V5080
    frames, V2020, V2025
    hearing aid, V5230
Glaucoma
    screening, G0117, G0118
Gloves, A4927
Glucagon HCl, J1610
Glucose
    monitor with integrated lancing/blood sample collection, E2101
    monitor with integrated voice synthesizer, E2100
    test strips, A4253, A4772
Gluteal pad, L2650
Glycopyrrolate, inhalation solution, concentrated, J7642
Glycopyrrolate, inhalation solution, unit dose, J7643
Gold
    foil dental restoration, D2410–D2430
        gold foil, one surface, D2410
        gold foil, two surfaces, D2420
        gold foli, three surfaces, D2430
    sodium thiomalate, J1600
Golimumab, J1602
Gomco drain bottle, A4912
Gonadorelin HCl, J1620
Goserelin acetate implant (*see also* Implant), J9202
Grab bar, trapeze, E0910, E0940
Gradient, compression stockings, *A6530–A6549*
    below knee, 18–30 mmHg, A6530
    below knee, 30–40 mmHg, A6531
    below knee, thigh length, 18–30 mmHg, A6533
    full length/chap style, 18–30 mmHg, A6536
    full length/chap style, 30–40 mmHg, A6537

Gradient, compression stockings *(Continued)*
    full length/chap style, 40–50 mmHg, A6538
    garter belt, A6544
    non-elastic below knee, 30–50 mmHg, A6545
    sleeve, NOS, A6549
    thigh length, 30–40 mmHg, A6534
    thigh length, 40–50 mmHg, A6535
    waist length, 18–30 mmHg, A6539
    waist length, 30–40 mmHg, A6540
    waist length, 40–50 mmHg, A6541
Grade-aid, wheelchair, E0974
Granisetron HCl, J1626
Gravity traction device, E0941
Gravlee jet washer, A4470
Guaiac, stool, *G0394*
Guidelines, practice, oncology, *G9056–G9062*

H

Hair analysis (excluding arsenic), P2031
Halaven, Injection, eribulin mesylate, 0.1 mg, J9179
Hallus-Valgus dynamic splint, L3100
Hallux prosthetic implant, L8642
Haloperidol, J1630
    decanoate, J1631
Halo procedures, L0810–L0861
    addition HALO procedure, MRI compatible systems, L0859
    addition HALO procedure, replacement liner, L0861
    cervical halo/jacket vest, L0810
    cervical halo/Milwaukee type orthosis, L0830
    cervical halo/plaster body jacket, L0820
Halter, cervical head, E0942
Hand finger orthosis, prefabricated, L3923
Hand restoration, L6900–L6915
    partial prosthesis, L6000–L6020
        partial hand, little and/or ring finger remaining, L6010
        partial hand, no finger, L6020
        partial hand, thumb remaining, L6000
        transcarpal/metacarpal or partial hand disarticulation prosthesis, L6025
    orthosis (WHFO), E1805, E1825, L3800–L3805, L3900–L3954
    rims, wheelchair, E0967
Handgrip (cane, crutch, walker), A4636
Harness, E0942, E0944, E0945
Headgear (for positive airway pressure device), K0185
Hearing
    aid, V5030–V5267, V5298
        aid-body worn, V5100
        assistive listening device, V5268–V5274, V5281–V5290
        battery, use in hearing device, V5266
        dispensing fee, binaural, V5160

◄ **New**   ⟳ **Revised**   ✔ **Reinstated**   ~~deleted~~ **Deleted**

Hearing (Continued)

    dispensing fee, monaural hearing aid, any type, V5241

    dispensing fee, unspecified hearing aid, V5090

    ear impression, each, V5275

    ear mold/insert, disposable, any type, V5265

    ear mold/insert, not disposable, V5264

    glasses, air conduction, V5070

    glasses, bone conduction

    hearing aid or assistive listening device/supplies/ accessories, NOS, V5267

    hearing aid, analog, binaural, CIC, V5248

    hearing aid, analog, binaural, ITC, V5249

    hearing aid, analog, monaural, CIC, V5242

    hearing aid, analog, monaural, ITC, V5243

    hearing aid, BICROS, V5210–V5240

    hearing aid, binaural, V5120–V5150

    hearing aid, CROS, V5170–V5200

    hearing aid, digital, V5254–V5261

    hearing aid, digitally programmable, V5244–V5247, V5250–V5253

    hearing aid, disposable, any type, binaural, V5263

    hearing aid, disposable, any type, monaural, V5262

    hearing aid, monaural, V5030–V5060

    hearing aid, NOC, V5298

    hearing service, miscellaneous, V5299

    semi-implantable, middle ear, V5095

    assessment, S0618, V5008, V5010

    devices, V5000–V5299, L8614

    services, V5000–V5999

Heat

    application, E0200–E0239

    lamp, E0200, E0205

    infrared heating pad system, A4639, E0221

    pad, A9273, E0210, E0215, E0237, E0249

Heater (nebulizer), E1372

Heavy duty, wheelchair, *E1280–E1298, K0006, K0007, K0801–K0886*

    detachable arms, elevating legrests, E1280

    detachable arms, swing away detachable footrest, E1290

    extra heavy duty wheelchair, K0007

    fixed full length arms, elevating legrest, E1295

    fixed full length arms, swing away detachable footrest, E1285

    heavy duty wheelchair, K0006

    power mobility device, not coded by DME PDAC or no criteria, K0900

    power operated vehicle, group 2, K0806–K0808

    power operated vehicle, NOC, K0812

    power wheelchair, group 1, K0813–K0816

    power wheelchair, group 2, K0820–K0843

    power wheelchair, group 3, K0848–K0864

    power wheelchair, group 4, K0868–K0886

    power wheelchair, group 5, pediatric, K0890–K0891

    power wheelchair, NOC, K0898

    power-operated vehicle, group 1, K0800–K0802

Heavy duty, wheelchair (Continued)

    special wheelchair seat depth and/or width, by construction, E1298

    special wheelchair seat depth, by upholstery, E1297

    special wheelchair seat height from floor, E1296

Heel

    elevator, air, E0370

    protector, E0191

    shoe, L3430–L3485

    stabilizer, L3170

Helicopter, ambulance (see also Ambulance**)**

Helmet

    cervical, L0100, L0110

    head, A8000–A8004

Hemin, J1640

Hemi-wheelchair, E1083–E1086

Hemipelvectomy prosthesis, L5280

Hemodialysis machine, E1590

Hemodialysis, vessel mapping, *G0365*

Hemodialyzer, portable, E1635

Hemofil M, J7190

    hemoglobin, level, G0908, G0910

Hemophilia clotting factor, J7190–J7198

    anti-inhibitor, per IU, J7198

    anti-thrombin III, human, per IU, J7197

    Factor IX, complex, per IU, J7194

    Factor IX, purified, non-recombinant, per IU, J7193

    Factor IX, recombinant, J7195

    Factor VIII, human, per IU

    Factor VIII, porcine, per IU, J7191

    Factor VIII, recombinant, per IU, NOS, J7192

    injection, antithrombin recombinant, 50 i.u., J7196

    NOC, J7199

Hemostats, A4850

Hemostix, A4773

Hepagam B

    IM, J1571

    IV, J1573

Heparin

    infusion pump, dialysis, E1520

    lock flush, J1642

    sodium, J1644

Hepatitis B, vaccine, administration, *G0010*

Hep-Lock (U/P), J1642

Hexalite, A4590

High osmolar contrast material, Q9958–Q9964

    HOCM 150–199 mg/ml iodine, Q9959

    HOCM 200–249 mg/ml iodine, Q9960

    HOCM up to 149 mg/ml iodine, Q9958

    HOCM, 250–299 mg/ml iodine, Q9961

    HOCM, 300–349 mg/ml iodine, Q9962

    HOCM, 350–399 mg/ml iodine, Q9963

    HOCM, 400 or greater mg/ml iodine, Q9964

Hip

    disarticulation prosthesis, L5250, L5270

    orthosis (HO), L1600–L1690

Hip-knee-ankle-foot orthosis (HKAFO), L2040–L2090

◀ **New** ↻ **Revised** ✔ **Reinstated** ~~deleted~~ **Deleted**

Histrelin
   acetate, J1675
   implant, J9225
HKAFO, L2040–L2090
Home
   certification, home health, G0180
   glucose, monitor, E0607, E2100, E2101,
      S1030, S1031
   health, aide, G0156, S9122, T1021
   health, aide, per visit, T1021
   health, aide, in home, per hour, S9122
   health, clinical, social worker, G0155
   health, hospice, each 15 min, G0156
   health, nursing, skilled, G0154
   health, occupational, therapist, G0152
   health, physical therapist, G0151
   health, physician, certification, G0179–G0182
   health, respiratory therapy, S5180, S5181
   recerticication, home health, G0179
   supervision, home health, G0181
   supervision, hospice, G0182
   therapist, speech, S9128
Home Health Agency Services, T0221
   care improvement home visit assessment, G9187
Home sleep study test, G0398–G0400
HOPPS, *C1000–C9999*
Hospice, evaluation, pre-election, G0337
Hospice care
   hospice facility, Q5010
   patient's home, Q5001
   assisted living facility, Q5002
   nursing long-term facility, Q5003
   skilled nursing facility, Q5004
   inpatient hospital, Q5005
   inpatient hospice facility, Q5006
   long term care facility, Q5007
   inpatient psychiatric facility, Q5008
Hospice physician supervision, G0182
Hospital
   bed, E0250–E0304, E0328, E0329
   observation, G0378, G0379
Hospital Outpatient Payment System,
   C1000–C9999
Hot water bottle, A9273
Human fibrinogen concentrate, J7178
Humidifier, A7046, E0550–E0563
   durable glass bottle type, for regulator, E0555
   durable, diring IPPB treatment, E0560
   durable, extensive, IPPB, E0550
   heated, used with positive airway pressure
     device, E0562
   non-heated, used with positive airway
     pressure, E0561
   water chamber, humidifier, replacement, positive air-
     way device, A7046
Hyalgan, J7321
Hyalomatrix, Q4117
Hyaluronan, J7326, J7327↺

Hyaluronate, sodium, J7317
Hyaluronidase, J3470
   ovine, J3471–J3473
Hydralazine HCl, J0360
Hydraulic patient lift, E0630
Hydrocollator, E0225, E0239
Hydrocolloid dressing, A6234–A6241
Hydrocortisone
   acetate, J1700
   sodium phosphate, J1710
   sodium succinate, J1720
Hydrogel dressing, A6242–A6248, A6231–A6233
Hydromorphone, J1170
Hydroxyprogesterone caproate, J1725
Hydroxyzine HCl, J3410
Hylan G-F 20, J7322
Hyoscyamine Sulfate, J1980
Hyperbaric oxygen chamber, topical, A4575
Hypertonic saline solution, J7130

I

Ibandronate sodium, J1740
Ibuprofen, J1741
Ibutilide Fumarate, J1742
Icatibant, J1744
Ice
   cap, E0230
   collar, E0230
Idarubicin HCl, J9211
Idursulfase, J1743
Ifosfamide, J9208
Iliac, artery, angiography, G0278
Iloprost, Q4074
Imaging, PET, G0219, G0235
   any site, NOS, G0235
   whole body, melanoma, non-covered
     indications, G0219
Imiglucerase, J1786
Immune globulin
   Bivigam, *500 mg,* J1556
   Flebogamma, J1572
   Gammagard liquid, J1569
   Gammaplex, J1557
   Gamunex, J1561
   HepaGam B, J1571
   Hizentra, J1559
   Intravenous services, supplies and
     accessories, Q2052
   NOS, J1566
   Octagam, J1568
   Privigen, J1459
   Rho(D), J2788, J2790
   Rhophylac, J2791
   Subcutaneous, J1562
Immunosuppressive drug, not otherwise
   classified, J7599

◀ New   ↺ Revised   ✔ Reinstated   ~~deleted~~ Deleted

Immunohistochemistry, *G0461, G0462*
Implant
  access system, A4301
  aqueous shunt, L8612
  breast, L8600
  cochlear, L8614, L8619
  collagen, urinary tract, L8603
  dental, D3460, D5925, D6010–D6067, D6075–D6199
    endodontic endosseous implant, D3460
    facial augmentation implant prosthesis, D5925
    implant supported prosthetics, D6055–D6067,
    D6075–D6079
    other implant services, D6080–D6199
    surgical placement, D6010–D6054
  dextranomer/hyaluronic acid copolymer, L8604
  ganciclovir, J7310
  hallux, L8642
  urinary tract, L8603, L8606
  infusion pump, programmable, E0783, E0786
    implantable, programmable, E0783
    implantable, programmable, replacement, E0786
  joint, L8630, L8641, L8658
    interphalangeal joint spacer, silicone or
    equal, L8658
    metacarpophalangeal joint implant, L8630
    metatarsal joint implant, L8641
  lacrimal duct, A4262, A4263
  maintenance procedures, D6080
  maxillofacial, D5913–D5937
    auricular prosthesis, D5914
    auricular prosthesis, replacement, D5927
    cranial prosthesis, D5924
    facial augmentation implant prosthesis, D5925
    facial prosthesis, D5919
    facial prosthesis, replacement, D5929
    mandibular resection prosthesis, with guide
    flange, D5934
    mandibular resection prosthesis, without guide
    flange, D5935
    nasal prosthesis, D5913
    nasal prosthesis, replacement, D5926
    nasal septal prosthesis, D5922
    obturator prosthesis, definitive, D5932
    obturator prosthesis, modification, D5933
    obturator prosthesis, surgical, D5931
    obturator/prosthesis, interim, D5936
    ocular prosthesis, D5916
    ocular prosthesis, interim, D5923
    orbital prosthesis, D5915
    orbital prosthesis, replacement, D5928
    trismus appliance, not for TM treatment, D5937
  metacarpophalangeal joint, L8630
  metatarsal joint, L8641
  neurostimulator pulse generator, L8679,
    L8681–L8688
  not otherwise specified, L8699
  ocular, L8610
  ossicular, L8613

Implant *(Continued)*
  osteogenesis stimulator, E0749
  percutaneous access system, A4301
  removal, dental, D6100
  repair, dental, D6090
  replacement implantable intraspinal catheter, E0785
  synthetic, urinary, L8606
  vascular graft, L8670
Implantable radiation dosimeter, A4650
Impregnated gauze dressing, A6222–A6230
Incobotulinumtoxin a, J0588
Incontinence
  appliances and supplies, A4310, A4360,
    A5071–A5075, A5102–A5114, K0280, K0281
  garment, A4520, T4521–T4543
    adult sized disposable incontinence product,
    T4522–T4528
    any type, e.g. brief, diaper, A4520
    pediatric sized disposable incontinence product,
    T4529–T4532
    youth sized disposable incontinence product,
    T4533–T4534
  supply, A4335, A4356–A4358
    bedside drainage bag, A4357
    disposable external urethral clamp/compression
    device, A4360
    external urethral clamp or compression
    device, A4356
    incontinence supply, miscellaneous, A4335
    urinary drainage bag, leg or abdomen, A4358
  treatment system, E0740
  urinary, documentation, G8063, G8067
Indium IN-111
  carpromab pendetide, A9507
  ibritumomab tiuxetan, A9542
  labeled autologous white blood cells, A9570
  labeled autologous platelets, A9571
  oxyquinoline, A9547
  pentetate, A9548
  pentetreotide, A9572
  satumomab, A4642
Infliximab injection, J1745
Influenza
  immunization, documentation, G8482–G8484
  vaccine, administration, G0008
  virus vaccine, Q2033–Q2039
  afluria, Q21035
  agriflu, Q2034
  flublock, Q2033
  flulaval, Q2036
  fluvirin, Q2037
  fluzone, Q2038
  not otherwise specified, Q2039
Infusion
  pump, ambulatory, with administrative equipment,
    E0781
  pump, heparin, dialysis, E1520
  pump, implantable, E0782, E0783

◄ **New**   ⊃ **Revised**   ✔ **Reinstated**   ~~deleted~~ **Deleted**

Infusion *(Continued)*
  pump, implantable, refill kit, A4220
  pump, insulin, E0784
  pump, mechanical, reusable, E0779, E0780
  pump, uninterrupted infusion of
    Epiprostenol, K0455
  replacement battery, A4602◄
  saline, J7030–J7060
  supplies, A4219, A4221, A4222, A4230–A4232,
    E0776–E0791
  therapy, other than chemotherapeutic
    drugs, Q0081
Inhalation solution (*see also* **drug name**),
  J7608–J7699, Q4074
Injection device, needle-free, *A4210*
Injections (*see also* **drug name**), J0120–J7320
  ado-trastuzumab emtansine, 1 mg, J9354
  arthrography, sacroiliac, joint, G0259, G0260
  aripiprazole, extended release, J0401
  carfilzomib, 1 mg, J9047
  certolizumab pegol, J0717
  filgrastim, J1442, J1446
  interferon beta-1a, IM, Q3027
  interferon beta-1a, SC, Q3028
  omacetaxine mepesuccinate, 0.01 mg, J9262
  pertuzumb, 1 mg, J9306
  sculptra, 0.5 mg, Q2028
  vincristine, 1 mg, J9371
  ziv-aflibercept, 1 mg, J9400
  dental service, D9610, D9630
    other drugs/medicaments, by report, D9630
    therapeutic parenteral drug, single
    administration, D9610
    therapeutic parenteral drugs, two or more adminis-
    trations, different medications, D9612
  dermal filler (LDS), G0429
  supplies for self-administered, A4211
Inlay/onlay dental restoration, *D2510–D2664*
INR, monitoring, *G0248–G0250*
  demonstration prior to initiation, home INR, G0248
  physician review and interpretation, home INR, G0250
  provision of test materials, home INR, G0249
Insertion tray, A4310–A4316
Insulin, J1815, J1817, S5550–S5571
  ambulatory, external, system, A9274
  treatment, outpatient, G9147
Integra flowable wound matrix, *Q4114*
Interferon
  Alpha, J9212–J9215
  Beta-1 a, J1826, Q3027, Q3028
  Beta-1 b, J1830
  Gamma, J9216
Intermittent
  assist device with continuous positive airway pres-
    sure device, E0470–E0472
  limb compression device, E0676
  peritoneal dialysis system, E1592
  positive pressure breathing (IPPB) machine,E0500

Interphalangeal joint, prosthetic implant, L8658,
  L8659
Interscapular thoracic prosthesis
  endoskeletal, L6570
  upper limb, L6350–L6370
Intervention, alcohol/substance (not tobacco),
  G0396–G0397
Intervention, tobacco, *G9016*
Intraconazole, J1835
Intraocular
  lenses, V2630–V2632
Intraoral radiographs, dental, *D0210–D0240*
  intraoral-complete series, D0210
  intraoral-occlusal image, D0420
  intraoral-periapical-each additional image, D0230
  intraoral-periapical-first radiographic
    image, D0220
Intrapulmonary percussive ventilation system, E0481
Intrauterine copper contraceptive, J7300
Iodine Iobenguane sulfate I-131, A9508
Iodine I-123
  iobenguane, A9582
  ioflupane, A9584
  sodium iodide, A9509, A9516
Iodine I-125
  serum albumin, A9532
  sodium iodide, A9527
  sodium iothalamate, A9554
Iodine I-131
  iodinated serum albumin, A9524
  sodium iodide capsule, A9517, A9528
  sodium iodide solution, A9529–A9531
  tositumomab, A9544–A9545
Iodine swabs/wipes, A4247
IPD
  system, E1592
Ipilimumab, J9228
IPPB machine, E0500
Ipratropium bromide, inhalation solution, unit
  dose, J7644, J7645
Irinotecan, J9206
Iron
  Dextran, J1750
  sucrose, J1756
Irrigation/evacuation system, bowel
  control unit, E0350
  disposable supplies for, E0352
  manual pump enema, A4459◄
Irrigation solution for bladder calculi, Q2004
Irrigation supplies, A4320–A4322, A4355,
  A4397–A4400
  irrigation supply, sleeve, each, A4397
  irrigation syringe, bulb, or piston, each, A4320
  irrigation tubing set, bladder irrigation, A4355
  ostomy irrigation set, A4400
  ostomy irrigation supply, bag, A4398
  ostomy irrigation supply, cone/catheter, A4399
Islet, transplant, *G0341–G0343, S2102*

◄ **New**   ↻ **Revised**   ✓ **Reinstated**   ~~deleted~~ **Deleted**

Isoetharine HCl, inhalation solution
    concentrated, J7647, J7648
    unit dose, J7649, J7650
Isolates, B4150, B4152
Isoproterenol HCl, inhalation solution
    concentrated, J7657, J7658
    unit dose, J7659, J7660
Isosulfan blue, Q9968
Item, non-covered, A9270
IUD, J7300, S4989
IV pole, each, E0776, K0105
Ixabepilone, J9207

J

Jacket
    scoliosis, L1300, L1310
Jaw, motion, rehabilitation system, E1700–E1702
Jenamicin, J1580
Jetria, (ocriplasmin), J7316

K

Kadcyla, ado-trastuzumab emtansine, 1 mg, J9354
Kanamycin sulfate, J1840, J1850
Kartop patient lift, toilet or bathroom (*see also* Lift), E0625
Ketorolac thomethamine, J1885
Kidney
    ESRD supply, A4650–A4927
    machine, accessories, E1500–E1699
    machine, E1500–E1699
    system, E1510
    wearable artificial, E1632
Kits
    enteral feeding supply (syringe) (pump) (gravity), B4034–B4036
    fistula cannulation (set), A4730
    parenteral nutrition, B4220–B4224
        administration kit, per day, B4224
        supply kit, home mix, per day, B422
        supply kit, premix, per day, B4220
    surgical dressing (tray), A4550
    tracheostomy, A4625
Knee
    arthroscopy, surgical, G0289, S2112, S2300
        knee, surgical, harvesting cartilage, S112
        knee, surgical, removal loose body, chondroplasty, different compartment, G0289
        shoulder, surgical, thermally-induced, capsulorraphy, S2300
    disarticulation, prosthesis, L5150, L5160
    joint, miniature, L5826
    orthosis (KO), E1810, K0901–K0902, L1800–L1885↻
    dynamic adjustable elbow entension/flexion device, E1800

Knee *(Continued)*
    dynamic adjustable knee extension/flexion device, E1810
    static-progressive devices, E1801, E1806, E1811, E1816–E1818, E1831, E1841
Knee-ankle-foot orthosis (KAFO), L2000–L2039, L2126–L2136
    base procedure, used with any knee joint, full plastic double upright, L2036
    base procedure, used with any knee joint, double upright, double bar, L2020
    base procedure, used with any knee joint, single upright, single bar, L2000
    foot orthrosis, double upright, double bar, without knee joint, L2030
    foot orthrosis, single upright, single bar, without knee joint, L2010
    addition, high strength, lightweight material, L2755
Kyphosis pad, L1020, L1025

L

Laboratory
    dental, D0415–D0999
        adjunctive pre-diagnostic tests, mucosal abnormalities, D0431
        analysis saliva sample, D0418
        caries risk assessment, low, D0601
        caries risk assessment, moderate
        caries susceptibility tests, D0425
        collection and preparation, saliva sample, D0417
        collection of microorganisms for culture and sensitivity, D0415
        diagnostic casts, D0470
        genetic test for susceptibility to oral diseases, D0421
        oral pathology laboratory, D0472–D0502
        pulp vitality tests, D0460
    viral culture, D0416
    services, P0000–P9999
Laboratory tests
    chemistry, P2028–P2038
        cephalin flocculation, blood, P2028
        congo red, blood, P2029
        hair analysis, excluding arsenic, P2031
        mucoprotein, blood, P2038
        thymol turbidity, blood, P2033
    microbiology, P7001
    miscellaneous, P9010–P9615, Q0111–Q0115
        blood, split unit, P9011
        blood, whole, transfusion, unit, P9010
        catheterization, collection specimen, multiple patients, P9615
        catheterization, collection specimen, single patient, P9612
        cryoprecipitate, each unit, P9012
        fern test, Q0114

◄ **New**   ↻ **Revised**   ✔ **Reinstated**   ~~deleted~~ **Deleted**

Laboratory tests (*Continued*)
fresh frozen plasma (single donor), frozen within 8 hours, P9017
fresh frozen plasma, donor retested, each unit, P9060
fresh frozen plasma, within 8–24 hours of collection, each unit, P9059
granulocytes, pheresis, each unit, P9050
infusion, albumin (human), 25%, 20 ml, P9046
infusion, albumin (human), 25%, 50 ml, P9047
infusion, albumin (human), 5%, 250 ml, P9045
infusion, albumin (human), 5%, 50 ml, P9041
infusion, plasma protein fraction, human, 5%, 250 ml, P9048
infusion, plasma protein fraction, human, 5%, 50 ml, P9043
KOH preparation, Q0112
pinworm examinations, Q0113
plasma, cryoprecipitate reduced, each unit, P9044
plasma, pooled, multiple donor, frozen, P9023
platelet rich plasma, each unit, P9020
platelets, each unit, P9019
platelets, HLA-matched leukocytes reduced, apheresis/pheresis, each unit, P9052
platelets, irradiated, each unit, P9032
platelets, leukocytes reduced, CMV-neg, aphresis/pheresis, each unit, P9055
platelets, leukocytes reduced, each unit, P9031
platelets, leukocytes reduced, irradiated, each unit, P9033
platelets, pheresis, each unit, P9034
platelets, pheresis, irradiated, each unit, P9036
platelets, pheresis, leukocytes reduced, CMV-neg, irradiated, each unit, P9053
platelets, pheresis, leukocytes reduced, each unit, P9035
platelets, pheresis, leukocytes reduced, irradiated, each unit P9037
post-coital, direct qualitative, vaginal or cervical mucous, Q0115
red blood cells, deglycerolized, each unit, P9039
red blood cells, each unit, P9021
red blood cells, frozen/deglycerolized/washed, leukocytes reduced, irradiated, each unit, P9057
red blood cells, irradiated, each unit, P9038
red blood cells, leukocytes reduced, CMV-neg, irradiated, each unit, P9058
red blood cells, leukocytes reduced, each unit, P9016
red blood cells, leukocytes reduced, irradiated, each unit, P9040
red blood cells, washed, each unit, P9022
travel allowance, one way, specimen collection, home/nursing home, P9603, P9604
wet mounts, vaginal, cervical, or skin, Q0111
whole blood or red blood cells, leukocytes reduced, CMV-neg, each unit, P9051
whole blood or red blood cells, leukocytes reduced, frozen, deglycerol, washed, each unit, P9054

Laboratory tests (*Continued*)
whole blood, leukocytes reduced, irradiated, each unit, P9056
toxicology, P3000–P3001, Q0091
Lacrimal duct, implant
permanent, A4263
temporary, A4262
Lactated Ringer's infusion, J7120
Laetrile, J3570
Lancet, A4258, A4259
Language, screening, V5363
Lanreotide, J1930
Laronidase, J1931
Larynx, artificial, L8500
Laser blood collection device and accessory, E0620, A4257
LASIK, S0800
Lead investigation, T1029
Lead wires, per pair, A4557
Leg
bag, A4358, A5105, A5112
leg or abdomen, vinyl, with/without tubes, straps, each, A4358
urinary drainage bag, leg bag, leg/abdomen, latex, with/without tube, straps, A5112
urinary suspensory, leg bag, with/without tube, each, A5105
extensions for walker, E0158
rest, elevating, K0195
rest, wheelchair, E0990
strap, replacement, A5113–A5114
Legg Perthes orthosis, L1700–L1755
Newington type, L1710
Patten bottom type, L1755
Scottish Rite type, L1730
Tachdjian type, L1720
Toronto type, L1700
Lens
aniseikonic, V2118, V2318
contact, V2500–V2599
gas permeable, V2510–V2513
hydrophilic, V2520–V2523
other type, V2599
PMMA, V2500–V2503
scleral, gas, V2530–V2531
eye, V2100–V2615, V2700–V2799
bifocal, glass or plastic, V2200–V2299
contact lenses, V2500–V2599
low vision aids, V2600–V2615
miscellaneous, V2700–V2799
single vision, glass or plastic, V2100–V2199
trifocal, glass or plastic, V2300–V2399
variable asphericity, V2410–V2499
intraocular, V2630–V2632, C1840, Q1004–Q1005
anterior chamber, V2630
iris supported, V2631
new technology, category 4, IOL, Q1004
new technology, category 5, IOL, Q1005

◄ **New** ↻ **Revised** ✔ **Reinstated** ~~deleted~~ **Deleted**

Lens (Continued)
   posterior chamber, V2632
   telescopic lens, C1840
  low vision, V2600–V2615
   hand held vision aids, V2600
   single lens spectacle mounted, V2610
   telescopic and other compound lens system, V2615
  progressive, V2781
Lepirudin, J1945
Lesion, destruction, choroid, *G0186*
Leucovorin calcium, J0640
Leukocyte poor blood, each unit, P9016
Leuprolide acetate, J9217, J9218, J9219, J1950
  for depot suspension, 7.5 mg, J9217
  implant, 65 mg, J9219
  injection, for depot suspension, per 3.75 mg, J1950
  per 1 mg, J9218
Levalbuterol, all formulations, inhalation solution
  concentrated, J7607, J7612
  unit dose, J7614, J7615
Levetiracetam, J1953
Levocarnitine, J1955
Levofloxacin, J1956
Levoleucovorin, J0641
Levonorgestrel, (contraceptive), implants and supplies, J7306
Levorphanol tartrate, J1960
Lexidronam, A9604
Lidocaine HCl, J2001
Lift
  patient (includes seat lift), E0621–E0635
   bathroom or toilet, E0625
   mechanism incorporated into a combination lift-chair, E0627
   patient lift, electric, E0635
   patient lift, hydraulic or mechanical, E0630
   separate seat lift mechanism, patient owned furniture, electric, E0628
   separate seat lift mechanism, patient owned furniture, non-electric, E0629
   sling or seat, canvas or nylon, E0621
  shoe, L3300–L3334
   lift, elevation, heel and sole, cork, L3320
   lift, elevation, heel and sole, Neoprene, L3310
   lift, elevation, heel, L3334
   lift, elevation, heel, tapered to metatarsals, L3300
   lift, elevation, inside shoe, L3332
   lift, elevation, metal extension, L3330
Lightweight, wheelchair, *E1087–E1090, E1240–E1270*
  detachable arms, swing away detachable footrest, E1260
  detachable arms, swing away detachable, elevating leg rests, E1240
  fixed full length arms, swing away detachable elevating legrests, E1270
  fixed full length arms, swing away detachable footrest, E1250

Lightweight, wheelchair (Continued)
  high strength, detachable arms desk or full length, E1090
  high strength, detachable arms desk, E1088
  high strength, fixed full length arms, E1087
  high strength, fixed length arms swing away footrest, E1089
Lincomycin HCl, J2010
Linezolid, J2020
Listening devices, assistive, *V5281–V5290*
  personal blue tooth FM/DM, V5286
  personal FM/DM adapter/boot coupling device for receiver, V5289
  personal FM/DM binaural, 2 receivers, V5282
  personal FM/DM monaural, 1 receiver, V5281
  personal FM/DM neck, loop induction receiver, V5283
  personal FM/DM transmitter assistive listening device, V5288
  personal FM/DM, direct audio input, V5285
  personal FM/DM, ear level receiver, V5284
  transmitter microphone, V5290
Liquid barrier, ostomy, A4363
Lodging, recipient, escort nonemergency transport, A0180, A0200
LOPS, *G0245–G0247*
  follow-up evaluation and management, G0246
  initial evaluation and management, G0245
  routine foot care, G0247
Lorazepam, J2060
Loss of protective sensation, *G0245–G0247*
Low osmolar contrast material, *Q9965–Q9967*
LSO, *L0621–L0640*
Lubricant, A4402, A4332
Lumbar flexion, L0540
Lumbar-sacral orthosis (LSO), L0621–L0640
LVRS, services, *G0302–G0305*
Lymphocyte immune globulin, J7504, J7511

M

Machine
  IPPB, E0500
  kidney, E1500–E1699
Magnesium sulphate, J3475
Maintenance contract, ESRD, A4890
Mammography, screening, *G0202*
Mannitol, J2150, J7665
Mapping, vessel, for hemodialysis access, *G0365*
Marker, tissue, *A4648*
Mask
  aerosol, K0180
  oxygen, A4620
Mastectomy
  bra, L8000
  form, L8020
  prosthesis, L8030, L8600
  sleeve, L8010

◀ **New** ↻ **Revised** ✔ **Reinstated** ~~deleted~~ **Deleted**

◄ New ↻ Revised ✔ Reinstated ~~deleted~~ Deleted

N

Nabilone, J8650
Nails, trimming, dystrophic, G0127
Nalbuphine HCl, J2300
Naloxone HCl, J2310
Naltrexone, J2315
Nandrolone
  decanoate, J2320
Narrowing device, wheelchair, E0969
Nasal
  application device, K0183
  pillows/seals (for nasal application
    device), K0184
  vaccine inhalation, J3530
Nasogastric tubing, B4081, B4082
Natalizumab, J2323
Nebulizer, E0570–E0585
  aerosol compressor, E0571
  aerosol mask, A7015
  corrugated tubing, disposable, A7010
  corrugated tubing, non-disposable, A7011
  filter, disposable, A7013
  filter, non-disposable, A7014
  heater, E1372
  large volume, disposable, prefilled, A7008
  large volume, disposable, unfilled, A7007
  not used with oxygen, durable, glass, A7017
  pneumatic, administration set, A7003,
    A7005, A7006
  pneumatic, nonfiltered, A7004
  portable, E0570
  small volume, A7003–A7005
  ultrasonic, E0575
  ultrasonic, dome and mouthpiece, A7016
  ultrasonic, reservoir bottle, non-disposable, A7009
  water collection device, large volume
    nebulizer, A7012
Needle, A4215
  bone marrow biopsy, C1830
  non-coring, A4212
  with syringe, A4206–A4209
**Negative pressure wound therapy
    pump,** E2402
  accessories, A6550
  therapy, G0456, G0457
Nelarabine, J9261
**Neonatal transport, ambulance, base
    rate,** A0225
Neostigmine methylsulfate, J2710
Nerve, conduction, sensory, test, G0255
Nerve stimulator with batteries, E0765
Nesiritide injection, J2324
Neupogen, injection, filgrastim, 1 mcg, J1442
*Neurophysiology, intraoperative,
    monitoring, G0453*
Neuromuscular stimulator, E0745

Neurostimulator
  battery recharging system, L8695
  external antenna, L8696◄
  implantable pulse generator, L8679
  pulse generator, L8681–L8688
    dual array, non-rechargeable, with extension, L8688
    dual array, rechargeable, with extension, L8687
    *patient programmer (external), replacement
      only, L8681*
    radiofrequency receiver, L8682
    *radiofrequency transmitter (external), sacral root
      receiver, bowel and bladder management, L8684*
    *radiofrequency transmitter (external), with im-
      plantable receiver, L8683*
    single array, rechargeable, with extension, L8686
Nitrogen N-13 ammonia, A9526
NMES, E0720–E0749
Nonchemotherapy drug, oral, NOS, J8499
Noncovered services, A9270
Nonemergency transportation, A0080–A0210
Nonimpregnated gauze dressing, A6216–A6221,
    A6402–A6404
Nonprescription drug, A9150
Not otherwise classified drug, J3490, J7599, J7699,
    J7799, J8499, J8999, J9999, Q0181
NPH, J1820
NPWT, pump, E2402
NTIOL category 3, Q1003
NTIOL category 4, Q1004
NTIOL category 5, Q1005
Nursing care, T1030–T1031
Nursing service, direct, skilled, outpatient, G0128
Nursing, skilled, home, health, G0154
Nutrition
  counseling, dental, D1310, D1320
  enteral infusion pump, B9000, B9002
  parenteral infusion pump, B9004, B9006
  parenteral solution, B4164–B5200
  therapy, medical, G0270, G0271

O

Observation
  admission, G0379
  hospital, G0378
  LPN or RN, G0163
Obturator prosthesis
  definitive, D5932
  interim, D5936
  surgical, D5931
Occipital/mandibular support, cervical, L0160
Occlusive device, placement, G0269
Occult, blood, G0394
Occupational, therapy, G0129, S9129
Ocriplasmin, J7316
Octafluoropropane, Q9956
Octagam, J1568

◄ New   ↻ Revised   ✔ Reinstated   ~~deleted~~ Deleted

Octreotide acetate, J2353, J2354
Ocular prosthetic implant, L8610
Ofatumumab, J9302
Olanzapine, J2358
Omacetaxine Mepesuccinate, J9262
Omalizumab, J2357
OnabotulinumtoxinA, J0585
Oncology
  disease status, G9063–G9139
  practice guidelines, G9056–G9062
  visit, G9050–G9055
Ondansetron HCl, J2405
Ondansetron oral, Q0162
One arm, drive attachment, K0101
Ophthalmological examination, refraction, S0621
Oprelvekin, J2355
O & P supply/accessory/service, L9900
Oral and maxillofacial surgery, D7111–D7999
  alveoloplasty, D7310–D7321
  complicated suturing, D7911–D7912
  excision of bone tissue, D7471–D7490
  extractions, local, D7111–D7140
  other repair procedures, D7920–D7999
  other surgical procedures, D7260–D7295
  reduction of dislocation/TMJ dysfunction,
    D7810–D7899
  repair of traumatic wounds, D7910
  surgical excision, intra-osseous lesions,
    D7440–D7465
  surgical excision, soft tissue lesions, D7410–D7415
  surgical extractions, D7210–D7251
  surgical incision, D7510–D7560
  treatment of fractures, compound, D7710–D7780
  treatment of fractures, simple, D7610–D7680
  vestibuloplasty, D7340–D7350
Oral device/appliance, E0485–E0486
Oral interface, A7047
Oral/nasal mask, A7027
  nasal pillows, A7029
  oral cushion, A7028
Oral, NOS, drug, J8499
Oropharyngeal suction catheter, A4628
Orphenadrine, J2360
Orthodontics, D8000–D8999
Orthopedic shoes
  arch support, L3040–L3100
  footwear, L3201–L3265, *L3000–L3649*
  insert, L3000–L3030
  lift, L3300–L3334
  miscellaneous additions, L3500–L3595
  positioning device, L3140–L3170
  transfer, L3600–L3649
  wedge, L3340–L3420
Orthotic additions
  carbon graphite lamination, L2755
  fracture, L2180–L2192, L3995
  halo, L0860
  lower extremity, L2200–L2999, L4320

Orthotic additions *(Continued)*
  ratchet lock, L2430
  scoliosis, L1010–L1120, L1210–L1290
  shoe, L3300–L3595, L3649
  spinal, L0970–L0984
  upper limb, L3810–L3890, *L3900, L3901,*
    L3970–L3974, L3995
Orthotic devices
  ankle-foot (AFO; *see also* Orthopedic shoes), E1815,
    E1816, E1830, L1900–L1990, L2102–L2116,
    L3160, L4361, L4397
  anterior-posterior-lateral, L0700, L0710
  cervical, L0100–L0200
  cervical-thoracic-lumbar-sacral (CTLSO), L0700,
    L0710
  elbow (EO), E1800, E1801, L3700–L3740
  fracture, L2102–L2136, L3980–L3986
  halo, L0810–L0830
  hand, finger, prefabricated, L3923
  hand, (WHFO), E1805, E1825, L3807,
    L3900–L3954
  hip (HO), L1600–L1690
  hip-knee-ankle-foot (HKAFO), L2040–L2090
  interface material, E1820
  knee (KO), E1810, E1811, L1800–L1885
  knee-ankle-foot (KAFO; *see also* Orthopedic shoes),
    L2000–L2038, L2126–L2136
  Legg Perthes, L1700–L1755
  lumbar, L0625–L0651
  multiple post collar, L0180–L0200
  not otherwise specified, L0999, L1499, L2999,
    L3999, L5999, L7499, L8039, L8239
  pneumatic splint, L4350–L4380
  pronation/supination, E1818
  repair or replacement, L4000–L4210
  replace soft interface material, L4390–L4394
  sacroiliac, L0600–L0620
  scoliosis, L1000–L1499
  shoe, *see* Orthopedic shoes
  shoulder (SO), L1840, L3650, L3674
  shoulder-elbow-wrist-hand (SEWHO), L3960–L3978
  side bar disconnect, L2768
  spinal, cervical, L0100–L0200
  spinal, DME, K0112–K0116
  thoracic, L0210
  thoracic-hip-knee-ankle (THKO), L1500–L1520
  toe, E1830
  wrist-hand-finger (WHFO), E1805, E1806, E1825,
    L3900–L3954, *L3806–L3809*
Orthovisc, J7324
Ossicula prosthetic implant, L8613
Osteogenesis stimulator, E0747–E0749, E0760
Osteoporosis
  documentation, G8401
Osteotomy, segmented or subapical, D7944
Ostomy
  accessories, A5093
  belt, A4396

◀ **New**   ↺ **Revised**   ✔ **Reinstated**   ~~deleted~~ **Deleted**

Ostomy *(Continued)*
   pouches, A4416–A4435, *A5056, A5057*
   skin barrier, A4401–A4449
   supplies, A4361–A4434, A5051–A5131, *A5200*
Otto Bock, prosthesis, *L7007*
Outpatient payment system, hospital,
   C1000–C9999
Overdoor, traction, *E0860*
Oxacillin sodium, J2700
Oxaliplatin, J9263
Oxygen
   ambulance, A0422
   battery charger, E1357
   battery pack/cartridge, E1356
   catheter, transtracheal, A7018
   chamber, hyperbaric, topical, A4575
   concentrator, E1390–E1391
   DC power adapter, E1358
   delivery system, topical NOS, E0446
   equipment, E0424–E0486, E1353–E1406
   Liquid oxygen system, E0433
   mask, A4620
   medication supplies, A4611–A4627
   rack/stand, E1355
   regulator, E1352, E1353
   respiratory equipment/supplies, A4611–A4627,
     E0424–E0480
   supplies and equipment, E0425–E0444, E0455
   tent, E0455
   tubing, A4616
   water vapor enriching system, E1405, E1406
   wheeled cart, E1354
Oxymorphone HCl, J2410
Oxytetracycline HCl, J2460
Oxytocin, J2590

P

Pacemaker monitor, E0610, E0615
Paclitaxel, J9267⮌
Paclitaxel protein-bound particles, J9264
Pad
   correction, CTLSO, L1020–L1060
   gel pressure, E0185, E0196
   heat, A9273, E0210, E0215, E0217, E0249
     electric heat pad, moist, E0215
     electric heat pad, standard, E0210
     hot water bottle, ice cap or collar, heat and/or cold
     wrap, A9273
     pad for water circulating heat unit, replacement
     only, E0249
     water circulating heat pad with pump, E0217
   orthotic device interface, E1820
   sheepskin, E0188, E0189
   water circulating cold with pump, E0218
   water circulating heat with pump, E0217
   water circulating heat unit, E0249

Pail, for use with commode chair, E0167
Pain assessment, *G8730, G8731*
Palate, prosthetic implant, L8618
Palifermin, J2425
Paliperidone palmitate, J2426
Palonosetron HCl, J2469
Pamidronate disodium, J2430
Pan, for use with commode chair, E0167
Panitumumab, J9303
Papanicolaou (Pap) screening smear, P3000,
   P3001, Q0091
   cervical or vaginal, up to 3 smears, by
     technician, P3000
   cervical or vaginal, up to 3 smears, physician inter-
     pretation, P3001
   obtaining, preparing and conveyance, Q0091
Papaverine HCl, J2440
Paraffin, A4265
   bath unit, E0235
Parenteral nutrition
   administration kit, B4224
   pump, B9004, B9006
   solution, B4164–B5200
     compounded amino acid and carbohydrates, with
     electrolytes, B4189–B4199, B5000–B5200
     nutrition additives, homemix, B4216
     nutrition administration kit, B4224
     nutrition solution, amino acid, B4168–B4178
     nutrition solution, carbohydrates, B4164, B4180
     nutrition solution, per 10 grams, liquid, B4185
     nutrition supply kit, homemix, B4222
   supply kit, B4220, B4222
Paricalcitol, J2501
Parking fee, nonemergency transport, A0170
Partial Hospitalization, OT, *G0129*
Paste, conductive, A4558
Pathology and laboratory tests, miscellaneous,
   P9010–P9615
Pathology, surgical, *G0416–G0419*
Patient support system, E0636
Patient transfer system, E1035–E1036
Pediculosis (lice) treatment, *A9180*
PEFR, peak expiratory flow rate meter, A4614
Pegademase bovine, J2504
Pegaptanib, J2503
Pegaspargase, J9266
Pegfilgrastim, J2505
Peginesatide, J0890
Pegloticase, J2507
Pelvic
   belt/harness/boot, E0944
   traction, E0890, E0900, E0947
Pemetrexed, J9305
Penicillin
   G benzathine/G benzathine and penicillin G
     procaine, J0558, J0561
   G potassium, J2540
   G procaine, aqueous, J2510

 ◀ **New**   ⮌ **Revised**   ✔ **Reinstated**   ~~deleted~~ **Deleted**

Pouch
fecal collection, A4330
ostomy, A4375–A4378, A5051–A5054, A5061–A5065
urinary, A4379–A4383, A5071–A5075
Pralatrexate, J9307
Practice, guidelines, oncology, G9056–G9062
Pralidoxime chloride, J2730
Prednisolone
acetate, J2650
oral, J7506, J7510
Prednisone, J7506
Prefabricated crown, D2930–D2933
Preparation kits, dialysis, A4914
Preparatory prosthesis, L5510–L5595
chemotherapy, J8999
nonchemotherapy, J8499
Pressure
alarm, dialysis, E1540
pad, A4640, E0180–E0199
Preventive dental procedures, D1000–D1999
Privigen, J1459
Procainamide HCl, J2690
Procedure
HALO, L0810–L0861
noncovered, G0293, G0294
scoliosis, L1000–L1499
Prochlorperazine, J0780
Prolotherapy, M0076
Promazine HCl, J2950
Promethazine
HCl, J2550
and meperdine, J2180
Prophylaxis
DVT, documentation, G8218
thrombosis, deep, vein, documentation, G8218
Propranolol HCl, J1800
Prostate, cancer, screening, G0102, G0103
Prosthesis
artificial larynx battery/accessory, L8505
auricular, D5914
breast, L8000–L8035, L8600
dental, D5911–D5960, D5999
eye, L8610, L8611, V2623–V2629
fitting, L5400–L5460, L6380–L6388
foot/ankle one piece system, L5979
hand, L6000–L6020, L6026↻
implants, L8600–L8690
larynx, L8500
lower extremity, L5700–L5999, L8640–L8642
mandible, L8617
maxilla, L8616
maxillofacial, provided by a non-physician,
  L8040–L8048
miscellaneous service, L8499
obturator, D5931–D5933, D5936
ocular, V2623–V2629
repair of, L7520, L8049
socks (shrinker, sheath, stump sock), L8400–L8485

Prosthesis *(Continued)*
taxes, orthotic/prosthetic/other, L9999
tracheo-esophageal, L8507–L8509
upper extremity, L6000–L6999
vacuum erection system, L7900
Prosthetic additions
lower extremity, L5610–L5999
upper extremity, L6600–L7405
Prosthetic, eye, V2623
Prosthodontic procedure
fixed, D6200–D6999
removable, D5000–D5899
Protamine sulfate, J2720
Protectant, skin, A6250
Protector, heel or elbow, E0191
Protein C Concentrate, J2724
Prosthodontics, removable, D5110–D5899
Protirelin, J2725
Psychotherapy, group, partial hospitalization,
  G0410–G0411
Pulp capping, D3110, D3120
Pulpotomy, D3220
partial, D3222
vitality test, D0460
Pulse generator, E2120
Pump
alternating pressure pad, E0182
ambulatory infusion, E0781
ambulatory insulin, E0784
blood, dialysis, E1620
breast, E0602–E0604
enteral infusion, B9000, B9002
external infusion, E0779
heparin infusion, E1520
implantable infusion, E0782, E0783
implantable infusion, refill kit, A4220
infusion, supplies, A4230, A4232
negative pressure wound therapy, E2402
parenteral infusion, B9004, B9006
suction, portable, E0600
water circulating pad, E0236
wound, negative, pressure, E2402
Purification system, E1610, E1615
Pyridoxine HCl, J3415

Q

Quad cane, E0105
Quinupristin/dalfopristin, J2770

R

Rack/stand, oxygen, E1355
Radiesse, Q2026
Radioelements for brachytherapy, Q3001
Radiograph, dental, D0210–D0340

◄ **New** ↻ **Revised** ✔ **Reinstated** ~~deleted~~ **Deleted**

Radiology service, R0070–R0076
Radiological, supplies, A4641, A4642
Radiopharmaceutical diagnostic and therapeutic imaging agent, A4641, A4642, A9500–A9699
Radiosurgery, robotic, G0339–G0340
Radiosurgery, stereotactic, G0173, G0251, G0339, G0340
Rail
  bathtub, E0241, E0242, E0246
  bed, E0305, E0310
  toilet, E0243
Ranibizumab, J2778
Rasburicase, J2783
Reaching/grabbing device, A9281
Reagent strip, A4252
Recement
  crown, D2920
  inlay, D2910
Reciprocating peritoneal dialysis system, E1630
Reclining, wheelchair, E1014, E1050–E1070, E1100–E1110
Reconstruction, angiography, G0288
Reclast, J3488
Red blood cells, P9021, P9022
Regadenoson, J2785
Regular insulin, J1820
Regulator, oxygen, E1353
Rehabilitation
  cardiac, S9472, S9473
  program, H2001
  psychosocial, H2017, H2018
  services, G8699–G8701
  system, jaw, motion, E1700–E1702
  vestibular, S9476
Removal, cerumen, G0268
Repair
  contract, ESRD, A4890
  durable medical equipment, E1340
  maxillofacial prosthesis, L8049
  orthosis, L4000–L4130
  prosthetic, L7500, L7510
Replacement
  battery, A4630
  pad (alternating pressure), A4640
  tanks, dialysis, A4880
  tip for cane, crutches, walker, A4637
  underarm pad for crutches, A4635
Reporting, asthma measures group, G8645, G8646
Resin dental restoration, D2330–D2387
RespiGam, *see* **Respiratory syncytial virus immune globulin**
Respiratory
  DME, A7000–A7527
  equipment, E0424–E0601
  function, therapeutic, procedure, G0237–G0239, S5180, S5181
  supplies, A4604–A4629
Restorative dental procedure, D2000–D2999

Restraint, any type, E0710
Reteplase, J2993
Revascularization, C9603–C9608
Rho(D) immune globulin, human, J2788, J2790, J2791, J2792
Rib belt, thoracic, A4572, L0220
Rilanocept, J2793
RimabotulinumtoxinB, J0587
Ringers lactate infusion, J7120
Ring, ostomy, A4404
Risk-adjusted functional status
  elbow, wrist or hand, G8667–G8670
  hip, G8651–G8654
  lower leg, foot or ankle, G8655–G8658
  lumbar spine, G8659–G8662
  neck, cranium, mandible, thoracic spine, ribs, or other, G8671–G8674
  shoulder, G8663–G8666
Risperidone, J2794
Rituximab, J9310
Robin-Aids, L6000, L6010, L6020, L6855, L6860
Rocking bed, E0462
Rollabout chair, E1031
Romidepsin, J9315
Romiplostim, J2796
Root canal therapy, D3310–D3353
Ropivacaine HCl, J2795
Rubidium Rb-82, A9555

S

Sacral nerve stimulation test lead, A4290
Safety equipment, E0700
  vest, wheelchair, E0980
Saline
  infusion, J7030–J7060
  hypertonic, J7130
  solution, J7030–J7050, A4216–A4218
Saliva
  analysis, A0418
  artificial, A9155
  collection and preparation, D0417
Samarium SM 153 Lexidronamm, A9605
Sargramostim (GM-CSF), J2820
Scoliosis, L1000–L1499
  additions, L1010–L1120, L1210–L1290
Screening
  alcohol misuse, G0442
  cancer, cervical or vaginal, G0101
  colorectal, cancer, G0104–G0106, G0120–G0122, G0328, S3890
  cytopathology cervical or vaginal, G0123, G0124, G0141–G0148
  depression, G0444
  dysphagia, documentation, G8232, V5364
  enzyme immunoassay, G0432
  glaucoma, G0117, G0118

◄ **New** ↻ **Revised** ✔ **Reinstated** ~~deleted~~ **Deleted**

Screening (*Continued*)
  infectious agent antibody detection, G0433, G0435
  language, V5363
  mammography, digital image, G0202
  prostate, cancer, G0102, G0103
  speech,V5362
Sculptra, Q2028
Sealant
  skin, A6250
  tooth, D1351
Seat
  attachment, walker, E0156
  insert, wheelchair, E0992
  lift (patient), E0621, E0627–E0629
  upholstery, wheelchair, E0975
Secretin, J2850
Semen analysis, G0027
Semi-reclining, wheelchair, *E1100, E1110*
Sensitivity study, P7001
Sensory nerve conduction test, *G0255*
Sermorelin acetate, Q0515
Serum clotting time tube, A4771
Service
  Allied Health, home health, hospice, G0151–G0161
  behavioral health and/or substance abuse,
    H0001–H9999
  hearing, V5000–V5999
  laboratory, P0000–P9999
  mental, health, training, G0177
  non-covered, A9270
  physician, for mobility device, G0372
  pulmonary, for LVRS, G0302–G0305
  skilled, RN/LPN, home health, hospice,
    G0162–G0164
  social, psychological, G0409–G0411
  speech-language, V5336–V5364
  vision, V2020–V2799
SEWHO, L3960–L3974
SEXA, *G0130*
Sheepskin pad, E0188, E0189
Shoes
  arch support, L3040–L3100
  for diabetics, A5500–A5508
  insert, L3000–L3030
  lift, L3300–L3334
  miscellaneous additions, L3500–L3595
  orthopedic, L3201–L3265
  positioning device, L3140–L3170
  transfer, L3600–L3649
  wedge, L3340–L3485
Shoulder
  disarticulation, prosthetic, L6300–L6320, L6550
  orthosis (SO), L3650–L3674
  spinal, cervical, L0100–L0200
Shoulder-elbow-wrist-hand orthosis (SEWHO),
  L3960–L3969
Shoulder sling, A4566

Shunt accessory for dialysis, A4740
  aqueous, L8612
Sigmoidoscopy, cancer screening, G0104, G0106
Silicate dental restoration, *D2210*
Sincalide, J2805
Sipuleucel-T, Q2043
Sirolimus, J7520
Sitz bath, E0160–E0162
Skin
  barrier, ostomy, A4362, A4363, A4369–A4373,
    A4385, A5120
  bond or cement, ostomy, A4364
  sealant, protectant, moisturizer, A6250
  substitute, Q4100–Q4160↵
Skyla, 13.5 mg, *J7301*
Sling, A4565
  patient lift, E0621, E0630, E0635
Smear, Papanicolaou, screening, *P3000,*
  P3001, Q0091
SNCT, *G0255*
Social work/psychological services, CORF, *G0409*
Social worker, clinical, home, health, *G0155*
Social worker, nonemergency transport, A0160
Sock
  body sock, L0984
  prosthetic sock, L8420–L8435, L8470,
    L8480, L8485
  stump sock, L8470–L8485
Sodium
  chloride injection, J2912
  ferric gluconate complex in sucrose, J2916
  fluoride F-18, A9580
  hyaluronate
    Euflexxa, J7323
    Hyalgan, J7321
    Orthovisc, J7324
    Supartz, J7321
    Synvisc and Synvisc-One, J7325
  phosphate P32, A9563
  succinate, J1720
Solution
  calibrator, A4256
  dialysate, A4760
  elliotts b, J9175
  enteral formulae, B4149–B4156
  parenteral nutrition, B4164–B5200
Solvent, adhesive remover, *A4455*
Somatrem, J2940
Somatropin, J2941
Sorbent cartridge, ESRD, E1636
Special size, wheelchair, *E1220–E1239*
Specialty absorptive dressing, A6251–A6256
Spectinomycin HCl, J3320
Spectacle lenses, *V2100–V2199*
Speech assessment, V5362–V5364
Speech generating device, E2500–E2599
Speech-Language pathology, services, *V5336–V5364*

◀ **New**   ⊋ **Revised**   ✔ **Reinstated**   ~~deleted~~ **Deleted**

Speech, pathologist, G0153
Spherocylinder, single vision, V2100–V2114
  bifocal, V2203–V2214
  trifocal, V2303–V2314
Spinal orthosis
  cervical, L0100, L0200
  cervical-thoracic-lumbar-sacral (CTLSO), L0700,
    L0710
  DME, K0112–K0116
  halo, L0810–L0830
  multiple post collar, L0180–L0200
  scoliosis, L1000–L1499
  torso supports, L0960
Splint, A4570, L3100, L4350–L4380
  ankle, L4390–L4398
  dynamic, E1800, E1805, E1810, E1815, E1825,
    E1830, E1840
  footdrop, L4398
  supplies, miscellaneous, Q4051
Standard, wheelchair, E1130, K0001
Static progressive stretch, E1801, E1806, E1811,
  E1816, E1818, E1821
Status
  disease, oncology, G9063–G9139
STELARA, ustekinumab, 1 mg, J3357
Stent, transcatheter, placement, C9600,
  C9601, S2211
Sterile cefuroxime sodium, J0697
Sterile water, A4216–A4217
Stereotactic, radiosurgery, G0173, G0251,
  G0339, G0340
Stimulation, electrical, non-attended, G0281–G0283
Stimulators
  neuromuscular, E0744, E0745
  osteogenesis, electrical, E0747–E0749
  ultrasound, E0760
  salivary reflex, E0755
  stoma absorptive cover, A5083
  transcutaneous, electric, nerve, A4595, E0720–E0749
Stockings
  gradient, compression, A6530–A6549
  surgical, A4490–A4510
Stoma, plug or seal, A5081
Stomach tube, B4083
Stool, guaiac, G0394
Streptokinase, J2995
Streptomycin, J3000
Streptozocin, J9320
Strip, blood glucose test, A4253, A4772
  urine reagent, A4250
Strontium-89 chloride, supply of, A9600
Study, bone density, G0130
Stump sock, L8470–L8485
Stylet, A4212
Substance/Alcohol, assessment, G0396, G0397,
  H0001, H0003, H0049
Succinylcholine chloride, J0330

Suction pump
  gastric, home model, E2000
  portable, E0600
  respiratory, home model, E0600
Sumatriptan succinate, J3030
Supartz, J7321
Supply/accessory/service, A9900
Supplies
  battery, A4233–A4236, A4601, A4611–A4613, A4638
  cast, A4580, A4590, Q4001–Q4051
  catheters, A4300–A4306
  contraceptive, A4267–A4269
  diabetic shoes, A5500–A5513
  dialysis, A4653–A4927
  DME, other, A4630–A4640
  dressings, A6000–A6513
  enteral, therapy, B4000–B9999
  incontinence, A4310–A4355, A5102–A5200
  infusion, A4221, A4222, A4230–A4232,
    E0776–E0791
  needle, A4212, A4215
  ostomy, A4361–A4434, A5051–A5093, A5120–A5200
  parenteral, therapy, B4000–B9999
  radiological, A4641, A4642
  refill kit, infusion pump, A4220
  respiratory, A4604–A4629
  self-administered injections, A4211
  splint, Q4051
  sterile water/saline and/or dextrose, A4216–A4218
  surgical, miscellaneous, A4649
  syringe, A4206–A4209, A4213, A4232
  syringe with needle, A4206–A4209
  needle-free device, A4210
  urinary, external, A4356–A4360
Support
  arch, L3040–L3090
  cervical, L0100–L0200
  spinal, L0960
  stockings, L8100–L8239
Surgery, oral, D7000–D7999
Surgical
  arthroscopy, knee, G0289, S2112, S2113
  boot, L3208–L3211
  brush, dialysis, A4910
  dressing, A6196–A6406
  procedure, noncovered, G0293, G0294
  stocking, A4490–A4510
  supplies, A4649
  tray, A4550
Swabs, betadine or iodine, A4247
Syringe, A4213
  with needle, A4206–A4209
Synvisc and Synvisc-One, J7325
System
  external, ambulatory insulin, A9274
  rehabilitation, jaw, motion, E1700–E1702
  transport, E1035–E1039

◄ **New**   ⮌ **Revised**   ✔ **Reinstated**   ~~deleted~~ **Deleted**

T

Tables, bed, E0274, E0315
Tacrolimus
  oral, J7507, J7508
  parenteral, J7525
Taliglucerace, J3060
Tape, A4450–A4452
Taxi, non emergency transportation, A0100
Team, conference, G0175, G9007, S0220, S0221
Technetium TC 99M
  Arcitumomab, A9568
  Bicisate, A9557
  Depreotide, A9536
  Disofenin, A9510
  Exametazine, A9521
  Exametazine labeled autologous white blood cells, A9569
  Fanolesomab, A9566
  Glucepatate, A9550
  Labeled red blood cells, A9560
  Macroaggregated albumin, A9540
  Mebrofenin, A9537
  Mertiatide, A9562
  Oxidronate, A9561
  Pentetate, A9539, A9567
  Pertechnetate, A9512
  Pyrophosphate, A9538
  Sestamibi, A9500
  Succimer, A9551
  Sulfur colloid, A9541
  Teboroxime, A9501
  Tetrofosmin, A9502
  Tilmanocept, A9520
TEEV, J0900
Telavancin, J3095
Telehealth, Q3014
Telehealth transmission, T1014
Temozolomide
  injection, J9328
  oral, J8700
Temporary codes, Q0000–Q9999, S0009–S9999
Temporomandibular joint, D0320, D0321
Temsirolimus, J9330
Tenecteplase, J3101
Teniposide, Q2017
TENS, A4595, E0720–E0749
Tent, oxygen, E0455
Terbutaline sulfate, J3105
  inhalation solution, concentrated, J7680
  inhalation solution, unit dose, J7681
Teriparatide, J3110
Terminal devices, L6700–L6895
Test
  occult, blood, G0394
  sensory, nerve, conduction, G0255

Testosterone
  aqueous, J3140✖
  cypionate and estradiol cypionate, J1071↻
  enanthate, J3121↻
  enanthate and estradiol valerate, J0900✖
  propionate, J3150✖
  suspension, J3140✖
  undecanoate, J3145◀
Tetanus immune globulin, human, J1670
Tetracycline, J0120
Thallous Chloride TL 201, A9505
Theophylline, J2810
Therapeutic lightbox, A4634, E0203
Therapy
  activity, G0176
  electromagnetic, G0295, G0329
  endodontic, D3222–D3330
  enteral, supplies, B4000–B9999
  medical, nutritional, G0270, G0271
  occupational, H5300, G0129, S9129
  occupational, health, G0152
  respiratory, function, procedure, G0237–G0239, S5180, S5181
  parenteral, supplies, B4000–B9999
  speech, home, G0153, S9128
  wound, negative, pressure, pump, E2402
Theraskin, Q4121
Thermometer, A4931–A4932
  dialysis, A4910
Thiamine HCl, J3411
Thiethylperazine maleate, J3280
Thiotepa, J9340
Thoracic-hip-knee-ankle (THKAO), L1500–L1520
Thoracic-lumbar-sacral orthosis (TLSO)
  scoliosis, L1200–L1290
  spinal, L0450–L0492
Thoracic orthosis, L0210
Thymol turbidity, blood, P2033
Thyrotropin Alfa, J3240
Tigecycline, J3243
Tinzarparin sodium, J1655
Tip (cane, crutch, walker) replacement, A4637
Tire, wheelchair, E0999
Tirofiban, J3246
Tissue marker, A4648
TLSO, L0450–L0492, L1200–L1290
Tobacco
  intervention, G9016
Tobramycin
  inhalation solution, unit dose, J7682, J7685
  sulfate, J3260
Tocilizumab, J2362
Toe device, E1831
Toilet accessories, E0167–E0179, E0243, E0244, E0625
Tolazoline HCl, J2670
Toll, non emergency transport, A0170

◀ **New**   ↻ **Revised**   ✓ **Reinstated**   ~~deleted~~ **Deleted**

Tomographic radiograph, dental, *D0322*
Topical hyperbaric oxygen chamber, A4575
Topotecan, J8705, J9351
Torsemide, J3265
Tositumomab, administration and supply, *G3001*
Tracheostoma heat moisture exchange system,
    A7501–A7509
Tracheostomy
    care kit, A4629
    filter, A4481
    speaking valve, L8501
    supplies, A4623, A4629, A7523–A7524
    tube, A7520–A7522
Tracheotomy mask or collar, A7525–A7526
Traction
    cervical, E0855, E0856
    extremity, E0870–E0880
    device, ambulatory, E0830
    equipment, E0840–E0948
    pelvic, E0890, E0900, E0947
Training
    diabetes, outpatient, G0108, G0109
    home health or hospice, G0164
    services, mental, health, G0177
Transcatheter, placement, stent, *S2211*
**Transcutaneous electrical nerve stimulator
    (TENS),** E0720–E0770
Transducer protector, dialysis, E1575
Transfer (shoe orthosis), L3600–L3640
Transfer system with seat, E1035
Transplant
    islet, G0341–G0343, S2102
Transparent film (for dressing), A6257–A6259
Transport
    chair, E1035–E1039
    system, E1035–E1039
    x-ray, R0070–R0076
Transportation
    ambulance, A0021–A0999, Q3019, Q3020
    corneal tissue, V2785
    EKG (portable), R0076
    handicapped, A0130
    non emergency, A0080–A0210, T2001–T2005
    service, including ambulance, A0021–A0999,
        T2006
    taxi, non emergency, A0100
    toll, non emergency, A0170
    volunteer, non emergency, A0080, A0090
    x-ray (portable), R0070, R0075 *R0076*
Transportation services
    air services, A0430, A0431, A0435, A0436
    ALS disposable supplies, A0398
    ALS mileage, A0390
    ALS specialized service, A0392, A0394, A0396
    ambulance oxygen, A0422
    ambulance, ALS, A0426, A0427, A0433
    ambulance, outside state, Medicaid, A0021
    ambulance, waiting time, A0420

Transportation services (Continued)
    ancillary, lodging, escort, A0200
    ancillary, lodging, recipient, A0180
    ancillary, meals, escort, A0210
    ancillary, meals, recipient, A0190
    ancillary, parking fees, tolls, A0170
    BLS disposable supplies, A0382
    BLS mileage, A0380
    BLS specialized service, A0384
    emergency, neonatal, one-way, A0225
    extra ambulance attendant, A0424
    ground mileage, A0425
    non-emergency, air travel, A0140
    non-emergency, bus, A0110
    non-emergency, case worker, A0160
    non-emergency, mini-bus, A0120
    non-emergency, no vested interest, A0080
    non-emergency, taxi, A0100
    non-emergency, wheelchair van, A0130
    non-emergency, with vested interest, A0090
    paramedic intercept, A0432
    response and treat, no transport, A0998
    specialty transport, A0434
Transtracheal oxygen catheter, A7018
Trapeze bar, E0910–E0912, E0940
Trauma, response, team, *G0390*
Tray
    insertion, A4310–A4316
    irrigation, A4320
    surgical (*see also* kits), A4550
    wheelchair, E0950
Treatment
    bone, G0412–G0415
    pediculosis (lice), A9180
    services, behavioral health, H0002–H2037
Treprostinil, J3285
Triamcinolone, J3301–J3303
    acetonide, J3300, J3301
    diacetate, J3302
    hexacetonide, J3303
    inhalation solution, concentrated, J7683
    inhalation solution, unit dose, J7684
Triflupromazine HCl, J3400
Trifocal, glass or plastic, V2300–V2399
    aniseikonic, V2318
    lenticular, V2315, V2321
    specialty trifocal, by report, V2399
    sphere, plus or minus, V2300–V2302
    spherocylinder, V2303–V2314
    trifocal add-over 3.25d, V2320
    trifocal, seg width over 28 mm, V2319
Trigeminal division block anesthesia,
    D9212
Trimethobenzamide HCl, J3250
Trimetrexate glucuoronate, J3305
Trimming, nails, dystrophic, *G0127*
Triptorelin pamoate, J3315
Trismus appliance, *D5937*

◄ **New**   ⊋ **Revised**   ✔ **Reinstated**   d̶e̶l̶e̶t̶e̶d̶ **Deleted**

Truss, L8300–L8330
  addition to standard pad, scrotal pad, L8330
  addition to standard pad, water pad, L8320
  double, standard pads, L8310
  single, standard pad, L8300
Tube/Tubing
  anchoring device, A5200
  blood, A4750, A4755
  drainage extension, A4331
  gastrostomy, B4087, B4088
  irrigation, A4355
  larynectomy, A4622
  nasogastric, B4081, B4082
  oxygen, A4616
  serum clotting time, A4771
  stomach, B4083
  suction pump, each, A7002
  tire, K0091, K0093, K0095, K0097
  tracheostomy, A4622
  urinary drainage, K0280

U

Ultrasonic nebulizer, E0575
Ultrasound, *G0389, S8055, S9024*
  B scan and/or real time (AAA), G0389
  paranasal sinus ultrasound, S9024
  ultrasound guidance, multifetal pregnancy reduction, technical component, S8055
Ultraviolet, cabinet/system, *E0691–E0694*
Ultraviolet light therapy system, A4633, E0691–E0694
  light therapy system in 6 foot cabinet, E0694
  replacement bulb/lamp, A4633
  therapy system panel, 4 foot, E0692
  therapy system panel, 6 foot, E0693
  treatment area 2 sq feet or less, E0691
Unclassified drug, J3490
Underpads, disposable, *A4554*
Unipuncture control system, dialysis, E1580
Upper extremity addition, locking elbow, L6693
Upper extremity fracture orthosis, L3980–L3999
Upper limb prosthesis, L6000–L7499
Urea, J3350
Ureterostomy supplies, A4454–A4590
Urethral suppository, Alprostadil, J0275
Urinal, E0325, E0326
Urinary
  catheter, A4338–A4346, A4351–A4353
    indwelling catheter, A4338–A4346
    intermittent urinary catheter, A4351–A4353
    male external catheter A4349
  collection and retention (supplies), A4310–A4360
    bedside drainage bag, A4357
    disposable external urethral clamp, A4360
    external urethral clamp, A4356
    female external urinary collection device, A4328

Urinary *(Continued)*
    insertion trays, A4310–A4316, A4354–A4355
    irrigation syringe, A4322
    irrigation tray, A4320
    male external catheter/integral collection chamber, A4326
    perianal fecal collection pouch, A4330
    therapeutic agent urinary catheter irrigation, A4321
    urinary drainage bag, leg/abdomen, A4358
  incontinence, documentation, G8063, G8067
  supplies, external, A4335, A4356–A4358
    bedside drainage bag, A4357
    external urethral clamp/compression device, A4356
    incontinence supply, A4335
    urinary drainage bag, leg or abdomen, A4358
  tract implant, collagen, L8603
  tract implant, synthetic, L8606
Urine
  sensitivity study, P7001
  tests, A4250
Urofollitropin, J3355
Urokinase, J3364, J3365
Ustekinumab, J3357
U-V lens, V2755

V

Vabra aspirator, A4480
Vaccination, administration
  flublok, Q2033
  hepatitis B, G0010
  influenza virus, G0008
  pneumococcal, G0009
Vaccine
  administration, influenza, G0008
  administration, pneumococcal, G0009
  hepatitis B, administration, G0010
Vaginal
  cancer, screening, G0101
  cytopathology, G0123, G0124, G0141–G0148
  screening cytopathology smears, automated, G0141–G0148
  screening, cervical/vaginal, thin-layer, cytopathologist, G0123
  screening, cervical/vaginal, thin-layer, physician interpretation, G0124
Vancomycin HCl, J3370
Vaporizer, E0605
Vascular
  catheter (appliances and supplies), A4300–A4306
    disposable drug delivery system, <50 ml/hr, A4306
    disposable drug delivery system, >50 ml/hr, A4305
    implantable access catheter, external, A4300
    implantable access total, catheter, A4301
  graft material, synthetic, L8670
Vasoxyl, J3390
Vehicle, power-operated, *K0800–K0899*

◀ **New**   ↻ **Revised**   ✔ **Reinstated**   ~~deleted~~ **Deleted**

Velaglucerase alfa, J3385
Venous pressure clamp, dialysis, A4918
Ventilator
    battery, A4611–A4613
    moisture exchanger, disposable, A4483
    negative pressure, E0460
    volume, stationary or portable, E0450, E0461–
      E0464
      rocking bed, E0462
      used with non-invasive interface, E0461
      volume control mode, invasive interface, E0463
      volume control mode, non-invasive
      interface, E0464
      without pressure support mode, invasive
      interface, E0450
Ventricular assist device, Q0478–Q0509
    battery clips, electric or electric/pneumatic, replace-
      ment, Q0497
    battery, lithium-ion, electric or electric/pneumatic, re-
      placement, Q0506
    battery, other than lithium-ion, electric or electric/
      pneumatic, replacement, Q0496
    battery, pneumatic, replacement, Q0503
    battery/power-pack charger, electric or electric/pneu-
      matic, replacement, Q0495
    belt/vest/bag, carry external components,
      replacement, Q0499
    driver, replacement, Q0480
    emergency hand pump, electric or electric/pneumatic,
      replacement, Q0494
    emergency power source, electric, replacement,
      Q0490
    emergency power source, electric/pneumatic,
      replacement, Q0491
    emergency power supply cable, electric,
      replacement, Q0492
    emergency power supply cable, electric/pneumatic,
      replacement, Q0493
    filters, electric or electric/pneumatic,
      replacement, Q0500
    holster, electric or electric/pneumatic,
      replacement, Q0498
    leads (pneumatic/electrical), replacement, Q0487
    microprocessor control unit, electric/pneumatic com-
      bination, replacement, Q0482
    microprocessor control unit, pneumatic,
      replacement, Q0481
    miscellaneous supply, external VAD, Q0507
    miscellaneous supply, implanted device, payment not
      made under Medicare Part A, A0509
    miscellaneous supply, implanted device, Q0508
    mobility cart, replacement, Q0502
    monitor control cable, electric, replacement, Q0485
    monitor control cable, electric/pneumatic, Q0486
    monitor/display module, electric,
      replacement, Q0483
    monitor/display module, electric/electric pneumatic,
      replacement, Q0484

Ventricular assist device *(Continued)*
    power adapter, pneumatic, replacement, vehicle
      type, Q0504
    power adapter, vehicle type, Q0478
    power module, replacement, Q0479
    power-pack base, electric, replacement, Q0488
    power-pack base, electric/pneumatic,
      replacement, Q0489
    shower cover, electric or electric/pneumatic,
      replacement, Q0501
Verteporfin, J3396
Vest, safety, wheelchair, E0980
Vinblastine sulfate, J9360
Vincristine sulfate, J9370, J9371
Vinorelbine tartrate, J9390
Vision service, V2020–V2799
    bifocal, glass or plastic, V2200–V2299
    contact lenses, V2500–V2599
    frames, V2020–V2025
    intraocular lenses, V2630–V2632
    low-vision aids, V2600–V2615
    miscellaneous, V2700–V2799
    prosthetic eye, V2623–V2629
    spectacle lenses, V2100–V2199
    trifocal, glass or plastic, V2300–V2399
    variable asphericity, V2410–V2499
Visit, emergency department, G0380–G0384
Visual, function, postoperative cataract surgery,
    G0915–G0918
Vitamin B-12 cyanocobalamin, J3420
Vitamin K, J3430
Voice
    amplifier, L8510
    prosthesis, L8511–L8514
Von Willebrand Factor Complex, human, J7183,
    J7187
Voriconazole, J3465

W

Waiver, T2012–T2050
    assessment/plan of care development, T2024
    case management, per month, T2022
    day habilitation, per 15 minutes, T2021
    day habilitation, per diem, T2020
    habilitation, educational, per diem, T2012
    habilitation, educational, per hour, T2013
    habilitation, prevocational, per diem, T2014
    habilitation, prevocational, per hour, T2015
    habilitation, residential, 15 minutes, T2017
    habilitation, residential, per diem, T2016
    habilitation, supported employment,
      15 minutes, T2019
    habilitation, supported employment, per diem,
      T2018
    targeted case management, per month, T2023
    waiver services NOS, T2025

◄ **New** ⊃ **Revised** ✔ **Reinstated** ~~deleted~~ **Deleted**

X

Y

Z

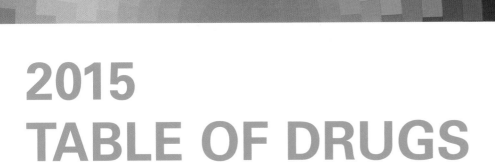

2015
TABLE OF DRUGS

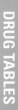

IA	Intra-arterial administration	
IU	International unit	
IV	Intravenous administration	
IM	Intramuscular administration	
IT	Intrathecal	
SC	Subcutaneous administration	
INH	Administration by inhaled solution	
VAR	Various routes of administration	
OTH	Other routes of administration	
ORAL	Administered orally	

Intravenous administration includes all methods, such as gravity infusion, injections, and timed pushes. The "VAR" posting denotes various routes of administration and is used for drugs that are commonly administered into joints, cavities, tissues, or topical applications, in addition to other parenteral administrations. Listings posted with "OTH" indicate other administration methods, such as suppositories or catheter injections.

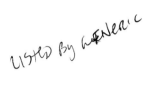

Blue typeface terms are added by publisher.

DRUG NAME	DOSAGE	METHOD OF ADMINISTRATION	HCPCS CODE
A			
Abatacept	10 mg	IV	**J0129**
Abbokinase	5,000 IU vial	IV	J3364
	250,000 IU vial	IV	J3365
Abbokinase, Open Cath	5,000 IU vial	IV	J3364
Abciximab	10 mg	IV	**J0130**
Abelcet	10 mg	IV	J0287
Abilify	0.25 mg		J0400
	1 mg		J0401
Ablavar	1 ml		A9583
ABLC	50 mg	IV	J0285
AbobotulinumtoxintypeA	5 units	IM	**J0586**
Abraxane	1 mg		J9264
Accuneb	1 mg		J7613
Acetadote	100 mg		J0132
Acetaminophen	10 mg	IV	**J0131**
Acetazolamide sodium	up to 500 mg	IM, IV	**J1120**
Acetylcysteine			
injection	100 mg	IV	**J0132**
unit dose form	per gram	INH	**J7604, J7608**
Achromycin	up to 250 mg	IM, IV	J0120
Actemra	1 mg		J3262
ACTH	up to 40 units	IV, IM, SC	J0800
Acthar	up to 40 units	IV, IM, SC	J0800
Acthib			J3490
Acthrel	1 mcg		J0795
Actimmune	0.25 mg	SC	J1830
	3 million units	SC	J9216
Activase	1 mg	IV	J2997

◄ New	↻ Revised	✔ Reinstated	~~deleted~~ Deleted

DRUG NAME	DOSAGE	METHOD OF ADMINISTRATION	HCPCS CODE
Acyclovir	5 mg		**J0133**
			J8499
Adagen	25 IU		J2504
Adalimumab	20 mg	SC	**J0135**
Adcetris	1 mg	IV	J9042
Adenocard	1 mg	IV	J0153
Adenoscan	1 mg	IV	J0151
Adenosine	~~6 mg~~	~~IV~~	~~J0150~~ ✖
	1 mg	IV	**J0153** ↻
Ado-trastuzumab Emtansine	1 mg	IV	**J9354**
Adrenalin Chloride	up to 1 ml ampule	SC, IM	J0171
Adrenalin, epinephrine	0.1 mg	SC, IM	**J0171**
Adriamycin, PFS, RDF	10 mg	IV	J9000
Adrucil	500 mg	IV	J9190
Advate	per IU		J7192
Aflibercept	1 mg	OTH	**J0178**
Agalsidase beta	1 mg	IV	**J0180**
Aggrastat	0.25 mg	IM, IV	J3246
Aglucosidase alfa	10 mg	IV	J0220
A-hydroCort	up to 50 mg	IV, IM, SC	J1710
	up to 100 m		J1720
Akineton	per 5 mg	IM, IV	J0190
Alatrofloxacin mesylate, injection	100 mg	IV	**J0200**
Albumin			P9041, P9045 P9046, P9047
Albuterol	0.5 mg	INH	**J7620**
concentrated form	1 mg	INH	**J7610, J7611**
unit dose form	1 mg	INH	**J7609, J7613**
Aldesleukin	per single use vial	IM, IV	**J9015**
Aldomet	up to 250 mg	IV	J0210
Aldurazyme	0.1 mg		J1931
Alefacept	0.5 mg	IM, IV	**J0215**
Alemtuzumab	10 mg	IV	**J9010**
Alferon N	250,000 IU	IM	J9215
Alglucerase	per 10 units	IV	**J0205**
Alglucosidase alfa	10 mg	IV	**J0220, J0221**
Alimta	10 mg	IV	J9305
Alkaban-AQ	1 mg	IV	J9360
Alkeran	2 mg	ORAL	J8600
	50 mg	IV	J9245
Allopurinol Sodium			J9999
Aloxi	25 mcg		J2469

◀ **New**   ↻ **Revised**   ✔ **Reinstated**   ~~deleted~~ **Deleted**

DRUG NAME	DOSAGE	METHOD OF ADMINISTRATION	HCPCS CODE
Alpha 1-proteinase inhibitor, human	10 mg	IV	J0256 , J0257
Alphanate			J7186
AlphaNine SD	per IU		J7193
Alprostadil			
injection	1.25 mcg	OTH	J0270
urethral suppository	EA	OTH	J0275
Alteplase recombinant	1 mg	IV	J2997
Alupent	per 10 mg	INH	J7667, J7668
noncompounded, unit dose	10 mg	INH	J7669
AmBisome	10 mg	IV	J0289
Amcort	per 5 mg	IM	J3302
A-methaPred	up to 40 mg	IM, IV	J2920
	up to 125 mg	IM, IV	J2930
Amevive	0.5 mg		J0215
Amgen	1 mcg	SC	J9212
Amifostine	500 mg	IV	J0207
Amikin	100 mg	IM, IV	J0278
Amikacin sulfate	100 mg	IM, IV	J0278
Aminocaproic Acid			J3490
Aminolevalinic acid HCl	unit dose (354 mg)	OTH	J7308
Aminolevulinate	1 g	OTH	J7309
Aminophylline	up to 250 mg	IV	J0280
Amiodarone HCl	30 mg	IV	J0282
Amitriptyline HCl	up to 20 mg	IM	J1320
Amobarbital	up to 125 mg	IM, IV	J0300
Amphocin	50 mg	IV	J0285
Amphotericin B	50 mg	IV	J0285
Amphotericin B, lipid complex	10 mg	IV	J0287–J0289
Ampicillin			
sodium	up to 500 mg	IM, IV	J0290
sodium/sulbactam sodium	per 1.5 g	IM, IV	J0295
Amygdalin			J3570
Amytal	up to 125 mg	IM, IV	J0300
Anabolin LA 100	up to 50 mg	IM	J2320
Anadulafungin	1 mg	IV	J0348
Anascorp	up to 120 mg	IV	J0716
Ancef	500 mg	IV, IM	J0690
Andrest 90-4	1 mg	IM	J3121
Andro-Cyp	1 mg		J1071
Andro-Cyp 200	1 mg		J1071
Andro L.A. 200	1 mg	IM	J3121
Andro-Estro 90-4	1 mg	IM	J3121

◄ New   ⊃ Revised   ✔ Reinstated   ~~deleted~~ Deleted

DRUG NAME	DOSAGE	METHOD OF ADMINISTRATION	HCPCS CODE
Andro/Fem	1 mg		J1071
Androgyn L.A	1 mg	IM	J3121
Androlone-50	up to 50 mg		J2320
Androlone-D 100	up to 50 mg	IM	J2320
Andronaq-50	up to 50 mg	IM	J3140
Andronaq-LA	1 mg		J1071
Andronate-200	1 mg		J1071
Andronate-100	1 mg		J1071
Andropository 100	1 mg		J3121
Andryl 200	1 mg		J3121
Anectine	up to 20 mg	IM, IV	J0330
Anergan 25	up to 50 mg	IM, IV	J2550
	12.5 mg	ORAL	Q0169
Anergan 50	up to 50 mg	IM, IV	J2550
	12.5 mg	ORAL	Q0169
Anestacaine	10 mg		J2001
Angiomax	1 mg		J0583
Anidulafungin	1 mg	IV	J0348
Anistreplase	30 units	IV	**J0350**
Antiflex	up to 60 mg		J2360
Anti-Inhibitor	per IU	IV	**J7198**
Antispas	up to 20 mg	IM	J0500
Antithrombin III (human)	per IU	IV	**J7197**
Antithrombin recombinant	50 IU	IV	**J7196**
Anzemet	10 mg	IV	J1260
	50 mg	ORAL	S0174
	100 mg	ORAL	Q0180
Apidra Solostar	per 50 units		J1817
A.P.L.	per 1,000 USP units	IM	J0725
Apomorphine Hydrochloride	1 mg	SC	**J0364**
Aprepitant	5 mg	ORAL	J8501
Apresoline	up to 20 mg	IV, IM	J0360
Aprotinin	10,000 kiu		**J0365**
AquaMEPHYTON	per 1 mg	IM, SC, IV	J3430
Aralast	10 mg	IV	J0256
Aralen	up to 250 mg	IM	J0390
Aramine	per 10 mg	IV, IM, SC	J0380
Aranesp			
ESRD use	1 mcg		J0882
Non-ESRD use	1 mcg		J0881
Arbutamine	1 mg	IV	**J0395**
Arcalyst	1 mg		J2793

◄ **New**   ↩ **Revised**   ✔ **Reinstated**   ~~deleted~~ **Deleted**

DRUG NAME	DOSAGE	METHOD OF ADMINISTRATION	HCPCS CODE
Aredia	per 30 mg	IV	J2430
Arfonad, see Trimethaphan camsylate			
Arformoterol tartrate	15 mcg	INH	**J7605**
Aridol	25% in 50 ml	IV	J2150
	5 mg	INH	J7665
Arimidex			J8999
Aripiprazole	0.25 mg	IM	**J0400**
Aripiprazole, extended release	1 mg	INJ	**J0401**
Aristocort Forte	per 5 mg	IM	J3302
Aristocort Intralesional	per 5 mg	IM	J3302
Aristopan	per 5 mg		J3303
Aristospan Intra-Articular	per 5 mg	VAR	J3303
Aristospan Intralesional	per 5 mg	VAR	J3303
Arixtra	per 0.5 m		J1652
Aromasin			J8999
Arranon	50 mg		J9261
Arrestin	up to 200 mg	IM	J3250
	250 mg	ORAL	Q0173
Arsenic trioxide	1 mg	IV	**J9017**
Arzerra	10 mg		J9302
Asparaginase	1,000 units	IV, IM	**J9019**
	10,000 units	IV, IM	**J9020**
Astagraf XL	0.1 mg		J7508
Astramorph PF	up to 10 mg	IM, IV, SC	J2270
Atgam	250 mg	IV	J7504
Ativan	2 mg	IM, IV	J2060
Atropine			
concentrated form	per mg	INH	**J7635**
unit dose form	per mg	INH	**J7636**
sulfate	0.01 mg, per mg	IV, IM, SC	J0461, J7636
Atrovent	per mg	INH	J7644, J7645
Atryn	50 IU		J7196
Aurothioglucose	up to 50 mg	IM	**J2910**
Autologous cultured chondrocytes implant		OTH	**J7330**
Autoplex T	per IU	IV	J7198, J7199
Avastin	10 mg		J9035
Avelox	100 mg		J2280
Avonex	30 mcg	IM	J1826
	1 mcg	IM	Q3027
	1 mcg	SC	Q3028
Azacitidine	1 mg	SC	**J9025**
Azasan	50 mg		J7500

◀ **New**　⟳ **Revised**　✔ **Reinstated**　~~deleted~~ **Deleted**

DRUG NAME	DOSAGE	METHOD OF ADMINISTRATION	HCPCS CODE
Azathioprine	50 mg	ORAL	J7500
Azathioprine			
parenteral	100 mg	IV	J7501
dihydrate	1 gm	ORAL	Q0144
injection	500 mg	IV	J0456
Azithromycin	500 mg		J0456
B			
Baci-RX			J3490
Baciim			J3490
Bacitracin			J3490
Baclofen	10 mg	IT	J0475
Baclofen for intrathecal trial	50 mcg	OTH	J0476
Bacteriostatic	10 ml		A4216
Bactocill	up to 250 mg	IM, IV	J2700
BAL in oil	per 100 mg	IM	J0470
Banflex	up to 60 mg	IV, IM	J2360
Basiliximab	20 mg	IV	J0480
Bayhep B			J3590
BayRho-D	50 mcg		J2788
BCG (Bacillus Calmette and Guérin), live	per vial	IV	J9031
Bebulin VH	per IU		J7194
Beclomethasone inhalation solution, unit dose form	per mg	INH	J7622, J7624
Belatacept	1 mg	IV	J0485
Belimumab	10 mg	IV	J0490
Bena-D 10	up to 50 mg	IV, IM	J1200
Bena-D 50	up to 50 mg	IV, IM	J1200
Benadryl	up to 50 mg	IV, IM	J1200
Benahist 10	up to 50 mg	IV, IM	J1200
Benahist 50	up to 50 mg	IV, IM	J1200
Ben-Allergin-50	up to 50 mg	IV, IM	J1200
	50 mg	ORAL	Q0163
Bendamustine HCl	1 mg	IV	J9033
Benefix	per IU	IV	J7195
Benlysta	10 mg		J0490
Benoject-10	up to 50 mg	IV, IM	J1200
Benoject-50	up to 50 mg	IV, IM	J1200
Bentyl	up to 20 mg	IM	J0500
Benzocaine			J3490
Benztropine mesylate	per 1 mg	IM, IV	J0515
Berinert, see C-1 esterase inhibitor			
Berubigen	up to 1,000 mcg	IM, SC	J3420
Beta amyloid	per study dose	OTH	A9599

◄ **New**   ⊋ **Revised**   ✔ **Reinstated**   ~~deleted~~ **Deleted**

DRUG NAME	DOSAGE	METHOD OF ADMINISTRATION	HCPCS CODE
Betalin 12	up to 1,000 mcg	IM, SC	J3420
Betameth.	per 3 mg	IM, IV	J0702
Betamethasone acetate & betamethasone sodium phosphate	per 3 mg	IM	J0702
Betamethasone inhalation solution, unit dose form	per mg	INH	J7624
Betaseron	0.25 mg	SC	J1830
Bethanechol chloride	up to 5 mg	SC	J0520
Bethkis	300 mg		J7682
Bevacizumab	10 mg	IV	J9035
Bicillin C-R	100,000 units		J0558
Bicillin C-R 900/300	100,000 units	IM	J0558, J0561
Bicillin L-A	100,000 units	IM	J0561
BiCNU	100 mg	IV	J9050
Biperiden lactate	per 5 mg	IM, IV	J0190
Bitolterol mesylate			
concentrated form	per mg	INH	J7628
unit dose form	per mg	INH	J7629
Bivalirudin	1 mg	IV	J0583
Blenoxane	15 units	IM, IV, SC	J9040
Bleomycin sulfate	15 units	IM, IV, SC	J9040
Boniva	1 mg		J1740
Bortezomib	0.1 mg	IV	J9041
Botox	1 unit		J0585
Bravelle	75 IU		J3355
Brentuximab Vedotin	1 mg	IV	J9042
Brethine			
concentrated form	per 1 mg	INH	J7680
unit dose	per 1 mg	INH	J7681
	up to 1 mg	SC, IV	J3105
Brevital Sodium			J3490
Bricanyl Subcutaneous	up to 1 mg	SC, IV	J3105
Brompheniramine maleate	per 10 mg	IM, SC, IV	J0945
Broncho Saline	10 ml		A4216
Bronkephrine, see Ethylnorepinephrine HCl			
Bronkosol			
concentrated form	per mg	INH	J7647, J7648
unit dose form	per mg	INH	J7649, J7650
Brovana			J7605, J7699
Budesonide inhalation solution			
concentrated form	0.25 mg	INH	J7633, J7634
unit dose form	0.5 mg	INH	J7626, J7627
Bumetanide			J3490
Bupivacaine			J3490

◀ **New**   ↻ **Revised**   ✔ **Reinstated**   ~~deleted~~ **Deleted**

DRUG NAME	DOSAGE	METHOD OF ADMINISTRATION	HCPCS CODE	
Buprenorphine Hydrochloride	0.1 mg	IM	**J0592**	
Buprenorphine/Naloxone	1 mg	ORAL	**J0571**	◄
	<= 3 mg	ORAL	**J0572**	◄
	> 3 mg but <= 6 mg	ORAL	**J0573**	◄
	> 6 mg but <= 10 mg	ORAL	**J0574**	◄
	> 10 mg	ORAL	**J0575**	◄
Busulfan	1 mg	IV	**J0594**	
	2 mg	ORAL	**J8510**	
Butorphanol tartrate	1 mg		**J0595**	
C				
C1 Esterase Inhibitor	10 units	IV	**J0597, J0598**	
Cabazitaxel	1 mg	IV	**J9043**	
Cabergoline	0.25 mg	ORAL	**J8515**	
Cafcit	5 mg	IV	J0706	
Caffeine citrate	5 mg	IV	**J0706**	
Caine-1	10 mg	IV	J2001	
Caine-2	10 mg	IV	J2001	
Calcijex	0.1 mcg	IM	J0636	
Calcimar	up to 400 units	SC, IM	J0630	
Calcitonin-salmon	up to 400 units	SC, IM	**J0630**	
Calcitriol	0.1 mcg	IM	**J0636**	
Calcitriol in almond oil	0.1 mcg		J0636	
Calcium Disodium Versenate	up to 1,000 mg	IV, SC, IM	J0600	
Calcium folinate (Hungarian import)	per 50 mg		J0640	
Calcium gluconate	per 10 ml	IV	**J0610**	
Calcium glycerophosphate and calcium lactate	per 10 ml	IM, SC	**J0620**	
Caldolor	100 mg	IV	J1741	
Calphosan	per 10 ml	IM, SC	J0620	
Camptosar	20 mg	IV	J9206	
Canakinumab	1 mg	SC	**J0638**	
Cancidas	5 mg		J0637	
Capecitabine	150 mg	ORAL	**J8520**	
	500 mg	ORAL	**J8521**	
Capsaicin patch	per sq cm	OTH	**J7336**	↻
Carbocaine with Neo-Cobefrin	per 10 ml	VAR	J0670	
Carbocaine	per 10 ml	VAR	J0670	
Carboplatin	50 mg	IV	**J9045**	
Carfilzomib	1 mg	IV	**J9047**	
Carimune	500 mg		J1566	
Carmustine	100 mg	IV	**J9050**	
Carnitor	per 1 g	IV	J1955	

◄ **New**   ↻ **Revised**   ✔ **Reinstated**   ~~deleted~~ **Deleted**

DRUG NAME	DOSAGE	METHOD OF ADMINISTRATION	HCPCS CODE
Carticel			J7330
Caspofungin acetate	5 mg	IV	J0637
Cathflo Activase	1 mg		J2997
Caverject	per 1.25 mcg		J0270
Cayston	500 mg		S0073
Cefadyl	up to 1 g	IV, IM	J0710
Cefazolin sodium	500 mg	IV, IM	J0690
Cefepime hydrochloride	500 mg	IV	J0692
Cefizox	per 500 mg	IM, IV.	J0715
Cefotaxime sodium	per 1 g	IV, IM	J0698
Cefotetan			J3490
Cefoxitin sodium	1 g	IV, IM	J0694
Ceftazidime	per 500 mg	IM, IV	J0713
Cefteroline fosamil	1 mg		J0712
Ceftizoxime sodium	per 500 mg	IV, IM	J0715
Ceftriaxone sodium	per 250 mg	IV, IM	J0696
Cefuroxime sodium, sterile	per 750 mg	IM, IV	J0697
Celestone Soluspan	per 3 mg	IM	J0702
	per mg	ORAL	J7624
CellCept	250 mg	ORAL	J7517
Cel-U-Jec	per 4 mg	IM, IV	Q0511
Cenacort A-40	per 10 mg	IM	J3301
	per 5 mg		J3302
Cenacort Forte	per 5 mg	IM	J3302
Centruroides Immune F(ab)	up to 120 mg	IV	J0716
Cephalothin sodium	up to 1 g	IM, IV	J1890
Cephapirin sodium	up to 1 g	IV, IM	J0710
Ceprotin	10 IU		J2724
Ceredase	per 10 units	IV	J0205
Cerezyme	10 units		J1786
Certolizumab pegol	1 mg	SC	J0717
Cerubidine	10 mg	IV	J9150
Cetuximab	10 mg	IV	J9055
Chealamide	per 150 mg	IV	J3520
Chirhostim	1 mcg	IV	J2850
Chloramphenicol sodium succinate	up to 1 g	IV	J0720
Chlordiazepoxide HCl	up to 100 mg	IM, IV	J1990
Chloromycetin Sodium Succinate	up to 1 g	IV	J0720
Chloroprocaine HCl	per 30 ml	VAR	J2400
	10 mg	ORAL	Q0171
	25 mg	ORAL	Q0172
	up to 50 mg	IM, IV	J3230

◀ **New**   ↻ **Revised**   ✔ **Reinstated**   ~~deleted~~ **Deleted**

DRUG NAME	DOSAGE	METHOD OF ADMINISTRATION	HCPCS CODE
Chloroquine HCl	up to 250 mg	IM	J0390
Chlorothiazide sodium	per 500 mg	IV	J1205
Chlorpromazine	5 mg	ORAL	Q0161
Chlorpromazine HCl	up to 50 mg	IM, IV	J3230
Cholografin Meglumine	per ml		Q9961
Chorex-5	per 1,000 USP units	IM	J0725
Chorex-10	per 1,000 USP units	IM	J0725
Chorignon	per 1,000 USP units	IM	J0725
Chorionic gonadotropin	per 1,000 USP units	IM	J0725
Choron 10	per 1,000 USP units	IM	J0725
Cidofovir	375 mg	IV	J0740
Cimzia	1 mg	SC	J0717
Cinryze	10 units		J0598
Cilastatin sodium, imipenem	per 250 mg	IV, IM	J0743
Cimetidine HCl			J3490
Cipro IV	200 mg	IV	J0706
Ciprofloxacin	200 mg	IV	J0706
			J3490
Cisplatin, powder or solution	per 10 mg	IV	J9060
Cladribine	per mg	IV	J9065
Claforan	per 1 gm	IM, IV	J0698
Cleocin Phosphate			J3490
Clinacort	per 5 mg		J3302
Clofarabine	1 mg	IV	J9027
Clolar	1 mg		J9027
Clonidine Hydrochloride	1 mg	epidural	J0735
Cobex	up to 1,000 mcg	IM, SC	J3420
Cobulin-M	up to 1,000 mcg		J3420
Codeine phosphate	per 30 mg	IM, IV, SC	J0745
Codimal-A	per 10 mg	IM, SC, IV	J0945
Cogentin	per 1 mg	IM, IV	J0515
Colchicine	per 1 mg	IV	J0760
Colistimethate sodium	up to 150 mg	IM, IV	J0770, S0142
Collagenase, Clostridium Histolyticum	0.01 mg	OTH	J0775
Coly-Mycin M	up to 150 mg	IM, IV	J0770
Compa-Z	up to 10 mg	IM, IV	J0780
Compazine	up to 10 mg	IM, IV	J0780
	5 mg	ORAL	Q0164
Compro			J8498
Comptosar	20 mg		J9206
Conray	per ml		Q9961
Conray 30	per ml		Q9958

◄ **New**   ⟳ **Revised**   ✔ **Reinstated**   ~~deleted~~ **Deleted**

DRUG NAME	DOSAGE	METHOD OF ADMINISTRATION	HCPCS CODE
Conray 43	per ml		Q9960
Copaxone	20 mg		J1595
Cophene-B	per 10 mg	IM, SC, IV	J0945
Copper contraceptive, intrauterine		OTH	**J7300**
Cordarone	30 mg	IV	J0282
Corgonject-5	per 1,000 USP units	IM	J0725
Corticorelin ovine triflutate	1 mcg		**J0795**
Corticotropin	up to 40 units	IV, IM, SC	**J0800**
Cortisone Acetate			J3490
Cortrosyn	per 0.25 mg	IM, IV	J0835
Corvert	1 mg		J1742
Cosmegen	0.5 mg	IV	J9120
Cosyntropin	per 0.25 mg	IM, IV	**J0833, J0834**
Cotolone	up to 1 ml		J2650
	per 5 mg		J7510
Cotranzine	up to 10 mg	IM, IV	J0780
Crofab	up to 1 gram		J0840
Cromolyn sodium, unit dose form	per 10 mg	INH	**J7631, J7632**
Crotalidae Polyvalent Immune Fab	up to 1 gram	IV	**J0840**
Crysticillin 300 A.S.	up to 600,000 units	IM, IV	J2510
Crysticillin 600 A.S.	up to 600,000 units	IM, IV	J2510
Cubicin	1 mg		J0878
Cyanocobalamin	up to 1,000 mcg		J3420
Cyclophosphamide	100 mg	IV	**J9070**
oral	25 mg	ORAL	**J8530**
Cyclosporine	25 mg	ORAL	J7515, J7516
	100 mg	ORAL	**J7502**
parenteral	250 mg	IV	**J7516**
Cymetra	1 cc		Q4112
Cyomin	up to 1,000 mcg		J3420
Cysto-Cornray LI	per ml		Q9958
Cystografin	per ml		Q9958
Cystografin-Dilute	per ml		Q9958
Cytarabine	100 mg	SC, IV	**J9100**
Cytarabine liposome	10 mg	IT	**J9098**
CytoGam	per vial		J0850
Cytomegalovirus immune globulin intravenous (human)	per vial	IV	**J0850**
Cytosar-U	100 mg	SC, IV	J9100
Cytovene	500 mg	IV	J1570
Cytoxan	100 mg	IV	J8530, J9070
D			
D-5-W, infusion	1000 cc	IV	**J7070**

◄ New   ↵ Revised   ✔ Reinstated   ~~deleted~~ Deleted

DRUG NAME	DOSAGE	METHOD OF ADMINISTRATION	HCPCS CODE
Dacarbazine	100 mg	IV	**J9130**
Daclizumab	25 mg	IV	**J7513**
Dactinomycin	0.5 mg	IV	**J9120**
Dalalone	1 mg	IM, IV, OTH	J1100
Dalalone L.A	1 mg	IM	J1094
Dalteparin sodium	per 2500 IU	SC	**J1645**
Daptomycin	1 mg	IV	**J0878**
Darbepoetin Alfa	1 mcg	IV, SC	**J0881, J0882**
Daunorubicin citrate, liposomal formulation	10 mg	IV	**J9151**
Daunorubicin HCl	10 mg	IV	**J9150**
Daunoxome	10 mg	IV	J9151
DDAVP	1 mcg	IV, SC	J2597
Decadron Phosphate	1 mg	IM, IV, OTH	J1100
Decadron	1 mg	IM, IV, OTH	J1100
	0.25 mg		J8540
Decadron-LA	1 mg	IM	J1094
Deca-Durabolin	up to 50 mg	IM	J2320
Decaject	1 mg	IM, IV, OTH	J1100
Decaject-L.A.	1 mg	IM	J1094
Decitabine	1 mg	IV	**J0894**
Decolone-50	up to 50 mg	IM	J2320
Decolone-100	up to 50 mg	IM	J2320
De-Comberol	1 mg		J1071
Deferoxamine mesylate	500 mg	IM, SC, IV	**J0895**
Definity	per ml		J3490, Q9957
Degarelix	1 mg	SC	**J9155**
Dehist	per 10 mg	IM, SC, IV	J0945
Deladumone OB	1 mg		J3121
Deladumone	1 mg		J3121
Delatest	1 mg		J3121
Delatestadiol	1 mg		J3121
Delatestryl	1 mg		J3121
Delta-Cortef	5 mg	ORAL	J7510
Delestrogen	up to 10 mg	IM	J1380
Demadex	10 mg/ml	IV	J3265
Demerol HCl	per 100 mg	IM, IV, SC	J2175
Denileukin diftitox	300 mcg	IV	**J9160**
Denosumab	1 mg	SC	**J0897**
DepAndro 100	1 mg		J1071
DepAndro 200	1 mg		J1071
DepAndrogyn	1 mg		J1071

◄ **New**   ⟳ **Revised**   ✔ **Reinstated**   deleted **Deleted**

DRUG NAME	DOSAGE	METHOD OF ADMINISTRATION	HCPCS CODE
DepGynogen	up to 5 mg	IM	J1000
DepoCyt	10 mg		J9098
DepMedalone 40	20 mg	IM	J1020
	40 mg	IM	J1030
	80 mg	IM	J1040
DepMedalone 80	20 mg	IM	J1020
	40 mg	IM	J1030
	80 mg	IM	J1040
Depo-estradiol cypionate	up to 5 mg	IM	**J1000**
Depogen	up to 5 mg	IM	J1000
Depoject	20 mg	IM	J1020
	40 mg	IM	J1030
	80 mg	IM	J1040
Depo-Medrol	20 mg	IM	J1020
	40 mg	IM	J1030
	80 mg	IM	J1040
Depopred-40	20 mg	IM	J1020
	40 mg	IM	J1030
	80 mg	IM	J1040
Depopred-80	20 mg	IM	J1020
	40 mg	IM	J1030
	80 mg	IM	J1040
Depotest	1 mg		J1071
Depo-Provera Contraceptive	1 mg		J1050
Depo-Testadiol	1 mg		J1071
Depotestrogen	1 mg		J1071
Depo-Testosterone	1 mg		J1071
Dermagraft	per square centimeter		Q4106
Desferal Mesylate	500 mg	IM, SC, IV	J0895
Desmopressin acetate	1 mcg	IV, SC	**J2597**
Dexacen LA-8	1 mg	IM	J1094
Dexacen-4	1 mg	IM, IV, OTH	J1100
Dexamethasone			
concentrated form	per mg	INH	**J7637**
intravitreal implant	0.1 mg	OTH	**J7312**
unit form	per mg	INH	**J7638**
oral	0.25 mg	ORAL	**J8540**
	1 mg		J1100
Dexamethasone acetate	1 mg	IM	**J1094**
Dexamethasone sodium phosphate	1 mg	IM, IV, OTH	J1100, J7638
Dexasone	1 mg	IM, IV, OTH	J1100

◀ **New** ↩ **Revised** ✔ **Reinstated** ~~deleted~~ **Deleted**

DRUG NAME	DOSAGE	METHOD OF ADMINISTRATION	HCPCS CODE
Dexasone L.A.	1 mg	IM	J1094
Dexferrum	50 mg		J1750
Dexone	0.25 mg	ORAL	J8540
	1 mg	IM, IV, OTH	J1100
Dexone LA	1 mg	IM	J1094
Dexpak	0.25 mg	ORAL	J8540
Dexrazoxane hydrochloride	250 mg	IV	J1190
Dextran 40	500 ml	IV	J7100
Dextran 75	500 ml	IV	J7110
Dextrose 5%/normal saline solution	500 ml = 1 unit	IV	J7042
Dextrose/water (5%)	500 ml = 1 unit	IV	J7060
D.H.E. 45	per 1 mg		J1110
Diamox	up to 500 mg	IM, IV	J1120
Diazepam	up to 5 mg	IM, IV	J3360
Diazoxide	up to 300 mg	IV	J1730
Dibent	up to 20 mg	IM	J0500
Dicyclocot	up to 20 mg		J0500
Dicyclomine HCl	up to 20 mg	IM	J0500
Didronel	per 300 mg	IV	J1436
Diethylstilbestrol diphosphate	250 mg	IV	J9165
Diflucan	200 mg	IV	J1450
Digibind	per vial		J1162
DigiFab	per vial		J1162
Digoxin	up to 0.5 mg	IM, IV	J1160
Digoxin immune fab (ovine)	per vial		J1162
Dihydrex	up to 50 mg	IV, IM	J1200
	50 mg	ORAL	Q0163
Dihydroergotamine mesylate	per 1 mg	IM, IV	J1110
Dilantin	per 50 mg	IM, IV	J1165
Dilaudid	up to 4 mg	SC, IM, IV	J1170
	250 mg	OTH	S0092
Dilocaine	10 mg	IV	J2001
Dilomine	up to 20 mg	IM	J0500
Dilor	up to 500 mg	IM	J1180
Dimenhydrinate	up to 50 mg	IM, IV	J1240
Dimercaprol	per 100 mg	IM	J0470
Dimethyl sulfoxide	50%, 50 ml	OTH	J1212
Dinate	up to 50 mg	IM, IV	J1240
Dioval	up to 10 mg	IM	J1380
Dioval 40	up to 10 mg	IM	J1380
Dioval XX	up to 10 mg	IM	J1380

◄ **New**   ↻ **Revised**   ✔ **Reinstated**   ~~deleted~~ **Deleted**

DRUG NAME	DOSAGE	METHOD OF ADMINISTRATION	HCPCS CODE
Diphenacen-50	up to 50 mg	IV, IM	J1200
	50 mg	ORAL	Q0163
Diphenhydramine HCl			
injection	up to 50 mg	IV, IM	**J1200**
oral	50 mg	ORAL	**Q0163**
Diprivan			J3490
Dipyridamole	per 10 mg	IV	**J1245**
Disotate	per 150 mg	IV	J3520
Di-Spaz	up to 20 mg	IM	J0500
Ditate-DS	1 mg		J3121
Diruril	per 500 mg	IV	J1205
Diuril Sodium	per 500 mg	IV	J1205
D-Med 80	20 mg	IM	J1020
	40 mg	IM	J1030
	80 mg	IM	J1040
DMSO, Dimethyl sulfoxide 50%	50 ml	OTH	**J1212**
Dobutamine HCl	per 250 mg	IV	**J1250**
Dobutrex	per 250 mg	IV	J1250
Docefrez	1 mg		J9171
Docetaxel	20 mg	IV	J9171
Dolasetron mesylate			
injection	10 mg	IV	**J1260**
tablets	100 mg	ORAL	**Q0180**
Dolophine HCl	up to 10 mg	IM, SC	J1230
Dommanate	up to 50 mg	IM, IV	J1240
Donbax	10 mg		J1267
Dopamine	40 mg		**J1265**
Dopamine HCl	40 mg		**J1265**
Doribax	10 mg		J1267
Doripenem	10 mg	IV	**J1267**
Dornase alpha, unit dose form	per mg	INH	**J7639**
Dotarem	0.1 ml		A9575
Doxercalciferol	1 mcg	IV	**J1270**
Doxil	10 mg	IV	Q2048
Doxorubicin HCl	10 mg	IV	**J9000**
Dramamine	up to 50 mg	IM, IV	J1240
Dramanate	up to 50 mg	IM, IV	J1240
Dramilin	up to 50 mg	IM, IV	J1240
Dramocen	up to 50 mg	IM, IV	J1240
Dramoject	up to 50 mg	IM, IV	J1240
Dronabinol	2.5 mg	ORAL	**Q0167**
Droperidol	up to 5 mg	IM, IV	**J1790**

◄ New   ↻ Revised   ✔ Reinstated   ~~deleted~~ Deleted

2015 TABLE OF DRUGS

DRUG NAME	DOSAGE	METHOD OF ADMINISTRATION	HCPCS CODE
Droxia		ORAL	J8999
Drug administered through a metered dose inhaler		INH	**J3535**
Droperidol and fentanyl citrate	up to 2 ml ampule	IM, IV	**J1810**
DTIC-Dome	100 mg	IV	J9130
Dua-Gen L.A.	1 mg		J3121
DuoNeb	up to 2.5 mg		J7620
	up to 0.5 mg		J7620
Duoval P.A.	1 mg		J3121
Durabolin	up to 50 mg	IM	J2320
Duraclon	1 mg	epidural	J0735
Dura-Estrin	up to 5 mg	IM	J1000
Duracillin A.S.	up to 600,000 units	IM, IV	J2510
Duragen-10	up to 10 mg	IM	J1380
Duragen-20	up to 10 mg	IM	J1380
Duragen-40	up to 10 mg	IM	J1380
Duralone-40	20 mg	IM	J1020
	40 mg	IM	J1030
	80 mg	IM	J1040
Duralone-80	20 mg	IM	J1020
	40 mg	IM	J1030
	80 mg	IM	J1040
Duralutin, see Hydroxyprogesterone Caproate			
Duramorph	up to 10 mg	IM, IV, SC	J2270
Duratest-100	1 mg		J1071
Duratest-200	1 mg		J1071
Duratestrin	1 mg		J1071
Durathate-200	1 mg		J3121
Dymenate	up to 50 mg	IM, IV	J1240
Dyphylline	up to 500 mg	IM	**J1180**
Dysport	5 units		J0586
E			
Ecallantide	1 mg	SC	**J1290**
Eculizumab	10 mg	IV	**J1300**
Edetate calcium disodium	up to 1,000 mg	IV, SC, IM	**J0600**
Edetate disodium	per 150 mg	IV	**J3520**
Elaprase	1 mg		J1743
Elavil	up to 20 mg	IM	J1320
Elelyso	10 units		J3060
Eligard	7.5 mg		J9217
Elitek	0.5 mg		J2783
Ellence	2 mg		J9178
Elliotts B solution	1 ml	OTH	**J9175**

◄ **New**   ↻ **Revised**   ✔ **Reinstated**   ~~deleted~~ **Deleted**

DRUG NAME	DOSAGE	METHOD OF ADMINISTRATION	HCPCS CODE
Elosulfase alfa	1 mg	IV	**J1322** ◄
Eloxatin	0.5 mg		J9263
Elspar	10,000 units	IV, IM	J9020
Emend	1 mg		J1453
Ememd	5 mg	ORAL	J8501
Emete-Con, see Benzquinamide			
Eminase	30 units	IV	J0350
Enbrel	25 mg	IM, IV	J1438
Endrate ethylenediamine-tetra-acetic acid	per 150 mg	IV	J3520
Enfuvirtide	1 mg	SC	**J1324**
Enovil	up to 20 mg	IM	J1320
Enoxaparin sodium	10 mg	SC	**J1650**
Eovist	1 ml		A9581
Epinephrine, adrenalin	0.1 mg	SC, IM	**J0171**
Epirubicin hydrochloride	2 mg		J9178, J7799
Epoetin alfa	1,000 units	IV, SC	J0885, J0886, Q4081
Epoetin beta, ESRD use	1 mcg	IV	**J0887** ◄
Epoetin beta, non-ESRD use	1 mcg	IV	**J0888** ◄
Epogen	1,000 units		J0885
			J0886
			Q4081
Epoprostenol	0.5 mg	IV	**J1325**
Eptifibatide, injection	5 mg	IM, IV	**J1327**
Eraxis	1 mg	IV	J0348
Erbitux	10 mg		J9055
Ergonovine maleate	up to 0.2 mg	IM, IV	**J1330**
Eribulin mesylate	0.1 mg	IV	**J9179**
Ertapenem sodium	500 mg	IM, IV	**J1335**
Erwinase	1,000 units	IV, IM	J9019
	10,000 units	IV, IM	J9020
Erythromycin lactobionate	500 mg	IV	**J1364**
Estra-D	up to 5 mg	IM	J1000
Estra-L 20	up to 10 mg	IM	J1380
Estra-L 40	up to 10 mg	IM	J1380
Estra-Testrin	1 mg		J3121
Estradiol Cypionate	up to 5 mg	IM	J1000
Estradiol			
L.A.	up to 10 mg	IM	J1380
L.A. 20	up to 10 mg	IM	J1380
L.A. 40	up to 10 mg	IM	J1380
Estradiol valerate	up to 10 mg	IM	**J1380**

◄ New   ↻ Revised   ✔ Reinstated   ~~deleted~~ Deleted

DRUG NAME	DOSAGE	METHOD OF ADMINISTRATION	HCPCS CODE
Estragyn 5	per 1 mg		J1435
Estro-Cyp	up to 5 mg	IM	J1000
Estrogen, conjugated	per 25 mg	IV, IM	**J1410**
Estroject L.A.	up to 5 mg	IM	J1000
Estrone	per 1 mg	IM	**J1435**
Estrone 5	per 1 mg	IM	J1435
Estrone Aqueous	per 1 mg	IM	J1435
Estronol	per 1 mg	IM	J1435
Estronol-L.A.	up to 5 mg	IM	J1000
Etanercept, injection	25 mg	IM, IV	**J1438**
Ethamolin	100 mg		J1430
Ethanolamine	100 mg		J1430, J3490
Ethyol	500 mg	IV	J0207
Etidronate disodium	per 300 mg	IV	**J1436**
Etonogestrel implant			**J7307**
Etopophos	10 mg	IV	J9181
Etoposide	10 mg	IV	**J9181**
oral	50 mg	ORAL	**J8560**
Euflexxa	per dose	OTH	**J7323**
Everolimus	0.25 mg	ORAL	**J7527**
Everone	1 mg		J3121
Eylea	1 mg		J0178
Eylen	1 mg	OTH	J0178
F			
Fabrazyme	1 mg	IV	J0180
Factor VIIa (coagulation factor, recombinant)	1 mcg	IV	**J7189**
Factor VIII (anti-hemophilic factor)			
human	per IU	IV	**J7190**
porcine	per IU	IV	**J7191**
recombinant	per IU	IV	**J7182, J7185, J7192**
Factor IX			
anti-hemophilic factor, purified, non-recombinant	per IU	IV	**J7193**
anti-hemophilic factor, recombinant	per IU	IV	**J7195, J7200– J7201**
complex	per IU	IV	**J7194**
Factor XIII A-subunit (recombinant)	per IU	IV	**J7181**
Factors, other hemophilia clotting	per IU	IV	**J7196**
Factrel	per 100 mcg	SC, IV	J1620
Famotidine			J3490
Faslodex	25 mg		J9395
Feiba VH Immuno	per IU	IV	J7196

◄ **New**   ↵ **Revised**   ✔ **Reinstated**   ~~deleted~~ **Deleted**

DRUG NAME	DOSAGE	METHOD OF ADMINISTRATION	HCPCS CODE
Fentanyl citrate	0.1 mg	IM, IV	J3010
Feraheme	1 mg		Q0138, Q0139
Ferric carboxymaltose	1 mg	IV	J1439
Ferrlecit	12.5 mg		J2916
Ferumoxytol	1 mg		Q0138, Q0139
Filgrastim			
(G-CSF)	1 mcg	SC, IV	J1442
(TBO)	5 mcg	SC, IV	J1446
Firazyr	1 mg	SC	J1744
Firmagon	1 mg		J9155
Flebogamma	500 mg	IV	J1572
	1 cc		J1460
Flexoject	up to 60 mg	IV, IM	J2360
Flexon	up to 60 mg	IV, IM	J2360
Flolan	0.5 mg	IV	J1325
Flo-Pred	5 mg		J7510
Floxuridine	500 mg	IV	J9200
Fluconazole	200 mg	IV	J1450
Fludara	1 mg	ORAL	J8562
	50 mg	IV	J9185
Fludarabine phosphate	50 mg	IV	J9185
Flunisolide inhalation solution, unit dose form	per mg	INH	J7641
Fluocinolone		OTH	J7311
Fluorouracil	500 mg	IV	J9190
Fluphenazine decanoate	up to 25 mg		J2680
Flutamide			J8999
Folex	5 mg	IA, IM, IT, IV	J9250
	50 mg	IA, IM, IT, IV	J9260
Folex PFS	5 mg	IA, IM, IT, IV	J9250
	50 mg	IA, IM, IT, IV	J9260
Follutein	per 1,000 USP units	IM	J0725
Folotyn	1 mg		J9307
Fomepizole	15 mg		J1451
Fomivirsen sodium	1.65 mg	Intraocular	J1452
Fondaparinux sodium	0.5 mg	SC	J1652
Formoterol	12 mcg	INH	J7640
Formoterol fumarate	20 mcg	INH	J7606
	12 mcg		J7640
Fortaz	per 500 mg	IM, IV	J0713
Forteo	10 mcg		J3110
Fosaprepitant	1 mg	IV	J1453
Foscarnet sodium	per 1,000 mg	IV	J1455

◄ **New**   ↻ **Revised**   ✔ **Reinstated**   deleted **Deleted**

DRUG NAME	DOSAGE	METHOD OF ADMINISTRATION	HCPCS CODE
Foscavir	per 1,000 mg	IV	J1455
Fosphenytoin	50 mg	IV	Q2009
Fragmin	per 2,500 IU		J1645
FUDR	500 mg	IV	J9200
Fulvestrant	25 mg	IM	J9395
Fungizone intravenous	50 mg	IV	J0285
Furomide M.D.	up to 20 mg	IM, IV	J1940
Furosemide	up to 20 mg	IM, IV	J1940
Fuzeon	1 mg		J1324
G			
Gablofen	10 mg		J0475
	50 mcg		J0476
Gadavist	0.1 ml		A9585
Gadoxetate disodium	1 ml	IV	A9581
Gallium nitrate	1 mg	IV	J1457
Galsulfase	1 mg	IV	J1458
Gamastan	1 cc	IM	J1460
	over 10 cc	IM	J1560
Gammagard Liquid	500 mg	IV	J1569
Gammagard S/D			J1566
Gamma globulin	1 cc	IM	J1460
	over 10 cc	IM	J1560
Gammaplex	500 mg	IV	J1557
GammaGraft	per square centimeter		Q4111
Gammar	1 cc	IM	J1460
	over 10 cc	IM	J1560
Gammar-IV, see Immune globin intravenous (human)			
Gamulin RH			
immune globulin, human	100 IU		J2791
	1 dose package, 300 mcg	IM	J2790
immune globulin, human, solvent detergent	100 IU	IV	J2792
Gamunex	500 mg	IV	J1561
Ganciclovir, implant	4.5 mg	OTH	J7310
Ganciclovir sodium	500 mg	IV	J1570
Ganirelix			J3490
Garamycin, gentamicin	up to 80 mg	IM, IV	J1580
Gastrografin	per ml		Q9963
Gatifloxacin	10 mg	IV	J1590
Gefitinib	250 mg	ORAL	J8565
Gel-One	per dose	OTH	J7326
Gemcitabine HCl	200 mg	IV	J9201

◄ **New**   ↻ **Revised**   ✔ **Reinstated**   ~~deleted~~ **Deleted**

DRUG NAME	DOSAGE	METHOD OF ADMINISTRATION	HCPCS CODE
Gemsar	200 mg	IV	J9201
Gemtuzumab ozogamicin	5 mg	IV	**J9300**
Gengraf	100 mg		J7502
	25 mg	ORAL	J7515
	250 mg		J7516
Gentamicin Sulfate	up to 80 mg	IM, IV	J1580, J7699
Gentran	500 ml	IV	J7100
Gentran 75	500 ml	IV	J7110
Gentropin	1 mg		J2941
Geodon	10 mg		J3486
Gesterol 50	per 50 mg		J2675
Glassia	10 mg	IV	**J0257**
Glatiramer Acetate	20 mg	SC	**J1595**
GlucaGen	per 1 mg		J1610
Glucagon HCl	per 1 mg	SC, IM, IV	**J1610**
Glukor	per 1,000 USP units	IM	J0725
Glycopyrrolate			
concentrated form	per 1 mg	INH	**J7642**
unit dose form	per 1 mg	INH	**J7643**
Gold sodium thiomalate	up to 50 mg	IM	**J1600**
Golimumab	1 mg	IV	**J1602**
Gonadorelin HCl	per 100 mcg	SC, IV	**J1620**
Gonal-F			J3490
Gonic	per 1,000 USP units	IM	J0725
Goserelin acetate implant	per 3.6 mg	SC	**J9202**
Graftjacket	per square centimeter		Q4107
Graftjacket express	1 cc		Q4113
Granisetron HCl			
injection	100 mcg	IV	**J1626**
oral	1 mg	ORAL	**Q0166**
Granix	5 mcg		J1446
Gynogen L.A. A10	up to 10 mg	IM	J1380
Gynogen L.A. A20	up to 10 mg	IM	J1380
Gynogen L.A. A40	up to 10 mg	IM	J1380
H			
Halaven	0.1 mg		J9179
Haldol	up to 5 mg	IM, IV	J1630
Haloperidol	up to 5 mg	IM, IV	**J1630**
Haloperidol decanoate	per 50 mg	IM	**J1631**
Haloperidol Lactate	up to 5 mg		J1630
Hectoral	1 mcg	IV	J1270
Helixate FS	per IU		J7192

◄ New   ⟳ Revised   ✔ Reinstated   ~~deleted~~ Deleted

DRUG NAME	DOSAGE	METHOD OF ADMINISTRATION	HCPCS CODE
Hemin	1 mg		**J1640**
Hemofil M	per IU	IV	J7190
Hemophilia clotting factors (e.g., anti-inhibitors)	per IU	IV	**J7198**
NOC	per IU	IV	**J7199**
Hepagam B	0.5 ml	IM	**J1571**
	0.5 ml	IV	**J1573**
Hep-Lock	10 units	IV	J1642
Hep-Lock U/P	10 units	IV	J1642
Heparin (Procine)	per 1,000 units		J1644
Heparin (Procine) Lock Flush	per 10 units		J1642
Heparin sodium	1,000 units	IV, SC	**J1644**
Heparin Sodium (Bovine)	per 1,000 units		J1644
Heparin Sodium Flush	per 10 units		J1642
Heparin sodium (heparin lock flush)	10 units	IV	**J1642**
Heparin Sodium (Procine)	per 1,000 units		J1644
Herceptin	10 mg	IV	J9355
Hexabrix 320	per ml		Q9967
Hexadrol Phosphate	1 mg	IM, IV, OTH	J1100
Histaject	per 10 mg	IM, SC, IV	J0945
Histerone 50	up to 50 mg	IM	J3140
Histerone 100	up to 50 mg	IM	J3140
Histrelin			
acetate	10 mcg		**J1675**
implant	50 mg	OTH	J9225, J9226
Hizentra, see Immune globulin			
Humalog	per 5 units		J1815
	per 50 units		J1817
Human fibrinogen concentrate	100 mg	IV	**J7178**
Humate-P	per IU		J7187
Humatrope	1 mg		J2941
Humira	20 mg		J0135
Humulin	per 5 units		J1815
	per 50 units		J1817
Hyalgan		OTH	**J7321**
Hyaluronan or derivative	per dose	IV	**J7327**
Hyaluronic Acid			J3490
Hyaluronidase	up to 150 units	SC, IV	**J3470**
Hyaluronidase			
ovine	up to 999 units	VAR	**J3471**
ovine	per 1000 units	VAR	**J3472**
recombinant	1 usp	SC	**J3473**
Hyate:C	per IU	IV	J7191

◄ **New**   ↻ **Revised**   ✔ **Reinstated**   ~~deleted~~ **Deleted**

DRUG NAME	DOSAGE	METHOD OF ADMINISTRATION	HCPCS CODE
Hybolin Improved, see Nandrolone phenpropionate			
Hybolin Decanoate	up to 50 mg	IM	J2320
Hycamtin	0.25 mg	ORAL	J8705
	4 mg	IV	J9351
Hydralazine HCl	up to 20 mg	IV, IM	J0360
Hydrate	up to 50 mg	IM, IV	J1240
Hydrea			J8999
Hydrocortisone acetate	up to 25 mg	IV, IM, SC	J1700
Hydrocortisone sodium phosphate	up to 50 mg	IV, IM, SC	J1710
Hydrocortisone succinate sodium	up to 100 mg	IV, IM, SC	J1720
Hydrocortone Acetate	up to 25 mg	IV, IM, SC	J1700
Hydrocortone Phosphate	up to 50 mg	IM, IV, SC	J1710
Hydromorphone HCl	up to 4 mg	SC, IM, IV	J1170
Hydroxocobalamin	up to 1,000 mcg		J3420
Hydroxyprogesterone Caproate	1 mg	IM	J1725
Hydroxyurea			J8999
Hydroxyzine HCl	up to 25 mg	IM	J3410
Hydroxyzine Pamoate	25 mg	ORAL	Q0177
Hylan G-F 20		OTH	J7325
Hyoscyamine sulfate	up to 0.25 mg	SC, IM, IV	J1980
Hyperhep B			J3590
Hyperrho S/D	300 mcg		J2790
	100 IU		J2792
Hyperstat IV	up to 300 mg	IV	J1730
Hyper-Tet	up to 250 units	IM	J1670
HypRho-D	300 mcg	IM	J2790
			J2791
	50 mcg		J2788
Hyrexin-50	up to 50 mg	IV, IM	J1200
Hyzine-50	up to 25 mg	IM	J3410
I			
Ibandronate sodium	1 mg	IV	J1740
Ibuprofen	100 mg	IV	J1741
Ibutilide fumarate	1 mg	IV	J1742
Icatibant	1 mg	SC	J1744
Idamycin	5 mg	IV	J9211
Idarubicin HCl	5 mg	IV	J9211
Idursulfase	1 mg	IV	J1743
Ifex	1 g	IV	J9208
Ifosfamide	1 g	IV	J9208
Ifosfumide/mesna			J9999
Ilaris	1 mg		J0638

◄ New   ⊃ Revised   ✔ Reinstated   ~~deleted~~ Deleted

DRUG NAME	DOSAGE	METHOD OF ADMINISTRATION	HCPCS CODE
Iloprost	20 mcg	INH	Q4074
Ilotycin, see Erythromycin gluceptate			
Imferon	50 mg		J1750, J1752
Imiglucerase	10 units	IV	J1786
Imitrex	6 mg	SC	J3030
Immune globulin			
Bivigam	500 mg	IV	J1556
Flebogamma	500 mg	IV	J1572
Gammagard Liquid	500 mg	IV	J1569
Gammaplex	500 mg	IV	J1557
Gamunex	500 mg	IV	J1561
HepaGam B	0.5 ml	IM	J1571
	0.5 ml	IV	J1573
Hizentra	100 mg	SC	J1559
NOS	500 mg	IV	J1566, J1599
Octagam	500 mg	IV	J1568
Privigen	500 mg	IV	J1459
Rhophylac	100 IU	IM	J2791
Subcutaneous	100 mg	SC	J1562
Immunosuppressive drug, not otherwise classified			J7599
Imuran	50 mg	ORAL	J7500
	100 mg		J7501
Inapsine	up to 5 mg	IM, IV	J1790
Incobotulinumtoxin type A	1 unit	IM	J0588
Increlex	1 mg		J2170
Inderal	up to 1 mg	IV	J1800
Infed	50 mg		J1750
Infergen	1 mcg	SC	J9212
Infliximab, injection	10 mg	IM, IV	J1745
Innohep	1,000 iu	SC	J1655
Innovar	up to 2 ml ampule	IM, IV	J1810
Insulin	5 units	SC	J1815
Insulin-Humalog	per 50 units		J1817
Insulin lispro	50 units	SC	J1817
Intal	per 10 mg	INH	J7631, J7632
Integrilin	5 mg	IM, IV	J1327
Integra			
Bilayer Matrix Wound Dressing (BMWD)	per square centimeter		Q4104
Dermal Regeneration Template (DRT)	per square centimeter		Q4105
Flowable Wound Matrix	1 cc		Q4114
Matrix	per square centimeter		Q4108
Interferon alphacon-1, recombinant	1 mcg	SC	J9212

◀ **New**   ↬ **Revised**   ✔ **Reinstated**   ~~deleted~~ **Deleted**

DRUG NAME	DOSAGE	METHOD OF ADMINISTRATION	HCPCS CODE
Interferon alfa-2a, recombinant	3 million units	SC, IM	J9213
Interferon alfa-2b, recombinant	1 million units	SC, IM	J9214
Interferon alfa-n3 (human leukocyte derived)	250,000 IU	IM	J9215
Interferon beta-1a	30 mcg	IM	J1826
	1 mcg	IM	Q3027
	1 mcg	SC	Q3028
Interferon beta-1b	0.25 mg	SC	J1830
Interferon gamma-1b	3 million units	SC	J9216
Intrauterine copper contraceptive		OTH	J7300
Intron-A	1 million units		J9214
Invanz	500 mg		J1335
Invega Sustenna	1 mg		J2426
Ipilimumab	1 mg	IV	J9228
Ipratropium bromide, unit dose form	per mg	INH	J7620, J7644, J7645, J3535
Iressa	250 mg	ORAL	J8565
Irinotecan	20 mg	IV	J9206
Iron dextran	50 mg	IV, IM	J1750
Iron sucrose	1 mg	IV	J1756
Irrigation solution for Tx of bladder calculi	per 50 ml	OTH	Q2004
Isocaine HCl	per 10 ml	VAR	J0670
Isoetharine HCl			
concentrated form	per mg	INH	J7647, J7648
unit dose form	per mg	INH	J7649, J7650
Isoproterenol HCl			
concentrated form	per mg	INH	J7657, J7658
unit dose form	per mg	INH	J7659, J7660
Isovue-200	per ml		Q9966, Q9967
Istodax	1 mg		J9315
Isuprel			
concentrated form	per mg	INH	J7657, J7658
unit dose form	per mg	INH	J7659, J7660
Itraconazole	50 mg	IV	J1835
Ixabepilone	1 mg	IV	J9207
Ixempra	1 mg		J9207
J			
Jenamicin	up to 80 mg	IM, IV	J1580
Jetrea	0.125 mg		J7316
Jevtana	1 mg		J9043
K			
Kabikinase	per 250,000 IU	IV	J2995
Kadcyla	1 mg		J9354

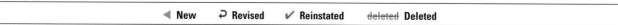

◄ **New**   ⟳ **Revised**   ✔ **Reinstated**   ~~deleted~~ **Deleted**

DRUG NAME	DOSAGE	METHOD OF ADMINISTRATION	HCPCS CODE
Kalbitor	1 mg		J1290
Kaleinate	per 10 ml	IV	J0610
Kanamycin sulfate	up to 75 mg	IM, IV	**J1850**
	up to 500 mg	IM, IV	**J1840**
Kantrex	up to 75 mg	IM, IV	J1850
	up to 500 mg	IM, IV	J1840
Kay-Pred	up to 1 ml		J2650
Keflin	up to 1 g	IM, IV	J1890
Kefurox	per 750 mg		J0697
Kefzol	500 mg	IV, IM	J0690
Kenaject-40	per 10 mg	IM	J3301
	1 mg		J3300
Kenalog-10	per 10 mg	IM	J3301
	1 mg		J3300
Kenalog-40	per 10 mg	IM	J3301
	1 mg		J3300
Kepivance	50 mcg		J2425
Keppra	10 mg		J1953
Kestrone 5	per 1 mg	IM	J1435
Ketorolac tromethamine	per 15 mg	IM, IV	**J1885**
Key-Pred 25	up to 1 ml	IM	J2650
Key-Pred 50	up to 1 ml	IM	J2650
Key-Pred-SP, see Prednisolone sodium phosphate			
K-Flex	up to 60 mg	IV, IM	J2360
Klebcil	up to 75 mg	IM, IV	J1850
	up to 500 mg	IM, IV	J1840
Koate-HP (anti-hemophilic factor)			
human	per IU	IV	J7190
porcine	per IU	IV	J7191
recombinant	per IU	IV	J7192
Kogenate			
human	per IU	IV	J7190
porcine	per IU	IV	J7191
recombinant	per IU	IV	J7192
Konakion	per 1 mg	IM, SC, IV	J3430
Konyne-80	per IU	IV	J7194, J7195
Krystexxa	1 mg		J2507
Kyprolis	1 mg		J9047
Kytril	1 mg	ORAL	Q0166
	1 mg	IV	S0091
	100 mcg	IV	J1626

◀ **New**   ↻ **Revised**   ✔ **Reinstated**   ~~deleted~~ **Deleted**

DRUG NAME	DOSAGE	METHOD OF ADMINISTRATION	HCPCS CODE
L			
Lactated Ringers	up to 1,000 cc		J7120
L.A.E. 20	up to 10 mg	IM	J1380
Laetrile, Amygdalin, vitamin B-17			**J3570**
Lanoxin	up to 0.5 mg	IM, IV	J1160
Lanreotide	1 mg	SC	**J1930**
Lantus	per 5 units		J1815
Largon, see Propiomazine HCl			
Laronidase	0.1 mg	IV	**J1931**
Lasix	up to 20 mg	IM, IV	J1940
L-Caine	10 mg	IV	J2001
L-Carnitine	per 1 gm		J1955
Lepirudin	50 mg		**J1945**
Leucovorin calcium	per 50 mg	IM, IV	**J0640**
Leukeran			J8999
Leukine	50 mcg	IV	J2820
Leuprolide acetate (for depot suspension)	per 3.75 mg	IM	**J1950**
	7.5 mg	IM	**J9217**
Leuprolide acetate	per 1 mg	IM	**J9218**
Leuprolide acetate implant	65 mg	OTH	**J9219**
Leustatin	per mg	IV	J9065
Levalbuterol HCl			
concentrated form	0.5 mg	INH	**J7607, J7612**
unit dose form	0.5 mg	INH	**J7614, J7615**
Levaquin I.U.	250 mg	IV	J1956
Levetiracetam	10 mg	IV	**J1953**
Levocarnitine	per 1 gm	IV	**J1955**
Levo-Dromoran	up to 2 mg	SC, IV	J1960
Levofloxacin	250 mg	IV	**J1956**
Levoleucovorin calcium	0.5 mg	IV	**J0641**
Levonorgestrel implant		OTH	**J7306**
Levonorgestrel-releasing intrauterine contraceptive system	52 mg	OTH	**J7302**
Levorphanol tartrate	up to 2 mg	SC, IV	**J1960**
Levsin	up to 0.25 mg	SC, IM, IV	J1980
Levulan Kerastick	unit dose (354 mg)	OTH	J7308
Lexiscan	0.1 mg		J2785
Librium	up to 100 mg	IM, IV	J1990
Lidocaine HCl	10 mg	IV	**J2001**
Lidoject-1	10 mg	IV	J2001
Lidoject-2	10 mg	IV	J2001
Lincocin	up to 300 mg	IV	J2010

◀ New   ↻ Revised   ✔ Reinstated   ~~deleted~~ Deleted

DRUG NAME	DOSAGE	METHOD OF ADMINISTRATION	HCPCS CODE
Lincomycin HCl	up to 300 mg	IV	J2010
Linezolid	200 mg	IV	J2020
Lipodox			Q2049
Liquaemin Sodium	1,000 units	IV, SC	J1644
Lioresal	10 mg	IT	J0475
			J0476
LMD (10%)	500 ml	IV	J7100
Lovenox	10 mg	SC	J1650
Lorazepam	2 mg	IM, IV	J2060
Lucentis	0.1 mg		J2778
Lufyllin	up to 500 mg	IM	J1180
Luminal Sodium	up to 120 mg	IM, IV	J2560
Lumizyme	10 mg		J0220, J0221
Lupon Depot	7.5 mg		J9217
	3.75 mg		J1950
Lupron	per 1 mg	IM	J9218
	per 3.75 mg	IM	J1950
	7.5 mg	IM	J9217
Lymphocyte immune globulin			
anti-thymocyte globulin, equine	250 mg	IV	J7504
anti-thymocyte globulin, rabbit	25 mg	IV	J7511
Lyophilized			J1566
M			
Macugen	0.3 mg		J2503
Magnesium sulfate	500 mg		J3475
Magnevist	per ml		A9579
Makena	1 mg		J1725
Malulane			J8999
Mannitol	25% in 50 ml	IV	J2150
	5 mg	INH	J7665, J7799
Marcaine			J3490
Marinol	2.5 mg	ORAL	Q0167
Marmine	up to 50 mg	IM, IV	J1240
Maxipime	500 mg	IV	J0692
MD-76R	per ml		Q9963
MD Gastroview	per ml		Q9963
Mecasermin	1 mg	SC	J2170
Mechlorethamine HCl (nitrogen mustard), HN2	10 mg	IV	J9230
Medralone 40	20 mg	IM	J1020
	40 mg	IM	J1030
	80 mg	IM	J1040

◀ **New** ↻ **Revised** ✓ **Reinstated** ~~deleted~~ **Deleted**

DRUG NAME	DOSAGE	METHOD OF ADMINISTRATION	HCPCS CODE
Medralone 80	20 mg	IM	J1020
	40 mg	IM	J1030
	80 mg	IM	J1040
Medrol	per 4 mg	ORAL	J7509
Medroxyprogesterone acetate	1 mg	IM	J1050
Mefoxin	1 g	IV, IM	J0694
Megace			J8999
Megestrol Acetate			J8999
Melphalan HCl	50 mg	IV	J9245
Melphalan, oral	2 mg	ORAL	J8600
Menoject LA	1 mg		J1071
Mepergan Injection	up to 50 mg	IM, IV	J2180
Meperidine HCl	per 100 mg	IM, IV, SC	J2175
Meperidine and promethazine HCl	up to 50 mg	IM, IV	J2180
Mepivacaine HCl	per 10 ml	VAR	J0670
Mercaptopurine			J8999
Meropenem	100 mg	IV	J2185
Merrem	100 mg		J2185
Mesna	200 mg	IV	J9209
Mesnex	200 mg	IV	J9209
Metaprel			
concentrated form	per 10 mg	INH	J7667, J7668
unit dose form	per 10 mg	INH	J7669, J7670
Metaproterenol sulfate			
concentrated form	per 10 mg	INH	J7667, J7668
unit dose form	per 10 mg	INH	J7669, J7670
Metaraminol bitartrate	per 10 mg	IV, IM, SC	J0380
Metastron	per millicurie		A9600
Methacholine chloride	1 mg	INH	J7674
Methadone HCl	up to 10 mg	IM, SC	J1230
Methergine	up to 0.2 mg		J2210
Methocarbamol	up to 10 ml	IV, IM	J2800
Methotrexate, oral	2.5 mg	ORAL	J8610
Methotrexate sodium	5 mg	IV, IM, IT, IA	J9250
	50 mg	IV, IM, IT, IA	J9260
Methotrexate LPF	5 mg	IV, IM, IT, IA	J9250
	50 mg	IV, IM, IT, IA	J9260
Methyldopate HCl	up to 250 mg	IV	J0210
Methylergonovine maleate	up to 0.2 mg		J2210
Methylnaltrexone	0.1 mg	SC	J2212

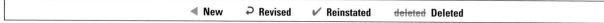

◀ **New**   ↻ **Revised**   ✔ **Reinstated**   ~~deleted~~ **Deleted**

DRUG NAME	DOSAGE	METHOD OF ADMINISTRATION	HCPCS CODE
Methylpred	20 mg		J1020
Methylpred DP	per 4 mg		J7509
Methylprednisolone, oral	per 4 mg	ORAL	J7509
Methylprednisolone acetate	20 mg	IM	J1020
	40 mg	IM	J1030
	80 mg	IM	J1040
Methylprednisolone sodium succinate	up to 40 mg	IM, IV	J2920
	up to 125 mg	IM, IV	J2930
Metoclopramide HCl	up to 10 mg	IV	J2765
Metrodin	75 IU		J3355
Metronidazole			J3490
Metvixia	1 g	OTH	J7309
Miacalcin	up to 400 units	SC, IM	J0630
Micafungin sodium	1 mg		J2248
MicRhoGAM	50 mcg		J2788
Midazolam HCl	per 1 mg	IM, IV	J2250
Milrinone lactate	5 mg	IV	J2260
Minocine	1 mg		J2265
Minocycline Hydrochloride	1 mg	IV	J2265
Mio-Rel	up to 60 mg		J2360
Mirena	52 mg	OTH	J7302
Mithracin	2,500 mcg	IV	J9270
Mitomycin	0.2 mg	Ophthalmic	J7315
	5 mg	IV	J9280
Mitosol	0.2 mg	Ophthalmic	J7315
	5 mg	IV	J9280
Mitoxantrone HCl	per 5 mg	IV	J9293
Monocid, see Cefonicic sodium			
Monoclate-P			
human	per IU	IV	J7190
porcine	per IU	IV	J7191
Monoclonal antibodies, parenteral	5 mg	IV	J7505
Monoject Prefill Advanced	10 ml		A4216
Mononine	per IU	IV	J7193
Morphine sulfate	up to 10 mg	IM, IV, SC	J2270
	~~100 mg~~	~~IM, IV, SC~~	~~J2271~~ ✗
preservative-free	10 mg	SC, IM, IV	J2274 ↻
Moxifloxacin	100 mg	IV	J2280
Mozobil	1 mg		J2562

◄ **New**   ↻ **Revised**   ✔ **Reinstated**   ~~deleted~~ **Deleted**

DRUG NAME	DOSAGE	METHOD OF ADMINISTRATION	HCPCS CODE
M-Prednisol-40	20 mg	IM	J1020
	40 mg	IM	J1030
	80 mg	IM	J1040
M-Prednisol-80	20 mg	IM	J1020
	40 mg	IM	J1030
	80 mg	IM	J1040
Mucomyst			
unit dose form	per gram	INH	J7604, J7608
Mucosol			
injection	100 mg		J0132
unit dose	per gram	INH	J7604, J7608
MultiHance	per ml		A9577
MultiHance Multipack	per ml		Aph78
Muromonab-CD3	5 mg	IV	**J7505**
Muse		OTH	J0275
	1.25 mcg	OTH	J0270
Mustargen	10 mg	IV	J9230
Mutamycin	5 mg	IV	J9280
Mycamine	1 mg		J2248
Mycophenolic acid	180 mg	ORAL	**J7518**
Mycophenolate Mofetil	250 mg	ORAL	**J7517**
Myfortic	180 mg		J7518
Myleran	1 mg		J0594
	2 mg	ORAL	J8510
Mylotarg	5 mg	IV	J9300
Myobloc	per 100 units	IM	J0587
Myochrysine	up to 50 mg	IM	J1600
Myolin	up to 60 mg	IV, IM	J2360
Myozyme	10 mg		J0221
N			
Nabi-HB			J3590
Nabilone	1 mg	ORAL	**J8650**
Nafcillin			J3490
Naglazyme	1 mg		J1458
Nalbuphine HCl	per 10 mg	IM, IV, SC	**J2300**
Nalojix	1 mg		J0485
Naloxone HCl	per 1 mg	IM, IV, SC	J2310, J3490
Naltrexone			J3490
Naltrexone, depot form	1 mg	IM	**J2315**
Nandrobolic L.A.	up to 50 mg	IM	J2320
Nandrolone decanoate	up to 50 mg	IM	**J2320**

◀ **New**   ⊃ **Revised**   ✔ **Reinstated**   deleted **Deleted**

DRUG NAME	DOSAGE	METHOD OF ADMINISTRATION	HCPCS CODE
Narcan	1 mg	IM, IV, SC	J2310
Naropin	1 mg		J2795
Nasahist B	per 10 mg	IM, SC, IV	J0945
Nasal vaccine inhalation		INH	**J3530**
Natalizumab	1 mg	IV	**J2323**
Natrecor	0.1 mg		J2325
Navane, see Thiothixene			
Navelbine	per 10 mg	IV	J9390
ND Stat	per 10 mg	IM, SC, IV	J0945
Nebcin	up to 80 mg	IM, IV	J3260
	per 300 mg		J7682
NebuPent	per 300 mg	INH	J2545, J7676
Nelarabine	50 mg	IV	**J9261**
Nembutal Sodium Solution	per 50 mg	IM, IV, OTH	J2515
Neocyten	up to 60 mg	IV, IM	J2360
Neo-Durabolic	up to 50 mg	IM	J2320
Neoral	100 mg		J7502
	25 mg		J7515
Neoquess	up to 20 mg	IM	J0500
Neosar	100 mg	IV	J9070
Neostigmine methylsulfate	up to 0.5 mg	IM, IV, SC	**J2710**
Neo-Synephrine	up to 1 ml	SC, IM, IV	J2370
Nervocaine 1%	10 mg	IV	J2001
Nervocaine 2%	10 mg	IV	J2001
Nesacaine	per 30 ml	VAR	J2400
Nesacaine-MPF	per 30 ml	VAR	J2400
Nesiritide	0.1 mg	IV	**J2325**
Neulasta	6 mg		J2505
Neumega	5 mg	SC	J2355
Neupogen			
(G-CSF)	1 mcg	SC, IV	J1442
(TBO)	5 mcg	SC, IV	J1446
Neuroforte-R	up to 1,000 mcg		J3420
Neutrexin	per 25 mg	IV	J3305
Nipent	per 10 mg	IV	J9268
Nolvadex			J8999
Nordryl	up to 50 mg	IV, IM	J1200
	50 mg	ORAL	Q0163
Norflex	up to 60 mg	IV, IM	J2360
Norzine	up to 10 mg	IM	J3280

◄ **New**   ↻ **Revised**   ✔ **Reinstated**   ~~deleted~~ **Deleted**

DRUG NAME	DOSAGE	METHOD OF ADMINISTRATION	HCPCS CODE
Not otherwise classified drugs			**J3490**
other than inhalation solution administered thru DME			**J7799**
inhalation solution administered thru DME			**J7699**
anti-neoplastic			**J9999**
chemotherapeutic		ORAL	**J8999**
immunosuppressive			**J7599**
nonchemotherapeutic		ORAL	**J8499**
Novantrone	per 5 mg	IV	J9293
Novarel	per 1,000 USP Units		J0725
Novolin	per 5 units		J1815
	per 50 units		J1817
Novolog	per 5 units		J1815
	per 50 units		J1817
Novo Seven	1 mcg	IV	J7189
NPH	5 units	SC	J1815
Nplate	100 units		J0587
	10 mcg		J2796
Nubain	per 10 mg	IM, IV, SC	J2300
Nulecit	12.5 mg		J2916
Nulicaine	10 mg	IV	J2001
Nulojix	1 mg	IV	J0485
Numorphan	up to 1 mg	IV, SC, IM	J2410
Numorphan H.P.	up to 1 mg	IV, SC, IM	J2410
Nutropin	1 mg		J2941
O			
Oasis Burn Matrix	per square centimeter		Q4103
Oasis Wound Matrix	per square centimeter		Q4102
Obinutuzumab	10 mg		J9301
Ocriplasmin	0.125 mg	IV	**J7316**
Octagam	500 mg	IV	**J1568**
Octreotide Acetate, injection	1 mg	IM	**J2353**
	25 mcg	IV, SQ	**J2354**
Oculinum	per unit	IM	J0585
Ofatumumab	10 mg		**J9302**
Ofirmev	10 mg	IV	J0131
O-Flex	up to 60 mg	IV, IM	J2360
Oforta	10 mg		J8562
Olanzapine	1 mg	IM	**J2358**
Omacetaxine Mepesuccinate	0.01 mg	IV	**J9262**
Omalizumab	5 mg	SC	**J2357**
Omnipaque	per ml		Q9965, Q9966, Q9967

◀ **New**   ↻ **Revised**   ✔ **Reinstated**   ~~deleted~~ **Deleted**

DRUG NAME	DOSAGE	METHOD OF ADMINISTRATION	HCPCS CODE
Omnipen-N	up to 500 mg	IM, IV	J0290
	per 1.5 gm	IM, IV	J0295
Omniscan	per ml		A9579
Omnitrope	1 mg		J2941
Omontys	0.1 mg	IV, SC	J0890
OnabotulinumtoxinA	1 unit	IM	J0585
Oncaspar	per single dose vial	IM, IV	J9266
Oncovin	1 mg	IV	J9370
Ondansetron HCl	1 mg	IV	J2405
	1 mg	ORAL	Q0162
Opana	up to 1 mg		J2410
Oprelvekin	5 mg	SC	J2355
Optimark	per ml		A9579
Optiray	per ml		Q9966, Q9967
Optison	per ml		Q9956
Oraminic II	per 10 mg	IM, SC, IV	J0945
Oraped	per 5 mg	ORAL	J7510
Orfro	up to 60 mg		J2360
Ormazine	up to 50 mg	IM, IV	J3230
Orphenadrine citrate	up to 60 mg	IV, IM	J2360
Orphenate	up to 60 mg	IV, IM	J2360
Orthovisc		OTH	J7324
Or-Tyl	up to 20 mg	IM	J0500
Osmitrol			J7799
Ovidrel			J3490
Oxacillin sodium	up to 250 mg	IM, IV	J2700
Oxaliplatin	0.5 mg	IV	J9263
Oxilan	per ml		Q9967
Oxymorphone HCl	up to 1 mg	IV, SC, IM	J2410
Oxytetracycline HCl	up to 50 mg	IM	J2460
Oxytocin	up to 10 units	IV, IM	J2590
Ozurdex	0.1 mg		J7312
P			
Paclitaxel	1 mg	IV	J9267
Paclitaxel protein-bound particles	1 mg	IV	J9264
Palifermin	50 mcg	IV	J2425
Paliperidone Palmitate	1 mg	IM	J2426
Palonosetron HCl	25 mcg	IV	J2469
Pamidronate disodium	per 30 mg	IV	J2430
Panhematin	1 mg		J1640
Panitumumab	10 mg	IV	J9303
Papaverine HCl	up to 60 mg	IV, IM	J2440

◄ **New**   ↻ **Revised**   ✔ **Reinstated**   ~~deleted~~ **Deleted**

DRUG NAME	DOSAGE	METHOD OF ADMINISTRATION	HCPCS CODE
Paragard T 380 A		OTH	J7300
Paraplatin	50 mg	IV	J9045
Paricalcitol, injection	1 mcg	IV, IM	**J2501**
Pediapred	per 5 mg	ORAL	**J7510**
Pegademase bovine	25 IU		**J2504**
Pegaptinib	0.3 mg	OTH	**J2503**
Pegaspargase	per single dose vial	IM, IV	**J9266**
Pegasys			J3490
Pegfilgrastim	6 mg	SC	**J2505**
Peginesatide	0.1 mg	IV, SC	**J0890**
Peg-Intron			J3490
Pegloticase	1 mg	IV	**J2507**
Pemetrexed	10 mg	IV	**J9305**
Penicillin G benzathine	up to 100,000 units	IM	**J0561**
Penicillin G benzathine and penicillin G procaine	100,000 units	IM	**J0558**
Penicillin G potassium	up to 600,000 units	IM, IV	**J2540**
Penicillin G procaine, aqueous	up to 600,000 units	IM, IV	**J2510**
Penicillin G Sodium			J3490
Pentam	per 300 mg		J7676
Pentamidine isethionate	per 300 mg	INH, IM	**J2545, J7676**
Pentastarch, 10%	100 ml		**J2513**
Pentazocine HCl	30 mg	IM, SC, IV	**J3070**
Pentobarbital sodium	per 50 mg	IM, IV, OTH	**J2515**
Pentostatin	per 10 mg	IV	**J9268**
Peforomist	20 mcg		J7606
Perjeta	1 mg		J9306
Permapen	up to 600,000	IM	J0561
Perphenazine			
injection	up to 5 mg	IM, IV	**J3310**
tablets	4 mg	ORAL	**Q0175**
Persantine IV	per 10 mg	IV	J1245
Pertuzumab	1 mg	IV	**J9306**
Pfizerpen	up to 600,000 units	IM, IV	J2540
Pfizerpen A.S.	up to 600,000 units	IM, IV	J2510
Phenadoz			J8498
Phenazine 25	up to 50 mg	IM, IV	J2550
	12.5 mg	ORAL	Q0169
Phenazine 50	up to 50 mg	IM, IV	J2550
	12.5 mg	ORAL	Q0169
Phenergan	12.5 mg	ORAL	Q0169
	up to 50 mg	IM, IV	J2550

◄ **New**   ↻ **Revised**   ✔ **Reinstated**   ~~deleted~~ **Deleted**

DRUG NAME	DOSAGE	METHOD OF ADMINISTRATION	HCPCS CODE
Phenobarbital sodium	up to 120 mg	IM, IV	**J2560**
Phentolamine mesylate	up to 5 mg	IM, IV	**J2760**
Phenylephrine HCl	up to 1 ml	SC, IM, IV	J2370, J7799
Phenytoin sodium	per 50 mg	IM, IV	**J1165**
Photofrin	75 mg	IV	J9600
Phytonadione (Vitamin K)	per 1 mg	IM, SC, IV	**J3430**
Piperacillin/Tazobactam Sodium, injection	1.125 g	IV	J2543, J3490
Pitocin	up to 10 units	IV, IM	J2590
Plantinol AQ	10 mg	IV	J9060
Plas+SD	each unit	IV	P9023
Plasma			
cryoprecipitate reduced	each unit	IV	**P9044**
pooled multiple donor, frozen	each unit	IV	**P9023**
Platinol	10 mg	IV, IM	J9060
Plerixafor	1 mg	SC	**J2562**
Plicamycin	2,500 mcg	IV	**J9270**
Polocaine	per 10 ml	VAR	J0670
Polycillin-N	up to 500 mg	IM, IV	J0290
	per 1.5 gm	IM, IV	J0295
Polygam	500 mg		J1566
Porfimer Sodium	75 mg	IV	**J9600**
Potassium chloride	per 2 mEq	IV	**J3480**
Pralatrexate	1 mg	IV	**J9307**
Pralidoxime chloride	up to 1 g	IV, IM, SC	**J2730**
Predalone-50	up to 1 ml	IM	J2650
Predcor-25	up to 1 ml	IM	J2650
Predcor-50	up to 1 ml	IM	J2650
Predicort-50	up to 1 ml	IM	J2650
Prelone	5 mg		J7510
Prednicot	5 mg		J7506, J7510
Prednisone	per 5 mg	ORAL	**J7506**
Prednisolone, oral	5 mg	ORAL	**J7510**
Prednisolone acetate	up to 1 ml	IM	**J2650**
Predoject-50	up to 1 ml	IM	J2650
Pregnyl	per 1,000 USP units	IM	J0725
Premarin Intravenous	per 25 mg	IV, IM	J1410
Prescription, chemotherapeutic, not otherwise specified		ORAL	**J8999**
Prescription, nonchemotherapeutic, not otherwise specified		ORAL	**J8499**
Prialt	1 mcg		J2278
Primacor	5 mg	IV	J2260

◀ **New**   ↻ **Revised**   ✔ **Reinstated**   ~~deleted~~ **Deleted**

DRUG NAME	DOSAGE	METHOD OF ADMINISTRATION	HCPCS CODE
Primatrix	per square centimeter		Q4110
Primaxin	per 250 mg	IV, IM	J0743
Priscoline HCl	up to 25 mg	IV	J2670
Privigen	500 mg	IV	**J1459**
Pro-Depo, see Hydroxyprogesterone Caproate			
Procainamide HCl	up to 1 g	IM, IV	**J2690**
Prochlorperazine	up to 10 mg	IM, IV	**J0780**
			J8498
Prochlorperazine maleate	5 mg	ORAL	**Q0164**
			S0183
Procrit			J0885
			J0886
			Q4081
Profasi HP	per 1,000 USP units	IM	J0725
Profilnine Heat-Treated			
non-recombinant	per IU	IV	J7193
recombinant	per IU	IV	J7195
complex	per IU	IV	J7194
Profilnine-SD	per IU		J7193, J7194, J7195
Progestaject	per 50 mg		J2675
Progesterone	per 50 mg	IM	**J2675**
Prograf			
oral	1 mg	ORAL	J7507
parenteral	5 mg		J7525
Prohance Multipack	per ml		A9576
Prokine	50 mcg	IV	J2820
Prolastin	10 mg	IV	J0256
Proleukin	per single use vial	IM, IV	J9015
Prolia	1 mg		J0897
Prolixin Decanoate	up to 25 mg	IM, SC	J2680
Promazine HCl	up to 25 mg	IM	**J2950**
Promethazine			J8498
Promethazine HCl			
injection	up to 50 mg	IM, IV	**J2550**
oral	12.5 mg	ORAL	**Q0169**
Promethegan			J8498
Pronestyl	up to 1 g	IM, IV	J2690
Proplex T			
non-recombinant	per IU	IV	**J7193**
recombinant	per IU	IV	**J7195**
complex	per IU	IV	**J7194**

◄ **New**   ↻ **Revised**   ✔ **Reinstated**   ~~deleted~~ **Deleted**

DRUG NAME	DOSAGE	METHOD OF ADMINISTRATION	HCPCS CODE
Proplex SX-T			
non-recombinant	per IU	IV	**J7193**
recombinant	per IU	IV	**J7195**
complex	per IU	IV	**J7194**
Propofol	10 mg	IV	**J2704** ◄
Propranolol HCl	up to 1 mg	IV	**J1800**
Prorex-25			
	up to 50 mg	IM, IV	J2550
	12.5 mg	ORAL	Q0169
Prorex-50			
	up to 50 mg	IM, IV	J2550
	12.5 mg	ORAL	Q0169
Prostaglandin E1	per 1.25 mcg		J0270
Prostaphlin	up to 1 g	IM, IV	J2690
Prostigmin	up to 0.5 mg	IM, IV, SC	J2710
Protamine sulfate	per 10 mg	IV	**J2720**
Protein C Concentrate	10 IU	IV	**J2724**
Protirelin	per 250 mcg	IV	**J2725**
Prothazine	up to 50 mg	IM, IV	J2550
	12.5 mg	ORAL	Q0169
Protonix			J3490
Protopam Chloride	up to 1 g	IV, IM, SC	J2730
Proventil			
concentrated form	1 mg	INH	J7610, J7611
unit dose form	1 mg	INH	J7609, J7613
Provocholine	per 1 mg		J7674
Prozine-50	up to 25 mg	IM	J2950
Pulmicort	0.25 mg	INH	J7633
Pulmicort Respules	0.5 mg	INH	J7627, J7626
	per 0.25 mg		J7633
noncompounded, concentrated	up to 0.5 mg	INH	J7626
Pulmozyme	per mg		J7639
Purinethol	50 mg		J8999
Pyridoxine HCl	100 mg		**J3415**
Q			
Quelicin	up to 20 mg	IV, IM	J0330
Quinupristin/dalfopristin	500 mg (150/350)	IV	**J2770**
Qutenza	per square cm		J7336
R			
Ranibizumab	0.1 mg	OTH	**J2778**

◄ New   ⮌ Revised   ✔ Reinstated   ~~deleted~~ Deleted

DRUG NAME	DOSAGE	METHOD OF ADMINISTRATION	HCPCS CODE
Ranitidine HCl, injection	25 mg	IV, IM	**J2780**
Rapamune	1 mg	ORAL	J7520
Rasburicase	0.5 mg	IV	**J2783**
Rebif	11 mcg		Q3026
Reclast	1 mg		J3489
Recombinate (anti-hemophilic factor)			
human	per IU	IV	J7190
porcine	per IU	IV	J7191
recombinant	per IU	IV	J7192
Recombivax			J3490
Redisol	up to 1,000 mcg	IM, SC	J3420
Regadenoson	0.1 mg	IV	**J2785**
Refacto	per IU		J7192
Refludan	50 mg		J1945
Regitine	up to 5 mg	IM, IV	J2760
Reglan	up to 10 mg	IV	J2765
Regular	5 units	SC	J1815
Relefact TRH	per 250 mcg	IV	J2725
Relistor	0.1 mg	SC	J2212
Remicade	10 mg	IM, IV	J1745
Remodulin	1 mg		J3285
Reno-60	per ml		Q9961
Reno-Dip	per ml		Q9958
ReoPro	10 mg	IV	J0130
Rep-Pred 40	20 mg	IM	J1020
	40 mg	IM	J1030
	80 mg	IM	J1040
Rep-Pred 80	20 mg	IM	J1020
	40 mg	IM	J1030
	80 mg	IM	J1040
Resectisol			J7799
Retavase	18.1 mg	IV	J2993
Reteplase	18.1 mg	IV	**J2993**
Retisert			J7311
Retrovir	10 mg	IV	J3485
Rheomacrodex	500 ml	IV	J7100
Rhesonativ	1 dose package/ 300 mcg	IM	J2790
	50 mg		J2788
Rheumatrex Dose Pack	2.5 mg	ORAL	J8610

◄ New   ⟳ Revised   ✔ Reinstated   ~~deleted~~ Deleted

DRUG NAME	DOSAGE	METHOD OF ADMINISTRATION	HCPCS CODE
Rho(D)			
immune globulin		IM, IV	**J2791**
immune globulin, human	1 dose package/ 300 mcg	IM	**J2790**
	50 mg	IM	**J2788**
immune globulin, human, solvent detergent	100	IU, IV	**J2792**
RhoGAM	1 dose package, 300 mcg	IM	J2790
	50 mg		J2788
Rhophylac	100 IU	IM, IV	**J2791**
Riastap	100 mg		J7178
Rifadin			J3490
Rifampin			J3490
Rilonacept	1 mg	SC	**J2793**
RimabotulinumtoxinB	100 units	IM	**J0587**
Rimso-50	50 ml		J1212
Ringers lactate infusion	up to 1,000 cc	IV	**J7120**
Risperdal Costa	0.5 mg		J2794
Risperidone	0.5 mg	IM	**J2794**
Rituxan	100 mg	IV	J9310
Rituximab	100 mg	IV	**J9310**
Robaxin	up to 10 ml	IV, IM	J2800
Robinul	per mg		J7643
Rocephin	per 250 mg	IV, IM	J0696
Rodex	100 mg		J3415
Roferon-A	3 million units	SC, IM	J9213
Romidepsin	1 mg	IV	**J9315**
Romiplostim	10 mcg	SC	**J2796**
Ropivacaine Hydrochloride	1 mg	OTH	**J2795**
Rubex	10 mg	IV	J9000
Rubramin PC	up to 1,000 mcg	IM, SC	J3420
S			
Saizen	1 mg		J2941
Saline solution	10 ml		A4216
5% dextrose	500 ml	IV	**J7042**
infusion	250 cc	IV	**J7050**
	1,000 cc	IV	**J7030**
sterile	500 ml = 1 unit	IV, OTH	**J7040**
Sandimmune	25 mg	ORAL	Jw7515
	100 mg	ORAL	J7502
	250 mg	OTH	J7516

◄ **New**   ↻ **Revised**   ✔ **Reinstated**   ~~deleted~~ **Deleted**

DRUG NAME	DOSAGE	METHOD OF ADMINISTRATION	HCPCS CODE
Sandoglobulin, see Immune globin intravenous (human)			
Sandostatin, Lar Depot	25 mcg		J2354
	1 mg	IM	J2353
Sargramostim (GM-CSF)	50 mcg	IV	**J2820**
Sculptra	0.5 mg	IV	**Q2028**
Selestoject	per 4 mg	IM, IV	J0702
Sensorcaine MPF			J3490
Sermorelin acetate	1 mcg	SC	**Q0515**
Serostim	1 mg		J2941
Simponi Aria	1 mg		J1602
Simulect	20 mg		J0480
Sincalide	5 mcg	IV	**J2805**
Sinografin	per ml		Q9963
Sinusol-B	per 10 mg	IM, SC, IV	J0945
Sirolimus	1 mg	ORAL	**J7520**
Skyla	13.5 mg	OTH	**J7301**
Smz-TMP			J3490
Sodium Chloride	1,000 cc		J7030
	10 ml		A4216
	500 ml 5 1 unit		J7040
	500 ml		A4217
	250 cc		J7050
inhalation solution			J7699
Sodium Chloride Bacteriostatic	10 ml		A4216
Sodium Chloride Concentrate			J7799
Sodium ferricgluconate in sucrose	12.5 mg		**J2916**
Sodium Hyaluronate			J3490
Euflexxa			**J7323**
Hyalgan			**J7321**
Orthovisc			**J7324**
Supartz			**J7321**
Solganal	up to 50 mg	IM	J2910
Soliris	10 mg		J1300
Solu-Cortef	up to 50 mg	IV, IM, SC	J1710
	100 mg		J1720
Solu-Medrol	up to 40 mg	IM, IV	J2920
	up to 125 mg	IM, IV	J2930
Solurex	1 mg	IM, IV, OTH	J1100
Solurex LA	1 mg	IM	J1094
Somatrem	1 mg	SC	**J2940**
Somatropin	1 mg	SC	**J2941**
Somatulin Depot	1 mg		J1930

◄ **New**   ⟳ **Revised**   ✔ **Reinstated**   ~~deleted~~ **Deleted**

DRUG NAME	DOSAGE	METHOD OF ADMINISTRATION	HCPCS CODE
Sparine	up to 25 mg	IM	J2950
Spasmoject	up to 20 mg	IM	J0500
Spectinomycin HCl	up to 2 g	IM	**J3320**
Sporanox	50 mg	IV	J1835
Stadol	1 mg		J0595
Staphcillin, see Methicillin sodium			
Stelara	1 mg		J3357
Sterapred DS	per 5 mg		J7506
Stilphostrol	250 mg	IV	J9165
Streptase	250,000 IU	IV	J2995
Streptokinase	per 250,000	IU, IV	**J2995**
Streptomycin Sulfate	up to 1 g	IM	J3000
Streptomycin	up to 1 g	IM	**J3000**
Streptozocin	1 gm	IV	**J9320**
Strontium-89 chloride	per millicurie		**A9600**
Sublimaze	0.1 mg	IM, IV	J3010
Succinylcholine chloride	up to 20 mg	IV, IM	**J0330**
Sufentanil Citrate			J3490
Sumarel Dosepro	6 mg		J3030
Sumatriptan succinate	6 mg	SC	**J3030**
Supartz		OTH	**J7321**
SurgiMend			C9358
Surostrin	up to 20 mg	IV, IM	**J0330**
Sus-Phrine	up to 1 ml ampule	SC, IM	J0171
Synercid	500 mg (150/350)	IV	J2770
Synkavite	per 1 mg	IM, SC, IV	J3430
Syntocinon	up to 10 units	IV, IM	J2590
Synvisc and Synvisc-One	1 mg	OTH	**J7325**
Syrex	10 ml		A4216
Sytobex	1,000 mcg	IM, SC	J3420
T			
Tacrolimus			
oral, extended release	0.1 mg	ORAL	**J7508**
oral, immediate release	1 mg	ORAL	**J7507**
parenteral	5 mg	IV	**J7525**
Taliglucerace Alfa	10 units	IV	**J3060**
Talwin	30 mg	IM, SC, IV	J3070
Tamoxifen Citrate			J8999
Taractan, see Chlorprothixene			
Taxol	1 mg	IV	J9267
Taxotere	20 mg	IV	J9171
Tazicef	per 500 mg		J0713

◀ **New**   ⮑ **Revised**   ✔ **Reinstated**   ~~deleted~~ **Deleted**

DRUG NAME	DOSAGE	METHOD OF ADMINISTRATION	HCPCS CODE
Tazidime, see Ceftazidime Technetium TC Sestambi	per dose		**A9500**
			J0713
TEEV	1 mg		J3121
Teflaro	1 mg		J0712
Telavancin	10 mg	IV	**J3095**
Temodar	5 mg	ORAL	J8700, J9328
Temozolomide	1 mg	IV	**J9328**
	5 mg	ORAL	**J8700**
Temsirolimus	1 mg	IV	**J9330**
Tenecteplase	1 mg	IV	**J3101**
Teniposide	50 mg		**Q2017**
Tequin	10 mg	IV	J1590
Terbutaline sulfate	up to 1 mg	SC, IV	**J3105**
concentrated form	per 1 mg	INH	**J7680**
unit dose form	per 1 mg	INH	**J7681**
Teriparatide	10 mcg	SC	**J3110**
Terramycin IM	up to 50 mg	IM	J2460
Testa-C	1 mg		J1071
Testadiate	1 mg		J3121
Testadiate-Depo	1 mg		J1071
Testaject-LA	1 mg		J1071
Testaqua	up to 50 mg	IM	J3140
Test-Estro Cypionates	1 mg		J1071
Test-Estro-C	1 mg		J1071
Testex	up to 100 mg	IM	J3150
Testo AQ	up to 50 mg		J3140
Testoject-50	up to 50 mg	IM	J3140
Testoject-LA	1 mg		J1071
Testone			
LA 200	1 mg		J3121
LA 100	1 mg		J3121
Testosterone Aqueous	up to 50 mg	IM	J3140
~~Testosterone enanthate and estradiol valerate~~	~~up to 1 cc~~	~~IM~~	~~J0900~~ ✖
Testosterone enanthate	1 mg	IM	**J3121** ↻
	~~up to 200 mg~~	~~IM~~	~~J3130~~ ✖
Testosterone cypionate	1 mg	IM	**J1071** ↻
	~~1 cc, 200 mg~~	~~IM~~	~~J1080~~ ✖
~~Testosterone cypionate and estradiol cypionate~~	~~up to 1 ml~~	~~IM~~	~~J1060~~ ✖
~~Testosterone propionate~~	~~up to 100 mg~~	~~IM~~	~~J3150~~ ✖
~~Testosterone suspension~~	~~up to 50 mg~~	~~IM~~	~~J3140~~ ✖
Testosterone undecanoate	1 mg	IM	**J3145** ◀
Testradiol 90/4	1 mg		J3121

◀ **New**   ↻ **Revised**   ✔ **Reinstated**   ~~deleted~~ **Deleted**

DRUG NAME	DOSAGE	METHOD OF ADMINISTRATION	HCPCS CODE
Testrin PA	1 mg		J3121
Testro AQ	up to 50 mg		J3140
Tetanus immune globulin, human	up to 250 units	IM	**J1670**
Tetracycline	up to 250 mg	IM, IV	**J0120**
Tev-Tropin	1 mg		J2941
Thallous Chloride TI–201	per MCI		**A9505**
Theelin Aqueous	per 1 mg	IM	J1435
Theophylline	per 40 mg	IV	**J2810**
TheraCys	per vial	IV	J9031
Thiamine HCl	100 mg		**J3411**
Thiethylenecthiophosphoramide/T	15 mg		J9340
Thiethylperazine maleate			
injection	up to 10 mg	IM	**J3280**
oral	10 mg	ORAL	**Q0174**
Thiotepa	15 mg	IV	**J9340**
Thorazine	up to 50 mg	IM, IV	J3230
Thrombate III	per IU		J7197
Thymoglobulin, see Immune globin, anti-thymocyte			
	25 mg		J7511
Thypinone	per 250 mcg	IV	J2725
Thyrogen	0.9 mg	IM, SC	J3240
Thyrotropin Alfa, injection	0.9 mg	IM, SC	**J3240**
Tice BCG	per vial	IV	J9031
Ticon			
injection	up to 200 mg	IM	J3250
oral	250 mg	ORAL	Q0173
Tigan			
injection	up to 200 mg	IM	J3250
oral	250 mg	ORAL	Q0173
Tigecycline	1 mg	IV	**J3243**
Tiject-20	up to 200 mg	IM	J3250
	250 mg	ORAL	Q0173
Timentin			J3490
Tinzaparin	1,000 IU	SC	**J1655**
Tirofiban Hydrochloride, injection	0.25 mg	IM, IV	**J3246**
TNKase	1 mg		**J3101**
Tobi	300 mg	INH	J7682, J7685
Tobramycin, inhalation solution	300 mg	INH	**J7682, J7685**
Tobramycin sulfate	up to 80 mg	IM, IV	J3260, J7685
Tocilizumab	1 mg	IV	**J3262**
Tofranil, see Imipramine HCl			
Tolazoline HCl	up to 25 mg	IV	**J2670**

◀ **New** ↩ **Revised** ✔ **Reinstated** ~~deleted~~ **Deleted**

DRUG NAME	DOSAGE	METHOD OF ADMINISTRATION	HCPCS CODE
Toposar	10 mg		J1981
Topotecan	0.25 mg	ORAL	**J8705**
	0.1 mg	IV	**J9351**
Toradol	per 15 mg	IM, IV	J1885
Torecan	10 mg	ORAL	Q0174
	up to 10 mg	IM	J3280
Torisel	1 mg		**J9330**
Tornalate			
concentrated form	per mg	INH	J7628
unit dose	per mg	INH	J7629
Torsemide	10 mg/ml	IV	**J3265**
Totacillin-N	up to 500 mg	IM, IV	J0290
	per 1.5 gm	IM, IV	J0295
Trastuzumab	10 mg	IV	**J9355**
Trasylol	10,000 KIU		J0365
Treanda	1 mg		J9033
Trelstar Depot	3.75 mg		J3315
Trelstar LA	3.75 mg		J3315
Treprostinil	1 mg		J3285, J7686
Trexall	2.5 mg	ORAL	J8610
Triethylenethosphoramide	15 mg		J9340
Tri-Kort	1 mg		J3300
	per 10 mg	IM	J3301
Triam-A	1 mg		J3300
	per 10 mg	IM	J3301
Triamcinolone			
concentrated form	per 1 mg	INH	**J7683**
unit dose	per 1 mg	INH	**J7684**
Triamcinolone acetonide	1 mg		J3300, J7684
	per 10 mg	IM	**J3301**
Triamcinolone diacetate	per 5 mg	IM	**J3302**
Triamcinolone hexacetonide	per 5 mg	VAR	**J3303**
Triamcot	per 5 mg		J3302
Triesence	1 mg		J3300
	per 10 mg	IM	J3301
Triflupromazine HCl	up to 20 mg	IM, IV	**J3400**
Trilafon	4 mg	ORAL	Q0175
	8 mg	ORAL	Q0176
	up to 5 mg	IM, IV	J3310
Trilog	1 mg		J3300
	per 10 mg	IM	J3301
Trilone	per 5 mg		J3302

◀ New   ⮌ Revised   ✔ Reinstated   ~~deleted~~ Deleted

DRUG NAME	DOSAGE	METHOD OF ADMINISTRATION	HCPCS CODE
Trimethobenzamide HCl			
injection	up to 200 mg	IM	**J3250**
oral	250 mg	ORAL	**Q0173**
Trimetrexate glucuronate	per 25 mg	IV	**J3305**
Triptorelin Pamoate	3.75 mg	SC	**J3315**
Trisenox	1 mg	IV	J9017
Trobicin	up to 2 g	IM	J3320
Trovan	100 mg	IV	J0200
Truxadryl	50 mg		J1200
Twinrix			J3490
Tysabri	1 mg		J2323
Tyvaso	1.74 mg		J7686
U			
Ultravist 150	per ml		Q9965
Ultravist 240	per ml		Q9966
Ultravist 300	per ml		Q9967
Ultravist 370	per ml		Q9967
Ultrazine-10	up to 10 mg	IM, IV	J0780
Unasyn	per 1.5 gm	IM, IV	J0295
Unclassified drugs (see also Not elsewhere classified)			**J3490**
Unspecified oral antiemetic			**Q0181**
Urea	up to 40 g	IV	**J3350**
Ureaphil	up to 40 g	IV	J3350
Urecholine	up to 5 mg	SC	J0520
Urofollitropin	75 IU		**J3355**
Urokinase	5,000 IU vial	IV	**J3364**
	250,000 IU vial	IV	**J3365**
Ustekinumab	1 mg	SC	**J3357**
V			
V-Gan 25	up to 50 mg	IM, IV	J2550
	12.5 mg	ORAL	Q0169
V-Gan 50	up to 50 mg	IM, IV	J2550
	12.5 mg	ORAL	Q0169
Valcyte			J3490
Valergen 10	10 mg	IM	J1380
Valergen 20	10 mg	IM	J1380
Valergen 40	up to 10 mg	IM	J1380
Valertest No. 1	1 mg		J3121
Valertest No. 2	1 mg		J3121
Valium	up to 5 mg	IM, IV	J3360
Valrubicin, intravesical	200 mg	OTH	**J9357**
Valstar	200 mg	OTH	J9357

◄ **New**   ⤵ **Revised**   ✔ **Reinstated**   d̶e̶l̶e̶t̶e̶d̶ **Deleted**

DRUG NAME	DOSAGE	METHOD OF ADMINISTRATION	HCPCS CODE
Vancocin	500 mg	IV, IM	J3370
Vancoled	500 mg	IV, IM	J3370
Vancomycin HCl	**500 mg**	**IV, IM**	**J3370**
Vantas	50 mg		J9226
Vasceze	per 10 mg		J1642
Vasceze Sodium Chloride	10 ml		A4216
Vasoxyl, see Methoxamine HCl			
Vectibix	10 mg		J9303
Velaglucerase alfa	**100 units**	**IV**	**J3385**
Velban	1 mg	IV	J9360
Velcade	0.1 mg		J9041
Veletri	0.5 mg		J1325
Velsar	1 mg	IV	J9360
Venofer	1 mg	IV	J1756
Ventavis	20 mcg		Q4074
Ventolin	0.5 mg	INH	J7620
concentrated form	1 mg	INH	J7610, J7611
unit dose form	1 mg	INH	J7609, J7613
VePesid			
	10 mg	IV	J9181
	50 mg	ORAL	J8560
Veritas Collagen Matrix			J3490
Versed	per 1 mg	IM, IV	J2250
Verteporfin	**0.1 mg**	**IV**	**J3396**
Vesprin	up to 20 mg	IM, IV	J3400
VFEND IV	10 mg		J3465
Viadur	65 mg		J9219
Vibativ	10 mg		J3095
Vidaza	1 mg		J9025
Vinblastine sulfate	**1 mg**	**IV**	**J9360**
Vincasar PFS	1 mg	IV	J9370
Vincristine sulfate	**1 mg**	**IV**	**J9370**
Vincristine sulfate Liposome	**1 mg**	**IV**	**J9371**
Vinorelbine tartrate	**per 10 mg**	**IV**	**J9390**
Vispaque	per ml		Q9966, Q9967
Vistacot	up to 25 mg		J3410
Vistaject-25	up to 25 mg	IM	J3410
Vistaril	up to 25 mg	IM	J3410
	25 mg	ORAL	Q0177
Vistide	375 mg	IV	J0740
Visudyne	0.1 mg	IV	J3396
Vita #12	up to 1,000 mcg		J3420

◄ **New**　↻ **Revised**　✔ **Reinstated**　deleted **Deleted**

DRUG NAME	DOSAGE	METHOD OF ADMINISTRATION	HCPCS CODE
Vitamin K, phytonadione, menadione, menadiol sodium diphosphate	per 1 mg	IM, SC, IV	**J3430**
Vitamin B-12 cyanocobalamin	up to 1,000 mcg	IM, SC	**J3420**
Vitrasert	4.5 mg		J7310
Vivaglobin	100 mg		J1562
Vivitrol	1 mg		J2315
Von Willebrand Factor Complex, human	per IU VWF:RCo	IV	**J7187**
	per IU VWF:RCo	IV	**J7183**
Voriconazole	10 mg	IV	**J3465**
Vpriv	100 units		J3385
W			
Water for injection bacteriostatic	10 ml		A4216
Wehamine	up to 50 mg	IM, IV	J1240
Wehdryl	up to 50 mg	IM, IV	J1200
	50 mg	ORAL	Q0163
Wellcovorin	per 50 mg	IM, IV	J0640
Wilate	per IU	IV	J7187
Win Rho SD	100 IU	IV	J2792
Wyamine Sulfate, see Mephentermine sulfate			
Wycillin	up to 600,000 units	IM, IV	J2510
Wydase	up to 150 units	SC, IV	J3470
X			
Xeloda	150 mg	ORAL	J8520
	500 mg	ORAL	J8521
Xeomin	1 unit		J0588
Xgera	1 mg		J0987
Xgeva	1 mg		J0897
Xiaflex	0.01 mg		J0775
Xolair	5 mg		J2357
Xopenex	0.5 mg	INH	J7620
concentrated form	1 mg	INH	J7610, J7611, J7612
unit dose form	1 mg	INH	J7609, J7613, J7614
Xylocaine HCl	10 mg	IV	J2001
Xyntha	per IU IV		J7185, J7192
Y			
Yervoy	1 mg		J9228
Z			
Zaltrap	1 mg		J9400
Zanosar	1 g	IV	J9320
Zantac	25 mg	IV, IM	J2780
Zemaira	10 mg	IV	J0256

◀ **New**   ↻ **Revised**   ✔ **Reinstated**   ~~deleted~~ **Deleted**

DRUG NAME	DOSAGE	METHOD OF ADMINISTRATION	HCPCS CODE
Zemplar	1 mcg	IM, IV	J2501
Zenapax	25 mg	IV	J7513
Zetran	up to 5 mg	IM, IV	J3360
Ziconotide	1 mcg	OTH	**J2278**
Zidovudine	10 mg	IV	**J3485**
Zinacef	per 750 mg	IM, IV	J0697
Zinecard	per 250 mg		J1190
Ziprasidone Mesylate	10 mg	IM	**J3486**
Zithromax	500 mg	ORAL	J0456
I.V.	500 mg	IV	J0456
Ziv-Aflibercept	1 mg	IV	**J9400**
Zmax	1 g		Q0144
Zofran	1 mg	IV	J2405
	1 mg	ORAL	Q0162
Zoladex	per 3.6 mg	SC	J9202
Zoledronic Acid	1 mg	IV	**J3489**
Zolicef	500 mg	IV, IM	J0690
Zometra	1 mg		J3489
Zorbtive	1 mg		J2941
Zortress	0.25 mg	ORAL	J7527
Zosyn	1.125 g	IV	J2543
Zovirax	5 mg		J8499
Zyprexa Relprevv	1 mg		J2358
Zyvox	200 mg	IV	J2020

◄ **New**   ↻ **Revised**   ✔ **Reinstated**   ~~deleted~~ **Deleted**

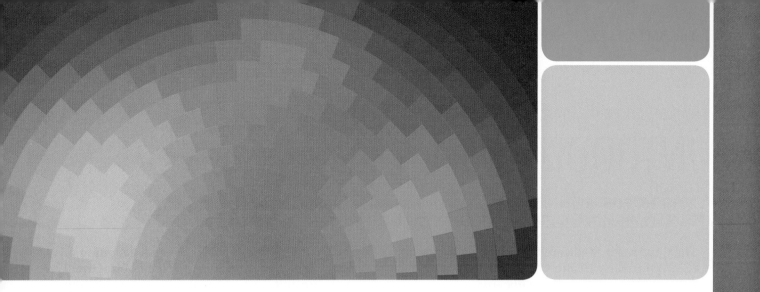

HCPCS 2015: LEVEL II NATIONAL CODES

2015 HCPCS quarterly updates available
on the companion website at:
http://www.codingupdates.com

DISCLAIMER

Every effort has been made to make this text complete and accurate,
but no guarantee, warranty, or representation is made for its
accuracy or completeness. This text is based on the Centers for
Medicare and Medicaid Services Healthcare Common Procedure
Coding System (HCPCS).

INTRODUCTION

2015 HCPCS quarterly updates available on the companion website at: www.codingupdates.com

The Centers for Medicare and Medicaid Services (CMS) (formerly Health Care Financing Administration [HCFA]) Healthcare Common Procedure Coding System (HCPCS) is a collection of codes and descriptors that represent procedures, supplies, products, and services that may be provided to Medicare beneficiaries and to individuals enrolled in private health insurance programs. The codes are divided as follows:

Level I: Codes and descriptors copyrighted by the American Medical Association's (AMA's) Current Procedural Terminology, ed. 4 (CPT-4). These are 5 position numeric codes representing physician and nonphysician services.

Level II: Includes codes and descriptors copyrighted by the American Dental Association's current dental terminology, seventh edition (CDT-7/8). These are 5 position alpha-numeric codes comprising the D series. All other Level II codes and descriptors are approved and maintained jointly by the alpha-numeric editorial panel (consisting of CMS, the Health Insurance Association of America, and the Blue Cross and Blue Shield Association). These are 5 position alpha-numeric codes representing primarily items and nonphysician services that are not represented in the Level I codes.

Level III: The CMS eliminated Level III local codes. See Program Memorandum AB-02-113.

Headings are provided as a means of grouping similar or closely related items. The placement of a code under a heading does not indicate additional means of classification, nor does it relate to any health insurance coverage categories.

HCPCS also contains modifiers, which are two-position codes and descriptors used to indicate that a service or procedure that has been performed has been altered by some specific circumstance but not changed in its definition or code. Modifiers are grouped by the levels. Level I modifiers and descriptors are copyrighted by the AMA. Level II modifiers are HCPCS modifiers. Modifiers in the D series are copyrighted by the ADA.

HCPCS is designed to promote uniform reporting and statistical data collection of medical procedures, supplies, products, and services.

HCPCS Disclaimer

Inclusion or exclusion of a procedure, supply, product, or service does not imply any health insurance coverage or reimbursement policy.

HCPCS makes as much use as possible of generic descriptions, but the inclusion of brand names to describe devices or drugs is intended only for indexing purposes; it is not meant to convey endorsement of any particular product or drug.

Updating HCPCS

The primary updates are made annually. Quarterly updates are also issued by CMS.

Legend

CMS Updates:

▶ New
↪ Revised
✔ Reinstated
✖ Deleted
☼ Special coverage instructions
⊘ Not covered or valid by Medicare
✷ Carrier discretion
ⓑ Bill local carrier
ⓓ Bill DME MAC

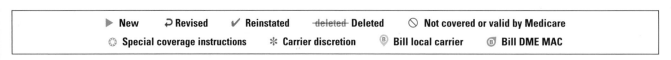

| ▶ New | ↪ Revised | ✔ Reinstated | deleted Deleted | ⊘ Not covered or valid by Medicare |
| ☼ Special coverage instructions | ✷ Carrier discretion | ⓑ Bill local carrier | ⓓ Bill DME MAC |

Publisher Updates:

⊛ PQRS

Qp Quantity Physician Appendix A

Qh Quantity Hospital Appendix B

♀ Female only

♂ Male only

A Age

& DMEPOS

A2-Z3 ASC Payment Indicator

A-Y ASC Status Indicator

Coding Clinic

Do not report HCPCS modifiers with PQRS CPT Category II codes, rather use Category II modifiers (i.e., 1P, 2P, 3P, or 8P) or the claim may be returned or denied.

LEVEL II NATIONAL MODIFIERS

⁎ **A1**   Dressing for one wound

⁎ **A2**   Dressing for two wounds

⁎ **A3**   Dressing for three wounds

⁎ **A4**   Dressing for four wounds

⁎ **A5**   Dressing for five wounds

⁎ **A6**   Dressing for six wounds

⁎ **A7**   Dressing for seven wounds

⁎ **A8**   Dressing for eight wounds

⁎ **A9**   Dressing for nine or more wounds

☺ **AA**   Anesthesia services performed personally by anesthesiologist

    IOM: 100-04, 12, 90.4

☺ **AD**   Medical supervision by a physician: more than four concurrent anesthesia procedures

    IOM: 100-04, 12, 90.4

⁎ **AE**   Registered dietician

⁎ **AF**   Specialty physician

⁎ **AG**   Primary physician

☺ **AH**   Clinical psychologist

    IOM: 100-04, 12, 170

⁎ **AI**   Principal physician of record

☺ **AJ**   Clinical social worker

    IOM: 100-04, 12, 170

    IOM: 100-04, 12, 150

⁎ **AK**   Nonparticipating physician

☺ **AM**   Physician, team member service

    Not assigned for Medicare

⁎ **AO**   Alternate payment method declined by provider of service

⁎ **AP**   Determination of refractive state was not performed in the course of diagnostic ophthalmological examination

⁎ **AQ**   Physician providing a service in an unlisted health professional shortage area (HPSA)

⁎ **AR**   Physician provider services in a physician scarcity area

⁎ **AS**   Physician assistant, nurse practitioner, or clinical nurse specialist services for assistant at surgery

⁎ **AT**   Acute treatment (this modifier should be used when reporting service 98940, 98941, 98942)

⁎ **AU**   Item furnished in conjunction with a urological, ostomy, or tracheostomy supply

⁎ **AV**   Item furnished in conjunction with a prosthetic device, prosthetic or orthotic

⁎ **AW**   Item furnished in conjunction with a surgical dressing

⁎ **AX**   Item furnished in conjunction with dialysis services

⁎ **AY**   Item or service furnished to an ESRD patient that is not for the treatment of ESRD

⊘ **AZ**   Physician providing a service in a dental health professional shortage area for the purpose of an electronic health record incentive payment

⁎ **BA**   Item furnished in conjunction with parenteral enteral nutrition (PEN) services

⁎ **BL**   Special acquisition of blood and blood products

⁎ **BO**   Orally administered nutrition, not by feeding tube

⁎ **BP**   The beneficiary has been informed of the purchase and rental options and has elected to purchase the item

⁎ **BR**   The beneficiary has been informed of the purchase and rental options and has elected to rent the item

⁎ **BU**   The beneficiary has been informed of the purchase and rental options and after 30 days has not informed the supplier of his/her decision

⊛ **PQRS**   Qp **Quantity Physician Appendix A**   Qh **Quantity Hospital Appendix B**   ♀ **Female only**
♂ **Male only**   A **Age**   & **DMEPOS**   A2-Z3 **ASC Payment Indicator**   A-Y **ASC Status Indicator**   Coding Clinic

LEVEL II NATIONAL MODIFIERS   A1 – BU

95

✳ **CA** Procedure payable only in the inpatient setting when performed emergently on an outpatient who expires prior to admission

✳ **CB** Service ordered by a renal dialysis facility (RDF) physician as part of the ESRD beneficiary's dialysis benefit, is not part of the composite rate, and is separately reimbursable

✳ **CC** Procedure code change (Use CC when the procedure code submitted was changed either for administrative reasons or because an incorrect code was filed)

⊛ **CD** AMCC test has been ordered by an ESRD facility or MCP physician that is part of the composite rate and is not separately billable

⊛ **CE** AMCC test has been ordered by an ESRD facility or MCP physician that is a composite rate test but is beyond the normal frequency covered under the rate and is separately reimbursable based on medical necessity

⊛ **CF** AMCC test has been ordered by an ESRD facility or MCP physician that is not part of the composite rate and is separately billable

✳ **CG** Policy criteria applied

⊛ **CH** 0 percent impaired, limited or restricted

⊛ **CI** At least 1 percent but less than 20 percent impaired, limited or restricted

⊛ **CJ** At least 20 percent but less than 40 percent impaired, limited or restricted

⊛ **CK** At least 40 percent but less than 60 percent impaired, limited or restricted

⊛ **CL** At least 60 percent but less than 80 percent impaired, limited or restricted

⊛ **CM** At least 80 percent but less than 100 percent impaired, limited or restricted

⊛ **CN** 100 percent impaired, limited or restricted

✳ **CR** Catastrophe/Disaster related

✳ **CS** Item or service related, in whole or in part, to an illness, injury, or condition that was caused by or exacerbated by the effects, direct or indirect, of the 2010 oil spill in the Gulf of Mexico, including but not limited to subsequent clean-up activities

✳ **DA** Oral health assessment by a licensed health professional other than a dentist

✳ **E1** Upper left, eyelid

✳ **E2** Lower left, eyelid

✳ **E3** Upper right, eyelid

Coding Clinic: 2011, Q3, P6

✳ **E4** Lower right, eyelid

⊛ **EA** Erythropoetic stimulating agent (ESA) administered to treat anemia due to anti-cancer chemotherapy

CMS requires claims for non-ESRD ESAs (J0881 and J0885) to include one of three modifiers: EA, EB, EC.

⊛ **EB** Erythropoetic stimulating agent (ESA) administered to treat anemia due to anti-cancer radiotherapy

CMS requires claims for non-ESRD ESAs (J0881 and J0885) to include one of three modifiers: EA, EB, EC.

⊛ **EC** Erythropoetic stimulating agent (ESA) administered to treat anemia not due to anti-cancer radiotherapy or anti-cancer chemotherapy

CMS requires claims for non-ESRD ESAs (J0881 and J0885) to include one of three modifiers: EA, EB, EC.

⊛ **ED** Hematocrit level has exceeded 39% (or hemoglobin level has exceeded 13.0 g/dl) for 3 or more consecutive billing cycles immediately prior to and including the current cycle

⊛ **EE** Hematocrit level has not exceeded 39% (or hemoglobin level has not exceeded 13.0 g/dl) for 3 or more consecutive billing cycles immediately prior to and including the current cycle

⊛ **EJ** Subsequent claims for a defined course of therapy, e.g., EPO, sodium hyaluronate, infliximab

⊛ **EM** Emergency reserve supply (for ESRD benefit only)

✳ **EP** Service provided as part of Medicaid early periodic screening diagnosis and treatment (EPSDT) program

✳ **ET** Emergency services

✳ **EY** No physician or other licensed health care provider order for this item or service

Items billed before a signed and dated order has been received by the supplier must be submitted with an EY modifier added to each related HCPCS code.

✳ **F1** Left hand, second digit

✳ **F2** Left hand, third digit

▶ **New**   ↻ **Revised**   ✔ **Reinstated**   ~~deleted~~ **Deleted**   ⊘ **Not covered or valid by Medicare**

⊛ **Special coverage instructions**   ✳ **Carrier discretion**   Ⓑ **Bill local carrier**   Ⓓ **Bill DME MAC**

❋ **F3**   Left hand, fourth digit

❋ **F4**   Left hand, fifth digit

❋ **F5**   Right hand, thumb

❋ **F6**   Right hand, second digit

❋ **F7**   Right hand, third digit

❋ **F8**   Right hand, fourth digit

❋ **F9**   Right hand, fifth digit

❋ **FA**   Left hand, thumb

⊘ **FB**   Item provided without cost to provider, supplier or practitioner, or full credit received for replaced device (examples, but not limited to, covered under warranty, replaced due to defect, free samples)

⊚ **FC**   Partial credit received for replaced device

❋ **FP**   Service provided as part of family planning program

❋ **G1**   Most recent URR reading of less than 60

IOM: 100-04, 8, 50.9

❋ **G2**   Most recent URR reading of 60 to 64.9

IOM: 100-04, 8, 50.9

❋ **G3**   Most recent URR reading of 65 to 69.9

IOM: 100-04, 8, 50.9

❋ **G4**   Most recent URR reading of 70 to 74.9

IOM: 100-04, 8, 50.9

❋ **G5**   Most recent URR reading of 75 or greater

IOM: 100-04, 8, 50.9

❋ **G6**   ESRD patient for whom less than six dialysis sessions have been provided in a month

IOM: 100-04, 8, 50.9

⊚ **G7**   Pregnancy resulted from rape or incest or pregnancy certified by physician as life threatening

IOM: 100-02, 15, 20.1; 100-03, 3, 170.3

❋ **G8**   Monitored anesthesia care (MAC) for deep complex, complicated, or markedly invasive surgical procedure

❋ **G9**   Monitored anesthesia care for patient who has history of severe cardiopulmonary condition

❋ **GA**   Waiver of liability statement issued as required by payer policy, individual case

An item/service is expected to be denied as not reasonable and necessary and an ABN is on file. Modifier GA can be used on either a specific or a miscellaneous HCPCS code. Modifiers GA and GY should never be reported together on the same line for the same HCPCS code.

❋ **GB**   Claim being resubmitted for payment because it is no longer covered under a global payment demonstration

⊚ **GC**   This service has been performed in part by a resident under the direction of a teaching physician.

IOM: 100-04, 12, 90.4, 100

❋ **GD**   Units of service exceeds medically unlikely edit value and represents reasonable and necessary services

⊚ **GE**   This service has been performed by a resident without the presence of a teaching physician under the primary care exception

❋ **GF**   Non-physician (e.g., nurse practitioner (NP), certified registered nurse anesthetist (CRNA), certified registered nurse (CRN), clinical nurse specialist (CNS), physician assistant (PA)) services in a critical access hospital

❋ **GG**   Performance and payment of a screening mammogram and diagnostic mammogram on the same patient, same day

❋ **GH**   Diagnostic mammogram converted from screening mammogram on same day

❋ **GJ**   "Opt out" physician or practitioner emergency or urgent service

❋ **GK**   Reasonable and necessary item/service associated with a GA or GZ modifier

An upgrade is defined as an item that goes beyond what is medically necessary under Medicare's coverage requirements. An item can be considered an upgrade even if the physician has signed an order for it. When suppliers know that an item will not be paid in full because it does not meet the coverage criteria stated in the LCD, the supplier can still obtain partial payment at the time of initial determination if the claim is billed using one of the upgrade modifiers (GK or GL). (https://www.cms.gov/manuals/downloads/clm104c01.pdf)

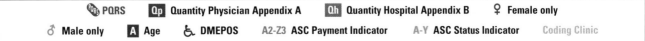

| PQRS | Qp Quantity Physician Appendix A | Qh Quantity Hospital Appendix B | ♀ Female only |
| ♂ Male only | A Age   & DMEPOS | A2-Z3 ASC Payment Indicator   A-Y ASC Status Indicator | Coding Clinic |

LEVEL II NATIONAL MODIFIERS   F3 — GK

97

✳ **GL** Medically unnecessary upgrade provided instead of non-upgraded item, no charge, no Advance Beneficiary Notice (ABN)

✳ **GM** Multiple patients on one ambulance trip

✳ **GN** Services delivered under an outpatient speech language pathology plan of care

✳ **GO** Services delivered under an outpatient occupational therapy plan of care

✳ **GP** Services delivered under an outpatient physical therapy plan of care

✳ **GQ** Via asynchronous telecommunications system

✳ **GR** This service was performed in whole or in part by a resident in a department of Veterans Affairs medical center or clinic, supervised in accordance with VA policy

❂ **GS** Dosage of EPO or erythropoietin-stimulating agent has been reduced and maintained in response to hematocrit or hemoglobin level

❂ **GT** Via interactive audio and video telecommunication systems

✳ **GU** Waiver of liability statement issued as required by payer policy, routine notice

❂ **GV** Attending physician not employed or paid under arrangement by the patient's hospice provider

❂ **GW** Service not related to the hospice patient's terminal condition

✳ **GX** Notice of liability issued, voluntary under payer policy

GX modifier must be submitted with non-covered charges only. This modifier differentiates from the required uses in conjunction with ABN. (https://www.cms.gov/manuals/downloads/clm104c01.pdf)

⊘ **GY** Item or service statutorily excluded, does not meet the definition of any Medicare benefit or, for non-Medicare insurers, is not a contract benefit

Examples of "statutorily excluded" include: Infusion drug not administered using a durable infusion pump, a wheelchair that is for use for mobility outside the home or hearing aids. GA and GY should never be coded together on the same line for the same HCPCS code. (https://www.cms.gov/manuals/downloads/clm104c01.pdf)

⊘ **GZ** Item or service expected to be denied as not reasonable or necessary

Used when an ABN is not on file and can be used on either a specific or a miscellaneous HCPCS code. It would never be correct to place any combination of GY, GZ or GA modifiers on the same claim line and will result in rejected or denied claim for invalid coding. (https://www.cms.gov/manuals/downloads/clm104c01.pdf)

⊘ **H9** Court-ordered

⊘ **HA** Child/adolescent program

⊘ **HB** Adult program, nongeriatric

⊘ **HC** Adult program, geriatric

⊘ **HD** Pregnant/parenting women's program

⊘ **HE** Mental health program

⊘ **HF** Substance abuse program

⊘ **HG** Opioid addiction treatment program

⊘ **HH** Integrated mental health/substance abuse program

⊘ **HI** Integrated mental health and intellectual disability/developmental disabilities program

⊘ **HJ** Employee assistance program

⊘ **HK** Specialized mental health programs for high-risk populations

⊘ **HL** Intern

⊘ **HM** Less than bachelor degree level

⊘ **HN** Bachelors degree level

⊘ **HO** Masters degree level

⊘ **HP** Doctoral level

⊘ **HQ** Group setting

⊘ **HR** Family/couple with client present

⊘ **HS** Family/couple without client present

⊘ **HT** Multi-disciplinary team

⊘ **HU** Funded by child welfare agency

⊘ **HV** Funded by state addictions agency

⊘ **HW** Funded by state mental health agency

⊘ **HX** Funded by county/local agency

⊘ **HY** Funded by juvenile justice agency

⊘ **HZ** Funded by criminal justice agency

✳ **J1** Competitive acquisition program no-pay submission for a prescription number

✳ **J2** Competitive acquisition program, restocking of emergency drugs after emergency administration

---

▶ **New**   ↻ **Revised**   ✔ **Reinstated**   ~~deleted~~ **Deleted**   ⊘ **Not covered or valid by Medicare**

❂ **Special coverage instructions**   ✳ **Carrier discretion**   Ⓑ **Bill local carrier**   Ⓑ **Bill DME MAC**

* **J3** Competitive acquisition program (CAP), drug not available through CAP as written, reimbursed under average sales price methodology

* **J4** DMEPOS item subject to DMEPOS competitive bidding program that is furnished by a hospital upon discharge

* **JA** Administered intravenously

  This modifier is informational only (not a payment modifier) and may be submitted with all injection codes. According to Medicare, reporting this modifier is voluntary. (CMS Pub. 100-04, chapter 8, section 60.2.3.1 and Pub. 100-04, chapter 17, section 80.11)

* **JB** Administered subcutaneously

* **JC** Skin substitute used as a graft

* **JD** Skin substitute not used as a graft

* **JE** Administered via dialysate

* **JW** Drug amount discarded/not administered to any patient

  Use JW to identify unused drugs or biologicals from single use vial/package that are appropriately discarded. Bill on separate line for payment of discarded drug/biological.

  IOM: 100-04, 17, 40

  Coding Clinic: 2010, Q3, P10

* **K0** Lower extremity prosthesis functional Level 0 - does not have the ability or potential to ambulate or transfer safely with or without assistance and a prosthesis does not enhance their quality of life or mobility.

* **K1** Lower extremity prosthesis functional Level 1 - has the ability or potential to use a prosthesis for transfers or ambulation on level surfaces at fixed cadence. Typical of the limited and unlimited household ambulator.

* **K2** Lower extremity prosthesis functional Level 2 - has the ability or potential for ambulation with the ability to traverse low level environmental barriers such as curbs, stairs or uneven surfaces. Typical of the limited community ambulator.

* **K3** Lower extremity prosthesis functional Level 3 - has the ability or potential for ambulation with variable cadence. Typical of the community ambulator who has the ability to traverse most environmental barriers and may have vocational, therapeutic, or exercise activity that demands prosthetic utilization beyond simple locomotion.

* **K4** Lower extremity prosthesis functional Level 4 - has the ability or potential for prosthetic ambulation that exceeds the basic ambulation skills, exhibiting high impact, stress, or energy levels, typical of the prosthetic demands of the child, active adult, or athlete.

* **KA** Add on option/accessory for wheelchair

* **KB** Beneficiary requested upgrade for ABN, more than 4 modifiers identified on claim

* **KC** Replacement of special power wheelchair interface

* **KD** Drug or biological infused through DME

* **KE** Bid under round one of the DMEPOS competitive bidding program for use with non-competitive bid base equipment

* **KF** Item designated by FDA as Class III device

* **KG** DMEPOS item subject to DMEPOS competitive bidding program number 1

* **KH** DMEPOS item, initial claim, purchase or first month rental

* **KI** DMEPOS item, second or third month rental

* **KJ** DMEPOS item, parenteral enteral nutrition (PEN) pump or capped rental, months four to fifteen

* **KK** DMEPOS item subject to DMEPOS competitive bidding program number 2

* **KL** DMEPOS item delivered via mail

* **KM** Replacement of facial prosthesis including new impression/moulage

* **KN** Replacement of facial prosthesis using previous master model

* **KO** Single drug unit dose formulation

* **KP** First drug of a multiple drug unit dose formulation

* **KQ** Second or subsequent drug of a multiple drug unit dose formulation

* **KR** Rental item, billing for partial month

○ **KS** Glucose monitor supply for diabetic beneficiary not treated with insulin

* **KT** Beneficiary resides in a competitive bidding area and travels outside that competitive bidding area and receives a competitive bid item

* **KU** DMEPOS item subject to DMEPOS competitive bidding program number 3

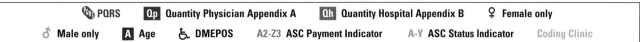

✳ **KV** DMEPOS item subject to DMEPOS competitive bidding program that is furnished as part of a professional service

✳ **KW** DMEPOS item subject to DMEPOS competitive bidding program number 4

✳ **KX** Requirements specified in the medical policy have been met

Used for physical, occupational, or speech-language therapy to request an exception to therapy payment caps and indicate the services are reasonable and necessary and that there is documentation of medical necessity in the patient's medical record. (Pub 100-04 Attachment-Business Requirements Centers for Medicare and Medicaid Services, Transmittal 2457, April 27, 2012)

✳ **KY** DMEPOS item subject to DMEPOS competitive bidding program number 5

✳ **KZ** New coverage not implemented by managed care

▶ ✳ **L1** Provider attestation that the hospital laboratory test(s) is not packaged under the hospital OPPS

✳ **LC** Left circumflex coronary artery

✳ **LD** Left anterior descending coronary artery

✳ **LL** Lease/rental (use the LL modifier when DME equipment rental is to be applied against the purchase price)

✳ **LM** Left main coronary artery

✳ **LR** Laboratory round trip

◎ **LS** FDA-monitored intraocular lens implant

✳ **LT** Left side (used to identify procedures performed on the left side of the body)

✳ **M2** Medicare secondary payer (MSP)

✳ **MS** Six month maintenance and servicing fee for reasonable and necessary parts and labor which are not covered under any manufacturer or supplier warranty

✳ **NB** Nebulizer system, any type, FDA-cleared for use with specific drug

✳ **NR** New when rented (use the NR modifier when DME which was new at the time of rental is subsequently purchased)

✳ **NU** New equipment

✳ **P1** A normal healthy patient

✳ **P2** A patient with mild systemic disease

✳ **P3** A patient with severe systemic disease

✳ **P4** A patient with severe systemic disease that is a constant threat to life

✳ **P5** A moribund patient who is not expected to survive without the operation

✳ **P6** A declared brain-dead patient whose organs are being removed for donor purposes

⊘ **PA** Surgical or other invasive procedure on wrong body part

⊘ **PB** Surgical or other invasive procedure on wrong patient

⊘ **PC** Wrong surgery or other invasive procedure on patient

✳ **PD** Diagnostic or related non diagnostic item or service provided in a wholly owned or operated entity to a patient who is admitted as an inpatient within 3 days

✳ **PI** Positron emission tomography (PET) or PET/computed tomography (CT) to inform the initial treatment strategy of tumors that are biopsy proven or strongly suspected of being cancerous based on other diagnostic testing

✳ **PL** Progressive addition lenses

✳ **PM** Post mortem

▶ ✳ **PO** Services, procedures and/or surgeries provided at off-campus provider-based outpatient departments

✳ **PS** Positron emission tomography (PET) or PET/computed tomography (CT) to inform the subsequent treatment strategy of cancerous tumors when the beneficiary's treating physician determines that the PET study is needed to inform subsequent anti-tumor strategy

✳ **PT** Colorectal cancer screening test; converted to diagnostic text or other procedure

Assign this modifier with the appropriate CPT procedure code for colonoscopy, flexible sigmoidoscopy, or barium enema when the service is initiated as a colorectal cancer screening service but then becomes a diagnostic service. (MLN Matters article MM7012 (PDF, 75 KB) Coding Clinic: 2011, Q1, P10

◎ **Q0** Investigational clinical service provided in a clinical research study that is in an approved clinical research study

◎ **Q1** Routine clinical service provided in a clinical research study that is in an approved clinical research study

✳ **Q2** HCFA/ORD demonstration project procedure/service

✳ **Q3** Live kidney donor surgery and related services

▶ New	↻ Revised	✔ Reinstated	̶d̶e̶l̶e̶t̶e̶d̶ Deleted	⊘ Not covered or valid by Medicare
◎ Special coverage instructions		✳ Carrier discretion	⑧ Bill local carrier	⑨ Bill DME MAC

✳ **Q4**   Service for ordering/referring physician qualifies as a service exemption

⚙ **Q5**   Service furnished by a substitute physician under a reciprocal billing arrangement

IOM: 100-04, 1, 30.2.10

⚙ **Q6**   Service furnished by a locum tenens physician

IOM: 100-04, 1, 30.2.11

✳ **Q7**   One Class A finding

✳ **Q8**   Two Class B findings

✳ **Q9**   One Class B and two Class C findings

✳ **QC**   Single channel monitoring

✳ **QD**   Recording and storage in solid state memory by a digital recorder

✳ **QE**   Prescribed amount of oxygen is less than 1 liter per minute (LPM)

✳ **QF**   Prescribed amount of oxygen exceeds 4 liters per minute (LPM) and portable oxygen is prescribed

✳ **QG**   Prescribed amount of oxygen is greater than 4 liters per minute (LPM)

✳ **QH**   Oxygen conserving device is being used with an oxygen delivery system

⚙ **QJ**   Services/items provided to a prisoner or patient in state or local custody, however, the state or local government, as applicable, meets the requirements in 42 CFR 411.4 (B)

⚙ **QK**   Medical direction of two, three, or four concurrent anesthesia procedures involving qualified individuals

IOM: 100-04, 12, 50K, 90

✳ **QL**   Patient pronounced dead after ambulance called

✳ **QM**   Ambulance service provided under arrangement by a provider of services

✳ **QN**   Ambulance service furnished directly by a provider of services

⚙ **QP**   Documentation is on file showing that the laboratory test(s) was ordered individually or ordered as a CPT-recognized panel other than automated profile codes 80002-80019, G0058, G0059, and G0060.

⚙ **QS**   Monitored anesthesia care service

IOM: 100-04, 12, 30.6, 501

✳ **QT**   Recording and storage on tape by an analog tape recorder

✳ **QW**   CLIA-waived test

✳ **QX**   CRNA service: with medical direction by a physician

⚙ **QY**   Medical direction of one certified registered nurse anesthetist (CRNA) by an anesthesiologist

IOM: 100-04, 12, 50K, 90

✳ **QZ**   CRNA service: without medical direction by a physician

✳ **RA**   Replacement of a DME, orthotic or prosthetic item

Contractors will deny claims for replacement parts when furnished in conjunction with the repair of a capped rental item and billed with modifier -RB, including claims for parts submitted using code E1399, that are billed during the capped rental period (i.e., the last day of the 13th month of continuous use or before). Repair includes all maintenance, servicing, and repair of capped rental DME because it is included in the allowed rental payment amounts. (Pub 100-20 One-Time Notification Centers for Medicare & Medicaid Services, Transmittal: 901, May 13, 2011)

✳ **RB**   Replacement of a part of a DME, orthotic or prosthetic item furnished as part of a repair

✳ **RC**   Right coronary artery

✳ **RD**   Drug provided to beneficiary, but not administered "incident-to"

✳ **RE**   Furnished in full compliance with FDA-mandated risk evaluation and mitigation strategy (REMS)

✳ **RI**   Ramus intermedius coronary artery

✳ **RR**   Rental (use the 'RR' modifier when DME is to be rented)

✳ **RT**   Right side (used to identify procedures performed on the right side of the body)

⊘ **SA**   Nurse practitioner rendering service in collaboration with a physician

⊘ **SB**   Nurse midwife

✳ **SC**   Medically necessary service or supply

⊘ **SD**   Services provided by registered nurse with specialized, highly technical home infusion training

⊘ **SE**   State and/or federally funded programs/services

✳ **SF**   Second opinion ordered by a professional review organization (PRO) per Section 9401, P.L. 99-272 (100% reimbursement - no Medicare deductible or coinsurance)

✳ **SG**   Ambulatory surgical center (ASC) facility service

⊘ **SH** Second concurrently administered infusion therapy

⊘ **SJ** Third or more concurrently administered infusion therapy

⊘ **SK** Member of high risk population (use only with codes for immunization)

⊘ **SL** State supplied vaccine

⊘ **SM** Second surgical opinion

⊘ **SN** Third surgical opinion

⊘ **SQ** Item ordered by home health

⊘ **SS** Home infusion services provided in the infusion suite of the IV therapy provider

⊘ **ST** Related to trauma or injury

⊘ **SU** Procedure performed in physician's office (to denote use of facility and equipment)

⊘ **SV** Pharmaceuticals delivered to patient's home but not utilized

✳ **SW** Services provided by a certified diabetic educator

⊘ **SY** Persons who are in close contact with member of high-risk population (use only with codes for immunization)

▶ ✳ **SZ** Habilitative services

✳ **T1** Left foot, second digit

✳ **T2** Left foot, third digit

✳ **T3** Left foot, fourth digit

✳ **T4** Left foot, fifth digit

✳ **T5** Right foot, great toe

✳ **T6** Right foot, second digit

✳ **T7** Right foot, third digit

✳ **T8** Right foot, fourth digit

✳ **T9** Right foot, fifth digit

✳ **TA** Left foot, great toe

✳ **TC** Technical component; Under certain circumstances, a charge may be made for the technical component alone; under those circumstances the technical component charge is identified by adding modifier TC to the usual procedure number; technical component charges are institutional charges and not billed separately by physicians; however, portable x-ray suppliers only bill for technical component and should utilize modifier TC; the charge data from portable x-ray suppliers will then be used to build customary and prevailing profiles.

⊘ **TD** RN

⊘ **TE** LPN/LVN

⊘ **TF** Intermediate level of care

⊘ **TG** Complex/high tech level of care

⊘ **TH** Obstetrical treatment/services, prenatal or postpartum

⊘ **TJ** Program group, child and/or adolescent

⊘ **TK** Extra patient or passenger, non-ambulance

⊘ **TL** Early intervention/individualized family service plan (IFSP)

⊘ **TM** Individualized education program (IEP)

⊘ **TN** Rural/outside providers' customary service area

⊘ **TP** Medical transport, unloaded vehicle

⊘ **TQ** Basic life support transport by a volunteer ambulance provider

⊘ **TR** School-based individual education program (IEP) services provided outside the public school district responsible for the student

✳ **TS** Follow-up service

⊘ **TT** Individualized service provided to more than one patient in same setting

⊘ **TU** Special payment rate, overtime

⊘ **TV** Special payment rates, holidays/weekends

⊘ **TW** Back-up equipment

⊘ **U1** Medicaid Level of Care 1, as defined by each State

⊘ **U2** Medicaid Level of Care 2, as defined by each State

⊘ **U3** Medicaid Level of Care 3, as defined by each State

⊘ **U4** Medicaid Level of Care 4, as defined by each State

⊘ **U5** Medicaid Level of Care 5, as defined by each State

⊘ **U6** Medicaid Level of Care 6, as defined by each State

⊘ **U7** Medicaid Level of Care 7, as defined by each State

⊘ **U8** Medicaid Level of Care 8, as defined by each State

⊘ **U9** Medicaid Level of Care 9, as defined by each State

⊘ **UA** Medicaid Level of Care 10, as defined by each State

⊘ **UB** Medicaid Level of Care 11, as defined by each State

⊘ **UC** Medicaid Level of Care 12, as defined by each State

▶ **New**   ↵ **Revised**   ✔ **Reinstated**   ~~deleted~~ **Deleted**   ⊘ **Not covered or valid by Medicare**

⊛ **Special coverage instructions**   ✳ **Carrier discretion**   ⑧ **Bill local carrier**   ⑧ **Bill DME MAC**

SH – UC   LEVEL II NATIONAL MODIFIERS

⊘ **UD**   Medicaid Level of Care 13, as defined by each State

✳ **UE**   Used durable medical equipment

⊘ **UF**   Services provided in the morning

⊘ **UG**   Services provided in the afternoon

⊘ **UH**   Services provided in the evening

⊘ **UJ**   Services provided at night

⊘ **UK**   Services provided on behalf of the client to someone other than the client (collateral relationship)

✳ **UN**   Two patients served

✳ **UP**   Three patients served

✳ **UQ**   Four patients served

✳ **UR**   Five patients served

✳ **US**   Six or more patients served

✳ **V5**   Vascular catheter (alone or with any other vascular access)

✳ **V6**   Arteriovenous graft (or other vascular access not including a vascular catheter)

✳ **V7**   Arteriovenous fistula only (in use with two needles)

✳ **VP**   Aphakic patient

▶ ✳ **XE**   Separate encounter, a service that is distinct because it occurred during a separate encounter

▶ ✳ **XP**   Separate practitioner, a service that is distinct because it was performed by a different practitioner

▶ ✳ **XS**   Separate structure, a service that is distinct because it was performed on a separate organ/structure

▶ ✳ **XU**   Unusual non-overlapping service, the use of a service that is distinct because it does not overlap usual components of the main service

Ambulance Modifiers

Modifiers that are used on claims for ambulance services are created by combining two alpha characters. Each alpha character, with the exception of X, represents an origin (source) code or a destination code. The pair of alpha codes creates one modifier. The first position alpha-code = origin; the second position alpha-code = destination. On form CMS-1500, used to report ambulance services, Item 12 should contain the origin code and Item 13 should contain the destination code. Origin and destination codes and their descriptions are as follows:

D   Diagnostic or therapeutic site other than P or H when these are used as origin codes

E   Residential, domiciliary, custodial facility (other than an 1819 facility)

G   Hospital-based dialysis facility (hospital or hospital related)

H   Hospital

I   Site of transfer (e.g., airport or helicopter pad) between modes of ambulance transport

J   Non–hospital-based dialysis facility

N   Skilled nursing facility (SNF) (1819 facility)

P   Physician's office (includes HMO non-hospital facility, clinic, etc.)

R   Residence

S   Scene of accident or acute event

X   Destination code only. Intermediate stop at physician's office en route to the hospital (includes non-hospital facility, clinic, etc.)

TRANSPORT SERVICES INCLUDING AMBULANCE (A0000-A0999)

⊘ **A0021**   Ambulance service, outside state per mile, transport (Medicaid only) ⓑ   E
Cross Reference A0030

⊘ **A0080**   Non-emergency transportation, per mile - vehicle provided by volunteer (individual or organization), with no vested interest ⓑ   E

⊘ **A0090**   Non-emergency transportation, per mile - vehicle provided by individual (family member, self, neighbor) with vested interest ⓑ   E

⊘ **A0100**   Non-emergency transportation; taxi ⓑ   E

⊘ **A0110**   Non-emergency transportation and bus, intra or inter state carrier ⓑ   E

⊘ **A0120**   Non-emergency transportation: mini-bus, mountain area transports, or other transportation systems ⓑ   E

⊘ **A0130**   Non-emergency transportation: wheel chair van ⓑ   E

⊘ **A0140**   Non-emergency transportation and air travel (private or commercial), intra or inter state ⓑ   E

⊘ **A0160**   Non-emergency transportation: per mile - caseworker or social worker ⓑ   E

⊘ **A0170**   Transportation: ancillary: parking fees, tolls, other ⓑ   E

⊘ **A0180**   Non-emergency transportation: ancillary: lodging - recipient ⓑ   E

⊘ **A0190**   Non-emergency transportation: ancillary: meals - recipient ⓑ   E

⊘ **A0200**   Non-emergency transportation: ancillary: lodging - escort ⓑ   E

⊘ **A0210**   Non-emergency transportation: ancillary: meals - escort ⓑ   E

⊘ **A0225**   Ambulance service, neonatal transport, base rate, emergency transport, one way ⓑ   E

⊘ **A0380**   BLS mileage (per mile) ⓑ   E
Cross Reference A0425

✱ **A0382**   BLS routine disposable supplies ⓑ Qp Qh   E

✱ **A0384**   BLS specialized service disposable supplies; defibrillation (used by ALS ambulances and BLS ambulances in jurisdictions where defibrillation is permitted in BLS ambulances) ⓑ Qp Qh   E

⊘ **A0390**   ALS mileage (per mile) ⓑ   E
Cross Reference A0425

⊘ **A0392**   ALS specialized service disposable supplies; defibrillation (to be used only in jurisdictions where defibrillation cannot be performed in BLS ambulances) ⓑ Qp Qh   E

⊘ **A0394**   ALS specialized service disposable supplies; IV drug therapy ⓑ Qp Qh   E

⊘ **A0396**   ALS specialized service disposable supplies; esophageal intubation ⓑ Qp Qh   E

⊘ **A0398**   ALS routine disposable supplies ⓑ Qp Qh   E

▶ **New**   ↻ **Revised**   ✔ **Reinstated**   ~~deleted~~ **Deleted**   ⊘ **Not covered or valid by Medicare**   ⊙ **Special coverage instructions**   ✱ **Carrier discretion**   ⓑ **Bill local carrier**   ⓑ **Bill DME MAC**

A0021 – A0398   TRANSPORT SERVICES INCLUDING AMBULANCE

104

⊘ **A0420** Ambulance waiting time (ALS or BLS), one half (½) hour increments Ⓑ Qp Qh   E

Waiting Time Table			
UNITS	**TIME**	**UNITS**	**TIME**
1	½ to 1 hr.	6	3 to 3½ hrs.
2	1 to 1½ hrs.	7	3½ to 4 hrs.
3	1½ to 2 hrs.	8	4 to 4½ hrs.
4	2 to 2½ hrs.	9	4½ to 5 hrs.
5	2½ to 3 hrs.	10	5 to 5½ hrs.

⊘ **A0422** Ambulance (ALS or BLS) oxygen and oxygen supplies, life sustaining situation Ⓑ Qp Qh   E

⊘ **A0424** Extra ambulance attendant, ground (ALS or BLS) or air (fixed or rotary winged); (requires medical review) Ⓑ Qp Qh   E

✳ **A0425** Ground mileage, per statute mile   A

✳ **A0426** Ambulance service, advanced life support, non-emergency transport, Level 1 (ALS1) Ⓑ Qp Qh   A

✳ **A0427** Ambulance service, advanced life support, emergency transport, Level 1 (ALS1-Emergency) Ⓑ Qp Qh   A

✳ **A0428** Ambulance service, basic life support, non-emergency transport (BLS) Ⓑ Qp Qh   A

✳ **A0429** Ambulance service, basic life support, emergency transport (BLS-Emergency) Ⓑ Qp Qh   A

✳ **A0430** Ambulance service, conventional air services, transport, one way (fixed wing) Ⓑ Qp Qh   A

✳ **A0431** Ambulance service, conventional air services, transport, one way (rotary wing) Ⓑ Qp Qh   A

✳ **A0432** Paramedic intercept (PI), rural area, transport furnished by a volunteer ambulance company, which is prohibited by state law from billing third party payers Ⓑ Qp Qh   A

✳ **A0433** Advanced life support, Level 2 (ALS2) Ⓑ Qp Qh   A

✳ **A0434** Specialty care transport (SCT) Ⓑ Qp Qh   A

✳ **A0435** Fixed wing air mileage, per statute mile Ⓑ Qp Qh   A

✳ **A0436** Rotary wing air mileage, per statute mile Ⓑ Qp Qh   A

⊘ **A0888** Noncovered ambulance mileage, per mile (e.g., for miles traveled beyond closest appropriate facility) Ⓑ   E

MCM 2125

⊘ **A0998** Ambulance response and treatment, no transport Ⓑ   E

IOM: 100-02, 10, 20

⊙ **A0999** Unlisted ambulance service Ⓑ   A

IOM: 100-02, 10, 20

MEDICAL AND SURGICAL SUPPLIES (A4000-A6513)

✳ **A4206** Syringe with needle, sterile 1cc or less, each Ⓑ   N

If "incident to" a physician's service, do not bill.

✳ **A4207** Syringe with needle, sterile 2cc, each Ⓑ   N

If "incident to" a physician's service, do not bill.

✳ **A4208** Syringe with needle, sterile 3cc, each Ⓑ   N

If "incident to" a physician's service, do not bill.

✳ **A4209** Syringe with needle, sterile 5cc or greater, each Ⓑ   N

If "incident to" a physician's service, do not bill.

⊘ **A4210** Needle-free injection device, each Ⓑ   E

IOM: 100-03, 4, 280.1

⊙ **A4211** Supplies for self-administered injections Ⓑ   N

If "incident to" a physician service, do not bill.

IOM: 100-02, 15, 50

✳ **A4212** Non-coring needle or stylet with or without catheter Ⓑ   N

✳ **A4213** Syringe, sterile, 20 cc or greater, each Ⓑ   N

If "incident to" a physician service, do not bill.

✳ **A4215** Needle, sterile, any size, each Ⓑ   N

If "incident to" a physician service, do not bill.

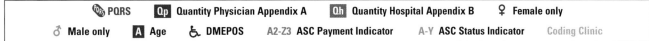

✪ **A4216**   Sterile water, saline and/or dextrose diluent/flush, 10 ml ⑧ &   N

If "incident to" a physician service, do not bill.

Other: Broncho Saline, Monoject Prefill advanced, Sodium Chloride, Sodium Chloride Bacteriostatic, Syrex, Vasceze Sodium Chloride, Water for Injection Bacteriostatic

IOM: 100-02, 15, 50

✪ **A4217**   Sterile water/saline, 500 ml ⑧ &   N

If "incident to" a physician service, do not bill.

Other: Sodium Chloride

IOM: 100-02, 15, 50

DMEPOS Modifier(s): AU

✪ **A4218**   Sterile saline or water, metered dose dispenser, 10 ml ⑧   N1 N

If "incident to" a physician service, do not bill.

Other: Sodium Chloride

✪ **A4220**   Refill kit for implantable infusion pump ⑧   N1 N

Do not report with 95990 or 95991 since Medicare payment for these codes includes the refill kit.

IOM: 100-03, 4, 280.1

✳ **A4221**   Supplies for maintenance of drug infusion catheter, per week (list drug separately) ⑧ Qp Qh &   N

If "incident to" a physician service, do not bill. Includes dressings for catheter site and flush solutions not directly related to drug infusion

✳ **A4222**   Infusion supplies for external drug infusion pump, per cassette or bag (list drug separately) ⑧ Qh &   N

If "incident to" physician service, do not bill. Includes cassette or bag, diluting solutions, tubing and/or administration supplies, port cap changes, compounding charges, and preparation charges.

✳ **A4223**   Infusion supplies not used with external infusion pump, per cassette or bag (list drugs separately) ⑧   N

If "incident to" physician service, do not bill.

IOM: 100-03, 4, 280.1

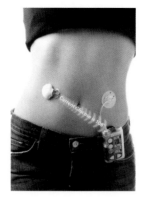

Figure 1   Insulin pump.

✪ **A4230**   Infusion set for external insulin pump, non-needle cannula type ⑧   N

If "incident to" physician service, do not bill. Requires prior authorization and copy of invoice

IOM: 100-03, 4, 280.1

✪ **A4231**   Infusion set for external insulin pump, needle type ⑧   N

If "incident to" physician service, do not bill. Requires prior authorization and copy of invoice

IOM: 100-03, 4, 280.1

⊘ **A4232**   Syringe with needle for external insulin pump, sterile, 3cc ⑧   E

If "incident to" physician service, do not bill. Reports insulin reservoir for use with external insulin infusion pump (E0784); may be glass or plastic; includes needle for drawing up insulin. Does not include insulin for use in reservoir

IOM: 100-03, 4, 280.1

✳ **A4233**   Replacement battery, alkaline (other than J cell), for use with medically necessary home blood glucose monitor owned by patient, each ⑧ Qh &   E

If "incident to" physician service, do not bill.

DMEPOS Modifier(s): NU   KL

✳ **A4234**   Replacement battery, alkaline, J cell, for use with medically necessary home blood glucose monitor owned by patient, each ⑧ Qh &   E

If "incident to" a physician's service, do not bill.

DMEPOS Modifier(s): NU   KL

▶ **New**   ↻ **Revised**   ✔ **Reinstated**   deleted **Deleted**   ⊘ **Not covered or valid by Medicare**
✪ **Special coverage instructions**   ✳ **Carrier discretion**   ⑧ **Bill local carrier**   ⑧ **Bill DME MAC**

106

* A4235 Replacement battery, lithium, for use with medically necessary home blood glucose monitor owned by patient, each Ⓑ **Qp** **Qh** ♿   E

If "incident to" a physician's service, do not bill.

DMEPOS Modifier(s): NU KL

* A4236 Replacement battery, silver oxide, for use with medically necessary home blood glucose monitor owned by patient, each Ⓑ **Qh** ♿   E

If "incident to" a physician's service, do not bill.

DMEPOS Modifier(s): NU KL

* A4244 Alcohol or peroxide, per pint Ⓑ   N

If "incident to" a physician's service, do not bill.

* A4245 Alcohol wipes, per box Ⓑ   N

If "incident to" a physician's service, do not bill.

* A4246 Betadine or pHisoHex solution, per pint Ⓑ   N

If "incident to" a physician's service, do not bill.

* A4247 Betadine or iodine swabs/wipes, per box Ⓑ   N

If "incident to" a physician's service, do not bill.

↻* A4248 Chlorhexidine containing antiseptic, 1 ml Ⓑ   N1 N

If "incident to" a physician's service, do not bill.

⊘ A4250 Urine test or reagent strips or tablets (100 tablets or strips) Ⓑ   E

If "incident to" a physician's service, do not bill.

IOM: 100-02, 15, 110

⊘ A4252 Blood ketone test or reagent strip, each Ⓑ   E

Medicare Statute 1861(n)

⊗ A4253 Blood glucose test or reagent strips for home blood glucose monitor, per 50 strips Ⓑ **Qp** **Qh** ♿   N

Test strips (1 unit = 50 strips); non-insulin treated (every 3 months) 100 test strips (1×/day testing), 100 lancets (1×/day testing); modifier KS

IOM: 100-03, 1, 40.2

DMEPOS Modifier(s): NU KL

⊗ A4255 Platforms for home blood glucose monitor, 50 per box Ⓑ **Qp** **Qh** ♿   N

IOM: 100-03, 1, 40.2

⊗ A4256 Normal, low and high calibrator solution/chips Ⓑ **Qh** ♿   N

IOM: 100-03, 1, 40.2

DMEPOS Modifier(s): KL

* A4257 Replacement lens shield cartridge for use with laser skin piercing device, each Ⓑ **Qp** **Qh** ♿   E

⊗ A4258 Spring-powered device for lancet, each Ⓑ **Qp** **Qh** ♿   N

IOM: 100-03, 1, 40.2

DMEPOS Modifier(s): KL

⊗ A4259 Lancets, per box of 100 Ⓑ **Qp** **Qh** ♿   N

IOM: 100-03, 1, 40.2

DMEPOS Modifier(s): KL

⊘ A4261 Cervical cap for contraceptive use Ⓑ   E

Medicare Statute 1862A1 ♀

⊗ A4262 Temporary, absorbable lacrimal duct implant, each Ⓑ **Qh**   N1 N

⊗ A4263 Permanent, long term, non-dissolvable lacrimal duct implant, each Ⓑ **Qh** N1 N

Bundled with insertion if performed in physician office.

IOM: 100-04, 12, 30.4

⊘ A4264 Permanent implantable contraceptive intratubal occlusion device(s) and delivery system ♀   E

Reports the Essure device.

⊗ A4265 Paraffin, per pound Ⓑ ♿   N

If "incident to" a physician's service, do not bill.

IOM: 100-03, 4, 280.1

⊘ A4266 Diaphragm for contraceptive use Ⓑ ♀   E

⊘ A4267 Contraceptive supply, condom, male, each Ⓑ ♂   E

⊘ A4268 Contraceptive supply, condom, female, each Ⓑ ♀   E

⊘ A4269 Contraceptive supply, spermicide (e.g., foam, gel), each Ⓑ ♀   E

* A4270 Disposable endoscope sheath, each Ⓑ   N1 N

* A4280 Adhesive skin support attachment for use with external breast prosthesis, each Ⓑ ♀ ♿   N

* A4281 Tubing for breast pump, replacement Ⓑ ♀   E

* **A4282** Adapter for breast pump, replacement ⑬ ♀   E

* **A4283** Cap for breast pump bottle, replacement ⑬ ♀   E

* **A4284** Breast shield and splash protector for use with breast pump, replacement ⑬ ♀   E

* **A4285** Polycarbonate bottle for use with breast pump, replacement ⑬ ♀   E

* **A4286** Locking ring for breast pump, replacement ⑬ ♀   E

* **A4290** Sacral nerve stimulation test lead, each ⑬   N

Vascular Catheters

⊘ **A4300** Implantable access catheter, (e.g., venous, arterial, epidural subarachnoid, or peritoneal, etc.) external access ⑬   N1 N

  IOM: 100-02, 15, 120

* **A4301** Implantable access total; catheter, port/reservoir (e.g., venous, arterial, epidural, subarachnoid, peritoneal, etc.) ⑬ **Qp** **Qh**   N1 N

* **A4305** Disposable drug delivery system, flow rate of 50 ml or greater per hour ⑬   N1 N

  If "incident to" a physician's service, do not bill.

* **A4306** Disposable drug delivery system, flow rate of less than 50 ml per hour ⑬   N1 N

  If "incident to" a physician's service, do not bill.

Incontinence Appliances and Care Supplies

A4310-A4355: If provided in the physician's office for a temporary condition, the item is incident to the physician's service and billed to the local carrier (⑬). If provided in the physician's office or other place of service for a permanent condition, the item is a prosthetic device and billed to the DME MAC (⑬).

⊘ **A4310** Insertion tray without drainage bag and without catheter (accessories only) ⑬ ⑬ ♿   N

  IOM: 100-02, 15, 120

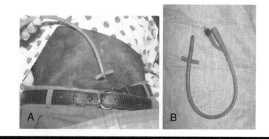

Figure 2 Foley catheter.

⊘ **A4311** Insertion tray without drainage bag with indwelling catheter, Foley type, two-way latex with coating (Teflon, silicone, silicone elastomer, or hydrophilic, etc.) ⑬ ⑬ ♿   N

  IOM: 100-02, 15, 120

⊘ **A4312** Insertion tray without drainage bag with indwelling catheter, Foley type, two-way, all silicone ⑬ ⑬ ♿   N

  Must meet criteria for indwelling catheter and medical record must justify need for:

  • Recurrent encrustation

  • Inability to pass a straight catheter

  • Sensitivity to latex

  Must be medically necessary.

  IOM: 100-02, 15, 120

⊘ **A4313** Insertion tray without drainage bag with indwelling catheter, Foley type, three-way, for continuous irrigation ⑬ ⑬ ♿   N

  Must meet criteria for indwelling catheter and medical record must justify need for:

  • Recurrent encrustation

  • Inability to pass a straight catheter

  • Sensitivity to latex

  Must be medically necessary.

  IOM: 100-02, 15, 120

⊘ **A4314** Insertion tray with drainage bag with indwelling catheter, Foley type, two-way latex with coating (Teflon, silicone, silicone elastomer or hydrophilic, etc.) ⑬ ⑬ ♿   N

  IOM: 100-02, 15, 120

⊘ **A4315** Insertion tray with drainage bag with indwelling catheter, Foley type, two-way, all silicone ⑬ ⑬ ♿   N

  IOM: 100-02, 15, 120

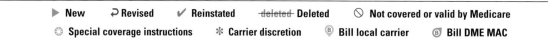

▶ **New**   ↻ **Revised**   ✔ **Reinstated**   ~~deleted~~ **Deleted**   ⊘ **Not covered or valid by Medicare**
⊘ **Special coverage instructions**   ✳ **Carrier discretion**   ⑬ **Bill local carrier**   ⑬ **Bill DME MAC**

⊘ **A4316**   Insertion tray with drainage bag with indwelling catheter, Foley type, three-way, for continuous irrigation Ⓑ Ⓞ ♿   N

IOM: 100-02, 15, 120

⊘ **A4320**   Irrigation tray with bulb or piston syringe, any purpose Ⓟ Ⓑ ♿   N

IOM: 100-02, 15, 120

⊘ **A4321**   Therapeutic agent for urinary catheter irrigation Ⓑ Ⓞ ♿   N

⊘ **A4322**   Irrigation syringe, bulb, or piston, each Ⓟ Ⓑ ♿   N

IOM: 100-02, 15, 120

⊘ **A4326**   Male external catheter with integral collection chamber, any type, each Ⓑ Ⓞ ♂ ♿   N

IOM: 100-02, 15, 120

⊘ **A4327**   Female external urinary collection device; meatal cup, each Ⓟ Ⓑ ♀ ♿   N

IOM: 100-02, 15, 120

⊘ **A4328**   Female external urinary collection device; pouch, each Ⓟ Ⓑ ♀ ♿   N

IOM: 100-02, 15, 120

⊘ **A4330**   Perianal fecal collection pouch with adhesive, each Ⓑ Ⓞ ♿   N

IOM: 100-02, 15, 120

⊘ **A4331**   Extension drainage tubing, any type, any length, with connector/adaptor, for use with urinary leg bag or urostomy pouch, each Ⓑ Ⓞ ♿   N

IOM: 100-02, 15, 120

⊘ **A4332**   Lubricant, individual sterile packet, each Ⓑ Ⓞ ♿   N

IOM: 100-02, 15, 120

⊘ **A4333**   Urinary catheter anchoring device, adhesive skin attachment, each Ⓟ Ⓑ ♿   N

IOM: 100-02, 15, 120

⊘ **A4334**   Urinary catheter anchoring device, leg strap, each Ⓟ Ⓑ ♿   N

IOM: 100-02, 15, 120

⊘ **A4335**   Incontinence supply; miscellaneous Ⓑ Ⓞ   N

IOM: 100-02, 15, 120

⊘ **A4336**   Incontinence supply, urethral insert, any type, each Ⓟ Ⓑ ♿   N1   N

⊘ **A4338**   Indwelling catheter; Foley type, two-way latex with coating (Teflon, silicone, silicone elastomer, or hydrophilic, etc.), each Ⓑ Ⓞ ♿   N

IOM: 100-02, 15, 120

⊘ **A4340**   Indwelling catheter; specialty type (e.g., coude, mushroom, wing, etc.), each Ⓑ Ⓞ ♿   N

Must meet criteria for indwelling catheter and medical record must justify need for:

• Recurrent encrustation

• Inability to pass a straight catheter

• Sensitivity to latex

Must be medically necessary.

IOM: 100-02, 15, 120

⊘ **A4344**   Indwelling catheter, Foley type, two-way, all silicone, each Ⓟ Ⓑ ♿   N

Must meet criteria for indwelling catheter and medical record must justify need for:

• Recurrent encrustation

• Inability to pass a straight catheter

• Sensitivity to latex

Must be medically necessary.

IOM: 100-02, 15, 120

⊘ **A4346**   Indwelling catheter; Foley type, three way for continuous irrigation, each Ⓑ Ⓞ ♿   N

IOM: 100-02, 15, 120

⊘ **A4349**   Male external catheter, with or without adhesive, disposable, each Ⓑ Ⓞ ♂ ♿   N

IOM: 100-02, 15, 120

⊘ **A4351**   Intermittent urinary catheter; straight tip, with or without coating (Teflon, silicone, silicone elastomer, or hydrophilic, etc.), each Ⓟ Ⓑ ♿   N

IOM: 100-02, 15, 120

⊘ **A4352**   Intermittent urinary catheter; coude (curved) tip, with or without coating (Teflon, silicone, silicone elastomeric, or hydrophilic, etc.), each Ⓑ Ⓞ ♿   N

IOM: 100-02, 15, 120

⊘ **A4353**   Intermittent urinary catheter, with insertion supplies Ⓑ Ⓞ ♿   N

IOM: 100-02, 15, 120

⊘ **A4354**   Insertion tray with drainage bag but without catheter Ⓑ Ⓞ ♿   N

IOM: 100-02, 15, 120

⒫ PQRS   Ⓠⓟ Quantity Physician Appendix A   Ⓠⓗ Quantity Hospital Appendix B   ♀ Female only
♂ Male only   Ⓐ Age   ♿ DMEPOS   A2-Z3 ASC Payment Indicator   A-Y ASC Status Indicator   Coding Clinic

⊗ **A4355** Irrigation tubing set for continuous bladder irrigation through a three-way indwelling Foley catheter, each Ⓑ Ⓓ ♿   N

IOM: 100-02, 15, 120

External Urinary Supplies

A4356-A4360: If provided in the physician's office for a temporary condition, the item is incident to the physician's service and billed to the local carrier (Ⓑ). If provided in the physician's office or other place of service for a permanent condition, the item is a prosthetic device and billed to the DME MAC (Ⓓ).

⊗ **A4356** External urethral clamp or compression device (not to be used for catheter clamp), each **Qp** **Qh** ♿   N

IOM: 100-02, 15, 120

⊗ **A4357** Bedside drainage bag, day or night, with or without anti-reflux device, with or without tube, each Ⓑ Ⓓ ♿   N

IOM: 100-02, 15, 120

⊗ **A4358** Urinary drainage bag, leg or abdomen, vinyl, with or without tube, with straps, each Ⓑ Ⓓ ♿   N

IOM: 100-02, 15, 120

⊗ **A4360** Disposable external urethral clamp or compression device, with pad and/or pouch, each Ⓑ Ⓓ ♿   N1   N

Ostomy Supplies

A4361-A4435: If provided in the physician's office for a temporary condition, the item is incident to the physician's service and billed to the local carrier (Ⓑ). If provided in the physician's office or other place of service for a permanent condition, the item is a prosthetic device and billed to the DME MAC (Ⓓ).

⊗ **A4361** Ostomy faceplate, each Ⓑ Ⓓ ♿   N

IOM: 100-02, 15, 120

⊗ **A4362** Skin barrier; solid, 4 × 4 or equivalent; each Ⓑ Ⓓ ♿   N

IOM: 100-02, 15, 120

⊗ **A4363** Ostomy clamp, any type, replacement only, each Ⓑ Ⓓ ♿   E

⊗ **A4364** Adhesive, liquid or equal, any type, per oz Ⓑ Ⓓ ♿   N

Fee schedule category: Ostomy, tracheostomy, and urologicals items.

IOM: 100-02, 15, 120

✳ **A4366** Ostomy vent, any type, each Ⓑ Ⓓ ♿   N

⊗ **A4367** Ostomy belt, each Ⓑ Ⓓ ♿   N

IOM: 100-02, 15, 120

✳ **A4368** Ostomy filter, any type, each Ⓑ Ⓓ ♿   N

⊗ **A4369** Ostomy skin barrier, liquid (spray, brush, etc), per oz Ⓑ Ⓓ ♿   N

IOM: 100-02, 15, 120

⊗ **A4371** Ostomy skin barrier, powder, per oz Ⓑ Ⓓ ♿   N

IOM: 100-02, 15, 120

⊗ **A4372** Ostomy skin barrier, solid 4 × 4 or equivalent, standard wear, with built-in convexity, each Ⓑ Ⓓ ♿   N

IOM: 100-02, 15, 120

⊗ **A4373** Ostomy skin barrier, with flange (solid, flexible, or accordian), with built-in convexity, any size, each Ⓑ Ⓓ ♿   N

IOM: 100-02, 15, 120

⊗ **A4375** Ostomy pouch, drainable, with faceplate attached, plastic, each Ⓑ Ⓓ ♿   N

IOM: 100-02, 15, 120

⊗ **A4376** Ostomy pouch, drainable, with faceplate attached, rubber, each Ⓑ Ⓓ ♿   N

IOM: 100-02, 15, 120

⊗ **A4377** Ostomy pouch, drainable, for use on faceplate, plastic, each Ⓑ Ⓓ ♿   N

IOM: 100-02, 15, 120

⊗ **A4378** Ostomy pouch, drainable, for use on faceplate, rubber, each Ⓑ Ⓓ ♿   N

IOM: 100-02, 15, 120

✳ **A4379** Ostomy pouch, urinary, with faceplate attached, plastic, each Ⓑ Ⓓ ♿   N

IOM: 100-02, 15, 120

⊗ **A4380** Ostomy pouch, urinary, with faceplate attached, rubber, each Ⓑ Ⓓ ♿   N

IOM: 100-02, 15, 120

⊗ **A4381** Ostomy pouch, urinary, for use on faceplate, plastic, each Ⓑ Ⓓ ♿   N

IOM: 100-02, 15, 120

⊗ **A4382** Ostomy pouch, urinary, for use on faceplate, heavy plastic, each Ⓑ Ⓓ ♿   N

IOM: 100-02, 15, 120

⊗ **A4383** Ostomy pouch, urinary, for use on faceplate, rubber, each Ⓑ Ⓓ ♿   N

IOM: 100-02, 15, 120

▶ **New**   ↻ **Revised**   ✔ **Reinstated**   ~~deleted~~ **Deleted**   ⊘ **Not covered or valid by Medicare**
⊗ **Special coverage instructions**   ✳ **Carrier discretion**   Ⓑ **Bill local carrier**   Ⓓ **Bill DME MAC**

⊚ **A4384** Ostomy faceplate equivalent, silicone ring, each Ⓑ Ⓑ ♿   N
IOM: 100-02, 15, 120

⊚ **A4385** Ostomy skin barrier, solid 4 × 4 or equivalent, extended wear, without built-in convexity, each Ⓑ Ⓑ ♿   N
IOM: 100-02, 15, 120

⊚ **A4387** Ostomy pouch closed, with barrier attached, with built-in convexity (1 piece), each Ⓑ Ⓑ ♿   N
IOM: 100-02, 15, 120

⊚ **A4388** Ostomy pouch, drainable, with extended wear barrier attached (1 piece), each Ⓑ Ⓑ ♿   N
IOM: 100-02, 15, 120

⊚ **A4389** Ostomy pouch, drainable, with barrier attached, with built-in convexity (1 piece), each Ⓑ Ⓑ ♿   N
IOM: 100-02, 15, 120

⊚ **A4390** Ostomy pouch, drainable, with extended wear barrier attached, with built-in convexity (1 piece), each Ⓑ Ⓑ ♿   N
IOM: 100-02, 15, 120

⊚ **A4391** Ostomy pouch, urinary, with extended wear barrier attached (1 piece), each Ⓑ Ⓑ ♿   N
IOM: 100-02, 15, 120

⊚ **A4392** Ostomy pouch, urinary, with standard wear barrier attached, with built-in convexity (1 piece), each Ⓑ Ⓑ ♿   N
IOM: 100-02, 15, 120

⊚ **A4393** Ostomy pouch, urinary, with extended wear barrier attached, with built-in convexity (1 piece), each Ⓑ Ⓑ ♿   N
IOM: 100-02, 15, 120

⊚ **A4394** Ostomy deodorant, with or without lubricant, for use in ostomy pouch, per fluid ounce Ⓑ Ⓑ ♿   N
IOM: 100-02, 15, 20

⊚ **A4395** Ostomy deodorant for use in ostomy pouch, solid, per tablet Ⓑ Ⓑ ♿   N
IOM: 100-02, 15, 20

⊚ **A4396** Ostomy belt with peristomal hernia support Ⓑ Ⓑ Qh ♿   N
IOM: 100-02, 15, 120

⊚ **A4397** Irrigation supply; sleeve, each Ⓑ Ⓑ ♿   N
IOM: 100-02, 15, 120

⊚ **A4398** Ostomy irrigation supply; bag, each Ⓑ Ⓑ ♿   N
IOM: 100-02, 15, 120

⊚ **A4399** Ostomy irrigation supply; cone/catheter, with or without brush Ⓑ Ⓑ Qh ♿   N
IOM: 100-02, 15, 120

⊚ **A4400** Ostomy irrigation set Ⓑ Ⓑ ♿   N
IOM: 100-02, 15, 120

⊚ **A4402** Lubricant, per ounce Ⓑ Ⓑ ♿   N
IOM: 100-02, 15, 120

⊚ **A4404** Ostomy ring, each Ⓑ Ⓑ ♿   N
IOM: 100-02, 15, 120

⊚ **A4405** Ostomy skin barrier, non-pectin based, paste, per ounce Ⓑ Ⓑ ♿   N
IOM: 100-02, 15, 120

⊚ **A4406** Ostomy skin barrier, pectin-based, paste, per ounce Ⓑ Ⓑ ♿   N
IOM: 100-02, 15, 120

⊚ **A4407** Ostomy skin barrier, with flange (solid, flexible, or accordion), extended wear, with built-in convexity, 4 × 4 inches or smaller, each Ⓑ Ⓑ ♿   N

⊚ **A4408** Ostomy skin barrier, with flange (solid, flexible, or accordion), extended wear, with built-in convexity, larger than 4 × 4 inches, each Ⓑ Ⓑ ♿   N
IOM: 100-02, 15, 120

⊚ **A4409** Ostomy skin barrier, with flange (solid, flexible, or accordion), extended wear, without built-in convexity, 4 × 4 inches or smaller, each Ⓑ Ⓑ ♿   N
IOM: 100-02, 15, 120

⊚ **A4410** Ostomy skin barrier, with flange (solid, flexible, or accordion), extended wear, without built-in convexity, larger than 4 × 4 inches, each Ⓑ Ⓑ ♿   N
IOM: 100-02, 15, 120

⊚ **A4411** Ostomy skin barrier, solid 4 × 4 or equivalent, extended wear, with built-in convexity, each Ⓑ Ⓑ ♿   N

⊚ **A4412** Ostomy pouch, drainable, high output, for use on a barrier with flange (2 piece system), without filter, each Ⓑ Ⓑ ♿   N

⊚ **A4413** Ostomy pouch, drainable, high output, for use on a barrier with flange (2 piece system), with filter, each Ⓑ Ⓑ ♿   N
IOM: 100-02, 15, 120

PQRS	Qp Quantity Physician Appendix A	Qh Quantity Hospital Appendix B	♀ Female only
♂ Male only	A Age	♿ DMEPOS	A2-Z3 ASC Payment Indicator	A-Y ASC Status Indicator	Coding Clinic

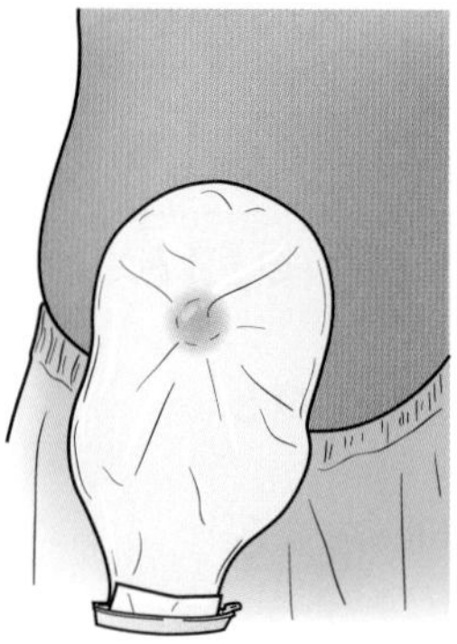

Figure 3 Ostomy pouch.

◌ **A4414** Ostomy skin barrier, with flange (solid, flexible, or accordion), without built-in convexity, 4 × 4 inches or smaller, each Ⓑ Ⓓ ♿ N

IOM: 100-02, 15, 120

◌ **A4415** Ostomy skin barrier, with flange (solid, flexible, or accordion), without built-in convexity, larger than 4 × 4 inches, each Ⓑ Ⓓ ♿ N

IOM: 100-02, 15, 120

* **A4416** Ostomy pouch, closed, with barrier attached, with filter (1 piece), each Ⓑ Ⓓ ♿ N

* **A4417** Ostomy pouch, closed, with barrier attached, with built-in convexity, with filter (1 piece), each Ⓑ Ⓓ ♿ N

* **A4418** Ostomy pouch, closed; without barrier attached, with filter (1 piece), each Ⓑ Ⓓ ♿ N

* **A4419** Ostomy pouch, closed; for use on barrier with non-locking flange, with filter (2 piece), each Ⓑ Ⓓ ♿ N

* **A4420** Ostomy pouch, closed; for use on barrier with locking flange (2 piece), each Ⓑ Ⓓ ♿ N

* **A4421** Ostomy supply; miscellaneous Ⓑ Ⓓ E

◌ **A4422** Ostomy absorbent material (sheet/pad/crystal packet) for use in ostomy pouch to thicken liquid stomal output, each Ⓑ Ⓓ ♿ N

IOM: 100-02, 15, 120

* **A4423** Ostomy pouch, closed; for use on barrier with locking flange, with filter (2 piece), each Ⓑ Ⓓ ♿ N

* **A4424** Ostomy pouch, drainable, with barrier attached, with filter (1 piece), each Ⓑ Ⓓ ♿ N

* **A4425** Ostomy pouch, drainable; for use on barrier with non-locking flange, with filter (2 piece system), each Ⓑ Ⓓ ♿ N

* **A4426** Ostomy pouch, drainable; for use on barrier with locking flange (2 piece system), each Ⓑ Ⓓ ♿ N

* **A4427** Ostomy pouch, drainable; for use on barrier with locking flange, with filter (2 piece system), each Ⓑ Ⓓ ♿ N

* **A4428** Ostomy pouch, urinary, with extended wear barrier attached, with faucet-type tap with valve (1 piece), each Ⓑ Ⓓ ♿ N

* **A4429** Ostomy pouch, urinary, with barrier attached, with built-in convexity, with faucet-type tap with valve (1 piece), each Ⓑ Ⓓ ♿ N

* **A4430** Ostomy pouch, urinary, with extended wear barrier attached, with built-in convexity, with faucet-type tap with valve (1 piece), each Ⓑ Ⓓ ♿ N

* **A4431** Ostomy pouch, urinary; with barrier attached, with faucet-type tap with valve (1 piece), each Ⓑ Ⓓ ♿ N

* **A4432** Ostomy pouch, urinary; for use on barrier with non-locking flange, with faucet-type tap with valve (2 piece), each Ⓑ Ⓓ ♿ N

* **A4433** Ostomy pouch, urinary; for use on barrier with locking flange (2 piece), each Ⓑ Ⓓ ♿ N

* **A4434** Ostomy pouch, urinary; for use on barrier with locking flange, with faucet-type tap with valve (2 piece), each Ⓑ Ⓓ ♿ N

* **A4435** Ostomy pouch, drainable, high output, with extended wear barrier (one-piece system), with or without filter, each Ⓑ Ⓓ ♿ N

Bill local carrier (Ⓑ) for a temporary condition.

Bill DME MAC (Ⓓ) for a permanent condition.

Miscellaneous Supplies

◌ **A4450** Tape, non-waterproof, per 18 square inches Ⓓ ♿ N

If "incident to" physician service, do not bill separately.

If used with surgical dressings, billed with AW modifier (in addition to appropriate A1-A9 modifier).

IOM: 100-02, 15, 120

DMEPOS Modifier(s): AU, AV, AW

▶ New ↻ Revised ✔ Reinstated ~~deleted~~ Deleted ⊘ Not covered or valid by Medicare
◌ Special coverage instructions * Carrier discretion Ⓑ Bill local carrier Ⓓ Bill DME MAC

⊛ **A4452** Tape, waterproof, per 18 square inches ⑧ ♿ N

If "incident to" physician service, do not bill separately.

If used with surgical dressings, billed with AW modifier (in addition to appropriate A1-A9 modifier).

IOM: 100-02, 15, 120

DMEPOS Modifier(s): AU, AV, AW

⊛ **A4455** Adhesive remover or solvent (for tape, cement or other adhesive), per ounce ⑧ ♿ N

If "incident to" a physician service, do not bill.

IOM: 100-02, 15, 120

⊛ **A4456** Adhesive remover, wipes, any type, each ♿ N

May be reimbursed for male or female clients to home health DME providers and DME medical suppliers in the home setting.

✳ **A4458** Enema bag with tubing, reusable ⑧ N

▶✳ **A4459** Manual pump-operated enema system, includes balloon, catheter and all accessories, reusable, any type N1 N

✳ **A4461** Surgical dressing holder, non-reusable, each ⑧ ♿ N

If "incident to" a physician's service, do not bill.

✳ **A4463** Surgical dressing holder, reusable, each ⑧ **Qh** ♿ N

If "incident to" a physician's service, do not bill.

✳ **A4465** Non-elastic binder for extremity ⑧ N

↻⊘ **A4466** Garment, belt, sleeve or other covering, elastic or similar stretchable material, any type, each N1 E

⊛ **A4470** Gravlee jet washer ⑧ **Qp** **Qh** N

Symptoms suggestive of endometrial disease must be present for this disposable diagnostic tool to be covered.

IOM: 100-02, 16, 90; 100-03, 4, 230.5

⊛ **A4480** VABRA aspirator ⑧ **Qp** **Qh** N

Symptoms suggestive of endometrial disease must be present for this disposable diagnostic tool to be covered.

IOM: 100-02, 16, 90; 100-03, 4, 230.6

⊛ **A4481** Tracheostoma filter, any type, any size, each ⑧ ♿ N

If "incident to" a physician's service, do not bill.

IOM: 100-02, 15, 120

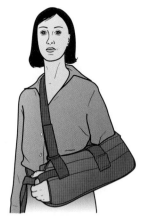

Figure 4 Arm sling.

⊛ **A4483** Moisture exchanger, disposable, for use with invasive mechanical ventilation ⑧ ♿ N

IOM: 100-02, 15, 120

⊘ **A4490** Surgical stockings above knee length, each ⑧ E

IOM: 100-02, 15, 100; 100-02, 15, 110; 100-03, 4, 280.1

⊘ **A4495** Surgical stockings thigh length, each ⑧ E

IOM: 100-02, 15, 100; 100-02, 15, 110; 100-03, 4, 280.1

⊘ **A4500** Surgical stockings below knee length, each ⑧ E

IOM: 100-02, 15, 100; 100-02, 15, 110; 100-03, 4, 280.1

⊘ **A4510** Surgical stockings full length, each ⑧ E

IOM: 100-02, 15, 100; 100-02, 15, 110; 100-03, 4, 280.1

⊘ **A4520** Incontinence garment, any type, (e.g. brief, diaper), each ⑧ E

IOM: 100-03, 4, 280.1

⊛ **A4550** Surgical trays ⑧ B

No longer payable by Medicare; included in practice expense for procedures. Some private payers may pay, most private payers follow Medicare guidelines

IOM: 100-04, 12, 20.3, 30.4

⊘ **A4554** Disposable underpads, all sizes ⑧ E

IOM: 100-02, 15, 120; 100-03, 4, 280.1

⊘ **A4555** Electrode/transducer for use with electrical stimulation device used for cancer treatment, replacement only **Qp** **Qh** E

⊚ PQRS　**Qp** Quantity Physician Appendix A　**Qh** Quantity Hospital Appendix B　♀ Female only　♂ Male only　**A** Age　♿ DMEPOS　A2-Z3 ASC Payment Indicator　A-Y ASC Status Indicator　Coding Clinic

* **A4556** Electrodes, (e.g., apnea monitor), per pair ⑧ 🦽   N

If "incident to" a physician's service, do not bill.

* **A4557** Lead wires, (e.g., apnea monitor), per pair ⑧ Qp Qh 🦽   N

If "incident to" a physician's service, do not bill.

* **A4558** Conductive gel or paste, for use with electrical device (e.g., TENS, NMES), per oz ⑧ 🦽   N

If "incident to" a physician's service, do not bill.

* **A4559** Coupling gel or paste, for use with ultrasound device, per oz ⑧ 🦽   N

If "incident to" a physician's service, do not bill.

* **A4561** Pessary, rubber, any type ⑧ Qp Qh ♀ 🦽   N

* **A4562** Pessary, non rubber, any type ⑧ Qp Qh ♀ 🦽   N

↻* **A4565** Slings ⑧ Qp Qh 🦽   N

⊘ **A4566** Shoulder sling or vest design, abduction restrainer, with or without swathe control, prefabricated, includes fitting and adjustment   E

⊘ **A4570** Splint ⑧   E

IOM: 100-02, 6, 10; 100-02, 15, 100; 100-04, 4, 240

⊘ **A4575** Topical hyperbaric oxygen chamber, disposable ⑧   E

IOM: 100-03, 1, 20.29

⊘ **A4580** Cast supplies (e.g. plaster) ⑧   E

IOM: 100-02, 6, 10; 100-02, 15, 100; 100-04, 4, 240

⊘ **A4590** Special casting material (e.g. fiberglass) ⑧   E

IOM: 100-02, 6, 10; 100-02, 15, 100; 100-04, 4, 240

⊛ **A4595** Electrical stimulator supplies, 2 lead, per month (e.g. TENS, NMES) ⑧ Qh 🦽   N

If "incident to" a physician's service, do not bill.

IOM: 100-03, 2, 160.13

* **A4600** Sleeve for intermittent limb compression device, replacement only, each ⑧   E

↻* **A4601** Lithium ion battery, rechargeable, for non-prosthetic use, replacement ⑧   E

▶* **A4602** Replacement battery for external infusion pump owned by patient, lithium, 1.5 volt, each   N1   N

* **A4604** Tubing with integrated heating element for use with positive airway pressure device ⑧ Qh 🦽   N

DMEPOS Modifier(s): NU

* **A4605** Tracheal suction catheter, closed system, each ⑧ Qh 🦽   N

DMEPOS Modifier(s): NU

* **A4606** Oxygen probe for use with oximeter device, replacement ⑧ Qp Qh   N

* **A4608** Transtracheal oxygen catheter, each ⑧ 🦽   N

Supplies for Respiratory and Oxygen Equipment

⊘ **A4611** Battery, heavy duty; replacement for patient owned ventilator ⑧ Qp Qh 🦽   E

Medicare Statute 1834(a)(3)(a)

DMEPOS Modifier(s): NU, RR, UE

⊘ **A4612** Battery cables; replacement for patient-owned ventilator ⑧ Qh 🦽   E

Medicare Statute 1834(a)(3)(a)

DMEPOS Modifier(s): NU, RR, UE

⊘ **A4613** Battery charger; replacement for patient-owned ventilator ⑧ Qh 🦽   E

Medicare Statute 1834(a)(3)(a)

DMEPOS Modifier(s): NU, RR, UE

* **A4614** Peak expiratory flow rate meter, hand held ⑧ Qp Qh 🦽   N

If "incident to" a physician's service, do not bill.

⊛ **A4615** Cannula, nasal ⑧ 🦽   N

If "incident to" a physician's service, do not bill.

IOM: 100-03, 2, 160.6; 100-04, 20, 100.2

⊛ **A4616** Tubing (oxygen), per foot ⑧ 🦽   N

If "incident to" a physician's service, do not bill.

IOM: 100-03, 2, 160.6; 100-04, 20, 100.2

⊛ **A4617** Mouth piece ⑧ 🦽   N

If "incident to" a physician's service, do not bill.

IOM: 100-03, 2, 160.6; 100-04, 20, 100.2

⊛ **A4618** Breathing circuits ⑧ Qh 🦽   N

If "incident to" a physician's service, do not bill.

IOM: 100-03, 2, 160.6; 100-04, 20, 100.2

DMEPOS Modifier(s): NU, RR, UE

▶ New   ↻ Revised   ✔ Reinstated   deleted Deleted   ⊘ Not covered or valid by Medicare
⊛ Special coverage instructions   * Carrier discretion   ⑧ Bill local carrier   ⑧ Bill DME MAC

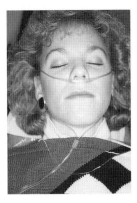

Figure 5 Nasal cannula.

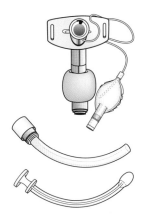

Figure 6 Tracheostomy cannula.

⚙ **A4619** Face tent ⓑ ♿ N

If "incident to" a physician's service, do not bill.

IOM: 100-03, 2, 160.6; 100-04, 20, 100.2

DMEPOS Modifier(s): NU

⚙ **A4620** Variable concentration mask ⓑ ♿ N

If "incident to" a physician's service, do not bill.

IOM: 100-03, 2, 160.6; 100-04, 20, 100.2

⚙ **A4623** Tracheostomy, inner cannula ⓑ Qh ♿ N

If "incident to" a physician's service, do not bill.

IOM: 100-02, 15, 120; 100-03, 1, 20.9

✳ **A4624** Tracheal suction catheter, any type, other than closed system, each ⓑ Qh ♿ N

If "incident to" a physician's service, do not bill.

DMEPOS Modifier(s): NU

Sterile suction catheters are medically necessary only for tracheostomy suctioning. Limitations include three suction catheters per day when covered for medically necessary tracheostomy suctioning. Assign DX V44.0 or V55.0 on the claim form. (CMS Manual System, Pub. 100-3, NCD manual, Chapter 1, Section 280-1)

⚙ **A4625** Tracheostomy care kit for new tracheostomy ⓑ Qp Qh ♿ N

If "incident to" a physician's service, do not bill.

IOM: 100-02, 15, 120

Dressings used with tracheostomies are included in the allowance for the code. This starter kit is covered after a surgical tracheostomy. (https://www.noridianmedicare.com/dme/coverage/docs/lcds/current_lcds/tracheostomy_care_supplies.htm)

⚙ **A4626** Tracheostomy cleaning brush, each ⓑ ♿ N

If "incident to" a physician's service, do not bill.

IOM: 100-02, 15, 120

⊘ **A4627** Spacer, bag, or reservoir, with or without mask, for use with metered dose inhaler ⓑ E

If "incident to" a physician's service, do not bill.

IOM: 100-02, 15, 110

✳ **A4628** Oropharyngeal suction catheter, each ⓑ Qh ♿ N

If "incident to" a physician's service, do not bill.

DMEPOS Modifier(s): NU

No more than three catheters per week are covered for medically necessary oropharyngeal suctioning because the catheters can be reused if cleansed and disinfected. (MS Manual System, Pub. 100-3, NCD manual, Chapter 1, Section 280-1)

⚙ **A4629** Tracheostomy care kit for established tracheostomy ⓑ ♿ N

If "incident to" a physician's service, do not bill.

IOM: 100-02, 15, 120

DMEPOS Modifier(s): NU

Supplies for Other Durable Medical Equipment

⚙ **A4630** Replacement batteries, medically necessary, transcutaneous electrical stimulator, owned by patient ⓑ ♿ E

IOM: 100-03, 3, 160.7

✳ **A4633** Replacement bulb/lamp for ultraviolet light therapy system, each ⓑ Qp Qh ♿ E

DMEPOS Modifier(s): NU

ⓆⓇⓈ PQRS	Qp Quantity Physician Appendix A	Qh Quantity Hospital Appendix B	♀ Female only
♂ Male only	Ⓐ Age	♿ DMEPOS	A2-Z3 ASC Payment Indicator	A-Y ASC Status Indicator	Coding Clinic

✳ **A4634** Replacement bulb for therapeutic light box, tabletop model Ⓑ   N

❂ **A4635** Underarm pad, crutch, replacement, each Ⓑ Qp Qh ♿   E

IOM: 100-03, 4, 280.1

DMEPOS Modifier(s): NU, RR, UE

❂ **A4636** Replacement, handgrip, cane, crutch, or walker, each Ⓑ Qh ♿   E

IOM: 100-03, 4, 280.1

DMEPOS Modifier(s): NU, KE, RR, UE

❂ **A4637** Replacement, tip, cane, crutch, walker, each Ⓑ Qh ♿   E

IOM: 100-03, 4, 280.1

DMEPOS Modifier(s): NU, KE, RR, UE

✳ **A4638** Replacement battery for patient-owned ear pulse generator, each Ⓑ Qp Qh ♿   E

DMEPOS Modifier(s): NU, RR, UE

↻✳ **A4639** Replacement pad for infrared heating pad system, each Ⓑ ♿   E

DMEPOS Modifier(s): RR

❂ **A4640** Replacement pad for use with medically necessary alternating pressure pad owned by patient Ⓑ Qp Qh ♿   E

IOM: 100-03, 4, 280.1; 100-08, 5, 5.2.3

DMEPOS Modifier(s): NU, RR, UE

Supplies for Radiological Procedures

✳ **A4641** Radiopharmaceutical, diagnostic, not otherwise classified Ⓑ   N1 N

Is not an applicable tracer for PET scans

✳ **A4642** Indium In-111 satumomab pendetide, diagnostic, per study dose, up to 6 millicuries Ⓑ Qp Qh   N1 N

Miscellaneous Supplies

✳ **A4648** Tissue marker, implantable, any type, each Ⓑ Qp Qh   N1 N

Coding Clinic: 2013, Q3, P9

✳ **A4649** Surgical supply; miscellaneous Ⓑ   N

Bill local carrier (Ⓑ) if incident to a physician's service (not separately payable) or if supply for implanted prosthetic device or implanted DME.

✳ **A4650** Implantable radiation dosimeter, each Ⓑ Qp Qh   N1 N

↻❂ **A4651** Calibrated microcapillary tube, each Ⓑ   N

IOM: 100-04, 3, 40.3

↻❂ **A4652** Microcapillary tube sealant Ⓑ   N

IOM: 100-04, 3, 40.3

Supplies for Dialysis

↻✳ **A4653** Peritoneal dialysis catheter anchoring device, belt, each Ⓑ   N

↻❂ **A4657** Syringe, with or without needle, each Ⓑ   N

IOM: 100-04, 8, 90.3.2

↻❂ **A4660** Sphygmomanometer/blood pressure apparatus with cuff and stethoscope Ⓑ Qh   N

IOM: 100-04, 8, 90.3.2

↻❂ **A4663** Blood pressure cuff only Ⓑ Qh   N

IOM: 100-04, 8, 90.3.2

↻⊘ **A4670** Automatic blood pressure monitor Ⓑ Qh   E

IOM: 100-04, 8, 90.3.2

↻❂ **A4671** Disposable cycler set used with cycler dialysis machine, each Ⓑ   B

IOM: 100-04, 8, 90.3.2

↻❂ **A4672** Drainage extension line, sterile, for dialysis, each Ⓑ   B

IOM: 100-04, 8, 90.3.2

↻❂ **A4673** Extension line with easy lock connectors, used with dialysis Ⓑ   B

IOM: 100-04, 8, 90.3.2

↻❂ **A4674** Chemicals/antiseptics solution used to clean/sterilize dialysis equipment, per 8 oz Ⓑ   B

IOM: 100-04, 8, 90.3.2

↻❂ **A4680** Activated carbon filters for hemodialysis, each Ⓑ   N

IOM: 100-04, 8, 90.3.2

↻❂ **A4690** Dialyzers (artificial kidneys), all types, all sizes, for hemodialysis, each Ⓑ   N

IOM: 100-04, 8, 90.3.2

↻❂ **A4706** Bicarbonate concentrate, solution, for hemodialysis, per gallon Ⓑ   N

IOM: 100-04, 8, 90.3.2

↻❂ **A4707** Bicarbonate concentrate, powder, for hemodialysis, per packet Ⓑ   N

IOM: 100-04, 8, 90.3.2

↻❂ **A4708** Acetate concentrate solution, for hemodialysis, per gallon Ⓑ   N

IOM: 100-04, 8, 90.3.2

▶ **New**   ↻ **Revised**   ✔ **Reinstated**   ~~deleted~~ **Deleted**   ⊘ **Not covered or valid by Medicare**
❂ **Special coverage instructions**   ✳ **Carrier discretion**   Ⓑ **Bill local carrier**   Ⓑ **Bill DME MAC**

⮌ ✿ **A4709** Acid concentrate, solution, for hemodialysis, per gallon Ⓑ   N

IOM: 100-04, 8, 90.3.2

⮌ ✿ **A4714** Treated water (deionized, distilled, or reverse osmosis) for peritoneal dialysis, per gallon Ⓑ   N

IOM: 100-03, 4, 230.7; 100-04, 3, 40.3

⮌ ✿ **A4719** "Y set" tubing for peritoneal dialysis Ⓑ   N

IOM: 100-04, 8, 90.3.2

⮌ ✿ **A4720** Dialysate solution, any concentration of dextrose, fluid volume greater than 249cc, but less than or equal to 999cc, for peritoneal dialysis Ⓑ   N

Do not use AX modifier

IOM: 100-04, 8, 90.3.2

⮌ ✿ **A4721** Dialysate solution, any concentration of dextrose, fluid volume greater than 999cc but less than or equal to 1999cc, for peritoneal dialysis Ⓑ   N

IOM: 100-04, 8, 90.3.2

⮌ ✿ **A4722** Dialysate solution, any concentration of dextrose, fluid volume greater than 1999cc but less than or equal to 2999cc, for peritoneal dialysis Ⓑ   N

IOM: 100-04, 8, 90.3.2

⮌ ✿ **A4723** Dialysate solution, any concentration of dextrose, fluid volume greater than 2999cc but less than or equal to 3999cc, for peritoneal dialysis Ⓑ   N

IOM: 100-04, 8, 90.3.2

⮌ ✿ **A4724** Dialysate solution, any concentration of dextrose, fluid volume greater than 3999cc but less than or equal to 4999cc for peritoneal dialysis Ⓑ   N

IOM: 100-04, 8, 90.3.2

⮌ ✿ **A4725** Dialysate solution, any concentration of dextrose, fluid volume greater than 4999cc but less than or equal to 5999cc, for peritoneal dialysis Ⓑ   N

IOM: 100-04, 8, 90.3.2

⮌ ✿ **A4726** Dialysate solution, any concentration of dextrose, fluid volume greater than 5999cc, for peritoneal dialysis Ⓑ   N

IOM: 100-04, 8, 90.3.2

⮌ ✳ **A4728** Dialysate solution, non-dextrose containing, 500 ml Ⓑ   B

⮌ ✿ **A4730** Fistula cannulation set for hemodialysis, each Ⓑ   N

IOM: 100-04, 8, 90.3.2

⮌ ✿ **A4736** Topical anesthetic, for dialysis, per gram Ⓑ   N

IOM: 100-04, 8, 90.3.2

⮌ ✿ **A4737** Injectable anesthetic, for dialysis, per 10 ml Ⓑ   N

IOM: 100-04, 8, 90.3.2

⮌ ✿ **A4740** Shunt accessory, for hemodialysis, any type, each Ⓑ   N

IOM: 100-04, 8, 90.3.2

⮌ ✿ **A4750** Blood tubing, arterial or venous, for hemodialysis, each Ⓑ   N

IOM: 100-04, 8, 90.3.2

⮌ ✿ **A4755** Blood tubing, arterial and venous combined, for hemodialysis, each Ⓑ   N

IOM: 100-04, 8, 90.3.2

⮌ ✿ **A4760** Dialysate solution test kit, for peritoneal dialysis, any type, each Ⓑ   N

IOM: 100-04, 8, 90.3.2

⮌ ✿ **A4765** Dialysate concentrate, powder, additive for peritoneal dialysis, per packet Ⓑ   N

IOM: 100-04, 8, 90.3.2

⮌ ✿ **A4766** Dialysate concentrate, solution, additive for peritoneal dialysis, per 10 ml Ⓑ   N

IOM: 100-04, 8, 90.3.2

⮌ ✿ **A4770** Blood collection tube, vacuum, for dialysis, per 50 Ⓑ   N

IOM: 100-04, 8, 90.3.2

⮌ ✿ **A4771** Serum clotting time tube, for dialysis, per 50 Ⓑ   N

IOM: 100-04, 8, 90.3.2

⮌ ✿ **A4772** Blood glucose test strips, for dialysis, per 50 Ⓑ   N

IOM: 100-04, 8, 90.3.2

⮌ ✿ **A4773** Occult blood test strips, for dialysis, per 50 Ⓑ   N

IOM: 100-04, 8, 90.3.2

⮌ ✿ **A4774** Ammonia test strips, for dialysis, per 50 Ⓑ   N

IOM: 100-04, 8, 90.3.2

⮌ ✿ **A4802** Protamine sulfate, for hemodialysis, per 50 mg Ⓑ   N

IOM: 100-04, 8, 90.3.2

⮌ ✿ **A4860** Disposable catheter tips for peritoneal dialysis, per 10 Ⓑ   N

IOM: 100-04, 8, 90.3.2

↩ ⊛ **A4870** Plumbing and/or electrical work for home hemodialysis equipment ⑧ N

IOM: 100-04, 8, 90.3.2

↩ ⊛ **A4890** Contracts, repair and maintenance, for hemodialysis equipment ⑧ N

IOM: 100-02, 15, 110.2

↩ ⊛ **A4911** Drain bag/bottle, for dialysis, each ⑧ N

↩ ⊛ **A4913** Miscellaneous dialysis supplies, not otherwise specified ⑧ N

Items not related to dialysis must not be billed with the miscellaneous codes A4913 or E1699.

↩ ⊛ **A4918** Venous pressure clamp, for hemodialysis, each ⑧ N

↩ ⊛ **A4927** Gloves, non-sterile, per 100 ⑧ N

↩ ⊛ **A4928** Surgical mask, per 20 ⑧ N

↩ ⊛ **A4929** Tourniquet for dialysis, each ⑧ N

↩ ⊛ **A4930** Gloves, sterile, per pair ⑧ N

↩ ✶ **A4931** Oral thermometer, reusable, any type, each ⑧ N

✶ **A4932** Rectal thermometer, reusable, any type, each ⑧ **Qh** N

Additional Ostomy Supplies

A5051-A5093: If provided in the physician's office for a temporary condition, the item is incident to the physician's service and billed to the local carrier (⑧). If provided in the physician's office or other place of service for a permanent condition, the item is a prosthetic device and billed to the DME MAC (⑧).

⊛ **A5051** Ostomy pouch, closed; with barrier attached (1 piece), each ⑧ ⑧ ♿ N

IOM: 100-02, 15, 120

⊛ **A5052** Ostomy pouch, closed; without barrier attached (1 piece), each ⑧ ⑧ ♿ N

IOM: 100-02, 15, 120

⊛ **A5053** Ostomy pouch, closed; for use on faceplate, each ⑧ ⑧ ♿ N

IOM: 100-02, 15, 120

⊛ **A5054** Ostomy pouch, closed; for use on barrier with flange (2 piece), each ⑧ ⑧ ♿ N

IOM: 100-02, 15, 120

⊛ **A5055** Stoma cap ⑧ ⑧ ♿ N

IOM: 100-02, 15, 120

⊛ **A5056** Ostomy pouch, drainable, with extended wear barrier attached, with filter, (1 piece), each ⑧ ⑧ **Qp** **Qh** ♿ N

IOM: 100-02, 15, 120

⊛ **A5057** Ostomy pouch, drainable, with extended wear barrier attached, with built in convexity, with filter, (1 piece), each ⑧ ⑧ **Qp** **Qh** ♿ N

IOM: 100-02, 15, 120

✶ **A5061** Ostomy pouch, drainable; with barrier attached, (1 piece), each ⑧ ⑧ ♿ N

IOM: 100-02, 15, 120

⊛ **A5062** Ostomy pouch, drainable; without barrier attached (1 piece), each ⑧ ⑧ ♿ N

IOM: 100-02, 15, 120

⊛ **A5063** Ostomy pouch, drainable; for use on barrier with flange (2 piece system), each ⑧ ⑧ ♿ N

IOM: 100-02, 15, 120

⊛ **A5071** Ostomy pouch, urinary; with barrier attached (1 piece), each ⑧ ⑧ ♿ N

IOM: 100-02, 15, 120

⊛ **A5072** Ostomy pouch, urinary; without barrier attached (1 piece), each ⑧ ⑧ ♿ N

IOM: 100-02, 15, 120

⊛ **A5073** Ostomy pouch, urinary; for use on barrier with flange (2 piece), each ⑧ ⑧ ♿ N

IOM: 100-02, 15, 120

⊛ **A5081** Stoma plug or seal, any type ⑧ ⑧ ♿ N

IOM: 100-02, 15, 120

⊛ **A5082** Continent device; catheter for continent stoma ⑧ ⑧ ♿ N

IOM: 100-02, 15, 120

✶ **A5083** Continent device, stoma absorptive cover for continent stoma ⑧ ⑧ ♿ N

⊛ **A5093** Ostomy accessory; convex insert ⑧ ⑧ ♿ N

IOM: 100-02, 15, 120

Additional Incontinence Appliances/Supplies

A5102-A5114: If provided in the physician's office for a temporary condition, the item is incident to the physician's service and billed to the local carrier (⑧). If provided in the physician's office or other place of service for a permanent condition, the item is a prosthetic device and billed to the DME MAC (⑧).

▶ **New** ↩ **Revised** ✔ **Reinstated** ~~deleted~~ **Deleted** ⊘ **Not covered or valid by Medicare**
⊛ **Special coverage instructions** ✶ **Carrier discretion** ⑧ **Bill local carrier** ⑧ **Bill DME MAC**

⊕ **A5102** Bedside drainage bottle with or without tubing, rigid or expandable, each Ⓑ Ⓓ **Qh** ᨒ N

IOM: 100-02, 15, 120

⊕ **A5105** Urinary suspensory, with leg bag, with or without tube, each Ⓑ Ⓓ ᨒ N

IOM: 100-02, 15, 120

⊕ **A5112** Urinary drainage bag, leg bag, leg or abdomen, latex, with or without tube, with straps, each Ⓑ Ⓓ ᨒ N

IOM: 100-02, 15, 120

⊕ **A5113** Leg strap; latex, replacement only, per set Ⓑ Ⓓ ᨒ E

IOM: 100-02, 15, 120

⊕ **A5114** Leg strap; foam or fabric, replacement only, per set Ⓑ Ⓓ ᨒ E

IOM: 100-02, 15, 120

Supplies for Either Incontinence or Ostomy Appliances

A5120-A5200: If provided in the physician's office for a temporary condition, the item is incident to the physician's service and billed to the local carrier (Ⓑ). If provided in the physician's office or other place of service for a permanent condition, the item is a prosthetic device and billed to the DME MAC (Ⓓ).

⊕ **A5120** Skin barrier, wipes or swabs, each Ⓑ Ⓓ **Qp** **Qh** ᨒ N

IOM: 100-02, 15, 120

DMEPOS Modifier(s): AU, AV

⊕ **A5121** Skin barrier; solid, 6 × 6 or equivalent, each Ⓑ Ⓓ ᨒ N

IOM: 100-02, 15, 120

⊕ **A5122** Skin barrier; solid, 8 × 8 or equivalent, each Ⓑ Ⓓ ᨒ N

IOM: 100-02, 15, 120

⊕ **A5126** Adhesive or non-adhesive; disk or foam pad Ⓑ Ⓓ ᨒ N

IOM: 100-02, 15, 120

⊕ **A5131** Appliance cleaner, incontinence and ostomy appliances, per 16 oz Ⓑ Ⓓ ᨒ N

IOM: 100-02, 15, 120

⊕ **A5200** Percutaneous catheter/tube anchoring device, adhesive skin attachment Ⓓ Ⓑ ᨒ N

IOM: 100-02, 15, 120

Diabetic Shoes, Fitting, and Modifications

⊕ **A5500** For diabetics only, fitting (including follow-up), custom preparation and supply of off-the-shelf depth-inlay shoe manufactured to accommodate multi-density insert(s), per shoe Ⓑ **Qp** **Qh** ᨒ Y

IOM: 100-02, 15, 140

⊕ **A5501** For diabetics only, fitting (including follow-up), custom preparation and supply of shoe molded from cast(s) of patient's foot (custom-molded shoe), per shoe Ⓓ **Qp** **Qh** ᨒ Y

The diabetic patient must have at least one of the following conditions: peripheral neuropathy with evidence of callus formation, pre-ulcerative calluses, previous ulceration, foot deformity, previous amputation or poor circulation

IOM: 100-02, 15, 140

⊕ **A5503** For diabetics only, modification (including fitting) of off-the-shelf depth-inlay shoe or custom-molded shoe with roller or rigid rocker bottom, per shoe Ⓓ **Qp** **Qh** ᨒ Y

IOM: 100-02, 15, 140

⊕ **A5504** For diabetics only, modification (including fitting) of off-the-shelf depth-inlay shoe or custom-molded shoe with wedge(s), per shoe Ⓓ **Qp** **Qh** ᨒ Y

IOM: 100-02, 15, 140

⊕ **A5505** For diabetics only, modification (including fitting) of off-the-shelf depth-inlay shoe or custom-molded shoe with metatarsal bar, per shoe Ⓓ **Qp** **Qh** ᨒ Y

IOM: 100-02, 15, 140

⊕ **A5506** For diabetics only, modification (including fitting) of off-the-shelf depth-inlay shoe or custom-molded shoe with off-set heel(s), per shoe Ⓓ **Qp** **Qh** ᨒ Y

IOM: 100-02, 15, 140

⊕ **A5507** For diabetics only, not otherwise specified modification (including fitting) of off-the-shelf depth-inlay shoe or custom-molded shoe, per shoe Ⓓ **Qp** **Qh** ᨒ Y

Only used for not otherwise specified therapeutic modifications to shoe or for repairs to a diabetic shoe(s)

IOM: 100-02, 15, 140

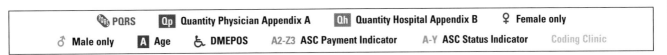

⚙ **A5508** For diabetics only, deluxe feature of off-the-shelf depth-inlay shoe or custom-molded shoe, per shoe ⓑ **Qp**   Y

⚙ **A5510** For diabetics only, direct formed, compression molded to patient's foot without external heat source, multiple-density insert(s) prefabricated, per shoe ⓑ **Qp**   N

IOM: 100-02, 15, 140

✳ **A5512** For diabetics only, multiple density insert, direct formed, molded to foot after external heat source of 230 degrees Fahrenheit or higher, total contact with patient's foot, including arch, base layer minimum of 1/4 inch material of shore a 35 durometer or 3/16 inch material of shore a 40 durometer (or higher), prefabricated, each ⓑ **Qp** **Qh** ♿   Y

✳ **A5513** For diabetics only, multiple density insert, custom molded from model of patient's foot, total contact with patient's foot, including arch, base layer minimum of 3/16 inch material of shore a 35 durometer (or higher), includes arch filler and other shaping material, custom fabricated, each ⓑ **Qp** **Qh** ♿   Y

Dressings

A6010-A6512: Bill local carrier (ⓑ) if incident to a physician's service (not separately payable) or if supply for implanted prosthetic device or implanted DME. If other, bill DME MAC (ⓓ).

⊘ **A6000** Non-contact wound warming wound cover for use with the non-contact wound warming device and warming card ⓓ   E

IOM: 100-02, 16, 20

⚙ **A6010** Collagen based wound filler, dry form, sterile, per gram of collagen ⓑ ⓓ ♿   N

IOM: 100-02, 15, 100

⚙ **A6011** Collagen based wound filler, gel/paste, per gram of collagen ⓑ ⓓ ♿   N

IOM: 100-02, 15, 100

⚙ **A6021** Collagen dressing, sterile, size 16 sq. in. or less, each ⓑ ⓓ ♿   N

IOM: 100-02, 15, 100

⚙ **A6022** Collagen dressing, sterile, size more than 16 sq. in. but less than or equal to 48 sq. in., each ⓑ ⓓ ♿   N

IOM: 100-02, 15, 100

⚙ **A6023** Collagen dressing, sterile, size more than 48 sq. in., each ⓑ ⓓ ♿   N

IOM: 100-02, 15, 100

⚙ **A6024** Collagen dressing wound filler, sterile, per 6 inches ⓑ ⓓ ♿   N

IOM: 100-02, 15, 100

✳ **A6025** Gel sheet for dermal or epidermal application, (e.g., silicone, hydrogel, other), each ⓑ ⓓ   N

If used for the treatment of keloids or other scars, a silicone gel sheet will not meet the definition of the surgical dressing benefit and will be denied as noncovered.

⚙ **A6154** Wound pouch, each ⓑ ⓓ ♿   N

Waterproof collection device with drainable port that adheres to skin around wound. Usual dressing change is up to 3 × per week.

IOM: 100-02, 15, 100

⚙ **A6196** Alginate or other fiber gelling dressing, wound cover, sterile, pad size 16 sq. in. or less, each dressing ⓑ ⓓ ♿   N

IOM: 100-02, 15, 100

⚙ **A6197** Alginate or other fiber gelling dressing, wound cover, sterile, pad size more than 16 sq. in., but less than or equal to 48 sq. in., each dressing ⓑ ⓓ ♿   N

IOM: 100-02, 15, 100

⚙ **A6198** Alginate or other fiber gelling dressing, wound cover, sterile, pad size more than 48 sq. in., each dressing ⓑ ⓓ   N

IOM: 100-02, 15, 100

⚙ **A6199** Alginate or other fiber gelling dressing, wound filler, sterile, per 6 inches ⓑ ⓓ ♿   N

IOM: 100-02, 15, 100

⚙ **A6203** Composite dressing, sterile, pad size 16 sq. in. or less, with any size adhesive border, each dressing ⓑ ⓓ ♿   N

Usual composite dressing change is up to 3 times per week, one wound cover per dressing change.

IOM: 100-02, 15, 100

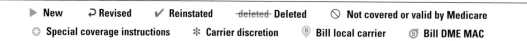

A6204   Composite dressing, sterile, pad size more than 16 sq. in. but less than or equal to 48 sq. in., with any size adhesive border, each dressing Ⓑ Ⓑ ♿   N

Usual composite dressing change is up to 3 times per week, one wound cover per dressing change.

IOM: 100-02, 15, 100

A6205   Composite dressing, sterile, pad size more than 48 sq. in., with any size adhesive border, each dressing Ⓑ Ⓑ   N

Usual composite dressing change is up to 3 times per week, one wound cover per dressing change.

IOM: 100-02, 15, 100

A6206   Contact layer, sterile, 16 sq. in. or less, each dressing Ⓑ Ⓑ   N

Contact layers are porous to allow wound fluid to pass through for absorption by separate overlying dressing and are not intended to be changed with each dressing change. Usual dressing change is up to once per week.

IOM: 100-02, 15, 100

A6207   Contact layer, sterile, more than 16 sq. in. but less than or equal to 48 sq. in., each dressing Ⓥ Ⓑ ♿   N

Contact layer dressings are used to line the entire wound; they are not intended to be changed with each dressing change. Usual dressing change is up to once per week.

IOM: 100-02, 15, 100

A6208   Contact layer, sterile, more than 48 sq. in., each dressing Ⓑ Ⓑ   N

Contact layer dressings are used to line the entire wound; they are not intended to be changed with each dressing change. Usual dressing change is up to once per week.

IOM: 100-02, 15, 100

A6209   Foam dressing, wound cover, sterile, pad size 16 sq. in. or less, without adhesive border, each dressing Ⓑ Ⓑ ♿   N

Made of open cell, medical grade expanded polymer; with nonadherent property over wound site

IOM: 100-02, 15, 100

A6210   Foam dressing, wound cover, sterile, pad size more than 16 sq. in. but less than or equal to 48 sq. in., without adhesive border, each dressing Ⓑ Ⓑ ♿   N

Foam dressings are covered items when used on full thickness wounds (e.g., stage III or IV ulcers) with moderate to heavy exudates. Usual dressing change for a foam wound cover when used as primary dressing is up to 3 times per week. When foam wound cover is used as a secondary dressing for wounds with very heavy exudates, dressing change may be up to 3 times per week. Usual dressing change for foam wound fillers is up to once per day (A6209-A6215).

IOM: 100-02, 15, 100

A6211   Foam dressing, wound cover, sterile, pad size more than 48 sq. in., without adhesive border, each dressing Ⓑ Ⓑ ♿   N

IOM: 100-02, 15, 100

A6212   Foam dressing, wound cover, sterile, pad size 16 sq. in. or less, with any size adhesive border, each dressing Ⓑ Ⓑ ♿   N

IOM: 100-02, 15, 100

A6213   Foam dressing, wound cover, sterile, pad size more than 16 sq. in. but less than or equal to 48 sq. in., with any size adhesive border, each dressing Ⓥ Ⓑ   N

IOM: 100-02, 15, 100

A6214   Foam dressing, wound cover, sterile, pad size more than 48 sq. in., with any size adhesive border, each dressing Ⓑ Ⓑ ♿   N

IOM: 100-02, 15, 100

A6215   Foam dressing, wound filler, sterile, per gram Ⓑ Ⓑ   N

IOM: 100-02, 15, 100

A6216   Gauze, non-impregnated, non-sterile, pad size 16 sq. in. or less, without adhesive border, each dressing Ⓑ Ⓑ ♿   N

IOM: 100-02, 15, 100

A6217   Gauze, non-impregnated, non-sterile, pad size more than 16 sq. in. but less than or equal to 48 sq. in., without adhesive border, each dressing Ⓑ Ⓑ ♿   N

IOM: 100-02, 15, 100

PQRS PQRS	**Qp** Quantity Physician Appendix A	**Qh** Quantity Hospital Appendix B	♀ **Female only**
♂ **Male only**	**A** Age	♿ DMEPOS	A2-Z3 **ASC Payment Indicator** A-Y **ASC Status Indicator** *Coding Clinic*

⊘ **A6218**   Gauze, non-impregnated, non-sterile, pad size more than 48 sq. in., without adhesive border, each dressing Ⓑ Ⓓ   N

IOM: 100-02, 15, 100

⊘ **A6219**   Gauze, non-impregnated, sterile, pad size 16 sq. in. or less, with any size adhesive border, each dressing Ⓑ Ⓓ ♿   N

IOM: 100-02, 15, 100

⊘ **A6220**   Gauze, non-impregnated, sterile, pad size more than 16 sq. in. but less than or equal to 48 sq. in., with any size adhesive border, each dressing Ⓑ Ⓓ ♿   N

IOM: 100-02, 15, 100

⊘ **A6221**   Gauze, non-impregnated, sterile, pad size more than 48 sq. in., with any size adhesive border, each dressing Ⓑ Ⓓ   N

IOM: 100-02, 15, 100

⊘ **A6222**   Gauze, impregnated with other than water, normal saline, or hydrogel, sterile, pad size 16 sq. in. or less, without adhesive border, each dressing Ⓑ Ⓓ ♿   N

Substances may have been incorporated into dressing material (i.e., iodinated agents, petrolatum, zinc paste, crystalline sodium chloride, chlorhexadine gluconate [CHG], bismuth tribromophenate [BTP], water, aqueous saline, hydrogel, or agents)

IOM: 100-02, 15, 100

⊘ **A6223**   Gauze, impregnated with other than water, normal saline, or hydrogel, sterile, pad size more than 16 sq. in. but less than or equal to 48 sq. in., without adhesive border, each dressing Ⓟ Ⓓ ♿   N

IOM: 100-02, 15, 100

⊘ **A6224**   Gauze, impregnated with other than water, normal saline, or hydrogel, sterile, pad size more than 48 square inches, without adhesive border, each dressing Ⓑ Ⓓ ♿   N

IOM: 100-02, 15, 100

⊘ **A6228**   Gauze, impregnated, water or normal saline, sterile, pad size 16 sq. in. or less, without adhesive border, each dressing Ⓟ Ⓓ   N

IOM: 100-02, 15, 100

⊘ **A6229**   Gauze, impregnated, water or normal saline, sterile, pad size more than 16 sq. in. but less than or equal to 48 sq. in., without adhesive border, each dressing Ⓑ Ⓓ ♿   N

IOM: 100-02, 15, 100

⊘ **A6230**   Gauze, impregnated, water or normal saline, sterile, pad size more than 48 sq. in., without adhesive border, each dressing Ⓑ Ⓑ   N

IOM: 100-02, 15, 100

⊘ **A6231**   Gauze, impregnated, hydrogel, for direct wound contact, sterile, pad size 16 sq. in. or less, each dressing Ⓑ Ⓟ ♿   N

IOM: 100-02, 15, 100

⊘ **A6232**   Gauze, impregnated, hydrogel, for direct wound contact, sterile, pad size greater than 16 sq. in., but less than or equal to 48 sq. in., each dressing Ⓑ Ⓓ ♿   N

IOM: 100-02, 15, 100

⊘ **A6233**   Gauze, impregnated, hydrogel, for direct wound contact, sterile, pad size more than 48 sq. in., each dressing Ⓑ Ⓓ ♿   N

IOM: 100-02, 15, 100

⊘ **A6234**   Hydrocolloid dressing, wound cover, sterile, pad size 16 sq. in. or less, without adhesive border, each dressing Ⓑ Ⓑ ♿   N

This type of dressing is usually used on wounds with light to moderate exudate with an average of three dressing changes a week.

IOM: 100-02, 15, 100

⊘ **A6235**   Hydrocolloid dressing, wound cover, sterile, pad size more than 16 sq. in. but less than or equal to 48 sq. in., without adhesive border, each dressing Ⓟ Ⓓ ♿   N

IOM: 100-02, 15, 100

⊘ **A6236**   Hydrocolloid dressing, wound cover, sterile, pad size more than 48 sq. in., without adhesive border, each dressing Ⓑ Ⓓ ♿   N

IOM: 100-02, 15, 100

⊘ **A6237**   Hydrocolloid dressing, wound cover, sterile, pad size 16 sq. in. or less, with any size adhesive border, each dressing Ⓑ Ⓓ ♿   N

IOM: 100-02, 15, 100

▶ New	↻ Revised	✔ Reinstated	~~deleted~~ Deleted	⊘ Not covered or valid by Medicare
⊘ Special coverage instructions		✳ Carrier discretion	Ⓟ Bill local carrier	Ⓑ Bill DME MAC

A6238   Hydrocolloid dressing, wound cover, sterile, pad size more than 16 sq. in. but less than or equal to 48 sq. in., with any size adhesive border, each dressing ⒷⒼ ♿   N

IOM: 100-02, 15, 100

A6239   Hydrocolloid dressing, wound cover, sterile, pad size more than 48 sq. in., with any size adhesive border, each dressing ⒷⒼ   N

IOM: 100-02, 15, 100

A6240   Hydrocolloid dressing, wound filler, paste, sterile, per ounce ⒷⒼ♿   N

IOM: 100-02, 15, 100

A6241   Hydrocolloid dressing, wound filler, dry form, sterile, per gram ⒷⒼ♿   N

IOM: 100-02, 15, 100

A6242   Hydrogel dressing, wound cover, sterile, pad size 16 sq. in. or less, without adhesive border, each dressing ⒷⒼ♿   N

Considered medically necessary when used on full thickness wounds with minimal or no exudate (e.g., stage III or IV ulcers)

Usually up to one dressing change per day is considered medically necessary, but if well documented and medically necessary, the payer may allow more frequent dressing changes.

IOM: 100-02, 15, 100

A6243   Hydrogel dressing, wound cover, sterile, pad size more than 16 sq. in. but less than or equal to 48 sq. in., without adhesive border, each dressing ⒷⒼ♿   N

IOM: 100-02, 15, 100

A6244   Hydrogel dressing, wound cover, sterile, pad size more than 48 sq. in., without adhesive border, each dressing ⒷⒼ♿   N

IOM: 100-02, 15, 100

A6245   Hydrogel dressing, wound cover, sterile, pad size 16 sq. in. or less, with any size adhesive border, each dressing ⒷⒼ♿   N

Coverage of a non-elastic gradient compression wrap is limited to one per 6 months per leg.

IOM: 100-02, 15, 100

A6246   Hydrogel dressing, wound cover, sterile, pad size more than 16 sq. in. but less than or equal to 48 sq. in., with any size adhesive border, each dressing   N

IOM: 100-02, 15, 100

A6247   Hydrogel dressing, wound cover, sterile, pad size more than 48 sq. in., with any size adhesive border, each dressing ⒷⒼ♿   N

IOM: 100-02, 15, 100

A6248   Hydrogel dressing, wound filler, gel, per fluid ounce ⒷⒼ♿   N

IOM: 100-02, 15, 100

A6250   Skin sealants, protectants, moisturizers, ointments, any type, any size ⒷⒼ   N

IOM: 100-02, 15, 100

A6251   Specialty absorptive dressing, wound cover, sterile, pad size 16 sq. in. or less, without adhesive border, each dressing ⒷⒼ♿   N

IOM: 100-02, 15, 100

A6252   Specialty absorptive dressing, wound cover, sterile, pad size more than 16 sq. in. but less than or equal to 48 sq. in., without adhesive border, each dressing ⒷⒼ♿   N

IOM: 100-02, 15, 100

A6253   Specialty absorptive dressing, wound cover, sterile, pad size more than 48 sq. in., without adhesive border, each dressing ⒷⒼ♿   N

IOM: 100-02, 15, 100

A6254   Specialty absorptive dressing, wound cover, sterile, pad size 16 sq. in. or less, with any size adhesive border, each dressing ⒷⒼ♿   N

IOM: 100-02, 15, 100

A6255   Specialty absorptive dressing, wound cover, sterile, pad size more than 16 sq. in. but less than or equal to 48 sq. in., with any size adhesive border, each dressing ⒷⒼ♿   N

IOM: 100-02, 15, 100

A6256   Specialty absorptive dressing, wound cover, sterile, pad size more than 48 sq. in., with any size adhesive border, each dressing ⒷⒼ   N

Considered medically necessary when used for moderately or highly exudative wounds (e.g., stage III or IV ulcers)

IOM: 100-02, 15, 100

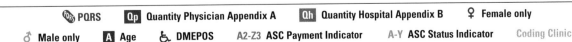

⊛ **A6257** Transparent film, sterile, 16 sq. in. or less, each dressing Ⓑ Ⓑ ♿ N

Considered medically necessary when used on open partial thickness wounds with minimal exudate or closed wounds

IOM: 100-02, 15, 100

⊛ **A6258** Transparent film, sterile, more than 16 sq. in. but less than or equal to 48 sq. in., each dressing Ⓑ Ⓑ ♿ N

IOM: 100-02, 15, 100

⊛ **A6259** Transparent film, sterile, more than 48 sq. in., each dressing Ⓑ Ⓑ ♿ N

IOM: 100-02, 15, 100

⊛ **A6260** Wound cleansers, any type, any size Ⓑ Ⓑ N

IOM: 100-02, 15, 100

⊛ **A6261** Wound filler, gel/paste, per fluid ounce, not otherwise specified Ⓑ Ⓑ N

Units of service for wound fillers are 1 gram, 1 fluid ounce, 6 inch length, or 1 yard depending on product

IOM: 100-02, 15, 100

⊛ **A6262** Wound filler, dry form, per gram, not otherwise specified Ⓑ Ⓑ N

Dry forms (e.g., powder, granules, beads) are used to eliminate dead space in an open wound.

IOM: 100-02, 15, 100

⊛ **A6266** Gauze, impregnated, other than water, normal saline, or zinc paste, sterile, any width, per linear yard Ⓑ Ⓑ ♿ N

IOM: 100-02, 15, 100

⊛ **A6402** Gauze, non-impregnated, sterile, pad size 16 sq. in. or less, without adhesive border, each dressing Ⓑ Ⓑ ♿ N

IOM: 100-02, 15, 100

⊛ **A6403** Gauze, non-impregnated, sterile, pad size more than 16 sq. in., less than or equal to 48 sq. in., without adhesive border, each dressing Ⓑ Ⓑ ♿ N

IOM: 100-02, 15, 100

⊛ **A6404** Gauze, non-impregnated, sterile, pad size more than 48 sq. in., without adhesive border, each dressing Ⓑ Ⓑ N

IOM: 100-02, 15, 100

✳ **A6407** Packing strips, non-impregnated, sterile, up to 2 inches in width, per linear yard Ⓑ Ⓑ ♿ N

IOM: 100-02, 15, 100

⊛ **A6410** Eye pad, sterile, each Ⓑ Ⓑ ♿ N

IOM: 100-02, 15, 100

⊛ **A6411** Eye pad, non-sterile, each Ⓑ Ⓑ ♿ N

IOM: 100-02, 15, 100

✳ **A6412** Eye patch, occlusive, each Ⓑ Ⓑ N

⊘ **A6413** Adhesive bandage, first-aid type, any size, each Ⓑ Ⓑ E

First aid type bandage is a wound cover with a pad size of less than 4 square inches. Does not meet the definition of the surgical dressing benefit and will be denied as non-covered.

Medicare Statute 1861(s)(5)

✳ **A6441** Padding bandage, non-elastic, non-woven/non-knitted, width greater than or equal to three inches and less than five inches, per yard Ⓑ Ⓑ ♿ N

✳ **A6442** Conforming bandage, non-elastic, knitted/woven, non-sterile, width less than three inches, per yard Ⓑ Ⓑ ♿ N

Non-elastic, moderate or high compression that is typically sustained for one week

✳ **A6443** Conforming bandage, non-elastic, knitted/woven, non-sterile, width greater than or equal to three inches and less than five inches, per yard Ⓑ Ⓑ ♿ N

✳ **A6444** Conforming bandage, non-elastic, knitted/woven, non-sterile, width greater than or equal to five inches, per yard Ⓑ Ⓑ ♿ N

✳ **A6445** Conforming bandage, non-elastic, knitted/woven, sterile, width less than three inches, per yard Ⓑ Ⓑ ♿ N

✳ **A6446** Conforming bandage, non-elastic, knitted/woven, sterile, width greater than or equal to three inches and less than five inches, per yard Ⓑ Ⓑ ♿ N

✳ **A6447** Conforming bandage, non-elastic, knitted/woven, sterile, width greater than or equal to five inches, per yard Ⓑ Ⓑ ♿ N

✳ **A6448** Light compression bandage, elastic, knitted/woven, width less than three inches, per yard Ⓑ Ⓑ ♿ N

Used to hold wound cover dressings in place over a wound. Example is an ACE type elastic bandage.

✳ **A6449** Light compression bandage, elastic, knitted/woven, width greater than or equal to three inches and less than five inches, per yard Ⓑ Ⓑ ♿ N

▶ New   ↻ Revised   ✔ Reinstated   ~~deleted~~ Deleted   ⊘ Not covered or valid by Medicare

⊛ Special coverage instructions   ✳ Carrier discretion   Ⓑ Bill local carrier   Ⓑ Bill DME MAC

✳ **A6450** Light compression bandage, elastic, knitted/woven, width greater than or equal to five inches, per yard Ⓑ Ⓑ 🦽   N

✳ **A6451** Moderate compression bandage, elastic, knitted/woven, load resistance of 1.25 to 1.34 foot pounds at 50% maximum stretch, width greater than or equal to three inches and less than five inches, per yard ⦿ Ⓑ Ⓑ 🦽   N

Elastic bandages that produce moderate compression that is typically sustained for one week

Medicare considers coverage if part of a multi-layer compression bandage system for the treatment of a venous stasis ulcer. Do not assign for strains or sprains.

✳ **A6452** High compression bandage, elastic, knitted/woven, load resistance greater than or equal to 1.35 foot pounds at 50% maximum stretch, width greater than or equal to three inches and less than five inches, per yard Ⓑ Ⓑ 🦽   N

Elastic bandages that produce high compression that is typically sustained for one week

✳ **A6453** Self-adherent bandage, elastic, non-knitted/non-woven, width less than three inches, per yard ⦿ Ⓑ Ⓑ 🦽   N

✳ **A6454** Self-adherent bandage, elastic, non-knitted/non-woven, width greater than or equal to three inches and less than five inches, per yard Ⓑ Ⓑ 🦽   N

✳ **A6455** Self-adherent bandage, elastic, non-knitted/non-woven, width greater than or equal to five inches, per yard Ⓑ Ⓑ 🦽   N

✳ **A6456** Zinc paste impregnated bandage, non-elastic, knitted/woven, width greater than or equal to three inches and less than five inches, per yard Ⓑ Ⓑ 🦽   N

✳ **A6457** Tubular dressing with or without elastic, any width, per linear yard Ⓑ Ⓑ 🦽   N

⦿ **A6501** Compression burn garment, bodysuit (head to foot), custom fabricated Ⓑ Ⓑ Qp Qh 🦽   N

Garments used to reduce hypertrophic scarring and joint contractures following burn injury

IOM: 100-02, 15, 100

⦿ **A6502** Compression burn garment, chin strap, custom fabricated Ⓑ Ⓑ Qp Qh 🦽   N

IOM: 100-02, 15, 100

⦿ **A6503** Compression burn garment, facial hood, custom fabricated Ⓑ Ⓑ Qp Qh 🦽   N

IOM: 100-02, 15, 100

⦿ **A6504** Compression burn garment, glove to wrist, custom fabricated Ⓑ Ⓑ Qp Qh 🦽   N

IOM: 100-02, 15, 100

⦿ **A6505** Compression burn garment, glove to elbow, custom fabricated Ⓑ Ⓑ Qp Qh 🦽   N

IOM: 100-02, 15, 100

⦿ **A6506** Compression burn garment, glove to axilla, custom fabricated Ⓑ Ⓑ Qp Qh 🦽   N

IOM: 100-02, 15, 100

⦿ **A6507** Compression burn garment, foot to knee length, custom fabricated Ⓑ Ⓑ Qp Qh 🦽   N

IOM: 100-02, 15, 100

⦿ **A6508** Compression burn garment, foot to thigh length, custom fabricated Ⓑ Ⓑ Qp Qh 🦽   N

IOM: 100-02, 15, 100

⦿ **A6509** Compression burn garment, upper trunk to waist including arm openings (vest), custom fabricated Ⓑ Ⓑ Qp Qh 🦽   N

IOM: 100-02, 15, 100

⦿ **A6510** Compression burn garment, trunk, including arms down to leg openings (leotard), custom fabricated Ⓑ Ⓑ Qp Qh 🦽   N

IOM: 100-02, 15, 100

⦿ **A6511** Compression burn garment, lower trunk including leg openings (panty), custom fabricated Ⓑ Ⓑ Qp Qh 🦽   N

IOM: 100-02, 15, 100

⦿ **A6512** Compression burn garment, not otherwise classified Ⓑ Ⓑ   N

IOM: 100-02, 15, 100

✳ **A6513** Compression burn mask, face and/or neck, plastic or equal, custom fabricated Ⓑ Qp Qh 🦽   B

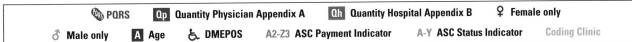

GRADIENT COMPRESSION STOCKINGS (A6530-A6549)

⊘ **A6530** Gradient compression stocking, below knee, 18–30 mmHg, each Ⓑ E

IOM: 100-03, 4, 280.1

✲ **A6531** Gradient compression stocking, below knee, 30–40 mmHg, each Ⓑ Qp & N

Covered when used in treatment of open venous stasis ulcer. Modifiers A1-A9 are not assigned. Must be billed with AW, RT, or LT

IOM: 100-02, 15, 100

DMEPOS Modifier(s): AW

✲ **A6532** Gradient compression stocking, below knee, 40–50 mmHg, each Ⓑ Qp & N

Covered when used in treatment of open venous stasis ulcer. Modifiers A1-A9 are not assigned. Must be billed with AW, RT, or LT

IOM: 100-02, 15, 100

DMEPOS Modifier(s): AW

⊘ **A6533** Gradient compression stocking, thigh length, 18–30 mmHg, each Ⓑ E

IOM: 100-02, 15, 130; 100-03, 4, 280.1

⊘ **A6534** Gradient compression stocking, thigh length, 30–40 mmHg, each Ⓑ E

IOM: 100-02, 15, 130; 100-03, 4, 280.1

⊘ **A6535** Gradient compression stocking, thigh length, 40–50 mmHg, each Ⓑ E

IOM: 100-02, 15, 130; 100-03, 4, 280.1

⊘ **A6536** Gradient compression stocking, full length/chap style, 18–30 mmHg, each Ⓑ E

IOM: 100-02, 15, 130; 100-03, 4, 280.1

⊘ **A6537** Gradient compression stocking, full length/chap style, 30–40 mmHg, each Ⓑ E

IOM: 100-02, 15, 130; 100-03, 4, 280.1

⊘ **A6538** Gradient compression stocking, full length/chap style, 40–50 mmHg, each Ⓑ E

IOM: 100-02, 15, 130; 100-03, 4, 280.1

⊘ **A6539** Gradient compression stocking, waist length, 18–30 mmHg, each Ⓑ E

IOM: 100-02, 15, 130; 100-03, 4, 280.1

⊘ **A6540** Gradient compression stocking, waist length, 30–40 mmHg, each Ⓑ E

IOM: 100-02, 15, 130; 100-03, 4, 280.1

⊘ **A6541** Gradient compression stocking, waist length, 40–50 mmHg, each Ⓑ E

IOM: 100-02, 15, 130; 100-03, 4, 280.1

⊘ **A6544** Gradient compression stocking, garter belt Ⓑ E

IOM: 100-02, 15, 130; 100-03, 4, 280.1

✲ **A6545** Gradient compression wrap, non-elastic, below knee, 30-50 mm hg, each Ⓑ Qp Qh & N

Modifiers RT and/or LT must be appended. When assigned for bilateral items (left/right) on the same date of service, bill both items on the same claim line using RT/LT modifiers and 2 units of service.

IOM: 10-02, 15, 100

DMEPOS Modifier(s): AW

⊘ **A6549** Gradient compression stocking/sleeve, not otherwise specified Ⓑ E

IOM: 100-02, 15, 130; 100-03, 4, 280.1

WOUND CARE (A6550)

✳ **A6550** Wound care set, for negative pressure wound therapy electrical pump, includes all supplies and accessories Ⓑ Qh & N

RESPIRATORY DURABLE MEDICAL EQUIPMENT, INEXPENSIVE AND ROUTINELY PURCHASED (A7000-A7509)

✳ **A7000** Canister, disposable, used with suction pump, each Ⓑ Qp Qh & Y

DMEPOS Modifier(s): NU, KE

✳ **A7001** Canister, non-disposable, used with suction pump, each Ⓑ Qh & Y

DMEPOS Modifier(s): NU

✳ **A7002** Tubing, used with suction pump, each Ⓑ Qh & Y

DMEPOS Modifier(s): NU

✳ **A7003** Administration set, with small volume nonfiltered pneumatic nebulizer, disposable Ⓑ Qp Qh & Y

DMEPOS Modifier(s): NU

✳ **A7004** Small volume nonfiltered pneumatic nebulizer, disposable Ⓑ Qh & Y

DMEPOS Modifier(s): NU

▶ New   ↻ Revised   ✔ Reinstated   ~~deleted~~ Deleted   ⊘ Not covered or valid by Medicare

✲ Special coverage instructions   ✳ Carrier discretion   Ⓑ Bill local carrier   Ⓓ Bill DME MAC

✳ **A7005** Administration set, with small volume nonfiltered pneumatic nebulizer, non-disposable ⑧ Qp Qh 🦽   Y

DMEPOS Modifier(s): NU

✳ **A7006** Administration set, with small volume filtered pneumatic nebulizer ⑧ Qp Qh 🦽   Y

DMEPOS Modifier(s): NU

✳ **A7007** Large volume nebulizer, disposable, unfilled, used with aerosol compressor ⑧ Qh 🦽   Y

DMEPOS Modifier(s): NU

✳ **A7008** Large volume nebulizer, disposable, prefilled, used with aerosol compressor ⑧ 🦽   Y

DMEPOS Modifier(s): NU

✳ **A7009** Reservoir bottle, nondisposable, used with large volume ultrasonic nebulizer ⑧ 🦽   Y

DMEPOS Modifier(s): NU

✳ **A7010** Corrugated tubing, disposable, used with large volume nebulizer, 100 feet ⑧ Qh 🦽   Y

DMEPOS Modifier(s): NU

✳ **A7011** Corrugated tubing, non-disposable, used with large volume nebulizer, 10 feet ⑧   Y

✳ **A7012** Water collection device, used with large volume nebulizer ⑧ Qh 🦽   Y

DMEPOS Modifier(s): NU

✳ **A7013** Filter, disposable, used with aerosol compressor or ultrasonic generator ⑧ Qp Qh 🦽   Y

DMEPOS Modifier(s): NU

✳ **A7014** Filter, non-disposable, used with aerosol compressor or ultrasonic generator ⑧ Qp Qh 🦽   Y

DMEPOS Modifier(s): NU

✳ **A7015** Aerosol mask, used with DME nebulizer ⑧ Qh 🦽   Y

DMEPOS Modifier(s): NU

✳ **A7016** Dome and mouthpiece, used with small volume ultrasonic nebulizer ⑧ Qp Qh 🦽   Y

DMEPOS Modifier(s): NU

◯ **A7017** Nebulizer, durable, glass or autoclavable plastic, bottle type, not used with oxygen ⑧ Qp Qh 🦽   Y

IOM: 100-03, 4, 280.1

DMEPOS Modifier(s): NU, RR, UE

✳ **A7018** Water, distilled, used with large volume nebulizer, 1000 ml ⑧ Qh 🦽   Y

✳ **A7020** Interface for cough stimulating device, includes all components, replacement only ⑧ Qp Qh 🦽   Y

DMEPOS Modifier(s): NU

↺ ✳ **A7025** High frequency chest wall oscillation system vest, replacement for use with patient owned equipment, each ⑧ Qp Qh 🦽   N

DMEPOS Modifier(s): RR

✳ **A7026** High frequency chest wall oscillation system hose, replacement for use with patient owned equipment, each ⑧ Qp Qh 🦽   Y

DMEPOS Modifier(s): NU

✳ **A7027** Combination oral/nasal mask, used with continuous positive airway pressure device, each ⑧ Qp Qh 🦽   Y

DMEPOS Modifier(s): NU

✳ **A7028** Oral cushion for combination oral/nasal mask, replacement only, each ⑧ Qp Qh 🦽   Y

DMEPOS Modifier(s): NU

✳ **A7029** Nasal pillows for combination oral/ nasal mask, replacement only, pair ⑧ Qp Qh 🦽   Y

DMEPOS Modifier(s): NU

✳ **A7030** Full face mask used with positive airway pressure device, each ⑧ Qh 🦽   Y

DMEPOS Modifier(s): NU

✳ **A7031** Face mask interface, replacement for full face mask, each ⑧ Qh 🦽   Y

DMEPOS Modifier(s): NU

✳ **A7032** Cushion for use on nasal mask interface, replacement only, each ⑧ Qp Qh 🦽   Y

DMEPOS Modifier(s): NU

✳ **A7033** Pillow for use on nasal cannula type interface, replacement only, pair ⑧ Qh 🦽   Y

DMEPOS Modifier(s): NU

✳ **A7034** Nasal interface (mask or cannula type) used with positive airway pressure device, with or without head strap ⑧ Qh 🦽   Y

DMEPOS Modifier(s): NU

✳ **A7035** Headgear used with positive airway pressure device ⑧ Qp Qh 🦽   Y

DMEPOS Modifier(s): NU

PQRS   Qp **Quantity Physician Appendix A**   Qh **Quantity Hospital Appendix B**   ♀ **Female only**

♂ **Male only**   A **Age**   🦽 **DMEPOS**   A2-Z3 **ASC Payment Indicator**   A-Y **ASC Status Indicator**   Coding Clinic

✳ A7036 Chinstrap used with positive airway pressure device Ⓑ Qp Qh ♿   Y

DMEPOS Modifier(s): NU

✳ A7037 Tubing used with positive airway pressure device Ⓑ Qp Qh ♿   Y

DMEPOS Modifier(s): NU

✳ A7038 Filter, disposable, used with positive airway pressure device Ⓑ Qh ♿   Y

DMEPOS Modifier(s): NU

✳ A7039 Filter, non disposable, used with positive airway pressure device Ⓑ Qp Qh ♿   Y

DMEPOS Modifier(s): NU

✳ A7040 One way chest drain valve Ⓑ Qp Qh ♿   N

✳ A7041 Water seal drainage container and tubing for use with implanted chest tube Ⓑ Qp Qh ♿   N

~~A7042~~ ~~Implanted pleural catheter, each~~   ✖

~~A7043~~ ~~Vacuum drainage bottle and tubing for use with implanted catheter~~   ✖

✳ A7044 Oral interface used with positive airway pressure device, each Ⓑ Qp Qh ♿   Y

DMEPOS Modifier(s): NU

✪ A7045 Exhalation port with or without swivel used with accessories for positive airway devices, replacement only Ⓑ Qh ♿   Y

IOM: 100-03, 4, 230.17

DMEPOS Modifier(s): NU, RR, UE

✪ A7046 Water chamber for humidifier, used with positive airway pressure device, replacement, each Ⓑ Qh ♿   Y

IOM: 100-03, 4, 230.17

DMEPOS Modifier(s): NU

✳ A7047 Oral interface used with respiratory suction pump, each Ⓑ Qp Qh   N

▶ **✳ A7048** Vacuum drainage collection unit and tubing kit, including all supplies needed for collection unit change, for use with implanted catheter, each   N1 N

✪ A7501 Tracheostoma valve, including diaphragm, each Ⓑ Qp ♿   N

IOM: 100-02, 15, 120

✪ A7502 Replacement diaphragm/faceplate for tracheostoma valve, each Ⓑ Qh ♿   N

IOM: 100-02, 15, 120

✪ A7503 Filter holder or filter cap, reusable, for use in a tracheostoma heat and moisture exchange system, each Ⓑ Qh ♿   N

IOM: 100-02, 15, 120

✪ A7504 Filter for use in a tracheostoma heat and moisture exchange system, each Ⓑ Qp Qh ♿   N

IOM: 100-02, 15, 120

✪ A7505 Housing, reusable without adhesive, for use in a heat and moisture exchange system and/or with a tracheostoma valve, each Ⓑ ♿   N

IOM: 100-02, 15, 120

✪ A7506 Adhesive disc for use in a heat and moisture exchange system and/or with tracheostoma valve, any type, each Ⓑ Qh ♿   N

IOM: 100-02, 15, 120

✪ A7507 Filter holder and integrated filter without adhesive, for use in a tracheostoma heat and moisture exchange system, each Ⓑ Qp Qh ♿   N

IOM: 100-02, 15, 120

✪ A7508 Housing and integrated adhesive, for use in a tracheostoma heat and moisture exchange system and/or with a tracheostoma valve, each Ⓑ Qh ♿   N

IOM: 100-02, 15, 120

✪ A7509 Filter holder and integrated filter housing, and adhesive, for use as a tracheostoma heat and moisture exchange system, each Ⓑ Qh ♿   N

IOM: 100-02, 15, 120

✳ A7520 Tracheostomy/laryngectomy tube, non-cuffed, polyvinylchloride (PVC), silicone or equal, each Ⓑ Qp ♿   N

✳ A7521 Tracheostomy/laryngectomy tube, cuffed, polyvinylchloride (PVC), silicone or equal, each Ⓑ ♿   N

✳ A7522 Tracheostomy/laryngectomy tube, stainless steel or equal (sterilizable and reusable), each Ⓑ Qh ♿   N

✳ A7523 Tracheostomy shower protector, each Ⓑ   N

✳ A7524 Tracheostoma stent/stud/button, each Ⓑ Qp Qh ♿   N

✳ A7525 Tracheostomy mask, each Ⓑ ♿   N

✳ A7526 Tracheostomy tube collar/holder, each Ⓑ Qh ♿   N

✳ A7527 Tracheostomy/laryngectomy tube plug/stop, each Ⓑ Qp ♿   N

▶ New ↻ Revised ✔ Reinstated ~~deleted~~ Deleted ⊘ Not covered or valid by Medicare
✪ Special coverage instructions ✳ Carrier discretion Ⓑ Bill local carrier Ⓑ Bill DME MAC

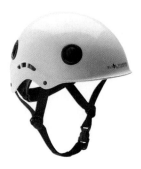

Figure 7 Helmet.

HELMETS (A8000-A8004)

✳ **A8000**   Helmet, protective, soft, prefabricated, includes all components and accessories ⑧ ♿   Y

     DMEPOS Modifier(s): NU, RR, UE

✳ **A8001**   Helmet, protective, hard, prefabricated, includes all components and accessories ⑧ ♿   Y

     DMEPOS Modifier(s): NU, RR, UE

✳ **A8002**   Helmet, protective, soft, custom fabricated, includes all components and accessories ⑧ ♿   Y

     DMEPOS Modifier(s): NU, RR, UE

✳ **A8003**   Helmet, protective, hard, custom fabricated, includes all components and accessories ⑧ ♿   Y

     DMEPOS Modifier(s): NU, RR, UE

✳ **A8004**   Soft interface for helmet, replacement only ⑧ ♿   Y

     DMEPOS Modifier(s): NU, RR, UE

ADMINISTRATIVE, MISCELLANEOUS, AND INVESTIGATIONAL (A9000-A9999)

NOTE: The following codes do not imply that codes in other sections are necessarily covered.

✪ **A9150**   Non-prescription drugs ⑧   B

     IOM: 100-02, 15, 50

⊘ **A9152**   Single vitamin/mineral/trace element, oral, per dose, not otherwise specified ⑧   E

⊘ **A9153**   Multiple vitamins, with or without minerals and trace elements, oral, per dose, not otherwise specified ⑧   E

✳ **A9155**   Artificial saliva, 30 ml ⑧   B

⊘ **A9180**   Pediculosis (lice infestation) treatment, topical, for administration by patient/caretaker ⑧   E

⊘ **A9270**   Non-covered item or service ⑧   E

     IOM: 100-02, 16, 20

↺ ⊘ **A9272**   Wound suction, disposable, includes dressing, all accessories and components, any type, each **Qp** **Qh**   E

     Medicare Statute 1861(n)

⊘ **A9273**   Hot water bottle, ice cap or collar, heat and/or cold wrap, any type   E

↺ ⊘ **A9274**   External ambulatory insulin delivery system, disposable, each, includes all supplies and accessories ⑧   E

     Medicare Statute 1861(n)

⊘ **A9275**   Home glucose disposable monitor, includes test strips ⑧   E

⊘ **A9276**   Sensor; invasive (e.g. subcutaneous), disposable, for use with interstitial continuous glucose monitoring system, one unit = 1 day supply ⑧   E

     Medicare Statute 1861(n)

⊘ **A9277**   Transmitter; external, for use with interstitial continuous glucose monitoring system ⑧   E

     Medicare Statute 1861(n)

⊘ **A9278**   Receiver (monitor); external, for use with interstitial continuous glucose monitoring system ⑧   E

     Medicare Statute 1861(n)

↺ ⊘ **A9279**   Monitoring feature/device, stand-alone or integrated, any type, includes all accessories, components and electronics, not otherwise classified ⑧   E

     Medicare Statute 1861(n)

⊘ **A9280**   Alert or alarm device, not otherwise classified ⑧   E

     Medicare Statute 1861

⊘ **A9281**   Reaching/grabbing device, any type, any length, each ⑧   E

     Medicare Statute 1862 SSA

⊘ **A9282**   Wig, any type, each ⑧   E

     Medicare Statute 1862 SSA

⊘ **A9283**   Foot pressure off loading/supportive device, any type, each ⑧   E

     Medicare Statute 1862A(i)13

✪ **A9284**   Spirometer, non-electronic, includes all accessories ⑧ **Qp** **Qh**   N

⊘ **A9300**   Exercise equipment ⑧   E

     IOM: 100-02, 15, 110.1; 100-03, 4, 280.1

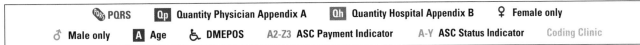

🄿🄿 PQRS	**Qp** Quantity Physician Appendix A	**Qh** Quantity Hospital Appendix B
♀ Female only	♂ Male only	**A** Age
♿ DMEPOS	A2-Z3 ASC Payment Indicator	A-Y ASC Status Indicator	Coding Clinic

Supplies for Radiology Procedures (Radiopharmaceuticals)

✳ **A9500** Technetium Tc-99m sestamibi, diagnostic, per study dose ⑧ **Qp** **Qh**   N1 N

Should be filed on same claim as procedure code reporting radiopharmaceutical. Verify with payer definition of a "study."

Coding Clinic: 2006, Q2, P5

✳ **A9501** Technetium Tc-99m teboroxime, diagnostic, per study dose ⑧ **Qp** **Qh**   N1 N

✳ **A9502** Technetium Tc-99m tetrofosmin, diagnostic, per study dose ⑧ **Qp** **Qh**   N1 N

Coding Clinic: 2006, Q2, P5

✳ **A9503** Technetium Tc-99m medronate, diagnostic, per study dose, up to 30 millicuries ⑧ **Qp** **Qh**   N1 N

✳ **A9504** Technetium Tc-99m apcitide, diagnostic, per study dose, up to 20 millicuries ⑧ **Qp** **Qh**   N1 N

✳ **A9505** Thallium Tl-201 thallous chloride, diagnostic, per millicurie ⑧   N1 N

✳ **A9507** Indium In-111 capromab pendetide, diagnostic, per study dose, up to 10 millicuries ⑧ **Qp** **Qh**   N1 N

✳ **A9508** Iodine I-131 iobenguane sulfate, diagnostic, per 0.5 millicurie ⑧ **Qp** **Qh**   N1 N

✳ **A9509** Iodine I-123 sodium iodide, diagnostic, per millicurie ⑧   N1 N

✳ **A9510** Technetium Tc-99m disofenin, diagnostic, per study dose, up to 15 millicuries ⑧ **Qp** **Qh**   N1 N

✳ **A9512** Technetium Tc-99m pertechnetate, diagnostic, per millicurie ⑧ **Qp** **Qh**   N1 N

✳ **A9516** Iodine I-123 sodium iodide, diagnostic, per 100 microcuries, up to 999 microcuries ⑧   N1 N

✳ **A9517** Iodine I-131 sodium iodide capsule(s), therapeutic, per millicurie ⑧   K

✳ **A9520** Technetium Tc-99m, tilmanocept, diagnostic, up to 0.5 millicuries ⑧ **Qp** **Qh**   K2 G

✳ **A9521** Technetium Tc-99m exametazime, diagnostic, per study dose, up to 25 millicuries ⑧ **Qp** **Qh**   N1 N

✳ **A9524** Iodine I-131 iodinated serum albumin, diagnostic, per 5 microcuries ⑧   N1 N

✳ **A9526** Nitrogen N-13 ammonia, diagnostic, per study dose, up to 40 millicuries ⑧ **Qp** **Qh**   N1 N

✳ **A9527** Iodine I-125, sodium iodide solution, therapeutic, per millicurie ⑧   H2 U

✳ **A9528** Iodine I-131 sodium iodide capsule(s), diagnostic, per millicurie ⑧   N1 N

✳ **A9529** Iodine I-131 sodium iodide solution, diagnostic, per millicurie ⑧   N1 N

✳ **A9530** Iodine I-131 sodium iodide solution, therapeutic, per millicurie ⑧   K

✳ **A9531** Iodine I-131 sodium iodide, diagnostic, per microcurie (up to 100 microcuries) ⑧   N1 N

✳ **A9532** Iodine I-125 serum albumin, diagnostic, per 5 microcuries ⑧   N1 N

✳ **A9536** Technetium Tc-99m depreotide, diagnostic, per study dose, up to 35 millicuries ⑧ **Qp** **Qh**   N1 N

✳ **A9537** Technetium Tc-99m mebrofenin, diagnostic, per study dose, up to 15 millicuries ⑧ **Qp** **Qh**   N1 N

✳ **A9538** Technetium Tc-99m pyrophosphate, diagnostic, per study dose, up to 25 millicuries ⑧ **Qp** **Qh**   N1 N

✳ **A9539** Technetium Tc-99m pentetate, diagnostic, per study dose, up to 25 millicuries ⑧ **Qp** **Qh**   N1 N

✳ **A9540** Technetium Tc-99m macroaggregated albumin, diagnostic, per study dose, up to 10 millicuries ⑧ **Qp** **Qh**   N1 N

✳ **A9541** Technetium Tc-99m sulfur colloid, diagnostic, per study dose, up to 20 millicuries ⑧ **Qp** **Qh**   N1 N

✳ **A9542** Indium In-111 ibritumomab tiuxetan, diagnostic, per study dose, up to 5 millicuries ⑧ **Qp** **Qh**   N1 N

Specifically for diagnostic use.

✳ **A9543** Yttrium Y-90 ibritumomab tiuxetan, therapeutic, per treatment dose, up to 40 millicuries ⑧ **Qp** **Qh**   K

Specifically for therapeutic use.

✳ **A9544** Iodine I-131 tositumomab, diagnostic, per study dose ⑧ **Qp** **Qh**   N1 N

✳ **A9545** Iodine I-131 tositumomab, therapeutic, per treatment dose ⑧ **Qp** **Qh**   E

✳ **A9546** Cobalt Co-57/58, cyanocobalamin, diagnostic, per study dose, up to 1 microcurie ⑧ **Qp** **Qh**   N1 N

✳ **A9547** Indium In-111 oxyquinoline, diagnostic, per 0.5 millicurie ⑧ **Qp** **Qh**   N1 N

✳ **A9548** Indium In-111 pentetate, diagnostic, per 0.5 millicurie ⑧   N1 N

▶ New   ↻ Revised   ✔ Reinstated   deleted Deleted   ⊘ Not covered or valid by Medicare
⟳ Special coverage instructions   ✳ Carrier discretion   ⑧ Bill local carrier   Ⓑ Bill DME MAC

＊ **A9550** Technetium Tc-99m sodium gluceptate, diagnostic, per study dose, up to 25 millicuries ⓑ Qp Qh N1 N

＊ **A9551** Technetium Tc-99m succimer, diagnostic, per study dose, up to 10 millicuries ⓑ Qp Qh N1 N

＊ **A9552** Fluorodeoxyglucose F-18 FDG, diagnostic, per study dose, up to 45 millicuries ⓑ Qp Qh N1 N

Coding Clinic: 2008, Q3, P7

＊ **A9553** Chromium Cr-51 sodium chromate, diagnostic, per study dose, up to 250 microcuries ⓑ Qp Qh N1 N

＊ **A9554** Iodine I-125 sodium Iothalamate, diagnostic, per study dose, up to 10 microcuries ⓑ Qp Qh N1 N

＊ **A9555** Rubidium Rb-82, diagnostic, per study dose, up to 60 millicuries ⓑ Qp Qh N1 N

＊ **A9556** Gallium Ga-67 citrate, diagnostic, per millicurie ⓑ Qp Qh N1 N

＊ **A9557** Technetium Tc-99m bicisate, diagnostic, per study dose, up to 25 millicuries ⓑ Qp Qh N1 N

＊ **A9558** Xenon Xe-133 gas, diagnostic, per 10 millicuries ⓑ N1 N

＊ **A9559** Cobalt Co-57 cyanocobalamin, oral, diagnostic, per study dose, up to 1 microcurie ⓑ Qp Qh N1 N

＊ **A9560** Technetium Tc-99m labeled red blood cells, diagnostic, per study dose, up to 30 millicuries ⓑ Qp Qh N1 N

Coding Clinic: 2008, Q3, P7

＊ **A9561** Technetium Tc-99m oxidronate, diagnostic, per study dose, up to 30 millicuries ⓑ Qp Qh N1 N

＊ **A9562** Technetium Tc-99m mertiatide, diagnostic, per study dose, up to 15 millicuries ⓑ Qp Qh N1 N

＊ **A9563** Sodium phosphate P-32, therapeutic, per millicurie ⓑ K

＊ **A9564** Chromic phosphate P-32 suspension, therapeutic, per millicurie ⓑ K

＊ **A9566** Technetium Tc-99m fanolesomab, diagnostic, per study dose, up to 25 millicuries ⓑ Qp Qh N1 N

＊ **A9567** Technetium Tc-99m pentetate, diagnostic, aerosol, per study dose, up to 75 millicuries ⓑ Qp Qh N1 N

＊ **A9568** Technetium TC-99m arcitumomab, diagnostic, per study dose, up to 45 millicuries ⓑ N1 N

＊ **A9569** Technetium Tc-99m exametazime labeled autologous white blood cells, diagnostic, per study dose ⓑ Qp Qh N1 N

＊ **A9570** Indium In-111 labeled autologous white blood cells, diagnostic, per study dose ⓑ Qp Qh N1 N

＊ **A9571** Indium In-111 labeled autologous platelets, diagnostic, per study dose ⓑ Qp Qh N1 N

＊ **A9572** Indium In-111 pentetreotide, diagnostic, per study dose, up to 6 millicuries ⓑ N1 N

＊ **A9575** Injection, gadoterate meglumine, 0.1 ml ⓑ N1 N

NDC: Dotarem

＊ **A9576** Injection, gadoteridol, (ProHance Multipack), per ml ⓑ N1 N

＊ **A9577** Injection, gadobenate dimeglumine (MultiHance), per ml ⓑ N1 N

＊ **A9578** Injection, gadobenate dimeglumine (MultiHance Multipack), per ml ⓑ N1 N

＊ **A9579** Injection, gadolinium-based magnetic resonance contrast agent, not otherwise specified (NOS), per ml ⓑ Qp Qh N1 N

NDC: Magnevist, Omniscan, Optimark, Prohance

＊ **A9580** Sodium fluoride F-18, diagnostic, per study dose, up to 30 millicuries ⓑ Qp Qh N1 N

＊ **A9581** Injection, gadoxetate disodium, 1 ml ⓑ N1 N

Local Medicare contractors may require the use of modifier JW to identify unused product from single-dose vials that are appropriately discarded.

NDC: Eovist

＊ **A9582** Iodine I-123 iobenguane, diagnostic, per study dose, up to 15 millicuries ⓑ Qp Qh N1 N

Molecular imaging agent that assists in the identification of rare neuroendocrine tumors.

＊ **A9583** Injection, gadofosveset trisodium, 1 ml ⓑ Qp Qh N1 N

NDC: Ablavar

＊ **A9584** Iodine 1-123 ioflupane, diagnostic, per study dose, up to 5 millicuries ⓑ Qp Qh N1 N

Coding Clinic: 2012, Q1, P9

| ⓆⓇⓈ PQRS | Qp Quantity Physician Appendix A | Qh Quantity Hospital Appendix B | ♀ Female only |
| ♂ Male only | A Age | ♿ DMEPOS | A2-Z3 ASC Payment Indicator | A-Y ASC Status Indicator | Coding Clinic |

* **A9585**   Injection, gadobutrol,
0.1 ml Ⓑ `Qp` `Qh`   N1 N

Coding Clinic: 2012, Q1, P8

NDC: Gadavist

↻ ✲ **A9586**   Florbetapir F18, diagnostic,
per study dose, up to
10 millicuries Ⓑ `Qp` `Qh`   K2 G

✲ **A9599**   Radiopharmaceutical, diagnostic,
for beta-amyloid positron emission
tomography (PET) imaging, per study
dose Ⓑ `Qp` `Qh`   N1 N

* **A9600**   Strontium Sr-89 chloride, therapeutic,
per millicurie Ⓑ `Qp` `Qh`   K

* **A9604**   Samarium SM-153 lexidronam,
therapeutic, per treatment dose, up to
150 millicuries Ⓑ `Qp` `Qh`   K

▶ * **A9606**   Radium Ra-223 dichloride, therapeutic,
per microcurie   K2 K

✲ **A9698**   Non-radioactive contrast imaging
material, not otherwise classified, per
study Ⓑ   N1 N

IOM: 100-04, 12, 70; 100-04, 13, 20

* **A9699**   Radiopharmaceutical, therapeutic, not
otherwise classified Ⓑ   N

✲ **A9700**   Supply of injectable contrast material
for use in echocardiography, per
study Ⓑ `Qp` `Qh`   N

IOM: 100-04, 12, 30.4

Miscellaneous Service Component

* **A9900**   Miscellaneous DME supply, accessory,
and/or service component of another
HCPCS code Ⓑ   Y

Local carrier (Ⓑ) if used with implanted
DME.

On DMEPOS fee schedule as a
payable replacement for miscellaneous
implanted or non-implanted items.

* **A9901**   DME delivery, set up, and/or dispensing
service component of another HCPCS
code Ⓑ   A

* **A9999**   Miscellaneous DME supply
or accessory, not otherwise
specified Ⓑ   Y

Local carrier (Ⓑ) if used with implanted
DME.

On DMEPOS fee schedule as a
payable replacement for miscellaneous
implanted or non-implanted items.

▶ **New**   ↻ **Revised**   ✔ **Reinstated**   deleted **Deleted**   ⊘ **Not covered or valid by Medicare**

✲ **Special coverage instructions**   * **Carrier discretion**   Ⓑ **Bill local carrier**   Ⓑ **Bill DME MAC**

ENTERAL AND PARENTERAL THERAPY
(B4000-B9999)

Enteral Formulae and Enteral Medical Supplies

⊛ **B4034** Enteral feeding supply kit; syringe fed, per day, includes but not limited to feeding/flushing syringe, administration set tubing, dressings, tape ⑧ **Qh**　Y

Dressings used with gastrostomy tubes for enteral nutrition (covered under the prosthetic device benefit) are included in the payment.

IOM: 100-02, 15, 120; 100-03, 3, 180.2; 100-04, 20, 100.2.2

PEN: On Fee Schedule

⊛ **B4035** Enteral feeding supply kit; pump fed, per day, includes but not limited to feeding/flushing syringe, administration set tubing, dressings, tape ⑧ **Qh**　Y

IOM: 100-02, 15, 120; 100-03, 3, 180.2; 100-04, 20, 100.2.2

PEN: On Fee Schedule

⊛ **B4036** Enteral feeding supply kit; gravity fed, per day, includes but not limited to feeding/flushing syringe, administration set tubing, dressings, tape ⑧ **Qh**　Y

IOM: 100-02, 15, 120; 100-03, 3, 180.2; 100-04, 20, 100.2.2

PEN: On Fee Schedule

⊛ **B4081** Nasogastric tubing with stylet ⑧ **Qh**　Y

More than 3 nasogastric tubes (B4081-B4083), or 1 gastrostomy/jejunostomy tube (B4087-B4088) every three months is rarely medically necessary

IOM: 100-02, 15, 120; 100-03, 3, 180.2; 100-04, 20, 100.2.2

PEN: On Fee Schedule

⊛ **B4082** Nasogastric tubing without stylet ⑧ **Qh**　Y

IOM: 100-02, 15, 120; 100-03, 3, 180.2; 100-04, 20, 100.2.2

PEN: On Fee Schedule

⊛ **B4083** Stomach tube - Levine type ⑧ **Qp** **Qh**　Y

IOM: 100-02, 15, 120; 100-03, 3, 180.2; 100-04, 20, 100.2.2

PEN: On Fee Schedule

✳ **B4087** Gastrostomy/jejunostomy tube, standard, any material, any type, each ⑧ **Qh**　A

PEN: On Fee Schedule

✳ **B4088** Gastrostomy/jejunostomy tube, low-profile, any material, any type, each ⑧　A

PEN: On Fee Schedule

⊘ **B4100** Food thickener, administered orally, per ounce ⑧　E

⊛ **B4102** Enteral formula, for adults, used to replace fluids and electrolytes (e.g. clear liquids), 500 ml = 1 unit ⑧ **A**　Y

IOM: 100-03, 3, 180.2

⊛ **B4103** Enteral formula, for pediatrics, used to replace fluids and electrolytes (e.g. clear liquids), 500 ml = 1 unit ⑧ **A**　Y

IOM: 100-03, 3, 180.2

⊛ **B4104** Additive for enteral formula (e.g. fiber) ⑧　E

IOM: 100-03, 3, 180.2

⊛ **B4149** Enteral formula, manufactured blenderized natural foods with intact nutrients, includes proteins, fats, carbohydrates, vitamins and minerals, may include fiber, administered through an enteral feeding tube, 100 calories = 1 unit ⑧ **Qp** **Qh**　Y

Produced to meet unique nutrient needs for specific disease conditions; medical record must document specific condition and need for special nutrient

IOM: 100-02, 15, 120; 100-03, 3, 180.2; 100-04, 20, 100.2.2

PEN: On Fee Schedule

⊛ **B4150** Enteral formulae, nutritionally complete with intact nutrients, includes proteins, fats, carbohydrates, vitamins, and minerals, may include fiber, administered through an enteral feeding tube, 100 calories = 1 unit ⑧ **Qh**　Y

IOM: 100-02, 15, 120; 100-03, 3, 180.2; 100-04, 20, 100.2.2

PEN: On Fee Schedule

⊛ **B4152** Enteral formula, nutritionally complete, calorically dense (equal to or greater than 1.5 kcal/ml) with intact nutrients, includes proteins, fats, carbohydrates, vitamins and minerals, may include fiber, administered through an enteral feeding tube, 100 calories = 1 unit ⑧ **Qh**　Y

IOM: 100-02, 15, 120; 100-03, 3, 180.2; 100-04, 20, 100.2.2

PEN: On Fee Schedule

PQRS PQRS	**Qp** Quantity Physician Appendix A	**Qh** Quantity Hospital Appendix B	♀ Female only
♂ Male only	**A** Age	♿ DMEPOS　A2-Z3 ASC Payment Indicator	A-Y ASC Status Indicator　Coding Clinic

⊛ **B4153** Enteral formula, nutritionally complete, hydrolyzed proteins (amino acids and peptide chain), includes fats, carbohydrates, vitamins and minerals, may include fiber, administered through an enteral feeding tube, 100 calories = 1 unit ⑬ **Qp** **Qh**   Y

If 2 enteral nutrition products described by same HCPCS code and provided at same time billed on single claim line with units of service reflecting total calories of both nutrients

IOM: 100-02, 15, 120; 100-03, 3, 180.2; 100-04, 20, 100.2.2

PEN: On Fee Schedule

⊛ **B4154** Enteral formula, nutritionally complete, for special metabolic needs, excludes inherited disease of metabolism, includes altered composition of proteins, fats, carbohydrates, vitamins and/or minerals, may include fiber, administered through an enteral feeding tube, 100 calories = 1 unit ⑬ **Qh**   Y

IOM: 100-02, 15, 120; 100-03, 3, 180.2; 100-04, 20, 100.2.2

PEN: On Fee Schedule

⊛ **B4155** Enteral formula, nutritionally incomplete/modular nutrients, includes specific nutrients, carbohydrates (e.g. glucose polymers), proteins/amino acids (e.g. glutamine, arginine), fat (e.g. medium chain triglycerides) or combination, administered through an enteral feeding tube, 100 calories = 1 unit ⑬ **Qh**   Y

IOM: 100-02, 15, 120; 100-03, 3, 180.2; 100-04, 20, 100.2.2

PEN: On Fee Schedule

⊛ **B4157** Enteral formula, nutritionally complete, for special metabolic needs for inherited disease of metabolism, includes proteins, fats, carbohydrates, vitamins and minerals, may include fiber, administered through an enteral feeding tube, 100 calories = 1 unit ⑬ **Qp** **Qh**   Y

IOM: 100-03, 3, 180.2

⊛ **B4158** Enteral formula, for pediatrics, nutritionally complete with intact nutrients, includes proteins, fats, carbohydrates, vitamins and minerals, may include fiber and/or iron, administered through an enteral feeding tube, 100 calories = 1 unit ⑬ **Qh** **A**   Y

IOM: 100-03, 3, 180.2

⊛ **B4159** Enteral formula, for pediatrics, nutritionally complete soy based with intact nutrients, includes proteins, fats, carbohydrates, vitamins and minerals, may include fiber and/or iron, administered through an enteral feeding tube, 100 calories = 1 unit ⑬ **Qh** **A**   Y

IOM: 100-03, 3, 180.2

⊛ **B4160** Enteral formula, for pediatrics, nutritionally complete calorically dense (equal to or greater than 0.7 kcal/ml) with intact nutrients, includes proteins, fats, carbohydrates, vitamins and minerals, may include fiber, administered through an enteral feeding tube, 100 calories = 1 unit ⑬ **Qp** **Qh** **A**   Y

IOM: 100-03, 3, 180.2

⊛ **B4161** Enteral formula, for pediatrics, hydrolyzed/amino acids and peptide chain proteins, includes fats, carbohydrates, vitamins and minerals, may include fiber, administered through an enteral feeding tube, 100 calories = 1 unit ⑬ **Qh** **A**   Y

IOM: 100-03, 3, 180.2

⊛ **B4162** Enteral formula, for pediatrics, special metabolic needs for inherited disease of metabolism, includes proteins, fats, carbohydrates, vitamins and minerals, may include fiber, administered through an enteral feeding tube, 100 calories = 1 unit ⑬ **Qh** **A**   Y

IOM: 100-03, 3, 180.2

Parenteral Nutritional Solutions and Supplies

⊛ **B4164** Parenteral nutrition solution: carbohydrates (dextrose), 50% or less (500 ml = 1 unit) - homemix ⑬ **Qp** **Qh**   Y

IOM: 100-02, 15, 120; 100-03, 3, 180.2; 100-04, 20, 100.2.2

PEN: On Fee Schedule

▶ New   ↩ Revised   ✔ Reinstated   ~~deleted~~ Deleted   ⊘ Not covered or valid by Medicare
⊛ Special coverage instructions   ✳ Carrier discretion   Ⓑ Bill local carrier   ⑬ Bill DME MAC

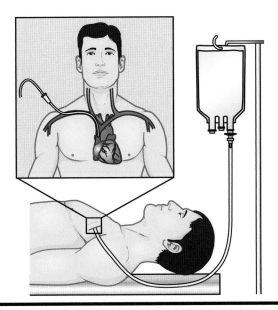

Figure 8 Total Parenteral Nutrition (TPN) involves percutaneous placement of central venous catheter into vena cava or right atrium.

⊛ **B4168** Parenteral nutrition solution; amino acid, 3.5%, (500 ml = 1 unit) - homemix Ⓑ Qh   Y

IOM: 100-02, 15, 120; 100-03, 3, 180.2; 100-04, 20, 100.2.2

PEN: On Fee Schedule

⊛ **B4172** Parenteral nutrition solution; amino acid, 5.5% through 7%, (500 ml = 1 unit) - homemix Ⓑ Qh   Y

IOM: 100-02, 15, 120; 100-03, 3, 180.2; 100-04, 20, 100.2.2

⊛ **B4176** Parenteral nutrition solution; amino acid, 7% through 8.5%, (500 ml = 1 unit) - homemix Ⓑ Qp Qh   Y

IOM: 100-02, 15, 120; 100-03, 3, 180.2; 100-04, 20, 100.2.2

PEN: On Fee Schedule

⊛ **B4178** Parenteral nutrition solution: amino acid, greater than 8.5% (500 ml = 1 unit) - homemix Ⓑ Qh   Y

IOM: 100-02, 15, 120; 100-03, 3, 180.2; 100-04, 20, 100.2.2

PEN: On Fee Schedule

⊛ **B4180** Parenteral nutrition solution; carbohydrates (dextrose), greater than 50% (500 ml = 1 unit) - home mix Ⓑ Qh   Y

IOM: 100-02, 15, 120; 100-03, 3, 180.2; 100-04, 20, 100.2.2

PEN: On Fee Schedule

⊛ **B4185** Parenteral nutrition solution, per 10 grams lipids Ⓑ   B

PEN: On Fee Schedule

⊛ **B4189** Parenteral nutrition solution; compounded amino acid and carbohydrates with electrolytes, trace elements, and vitamins, including preparation, any strength, 10 to 51 grams of protein - premix Ⓑ Qp Qh   Y

IOM: 100-02, 15, 120; 100-03, 3, 180.2; 100-04, 20, 100.2.2

PEN: On Fee Schedule

⊛ **B4193** Parenteral nutrition solution; compounded amino acid and carbohydrates with electrolytes, trace elements, and vitamins, including preparation, any strength, 52 to 73 grams of protein - premix Ⓑ Qh   Y

IOM: 100-02, 15, 120; 100-03, 3, 180.2; 100-04, 20, 100.2.2

PEN: On Fee Schedule

⊛ **B4197** Parenteral nutrition solution; compounded amino acid and carbohydrates with electrolytes, trace elements and vitamins, including preparation, any strength, 74 to 100 grams of protein - premix Ⓑ Qh   Y

IOM: 100-02, 15, 120; 100-03, 3, 180.2; 100-04, 20, 100.2.2

PEN: On Fee Schedule

⊛ **B4199** Parenteral nutrition solution; compounded amino acid and carbohydrates with electrolytes, trace elements and vitamins, including preparation, any strength, over 100 grams of protein - premix Ⓑ Qp Qh   Y

IOM: 100-02, 15, 120; 100-03, 3, 180.2; 100-04, 20, 100.2.2

PEN: On Fee Schedule

⊛ **B4216** Parenteral nutrition; additives (vitamins, trace elements, heparin, electrolytes) homemix per day Ⓑ Qh   Y

IOM: 100-02, 15, 120; 100-03, 3, 180.2; 100-04, 20, 100.2.2

PEN: On Fee Schedule

⊛ **B4220** Parenteral nutrition supply kit; premix, per day Ⓑ Qh   Y

IOM: 100-02, 15, 120; 100-03, 3, 180.2; 100-04, 20, 100.2.2

PEN: On Fee Schedule

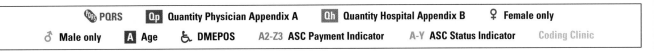

| ⟨PQRS⟩ PQRS | Qp Quantity Physician Appendix A | Qh Quantity Hospital Appendix B | ♀ Female only |
| ♂ Male only | Ⓐ Age | ⅗ DMEPOS | A2-Z3 ASC Payment Indicator | A-Y ASC Status Indicator | Coding Clinic |

⚙ **B4222** Parenteral nutrition supply kit; home mix, per day Ⓑ Qh Y

IOM: 100-02, 15, 120; 100-03, 3, 180.2; 100-04, 20, 100.2.2

PEN: On Fee Schedule

⚙ **B4224** Parenteral nutrition administration kit, per day Ⓑ Qh Y

Dressings used with parenteral nutrition (covered under the prosthetic device benefit) are included in the payment. (www.cms.gov/medicare-coverage-database/)

IOM: 100-02, 15, 120; 100-03, 3, 180.2; 100-04, 20, 100.2.2

PEN: On Fee Schedule

⚙ **B5000** Parenteral nutrition solution: compounded amino acid and carbohydrates with electrolytes, trace elements, and vitamins, including preparation, any strength, renal - Amirosyn-RF, NephrAmine, RenAmine - premix Ⓑ Qh Y

IOM: 100-02, 15, 120; 100-03, 3, 180.2; 100-04, 20, 100.2.2

PEN: On Fee Schedule

⚙ **B5100** Parenteral nutrition solution: compounded amino acid and carbohydrates with electrolytes, trace elements, and vitamins, including preparation, any strength, hepatic - FreAmine HBC, HepatAmine - premix Ⓑ Qh Y

IOM: 100-02, 15, 120; 100-03, 3, 180.2; 100-04, 20, 100.2.2

PEN: On Fee Schedule

⚙ **B5200** Parenteral nutrition solution; compounded amino acid and carbohydrates with electrolytes, trace elements, and vitamins, including preparation, any strength, stress - branch chain amino acids - premix Ⓑ Qp Qh Y

IOM: 100-02, 15, 120; 100-03, 3, 180.2; 100-04, 20, 100.2.2

Enteral and Parenteral Pumps

⚙ **B9000** Enteral nutrition infusion pump - without alarm Ⓑ Qh Y

Pump will be denied as not medically necessary if medical necessity of pump is not documented

IOM: 100-02, 15, 120; 100-03, 3, 180.2; 100-04, 20, 100.2.2

PEN: On Fee Schedule, DMEPOS Modifier(s): NU, RR, UE

⚙ **B9002** Enteral nutrition infusion pump - with alarm Ⓑ Qh Y

IOM: 100-02, 15, 120; 100-03, 3, 180.2; 100-04, 20, 100.2.2

PEN: On Fee Schedule, DMEPOS Modifier(s): NU, RR, UE

⚙ **B9004** Parenteral nutrition infusion pump, portable Ⓑ Qh Y

IOM: 100-02, 15, 120; 100-03, 3, 180.2; 100-04, 20, 100.2.2

PEN: On Fee Schedule, DMEPOS Modifier(s): NU, RR, UE

⚙ **B9006** Parenteral nutrition infusion pump, stationary Ⓑ Qh Y

IOM: 100-02, 15, 120; 100-03, 3, 180.2; 100-04, 20, 100.2.2

PEN: On Fee Schedule, DMEPOS Modifier(s): NU, RR, UE

⚙ **B9998** NOC for enteral supplies Ⓑ Y

IOM: 100-02, 15, 120; 100-03, 3, 180.2; 100-04, 20, 100.2.2

⚙ **B9999** NOC for parenteral supplies Ⓑ Y

Determine if an alternative HCPCS Level II or a CPT code better describes the service being reported. This code should be reported only if a more specific code is unavailable.

IOM: 100-02, 15, 120; 100-03, 3, 180.2; 100-04, 20, 100.2.2

▶ New   ↩ Revised   ✔ Reinstated   ~~deleted~~ Deleted   ⊘ Not covered or valid by Medicare
⚙ Special coverage instructions   ✳ Carrier discretion   Ⓑ Bill local carrier   Ⓓ Bill DME MAC

CMS HOSPITAL OUTPATIENT PAYMENT SYSTEM (C1000-C9999)

NOTE: C-codes are used on Medicare Ambulatory Surgical Center (ASC) and Hospital Outpatient Prospective Payment System (OPPS) claims, but may also be recognized on claims from other providers or by other payment systems. As of 10/01/2006, the following non-OPPS providers have been able to bill Medicare using the C-codes, or an appropriate CPT code on Types of Bill (TOBs) 12X, 13X, or 85X:

- Critical Access Hospitals (CAHs);
- Indian Health Service Hospitals (IHS);
- Hospitals located in American Samoa, Guam, Saipan or the Virgin Islands; and
- Maryland waiver hospitals.

The billing of C-codes by Method I and Method II Critical Access Hospitals (CAHs) is limited to the billing for facility (technical) services. The C-codes shall not be billed by Method II CAHs for professional services with revenue codes (RCs) 96X, 97X, or 98X.

C codes are updated quarterly by the Centers for Medicare and Medicaid Services (CMS).

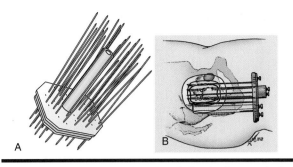

Figure 9 **A.** Brachytherapy device. **B.** Brachytherapy device inserted.

~~C1300~~	~~Hyperbaric oxygen under pressure, full body chamber, per 30-minute interval~~		✖

⊚ **C1713** Anchor/Screw for opposing bone-to-bone or soft tissue-to-bone (implantable)   N1   N

Medicare Statute 1833(t)

Coding Clinic: 2010, Q2, P3

⊚ **C1714** Catheter, transluminal atherectomy, directional   N1   N

Medicare Statute 1833(t)

⊚ **C1715** Brachytherapy needle   N1   N

Medicare Statute 1833(t)

⊚ **C1716** Brachytherapy source, non-stranded, gold-198, per source   H2   U

Medicare Statute 1833(t)

⊚ **C1717** Brachytherapy source, non-stranded, high dose rate iridium 192, per source   H2   U

Medicare Statute 1833(t)

⊚ **C1719** Brachytherapy source, non-stranded, non-high dose rate iridium-192, per source   H2   U

Medicare Statute 1833(t)

⊚ **C1721** Cardioverter-defibrillator, dual chamber (implantable) **Qh**   N1   N

Related CPT codes: 33224, 33240, 33249.

Medicare Statute 1833(t)

⊚ **C1722** Cardioverter-defibrillator, single chamber (implantable) **Qp** **Qh**   N1   N

Related CPT codes: 33240, 33249.

Medicare Statute 1833(t)

Coding Clinic: 2006, Q2, P9

⊚ **C1724** Catheter, transluminal atherectomy, rotational   N1   N

Medicare Statute 1833(t)

⊚ **C1725** Catheter, transluminal angioplasty, non-laser (may include guidance, infusion/perfusion capability)   N1   N

Medicare Statute 1833(t)

⊚ **C1726** Catheter, balloon dilatation, non-vascular   N1   N

Medicare Statute 1833(t)

⊚ **C1727** Catheter, balloon tissue dissector, non-vascular (insertable)   N1   N

Medicare Statute 1833(t)

⊚ **C1728** Catheter, brachytherapy seed administration   N1   N

Medicare Statute 1833(t)

⊚ **C1729** Catheter, drainage   N1   N

Medicare Statute 1833(t)

⊚ **C1730** Catheter, electrophysiology, diagnostic, other than 3D mapping (19 or fewer electrodes)   N1   N

Medicare Statute 1833(t)

⊚ **C1731** Catheter, electrophysiology, diagnostic, other than 3D mapping (20 or more electrodes) **Qh**   N1   N

Medicare Statute 1833(t)

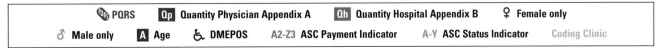

🅟 PQRS	**Qp** Quantity Physician Appendix A	**Qh** Quantity Hospital Appendix B	♀ Female only
♂ Male only	**A** Age	♿ DMEPOS	A2-Z3 ASC Payment Indicator A-Y ASC Status Indicator Coding Clinic

⊛ **C1732**   Catheter, electrophysiology, diagnostic/ablation, 3D or vector mapping `Qh`   N1 N

Medicare Statute 1833(t)

⊛ **C1733**   Catheter, electrophysiology, diagnostic/ablation, other than 3D or vector mapping, other than cool-tip `Qh`   N1 N

Medicare Statute 1833(t)

⊛ **C1749**   Endoscope, retrograde imaging/illumination colonoscope device (implantable) `Qp` `Qh`   N1 N

Medicare Statute 1833(t)

⊛ **C1750**   Catheter, hemodialysis/peritoneal, long-term `Qh`   N1 N

Medicare Statute 1833(t)

⊛ **C1751**   Catheter, infusion, inserted peripherally, centrally, or midline (other than hemodialysis) `Qh`   N1 N

Medicare Statute 1833(t)

⊛ **C1752**   Catheter, hemodialysis/peritoneal, short-term `Qh`   N1 N

Medicare Statute 1833(t)

⊛ **C1753**   Catheter, intravascular ultrasound `Qh`   N1 N

Medicare Statute 1833(t)

⊛ **C1754**   Catheter, intradiscal `Qh`   N1 N

Medicare Statute 1833(t)

⊛ **C1755**   Catheter, instraspinal `Qh`   N1 N

Medicare Statute 1833(t)

⊛ **C1756**   Catheter, pacing, transesophageal `Qh`   N1 N

Medicare Statute 1833(t)

⊛ **C1757**   Catheter, thrombectomy/embolectomy   N1 N

Medicare Statute 1833(t)

⊛ **C1758**   Catheter, ureteral `Qh`   N1 N

Medicare Statute 1833(t)

⊛ **C1759**   Catheter, intracardiac echocardi-ography `Qh`   N1 N

Medicare Statute 1833(t)

⊛ **C1760**   Closure device, vascular (implantable/insertable)   N1 N

Medicare Statute 1833(t)

⊛ **C1762**   Connective tissue, human (includes fascia lata)   N1 N

Medicare Statute 1833(t)

Coding Clinic: 2003, Q3, P12

⊛ **C1763**   Connective tissue, non-human (includes synthetic)   N1 N

Medicare Statute 1833(t)

Coding Clinic: 2010, Q4, P3; Q2, P3; 2003, Q3, P12

⊛ **C1764**   Event recorder, cardiac (implantable) `Qh`   N1 N

Medicare Statute 1833(t)

⊛ **C1765**   Adhesion barrier   N1 N

Medicare Statute 1833(t)

⊛ **C1766**   Introducer/sheath, guiding, intracardiac electrophysiological, steerable, other than peel-away   N1 N

Medicare Statute 1833(t)

⊛ **C1767**   Generator, neurostimulator (implantable), nonrechargeable `Qp` `Qh`   N1 N

Related CPT codes: 61885, 61886, 63685, 64590.

Medicare Statute 1833(t)

Coding Clinic: 2007, Q1, P8

⊛ **C1768**   Graft, vascular `Qh`   N1 N

Medicare Statute 1833(t)

⊛ **C1769**   Guide wire   N1 N

Medicare Statute 1833(t)

Coding Clinic: 2007, Q2, P7-8

⊛ **C1770**   Imaging coil, magnetic reasonance (insertable) `Qh`   N1 N

Medicare Statute 1833(t)

⊛ **C1771**   Repair device, urinary, incontinence, with sling graft `Qh`   N1 N

Medicare Statute 1833(t)

Coding Clinic: 2008, Q3, P7

⊛ **C1772**   Infusion pump, programmable (implantable) `Qp` `Qh`   N1 N

Medicare Statute 1833(t)

⊛ **C1773**   Retrieval device, insertable (used to retrieve fractured medical devices) `Qh`   N1 N

Medicare Statute 1833(t)

⊛ **C1776**   Joint device (implantable)   N1 N

Medicare Statute 1833(t)

Coding Clinic: 2010, Q3, P6; 2008, Q4, P10

⊛ **C1777**   Lead, cardioverter-defibrillator, endocardial single coil (implantable) `Qh`   N1 N

Related CPT codes: 33216, 33217, 33249.

Medicare Statute 1833(t)

Coding Clinic: 2006, Q2, P9

▶ **New**   ↻ **Revised**   ✔ **Reinstated**   ~~deleted~~ **Deleted**   ⊘ **Not covered or valid by Medicare**
⊛ **Special coverage instructions**   ✳ **Carrier discretion**   ⑧ **Bill local carrier**   ⑧ **Bill DME MAC**

⚙ **C1778**   Lead, neurostimulator
(implantable)   N1   N

Related CPT codes: 43647, 63650,
63655, 63663, 63664, 64553, 64555,
64560, 64561, 64565, 64573, 64575,
64577, 64580, 64581.

Medicare Statute 1833(t)

Coding Clinic: 2007, Q1, P8

⚙ **C1779**   Lead, pacemaker, trasvenous VDD
single pass **Qh**   N1   N

Related CPT codes: 33206, 33207,
33208, 33210, 33211, 33214, 33216,
33217, 33249.

Medicare Statute 1833(t)

⚙ **C1780**   Lens, intraocular (new
technology) **Qh**   N1   N

Medicare Statute 1833(t)

⚙ **C1781**   Mesh (implantable)   N1   N

Medicare Statute 1833(t)

Coding Clinic: 2012, Q2, P3; 2010, Q2, P2-3

⚙ **C1782**   Morcellator **Qh**   N1   N

Medicare Statute 1833(t)

⚙ **C1783**   Ocular implant, aqueous drainage
assist device **Qh**   N1   N

Medicare Statute 1833(t)

⚙ **C1784**   Ocular device, intraoperative, detached
retina **Qh**   N1   N

Medicare Statute 1833(t)

⚙ **C1785**   Pacemaker, dual
chamber, rate-responsive
(implantable) **Qp** **Qh**   N1   N

Related CPT codes: 33206, 33207,
33208, 33213, 33214, 33224.

Medicare Statute 1833(t)

⚙ **C1786**   Pacemaker, single chamber, rate-
responsive (implantable) **Qh**   N1   N

Related CPT codes: 33206, 33207, 33212.

Medicare Statute 1833(t)

⚙ **C1787**   Patient programmer,
neurostimulator **Qh**   N1   N

Medicare Statute 1833(t)

⚙ **C1788**   Port, indwelling
(implantable) **Qh**   N1   N

Medicare Statute 1833(t)

⚙ **C1789**   Prosthesis, breast
(implantable) ♀ **Qh**   N1   N

Medicare Statute 1833(t)

⚙ **C1813**   Prosthesis, penile,
inflatable ♂ **Qp** **Qh**   N1   N

Medicare Statute 1833(t)

⚙ **C1814**   Retinal tamponade device, silicone
oil **Qh**   N1   N

Medicare Statute 1833(t)

Coding Clinic: 2006, Q2, P9

⚙ **C1815**   Prosthesis, urinary sphincter
(implantable) **Qh**   N1   N

Medicare Statute 1833(t)

⚙ **C1816**   Receiver and/or transmitter,
neurostimulator
(implantable) **Qh**   N1   N

Medicare Statute 1833(t)

⚙ **C1817**   Septal defect implant system,
intracardiac **Qh**   N1   N

Medicare Statute 1833(t)

⚙ **C1818**   Integrated
keratoprosthesic **Qh**   N1   N

Medicare Statute 1833(t)

⚙ **C1819**   Surgical tissue localization and excision
device (implantable)   N1   N

Medicare Statute 1833(t)

⚙ **C1820**   Generator, neurostimulator
(implantable), with rechargeable
battery and charging
system **Qp** **Qh**   N1   N

Related CPT codes: 61885, 61886,
63685, 64590.

Medicare Statute 1833(t)

⚙ **C1821**   Interspinous process distraction device
(implantable)   N1   N

Medicare Statute 1833(t)

⚙ **C1830**   Powered bone marrow biopsy
needle **Qp** **Qh**   N1   N

Medicare Statute 1833(t)

⚙ **C1840**   Lens, intraocular
(telescopic) **Qp** **Qh**   N1   N

Medicare Statute 1833(t)

Coding Clinic: 2012, Q3, P10

⚙ **C1841**   Retinal prosthesis, includes
all internal and external
components **Qp** **Qh**   J7   H

Medicare Statute 1833(t)

⚙ **C1874**   Stent, coated/covered, with delivery
system   N1   N

Medicare Statute 1833(t)

⚙ **C1875**   Stent, coated/covered, without delivery
system   N1   N

Medicare Statute 1833(t)

⚙ **C1876**   Stent, non-coated/non-covered, with
delivery system   N1   N

Medicare Statute 1833(t)

PQRS PQRS   **Qp** Quantity Physician Appendix A   **Qh** Quantity Hospital Appendix B   ♀ Female only

♂ **Male only**   **A** Age   ♿ DMEPOS   **A2-Z3** ASC Payment Indicator   **A-Y** ASC Status Indicator   Coding Clinic

⊛ **C1877** Stent, non-coated/non-covered, without delivery system **N1 N**

Medicare Statute 1833(t)

⊛ **C1878** Material for vocal cord medialization, synthetic (implantable) **Qh** **N1 N**

Medicare Statute 1833(t)

⊛ **C1880** Vena cava filter **Qh** **N1 N**

Medicare Statute 1833(t)

⊛ **C1881** Dialysis access system (implantable) **Qh** **N1 N**

Medicare Statute 1833(t)

⊛ **C1882** Cardioverter-defibrillator, other than single or dual chamber (implantable) **Qh** **N1 N**

Related CPT codes: 33224, 33240, 33249.

Medicare Statute 1833(t)

Coding Clinic: 2012, Q2, P9; 2006, Q2, P9

⊛ **C1883** Adaptor/Extension, pacing lead or neurostimulator lead (implantable) **N1 N**

Medicare Statute 1833(t)

Coding Clinic: 2007, Q1, P8

⊛ **C1884** Embolization protective system **N1 N**

Medicare Statute 1833(t)

⊛ **C1885** Catheter, transluminal angioplasty, laser **N1 N**

Medicare Statute 1833(t)

⊛ **C1886** Catheter, extravascular tissue ablation, any modality (insertable) **Qp** **Qh** **N1 N**

Medicare Statute 1833(t)

⊛ **C1887** Catheter, guiding (may include infusion/perfusion capability) **N1 N**

Medicare Statute 1833(t)

⊛ **C1888** Catheter, ablation, non-cardiac, endovascular (implantable) **Qh** **N1 N**

Medicare Statute 1833(t)

⊛ **C1891** Infusion pump, non-programmable, permanent (implantable) **Qh** **N1 N**

Medicare Statute 1833(t)

⊛ **C1892** Introducer/sheath, guiding, intracardiac electrophysiological, fixed-curve, peel-away **N1 N**

Medicare Statute 1833(t)

⊛ **C1893** Introducer/sheath, guiding, intracardiac electrophysiological, fixed-curve, other than peel-away **N1 N**

Medicare Statute 1833(t)

⊛ **C1894** Introducer/sheath, other than guiding, other than intracardiac electrophysiological, non-laser **N1 N**

Medicare Statute 1833(t)

⊛ **C1895** Lead, cardioverter-defibrillator, endocardial dual coil (implantable) **Qh** **N1 N**

Related CPT codes: 33216, 33217, 33249.

Medicare Statute 1833(t)

Coding Clinic: 2006, Q2, P9

⊛ **C1896** Lead, cardioverter-defibrillator, other than endocardial single or dual coil (implantable) **Qh** **N1 N**

Related CPT codes: 33216, 33217, 33249.

Medicare Statute 1833(t)

⊛ **C1897** Lead, neurostimulator test kit (implantable) **Qh** **N1 N**

Related CPT codes: 43647, 63650, 63655, 63663, 63664, 64553, 64555, 64560, 64561, 64565, 64575, 64577, 64580, 64581.

Medicare Statute 1833(t)

Coding Clinic: 2007, Q1, P8

A. Pacemaker lead in the right atrium — Pulse generator (+)

B. Pacemaker leads in the right atrium and right ventricle — Pulse generator (+)

C. Biventricular pacemaker — Leads — Pulse generator (+) — ✳ = Electrical impulse

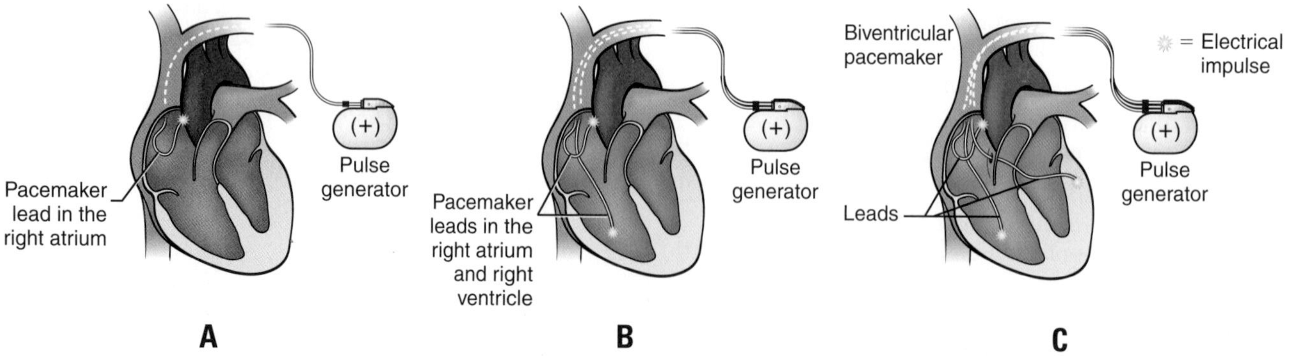

Figure 10 **A.** Single pacemaker. **B.** Dual pacemaker. **C.** Biventricular pacemaker.

▶ New ↻ Revised ✔ Reinstated ~~deleted~~ Deleted ⊘ Not covered or valid by Medicare
⊛ Special coverage instructions ✳ Carrier discretion Ⓑ Bill local carrier Ⓑ Bill DME MAC

⊕ **C1898** Lead, pacemaker, other than transvenous VDD single pass `Qh` N1 N

Related CPT codes: 33206, 33207, 33208, 33210, 33211, 33214, 33216, 33217, 33249.

Medicare Statute 1833(t)

Coding Clinic: 2002, Q3, P8

⊕ **C1899** Lead, pacemaker/cardioverter-defibrillator combination (implantable) `Qh` N1 N

Related CPT codes: 33216, 33217, 33249.

Medicare Statute 1833(t)

⊕ **C1900** Lead, left ventricular coronary venous system `Qh` N1 N

Related CPT codes: 33224, 33225.

Medicare Statute 1833(t)

⊕ **C2614** Probe, percutaneous lumbar discectomy `Qh` N1 N

Medicare Statute 1833(t)

⊕ **C2615** Sealant, pulmonary, liquid `Qh` N1 N

Medicare Statute 1833(t)

⊕ **C2616** Brachytherapy source, non-stranded, yttrium-90, per source `Qp` `Qh` H2 U

Medicare Statute 1833(t)

⊕ **C2617** Stent, non-coronary, temporary, without delivery system N1 N

Medicare Statute 1833(t)

⊕ **C2618** Probe/needle, cryoablation N1 N

Medicare Statute 1833(t)

⊕ **C2619** Pacemaker, dual chamber, non rate-responsive (implantable) `Qh` N1 N

Related CPT codes: 33206, 33207, 33208, 33213, 33214, 33224.

Medicare Statute 1833(t)

⊕ **C2620** Pacemaker, single chamber, non rate-responsive (implantable) `Qh` N1 N

Related CPT codes: 33206, 33207, 33212, 33224.

Medicare Statute 1833(t)

⊕ **C2621** Pacemaker, other than single or dual chamber (implantable) `Qh` N1 N

Related CPT codes: 33206, 33207, 33208, 33212, 33213, 33214, 33224.

Medicare Statute 1833(t)

Coding Clinic: 2002, Q3, P8

⊕ **C2622** Prosthesis, penile, non-inflatable ♂ `Qh` N1 N

Medicare Statute 1833(t)

▶ ⊕ **C2624** Implantable wireless pulmonary artery pressure sensor with delivery catheter, including all system components

Medicare Statute 1833(t) J7 H

⊕ **C2625** Stent, non-coronary, temporary, with delivery system N1 N

Medicare Statute 1833(t)

⊕ **C2626** Infusion pump, non-programmable, temporary (implantable) `Qh` N1 N

Medicare Statute 1833(t)

⊕ **C2627** Catheter, suprapubic/cystoscopic `Qh` N1 N

Medicare Statute 1833(t)

⊕ **C2628** Catheter, occlusion N1 N

Medicare Statute 1833(t)

⊕ **C2629** Introducer/Sheath, other than guiding, other than intracardiac electrophysiological, laser N1 N

Medicare Statute 1833(t)

⊕ **C2630** Catheter, electrophysiology, diagnostic/ablation, other than 3D or vector mapping, cool-tip N1 N

Medicare Statute 1833(t)

⊕ **C2631** Repair device, urinary, incontinence, without sling graft `Qh` N1 N

Medicare Statute 1833(t)

⊕ **C2634** Brachytherapy source, non-stranded, high activity, iodine-125, greater than 1.01 mci (NIST), per source H2 U

Medicare Statute 1833(t)

⊕ **C2635** Brachytherapy source, non-stranded, high activity, paladium-103, greater than 2.2 mci (NIST), per source H2 U

Medicare Statute 1833(t)

⊕ **C2636** Brachytherapy linear source, non-stranded, paladium-103, per 1 mm H2 U

⊕ **C2637** Brachytherapy source, non-stranded, Ytterbium-169, per source B

Medicare Statute 1833(t)

⊕ **C2638** Brachytherapy source, stranded, iodine-125, per source H2 U

Medicare Statute 1833(t)(2)

⊕ **C2639** Brachytherapy source, non-stranded, iodine-125, per source H2 U

Medicare Statute 1833(t)(2)

⊕ **C2640** Brachytherapy source, stranded, palladium-103, per source H2 U

Medicare Statute 1833(t)(2)

⊛ **C2641** Brachytherapy source, non-stranded, palladium-103, per source   **H2** **U**

Medicare Statute 1833(t)(2)

⊛ **C2642** Brachytherapy source, stranded, cesium-131, per source   **H2** **U**

Medicare Statute 1833(t)(2)

⊛ **C2643** Brachytherapy source, non-stranded, cesium-131, per source   **H2** **U**

Medicare Statute 1833(t)(2)

▶ ⊛ **C2644** Brachytherapy source, Cesium-131 chloride solution, per millicurie

Medicare Statute 1833(t)

⊛ **C2698** Brachytherapy source, stranded, not otherwise specified, per source   **H2** **U**

Medicare Statute 1833(t)(2)

⊛ **C2699** Brachytherapy source, non-stranded, not otherwise specified, per source   **H2** **U**

Medicare Statute 1833(t)(2)

⊛ **C5271** Application of low cost skin substitute graft to trunk, arms, legs, total wound surface area up to 100 sq cm; first 25 sq cm or less wound surface area **Qp** **Qh**   **T**

Medicare Statute 1833(t)

⊛ **C5272** Application of low cost skin substitute graft to trunk, arms, legs, total wound surface area up to 100 sq cm; each additional 25 sq cm wound surface area, or part thereof (list separately in addition to code for primary procedure) **Qp** **Qh**   **N**

Medicare Statute 1833(t)

⊛ **C5273** Application of low cost skin substitute graft to trunk, arms, legs, total wound surface area greater than or equal to 100 sq cm; first 100 sq cm wound surface area, or 1% of body area of infants and children **Qp** **Qh** **A**   **T**

Medicare Statute 1833(t)

⊛ **C5274** Application of low cost skin substitute graft to trunk, arms, legs, total wound surface area greater than or equal to 100 sq cm; each additional 100 sq cm wound surface area, or part thereof, or each additional 1% of body area of infants and children, or part thereof (list separately in addition to code for primary procedure) **Qp** **Qh** **A**   **N**

Medicare Statute 1833(t)

⊛ **C5275** Application of low cost skin substitute graft to face, scalp, eyelids, mouth, neck, ears, orbits, genitalia, hands, feet, and/or multiple digits, total wound surface area up to 100 sq cm; first 25 sq cm or less wound surface area **Qp** **Qh**   **T**

Medicare Statute 1833(t)

⊛ **C5276** Application of low cost skin substitute graft to face, scalp, eyelids, mouth, neck, ears, orbits, genitalia, hands, feet, and/or multiple digits, total wound surface area up to 100 sq cm; each additional 25 sq cm wound surface area, or part thereof (list separately in addition to code for primary procedure) **Qp** **Qh**   **N**

Medicare Statute 1833(t)

⊛ **C5277** Application of low cost skin substitute graft to face, scalp, eyelids, mouth, neck, ears, orbits, genitalia, hands, feet, and/or multiple digits, total wound surface area greater than or equal to 100 sq cm; first 100 sq cm wound surface area, or 1% of body area of infants and children **Qp** **Qh** **A**   **T**

Medicare Statute 1833(t)

⊛ **C5278** Application of low cost skin substitute graft to face, scalp, eyelids, mouth, neck, ears, orbits, genitalia, hands, feet, and/or multiple digits, total wound surface area greater than or equal to 100 sq cm; each additional 100 sq cm wound surface area, or part thereof, or each additional 1% of body area of infants and children, or part thereof (list separately in addition to code for primary procedure) **Qp** **Qh** **A**   **N**

Medicare Statute 1833(t)

⊛ **C8900** Magnetic resonance angiography with contrast, abdomen **Qh**   **Z2** **Q3**

Medicare Statute 1833(t)(2)

⊛ **C8901** Magnetic resonance angiography without contrast, abdomen **Qh**   **Z2** **Q3**

Medicare Statute 1833(t)(2)

⊛ **C8902** Magnetic resonance angiography without contrast followed by with contrast, abdomen **Qh**   **Z2** **Q3**

Medicare Statute 1833(t)(2)

⊛ **C8903** Magnetic resonance imaging with contrast, breast; unilateral **Qh**   **Z2** **Q3**

Medicare Statute 1833(t)(2)

⊛ **C8904** Magnetic resonance imaging without contrast, breast; unilateral **Qh**   **Z2** **Q3**

Medicare Statute 1833(t)(2)

⊛ **C8905** Magnetic resonance imaging without contrast followed by with contrast, breast; unilateral **Qh**   **Z2** **Q3**

Medicare Statute 1833(t)(2)

⊛ **C8906** Magnetic resonance imaging with contrast, breast; bilateral **Qh**   **Z2** **Q3**

Medicare Statute 1833(t)(2)

▶ **New**   ↻ **Revised**   ✔ **Reinstated**   ~~deleted~~ **Deleted**   ⊘ **Not covered or valid by Medicare**

⊛ **Special coverage instructions**   ✳ **Carrier discretion**   Ⓑ **Bill local carrier**   Ⓑ **Bill DME MAC**

◎ **C8907** Magnetic resonance imaging without contrast, breast; bilateral `Qh`   Z2 Q3

Medicare Statute 1833(t)(2)

◎ **C8908** Magnetic resonance imaging without contrast followed by with contrast, breast; bilateral `Qh`   Z2 Q3

Medicare Statute 1833(t)(2)

◎ **C8909** Magnetic resonance angiography with contrast, chest (excluding myocardium) `Qh`   Z2 Q3

Medicare Statute 1833(t)(2)

◎ **C8910** Magnetic resonance angiography without contrast, chest (excluding myocardium) `Qh`   Z2 Q3

Medicare Statute 1833(t)(2)

◎ **C8911** Magnetic resonance angiography without contrast followed by with contrast, chest (excluding myocardium) `Qh`   Z2 Q3

Medicare Statute 1833(t)(2)

◎ **C8912** Magnetic resonance angiography with contrast, lower extremity `Qh`   Z2 Q3

Medicare Statute 1833(t)(2)

◎ **C8913** Magnetic resonance angiography without contrast, lower extremity `Qh`   Z2 Q3

Medicare Statute 1833(t)(2)

◎ **C8914** Magnetic resonance angiography without contrast followed by with contrast, lower extremity `Qh`   Z2 Q3

Medicare Statute 1833(t)(2)

◎ **C8918** Magnetic resonance angiography with contrast, pelvis `Qh`   Z2 Q3

Medicare Statute 1833(t)(2)

◎ **C8919** Magnetic resonance angiography without contrast, pelvis `Qh`   Z2 Q3

Medicare Statute 1833(t)(2)

◎ **C8920** Magnetic resonance angiography without contrast followed by with contrast, pelvis `Qh`   Z2 Q3

Medicare Statute 1833(t)(2)

◎ **C8921** Transthoracic echocardiography with contrast, or without contrast followed by with contrast, for congenital cardiac anomalies; complete `Qh`   S

Medicare Statute 1833(t)(2)

Coding Clinic: 2012, Q3, P8

◎ **C8922** Transthoracic echocardiography with contrast, or without contrast followed by with contrast, for congenital cardiac anomalies; follow-up or limited study `Qh`   S

Medicare Statute 1833(t)(2)

Coding Clinic: 2012, Q3, P8

◎ **C8923** Transthoracic echocardiography with contrast, or without contrast followed by with contrast, real-time with image documentation (2D), includes M-mode recording, when performed, complete, without spectral or color Doppler echocardiography `Qh`   S

Medicare Statute 1833(t)(2)

Coding Clinic: 2012, Q3, P8

◎ **C8924** Transthoracic echocardiography with contrast, or without contrast followed by with contrast, real-time with image documentation (2D), includes M-mode recording, when performed, follow-up or limited study `Qh`   S

Medicare Statute 1833(t)(2)

Coding Clinic: 2012, Q3, P8

◎ **C8925** Transesophageal echocardiography (TEE) with contrast, or without contrast followed by with contrast, real time with image documentation (2D) (with or without M-mode recording); including probe placement, image acquisition, interpretation and report `Qh`   S

Medicare Statute 1833(t)(2)

Coding Clinic: 2012, Q3, P8

◎ **C8926** Transesophageal echocardiography (TEE) with contrast, or without contrast followed by with contrast, for congenital cardiac anomalies; including probe placement, image acquisition, interpretation and report `Qh`   S

Medicare Statute 1833(t)(2)

Coding Clinic: 2012, Q3, P8

◎ **C8927** Transesophageal echocardiography (TEE) with contrast, or without contrast followed by with contrast, for monitoring purposes, including probe placement, real time 2-dimensional image acquisition and interpretation leading to ongoing (continuous) assessment of (dynamically changing) cardiac pumping function and to therapeutic measures on an immediate time basis `Qh`   S

Medicare Statute 1833(t)(2)

Coding Clinic: 2012, Q3, P8

⊛ **C8928** Transthoracic echocardiography with contrast, or without contrast followed by with contrast, real-time with image documentation (2D), includes M-mode recording, when performed, during rest and cardiovascular stress test using treadmill, bicycle exercise and/or pharmacologically induced stress, with interpretation and report `Qh`   S

Medicare Statute 1833(t)(2)

Coding Clinic: 2012, Q3, P8

⊛ **C8929** Transthoracic echocardiography with contrast, or without contrast followed by with contrast, real-time with image documentation (2D), includes M-mode recording, when performed, complete, with spectral Doppler echocardiography, and with color flow Doppler echocardiography `Qh`   S

Medicare Statute 1833(t)(2)

Coding Clinic: 2012, Q3, P8

⊛ **C8930** Transthoracic echocardiography, with contrast, or without contrast followed by with contrast, real-time with image documentation (2D), includes M-mode recording, when performed, during rest and cardiovascular stress test using treadmill, bicycle exercise and/or pharmacologically induced stress, with interpretation and report; including performance of continuous electrocardiographic monitoring, with physician supervision `Qh`   S

Medicare Statute 1833(t)(2)

Coding Clinic: 2012, Q3, P8

⊛ **C8931** Magnetic resonance angiography with contrast, spinal canal and contents `Qh`   Z2   Q3

Medicare Statute 1833(t)

⊛ **C8932** Magnetic resonance angiography without contrast, spinal canal and contents `Qh`   Z2   Q3

Medicare Statute 1833(t)

⊛ **C8933** Magnetic resonance angiography without contrast followed by with contrast, spinal canal and contents `Qh`   Z2   Q3

Medicare Statute 1833(t)

⊛ **C8934** Magnetic resonance angiography with contrast, upper extremity `Qh`   Z2   Q3

Medicare Statute 1833(t)

⊛ **C8935** Magnetic resonance angiography without contrast, upper extremity `Qh`   Z2   Q3

Medicare Statute 1833(t)

⊛ **C8936** Magnetic resonance angiography without contrast followed by with contrast, upper extremity `Qh`   Z2   Q3

Medicare Statute 1833(t)

⊛ **C8957** Intravenous infusion for therapy/diagnosis; initiation of prolonged infusion (more than 8 hours), requiring use of portable or implantable pump `Qh`   S

Medicare Statute 1833(t)

Coding Clinic: 2008, Q3, P8

~~C9021~~   ~~Injection, obinutuzumab, 10 mg~~   ✖

~~C9022~~   ~~Injection, elosulfase alfa, 1 mg~~   ✖

Cross Reference J1322

~~C9023~~   ~~Injection, testosterone undecanoate, 1 mg~~   ✖

Cross Reference J3145

▶ ⊛ **C9025** Injection, Ramucirumab, 5 mg

Medicare Statute 1833(t)   G

▶ ⊛ **C9026** Injection, Vedolizumab, 1 mg

Medicare Statute 1833(t)   G

▶ ⊛ **C9027** Injection, Pembrolizumab, 1 mg

Medicare Statute 1833(t)   K2   G

⊛ **C9113** Injection, pantoprazole sodium, per vial   N1   N

Medicare Statute 1833(t)

⊛ **C9121** Injection, argatroban, per 5 mg   K2   K

Medicare Statute 1833(t)

⊛ **C9132** Prothrombin complex concentrate (human), Kcentra, per i.u. of Factor IX activity   K2   G

Medicare Statute 1833(t)

~~C9133~~   ~~Factor ix (antihemophilic factor, recombinant), Rixibus, per i.u.~~   ✖

~~C9134~~   ~~Factor XIII (antihemophilic factor, recombinant), tretten, per 10 i.u.~~   ✖

Cross Reference J7181

~~C9135~~   ~~Factor IX (antihemophilic factor, recombinant), alprolix, per i.u.~~   ✖

Cross Reference J7201

▶ ⊛ **C9136** Injection, factor VIII, Fc fusion protein, (recombinant), per i.u.

Medicare Statute 1833(t)   K2   G

↻ ✳ **C9248** Injection, clevidipine butyrate, 1 mg   K2   K

Medicare Statute 1833(t)

▶ **New**   ↻ **Revised**   ✔ **Reinstated**   ~~deleted~~ **Deleted**   ⊘ **Not covered or valid by Medicare**   ⊛ **Special coverage instructions**   ✳ **Carrier discretion**   Ⓑ **Bill local carrier**   Ⓑ **Bill DME MAC**

↻ ⊛ **C9250** Human plasma fibrin sealant, vapor-heated, solvent-detergent (ARTISS), 2 ml   N1 N

Example of diagnosis codes to be reported with C9250: 941.00–949.5.

Medicare Statute 621MMA

⊛ **C9254** Injection, lacosamide, 1 mg `Qp` `Qh`   N1 N

Medicare Statute 621MMA

⊛ **C9257** injection, bevacizumab, 0.25 mg   K2 K

Medicare Statute 1833(t)

⊛ **C9275** Injection, hexaminolevulinate hydrochloride, 100 mg, per study dose `Qp` `Qh`   N1 N

Medicare Statute 1833(t)

Coding Clinic: 2011, Q1, P6

⊛ **C9285** Lidocaine 70 mg/tetracaine 70 mg, per patch `Qp` `Qh`   N1 N

Medicare Statute 1833(t)

Coding Clinic: 2011, Q3, P9

↻ ⊛ **C9290** Injection, bupivacine liposome, 1 mg `Qp` `Qh`   N1 N

Medicare Statute 1833(t)

⊛ **C9293** Injection, glucarpidase, 10 units `Qp` `Qh`   K

Medicare Statute 1833(t)

▶ ⊛ **C9349** FortaDerm, and FortaDerm Antimicrobial, any type, per square centimeter   K2

Medicare Statute 1833(t)

⊛ **C9352** Microporous collagen implantable tube (NeuraGen Nerve Guide), per centimeter length `Qp` `Qh`   N1 N

Medicare Statute 621MMA

⊛ **C9353** Microporous collagen implantable slit tube (NeuraWrap Nerve Protector), per centimeter length `Qp` `Qh`   N1 N

Medicare Statute 621MMA

⊛ **C9354** Acellular pericardial tissue matrix of non-human origin (Veritas), per square centimeter `Qp` `Qh`   N1 N

Medicare Statute 621MMA

⊛ **C9355** Collagen nerve cuff (NeuroMatrix), per 0.5 centimeter length `Qp` `Qh`   N1 N

Medicare Statute 621MMA

⊛ **C9356** Tendon, porous matrix of cross-linked collagen and glycosaminoglycan matrix (TenoGlide Tendon Protector Sheet), per square centimeter `Qp` `Qh`   N1 N

Medicare Statute 621MMA

⊛ **C9358** Dermal substitute, native, non-denatured collagen, fetal bovine origin (SurgiMend Collagen Matrix), per 0.5 square centimeters `Qp` `Qh`   N1 N

Medicare Statute 621MMA

Coding Clinic: 2013, Q3, P9; 2012, Q2, P7

⊛ **C9359** Porous purified collagen matrix bone void filler (Integra Mozaik Osteoconductive Scaffold Putty, Integra OS Osteoconductive Scaffold Putty), per 0.5 cc `Qp` `Qh`   N1 N

Medicare Statute 1833(t)

⊛ **C9360** Dermal substitute, native, non-denatured collagen, neonatal bovine origin (SurgiMend Collagen Matrix), per 0.5 square centimeters `Qp` `Qh`   N1 N

Medicare Statute 621MMA

Coding Clinic: 2012, Q2, P7

⊛ **C9361** Collagen matrix nerve wrap (NeuroMend Collagen Nerve Wrap), per 0.5 centimeter length `Qp` `Qh`   N1 N

Medicare Statute 621MMA

⊛ **C9362** Porous purified collagen matrix bone void filler (Integra Mozaik Osteoconductive Scaffold Strip), per 0.5 cc `Qp` `Qh`   N1 N

Medicare Statute 621MMA

Coding Clinic: 2010, Q2, P8

⊛ **C9363** Skin substitute, Integra Meshed Bilayer Wound Matrix, per square centimeter `Qp` `Qh`   N1 N

Medicare Statute 621MMA

Coding Clinic: 2012, Q2, P7; 2010, Q2, P8

⊛ **C9364** Porcine implant, Permacol, per square centimeter `Qp` `Qh`   N1 N

Medicare Statute 621MMA

⊛ **C9399** Unclassified drugs or biologicals   K7 A

Medicare Statute 621MMA

Coding Clinic: 2014, Q2, P8; 2013, Q2, P3; 2010, Q3, P8

~~C9441~~ ~~Injection, ferric carboxymaltose, 1 mg~~ ✖

▶ ⊛ **C9442** Injection, Belinostat, 10 mg

Medicare Statute 1833(t)   K2

▶ ⊛ **C9443** Injection, Dalbavancin, 10 mg

Medicare Statute 1833(t)   K2 G

▶ ⊛ **C9444** Injection, Oritavancin, 10 mg

Medicare Statute 1833(t)   K2 G

▶ ⊛ **C9446** Injection, Tedizolid phosphate, 1 mg

Medicare Statute 1833(t)   K2 G

PQRS   `Qp` Quantity Physician Appendix A   `Qh` Quantity Hospital Appendix B   ♀ Female only   ♂ Male only   `A` Age   DMEPOS   A2-Z3 ASC Payment Indicator   A-Y ASC Status Indicator   Coding Clinic

▶ ✪ **C9447** Injection, phenylephrine and ketorolac, 4 ml vial

Medicare Statute 1833(t) K2 G

✪ **C9497** Loxapine, inhalation powder, 10 mg K2 G

Medicare Statute 1833(t)

✪ **C9600** Percutaneous transcatheter placement of drug eluting intracoronary stent(s), with coronary angioplasty when performed; a single major coronary artery or branch **Qp** **Qh** J1

Medicare Statute 1833(t)

✪ **C9601** Percutaneous transcatheter placement of drug-eluting intracoronary stent(s), with coronary angioplasty when performed; each additional branch of a major coronary artery (list separately in addition to code for primary procedure) **Qp** **Qh** N

Medicare Statute 1833(t)

✪ **C9602** Percutaneous transluminal coronary atherectomy, with drug eluting intracoronary stent, with coronary angioplasty when performed; a single major coronary artery or branch **Qp** **Qh** J1

Medicare Statute 1833(t)

✪ **C9603** Percutaneous transluminal coronary atherectomy, with drug-eluting intracoronary stent, with coronary angioplasty when performed; each additional branch of a major coronary artery (list separately in addition to code for primary procedure) **Qp** **Qh** N

Medicare Statute 1833(t)

✪ **C9604** Percutaneous transluminal revascularization of or through coronary artery bypass graft (internal mammary, free arterial, venous), any combination of drug-eluting intracoronary stent, atherectomy and angioplasty, including distal protection when performed; a single vessel **Qp** **Qh** J1

✪ **C9605** Percutaneous transluminal revascularization of or through coronary artery bypass graft (internal mammary, free arterial, venous), any combination of drug-eluting intracoronary stent, atherectomy and angioplasty, including distal protection when performed; each additional branch subtended by the bypass graft (list separately in addition to code for primary procedure) **Qp** **Qh** N

Medicare Statute 1833(t)

✪ **C9606** Percutaneous transluminal revascularization of acute total/subtotal occlusion during acute myocardial infarction, coronary artery or coronary artery bypass graft, any combination of drug-eluting intracoronary stent, atherectomy and angioplasty, including aspiration thrombectomy when performed, single vessel **Qp** **Qh** J1

Medicare Statute 1833(t)

✪ **C9607** Percutaneous transluminal revascularization of chronic total occlusion, coronary artery, coronary artery branch, or coronary artery bypass graft, any combination of drug-eluting intracoronary stent, atherectomy and angioplasty; single vessel **Qp** **Qh** J1

Medicare Statute 1833(t)

✪ **C9608** Percutaneous transluminal revascularization of chronic total occlusion, coronary artery, coronary artery branch, or coronary artery bypass graft, any combination of drug-eluting intracoronary stent, atherectomy and angioplasty; each additional coronary artery, coronary artery branch, or bypass graft (list separately in addition to code for primary procedure) **Qp** **Qh** N

Medicare Statute 1833(t)

✪ **C9724** Endoscopic full-thickness plication of the stomach using endoscopic plication system (EPS); includes endoscopy **Qh** G2 T

Medicare Statute 1833(t)

✪ **C9725** Placement of endorectal intracavitary applicator for high intensity brachytherapy **Qh** G2 T

Medicare Statute 1833(t)

✪ **C9726** Placement and removal (if performed) of applicator into breast for intraoperative radiation therapy, add-on to primary breast procedure **Qh** G2 N

Medicare Statute 1833(t)

✪ **C9727** Insertion of implants into the soft palate; minimum of three implants **Qh** G2 T

Medicare Statute 1833(t)

▶ **New** ↻ **Revised** ✔ **Reinstated** ~~deleted~~ **Deleted** ⊘ **Not covered or valid by Medicare**
✪ **Special coverage instructions** ✳ **Carrier discretion** ⑧ **Bill local carrier** ⑧ **Bill DME MAC**

✳ **C9728** Placement of interstitial device(s) for radiation therapy/surgery guidance (e.g., fiducial markers, dosimeter), for other than the following sites (any approach): abdomen, pelvis, prostate, retroperitoneum, thorax, single or multiple `Qh`   R2   S

Medicare Statute 1833(t)

⊛ **C9733** Non-ophthalmic fluorescent vascular angiography `Qp` `Qh`   N1   Q2

Medicare Statute 1833(t)

Coding Clinic: 2012, Q1, P7

⊛ **C9734** Focused ultrasound ablation/ therapeutic intervention, other than uterine leiomyomata, with magnetic resonance (MR) guidance `Qp` `Qh`   S

Medicare Statute 1833(t)

~~C9735~~ ~~Anoscopy; with directed submucosal~~ ✖
~~injection(s), any substance~~

⊛ **C9737** Laparoscopy, surgical, esophageal sphincter augmentation with device (e.g., magnetic band) `Qp` `Qh`   T

Medicare Statute 1833(t)

▶ ⊛ **C9739** Cystourethroscopy, with insertion of transprostatic implant; 1 to 3 implants `Qp` `Qh`   T

Medicare Statute 1833(t)

Coding Clinic: 2014, Q2, P6

▶ ⊛ **C9740** Cystourethroscopy, with insertion of transprostatic implant; 4 or more implants `Qp` `Qh`   T

Medicare Statute 1833(t)

Coding Clinic: 2014, Q2, P6

↺ ⊛ **C9741** Right heart catheterization with implantation of wireless pressure sensor in the pulmonary artery, including any type of measurement, angiography, imaging supervision, interpretation, and report   T

Medicare Statute 1833(t)

▶ ⊛ **C9742** Laryngoscopy, flexible fiberoptic, with injection into vocal cord(s), therapeutic, including diagnostic laryngoscopy, if performed   T

Medicare Statute 1833(t)

⊛ **C9800** Dermal injection procedure(s) for facial lipodystrophy syndrome (LDS) and provision of radiesse or sculptra dermal filler, including all items and supplies `Qh`   R2   T

Temporary office-based destination

Medicare Statute 1833(t)

Coding Clinic: 2010, Q3, P8, 10

⊛ **C9898** Radiolabeled product provided during a hospital inpatient stay `Qh`   N

⊛ **C9899** Implanted prosthetic device, payable only for inpatients who do not have inpatient coverage   A

Medicare Statute 1833(t)

PQRS PQRS	`Qp` Quantity Physician Appendix A	`Qh` Quantity Hospital Appendix B	♀ Female only
♂ Male only `A` Age ♿ DMEPOS	A2-Z3 ASC Payment Indicator	A-Y ASC Status Indicator	Coding Clinic

DENTAL PROCEDURES (D0000-D9999)

Diagnostic

Clinical Oral Evaluations

⊘ **D0120**   Periodic oral evaluation Ⓑ   E

Medicare Statute 1862A(12)

⊘ **D0140**   Limited oral evaluation - problem focused Ⓑ   E

Medicare Statute 1862A(12)

⊘ **D0145**   Oral evaluation for a patient under three years of age and counseling with primary caregiver Ⓑ 🅰   E

Medicare Statute 1862A(12)

✹ **D0150**   Comprehensive oral evaluation - new or established patient Ⓑ   S

IOM: 100-02, 15, 150; 100-02, 16, 140; 100-03, 4, 260.6

⊘ **D0160**   Detailed and extensive oral evaluation - problem focused, by report Ⓑ   E

Medicare Statute 1862A(12)

⊘ **D0170**   Re-evaluation-limited, problem focused (established patient; not post-operative visit) Ⓑ   E

Medicare Statute 1862A(12)

▶ **D0171**   Re-evaluation – post-operative office visit   E

⊘ **D0180**   Comprehensive periodontal evaluation - new or established patient Ⓑ   E

Medicare Statute 1862A(12)

Pre-Diagnostic Services

D0190   Screening of a patient Ⓑ   E

D0191   Assessment of a patient Ⓑ   E

Diagnostic Imaging

Image Capture with Interpretation

⊘ **D0210**   Intraoral-complete series (radiographic image) Ⓑ   E

Cross Reference CPT 70320

⊘ **D0220**   Intraoral-periapical-first radiographic image Ⓑ   E

Cross Reference CPT 70300

⊘ **D0230**   Intraoral-periapical-each additional radiographic image Ⓑ   E

Cross Reference CPT 70310

✹ **D0240**   Intraoral-occlusal radiographic image Ⓑ   S

IOM: 100-02, 15, 150; 100-02, 16, 140

✹ **D0250**   Extraoral-first radiographic image Ⓑ   S

IOM: 100-02, 15, 150; 100-02, 16, 140

✹ **D0260**   Extraoral-each additional radiographic image Ⓑ   S

IOM: 100-02, 15, 150; 100-02, 16, 140

✹ **D0270**   Bitewing-single radiographic image Ⓑ   S

IOM: 100-02, 15, 150; 100-02, 16, 140

✹ **D0272**   Bitewings-two radiographic images Ⓑ   S

IOM: 100-02, 15, 150; 100-02, 16, 140

⊘ **D0273**   Bitewings - three radiographic images Ⓑ   E

Medicare Statute 1862A(12)

✹ **D0274**   Bitewings-four radiographic images Ⓑ   S

IOM: 100-02, 15, 150; 100-02, 16, 140

✹ **D0277**   Vertical bitewings - 7 to 8 radiographic images Ⓑ   S

IOM: 100-02, 15, 150; 100-02, 16, 140

⊘ **D0290**   Posterior-anterior or lateral skull and facial bone survey radiographic image Ⓑ   E

Cross Reference 70150

⊘ **D0310**   Sialography Ⓑ   E

Cross Reference 70390

⊘ **D0320**   Temporomandibular joint arthrogram, including injection Ⓑ   E

Cross Reference 70332

⊘ **D0321**   Other temporomandibular joint radiographic image, by report Ⓑ   E

Cross Reference 76499

⊘ **D0322**   Tomographic survey Ⓑ   E

Cross Reference CPT

IOM: 100-03, 4, 260.6

⊘ **D0330**   Panoramic radiographic image Ⓑ   E

Cross Reference 70320

⊘ **D0340**   Cephalometric radiographic image Ⓑ   E

Cross Reference 70350

↻ ⊘ **D0350**   2D oral/facial photographic image obtained intra-orally or extra-orally Ⓑ   E

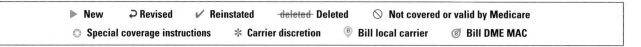

▶ **New**   ↻ **Revised**   ✔ **Reinstated**   ~~deleted~~ **Deleted**   ⊘ **Not covered or valid by Medicare**
✹ **Special coverage instructions**   ✲ **Carrier discretion**   Ⓛ **Bill local carrier**   Ⓑ **Bill DME MAC**

▶ **D0351** 3D photographic image E

D0364 Cone beam CT capture and interpretation with limited field of view – less than one whole jaw ⓑ E

D0365 Cone beam CT capture and interpretation with field of view of one full dental arch – mandible ⓑ E

D0366 Cone beam CT capture and interpretation with field of view of one full dental arch – maxilla, with or without cranium ⓑ E

D0367 Cone beam CT capture and interpretation with field of view of both jaws, with or without cranium ⓑ E

D0368 Cone beam CT capture and interpretation for TMJ series including two or more exposures ⓑ E

D0369 Maxillofacial MRI capture and interpretation ⓑ E

D0370 Maxillofacial ultrasound capture and interpretation ⓑ E

D0371 Sialoendoscopy capture and interpretation ⓑ E

Image Capture Only

D0380 Cone beam CT image capture with limited field of view – less than one whole jaw ⓑ E

D0381 Cone beam CT image capture with field of view of one full dental arch – mandible ⓑ E

D0382 Cone beam CT image capture with field of view of one full dental arch – maxilla, with or without cranium ⓑ E

D0383 Cone beam CT image capture with field of view of both jaws, with or without cranium ⓑ E

D0384 Cone beam CT image capture for TMJ series including two or more exposures ⓑ E

D0385 Maxillofacial MRI image capture ⓑ E

D0386 Maxillofacial ultrasound image capture ⓑ E

Interpretation and Report Only

D0391 Interpretation of diagnostic image by a practitioner not associated with capture of the image, including report ⓑ E

Post Processing of Image or Image Sets

D0393 Treatment simulation using 3D image volume ⓑ E

D0394 Digital subtraction of two or more images or image volumes of the same modality ⓑ E

D0395 Fusion of two or more 3D image volumes of one or more modalities ⓑ E

Tests and Examinations

⊘ **D0415** Collection of microorganisms for culture and sensitivity ⓑ E

Medicare Statute 1862A(12)

Cross Reference D0410

⊛ **D0416** Viral culture ⓑ B

⊘ **D0417** Collection and preparation of saliva sample for laboratory diagnostic testing ⓑ E

⊘ **D0418** Analysis of saliva sample ⓑ E

⊛ **D0421** Genetic test for susceptibility to oral diseases ⓑ B

⊘ **D0425** Caries susceptibility tests ⓑ E

Medicare Statute 1862A(12)

Cross Reference D0420

⊛ **D0431** Adjunctive pre-diagnostic test that aids in detection of mucosal abnormalities including premalignant and malignant lesions, not to include cytology or biopsy procedures ⓑ B

⊛ **D0460** Pulp vitality tests ⓑ S

IOM: 100-02, 15, 150; 100-02, 16, 140; 100-03, 4, 260.6

⊘ **D0470** Diagnostic casts ⓑ E

Medicare Statute 1862A(12)

Oral Pathology Laboratory (Use Codes D0472–D0502)

⊛ **D0472** Accession of tissue, gross examination, preparation and transmission of written report ⓑ B

IOM: 100-02, 15, 150; 100-02, 16, 140; 100-03, 4, 260.6

⊛ **D0473** Accession of tissue, gross and microscopic examination, preparation and transmission of written report ⓑ B

IOM: 100-02, 15, 150; 100-02, 16, 140; 100-03, 4, 260.6

⊙ **D0474** Accession of tissue, gross and microscopic examination, including assessment of surgical margins for presence of disease, preparation and transmission of written report ⑧ B

IOM: 100-02, 15, 150; 100-02, 16, 140; 100-03, 4, 260.6

⊙ **D0475** Decalcification procedure ⑧ B

⊙ **D0476** Special stains for microorganisms ⑧ B

⊙ **D0477** Special stains, not for microorganisms ⑧ B

⊙ **D0478** Immunohistochemical stains ⑧ B

⊙ **D0479** Tissue in-situ hybridization, including interpretation ⑧ B

⊙ **D0480** Accession of exfoliative cytologic smears, microscopic examination, preparation and transmission of written report ⑧ B

IOM: 100-02, 15, 150; 100-02, 16, 140; 100-03, 4, 260.6

↻ ⊙ **D0481** Electron microscopy ⑧ B

⊙ **D0482** Direct immunofluorescence ⑧ B

⊙ **D0483** Indirect immunofluorescence ⑧ B

⊙ **D0484** Consultation on slides prepared elsewhere ⑧ B

⊙ **D0485** Consultation, including preparation of slides from biopsy material supplied by referring source ⑧ B

⊘ **D0486** Laboratory accession of transepithelial cytologic sample, microscopic examination, preparation and transmission of written report ⑧ E

Medicare Statute 1862A(12)

⊙ **D0502** Other oral pathology procedures, by report ⑧ B

IOM: 100-02, 15, 150; 100-02, 16, 140; 100-03, 4, 260.6

D0601 Caries risk assessment and documentation, with a finding of low risk ⑧ E

D0602 Caries risk assessment and documentation, with a finding of moderate risk ⑧ E

D0603 Caries risk assessment and documentation, with a finding of high risk ⑧ E

⊙ **D0999** Unspecified diagnostic procedure, by report ⑧ B

IOM: 100-02, 15, 150; 100-02, 16, 140; 100-03, 4, 260.6

Preventative

Dental Prophylaxis

⊘ **D1110** Prophylaxis-adult ⑧ **A** E

Medicare Statute 1862A(12)

⊘ **D1120** Prophylaxis-child ⑧ **A** E

Medicare Statute 1862A(12)

Topical Fluoride Treatment (Office Procedure)

⊘ **D1206** Topical application of fluoride varnish ⑧ E

Medicare Statute 1862A(12)

↻ ⊘ **D1208** Topical application of fluoride — excluding varnish ⑧ E

Medicare Statute 1862A(12)

Other Preventative Services

⊘ **D1310** Nutritional counseling for the control of dental disease ⑧ E

IOM: 100-02, 16, 10

⊘ **D1320** Tobacco counseling for the control and prevention of oral disease ⑧ E

IOM: 100-02, 16, 10

⊘ **D1330** Oral hygiene instruction ⑧ E

IOM: 100-02, 16, 10

⊘ **D1351** Sealant-per tooth ⑧ E

Medicare Statute 1862A(12)

⊘ **D1352** Preventive resin restoration in a moderate to high caries risk patient — permanent tooth ⑧ E

▶ **D1353** Sealant repair–per tooth E

Space Maintenance (Passive Appliances)

⊙ **D1510** Space maintainer-fixed unilateral ⑧ S

IOM: 100-02, 16, 140; 100-04, 4, 20.5

⊙ **D1515** Space maintainer-fixed bilateral ⑧ S

IOM: 100-02, 15, 150; 100-02, 16, 140

⊙ **D1520** Space maintainer-removable unilateral ⑧ S

IOM: 100-02, 15, 150; 100-02, 16, 140

⊙ **D1525** Space maintainer-removable bilateral ⑧ S

IOM: 100-02, 15, 150; 100-02, 16, 140

↻ ⊙ **D1550** Re-cement or re-bond space maintainer ⑧ S

IOM: 100-02, 15, 150; 100-02, 16, 140

▶ **New**   ↻ **Revised**   ✔ **Reinstated**   ~~deleted~~ **Deleted**   ⊘ **Not covered or valid by Medicare**

⊙ **Special coverage instructions**   ✳ **Carrier discretion**   ⑧ **Bill local carrier**   ⑧ **Bill DME MAC**

⊘ **D1555** Removal of fixed space
maintainer ⓑ   E
Medicare Statute 1862A(12)

D1999 Unspecified preventive procedure, by
report ⓑ   E

Restorative

Amalgam Restorations (Including Polishing)

⊘ **D2140** Amalgam-one surface, primary or
permanent ⓑ   E
Medicare Statute 1862A(12)

⊘ **D2150** Amalgam-two surfaces, primary or
permanent ⓑ   E
Medicare Statute 1862A(12)

⊘ **D2160** Amalgam-three surfaces, primary or
permanent ⓑ   E
Medicare Statute 1862A(12)

⊘ **D2161** Amalgam-four or more surfaces,
primary or permanent ⓑ   E
Medicare Statute 1862A(12)

Resin-Based Composite Restorations—Direct

⊘ **D2330** Resin-one surface, anterior ⓑ   E
Medicare Statute 1862A(12)

⊘ **D2331** Resin-two surfaces, anterior ⓑ   E
Medicare Statute 1862A(12)

⊘ **D2332** Resin-three surfaces, anterior ⓑ   E
Medicare Statute 1862A(12)

⊘ **D2335** Resin-four or more surfaces or
involving incisal angle (anterior) ⓑ   E
Medicare Statute 1862A(12)

⊘ **D2390** Resin-based composite crown,
anterior ⓑ   E
Medicare Statute 1862A(12)

⊘ **D2391** Resin-based composite - one surface,
posterior ⓑ   E
Medicare Statute 1862A(12)

⊘ **D2392** Resin-based composite - two surfaces,
posterior ⓑ   E
Medicare Statute 1862A(12)

⊘ **D2393** Resin-based composite - three surfaces,
posterior ⓑ   E
Medicare Statute 1862A(12)

⊘ **D2394** Resin-based composite - four or more
surfaces, posterior ⓑ   E
Medicare Statute 1862A(12)

Gold Foil Restorations

⊘ **D2410** Gold foil-one surface ⓑ   E
Medicare Statute 1862A(12)

⊘ **D2420** Gold foil-two surfaces ⓑ   E
Medicare Statute 1862A(12)

⊘ **D2430** Gold foil-three surfaces ⓑ   E
Medicare Statute 1862A(12)

Inlay/Onlay Restorations

⊘ **D2510** Inlay-metallic-one surface ⓑ   E
Medicare Statute 1862A(12)

⊘ **D2520** Inlay-metallic-two surfaces ⓑ   E
Medicare Statute 1862A(12)

⊘ **D2530** Inlay-metallic-three or more
surfaces ⓑ   E
Medicare Statute 1862A(12)

⊘ **D2542** Onlay-metallic-two surfaces ⓑ   E
Medicare Statute 1862A(12)

⊘ **D2543** Onlay - metallic - three surfaces ⓑ   E
Medicare Statute 1862A(12)

⊘ **D2544** Onlay - metallic - four or more
surfaces ⓑ   E
Medicare Statute 1862A(12)

⊘ **D2610** Inlay-porcelain/ceramic-one
surface ⓑ   E
Medicare Statute 1862A(12)

⊘ **D2620** Inlay-porcelain/ceramic-two
surfaces ⓑ   E
Medicare Statute 1862A(12)

⊘ **D2630** Inlay-porcelain/ceramic-three or more
surfaces ⓑ   E
Medicare Statute 1862A(12)

⊘ **D2642** Onlay - porcelain/ceramic - two
surfaces ⓑ   E
Medicare Statute 1862A(12)

⊘ **D2643** Onlay - porcelain/ceramic - three
surfaces ⓑ   E
Medicare Statute 1862A(12)

⊘ **D2644** Onlay - porcelain/ceramic - four or
more surfaces ⓑ   E
Medicare Statute 1862A(12)

⊘ **D2650** Inlay - resin-based composite - one
surface ⓑ   E
Medicare Statute 1862A(12)

⊘ **D2651** Inlay - resin-based composite - two
surfaces ⓑ   E
Medicare Statute 1862A(12)

🄟 PQRS   Qp Quantity Physician Appendix A   Qh Quantity Hospital Appendix B   ♀ Female only
♂ Male only   A Age   ♿ DMEPOS   A2-Z3 ASC Payment Indicator   A-Y ASC Status Indicator   Coding Clinic

DENTAL PROCEDURES   D1555 – D2651

151

⊘ **D2652** Inlay - resin-based composite - three or more surfaces Ⓑ   E

Medicare Statute 1862A(12)

⊘ **D2662** Onlay - resin-based composite - two surfaces Ⓑ   E

Medicare Statute 1862A(12)

⊘ **D2663** Onlay - resin-based composite - three surfaces Ⓑ   E

Medicare Statute 1862A(12)

⊘ **D2664** Onlay - resin-based composite - four or more surfaces Ⓑ   E

Medicare Statute 1862A(12)

Crowns—Single Restoration Only

⊘ **D2710** Crown - resin-based composite (indirect) Ⓑ   E

Medicare Statute 1862A(12)

⊘ **D2712** Crown - 3/4 resin-based composite (indirect) Ⓑ   E

Medicare Statute 1862A(12)

⊘ **D2720** Crown-resin with high noble metal Ⓑ   E

Medicare Statute 1862A(12)

⊘ **D2721** Crown-resin with predominantly base metal Ⓑ   E

Medicare Statute 1862A(12)

⊘ **D2722** Crown-resin with noble metal Ⓑ   E

Medicare Statute 1862A(12)

⊘ **D2740** Crown-porcelain/ceramic substrate Ⓑ   E

Medicare Statute 1862A(12)

⊘ **D2750** Crown-porcelain fused to high noble metal Ⓑ   E

Medicare Statute 1862A(12)

⊘ **D2751** Crown-porcelain fused to predominantly base metal Ⓑ   E

Medicare Statute 1862A(12)

⊘ **D2752** Crown-porcelain fused to noble metal Ⓑ   E

Medicare Statute 1862A(12)

⊘ **D2780** Crown - 3/4 cast high noble metal Ⓑ   E

Medicare Statute 1862A(12)

⊘ **D2781** Crown - 3/4 cast predominantly base metal Ⓑ   E

Medicare Statute 1862A(12)

⊘ **D2782** Crown - 3/4 cast noble metal Ⓑ   E

Medicare Statute 1862A(12)

⊘ **D2783** Crown - 3/4 porcelain/ceramic Ⓑ   E

Medicare Statute 1862A(12)

⊘ **D2790** Crown-full cast high noble metal Ⓑ   E

Medicare Statute 1862A(12)

⊘ **D2791** Crown-full cast predominantly base metal Ⓑ   E

Medicare Statute 1862A(12)

⊘ **D2792** Crown-full cast noble metal Ⓑ   E

Medicare Statute 1862A(12)

⊘ **D2794** Crown-titanium Ⓑ   E

Medicare Statute 1862A(12)

⊘ **D2799** Provisional crown - further treatment or completion of diagnosis necessary prior to final impression Ⓑ   E

Medicare Statute 1862A(12)

↻ ⊘ **D2910** Re-cement or re-bond inlay, onlay, veneer or partial coverage restoration Ⓑ   E

Medicare Statute 1862A(12)

↻ ⊘ **D2915** Re-cement or re-bond indirectly fabricated cast or prefabricated post and core Ⓑ   E

Medicare Statute 1862A(12)

↻ ⊘ **D2920** Re-cement or re-bond crown Ⓑ   E

Medicare Statute 1862A(12)

D2921 Reattachment of tooth fragment, incisal edge or cusp Ⓑ   E

D2929 Prefabricated porcelain/ceramic crown – primary tooth Ⓑ   E

⊘ **D2930** Prefabricated stainless steel crown-primary tooth Ⓑ   E

Medicare Statute 1862A(12)

⊘ **D2931** Prefabricated stainless steel crown-permanent tooth Ⓑ   E

Medicare Statute 1862A(12)

⊘ **D2932** Prefabricated resin crown Ⓑ   E

Medicare Statute 1862A(12)

⊘ **D2933** Prefabricated stainless steel crown with resin window Ⓑ   E

Medicare Statute 1862A(12)

⊘ **D2934** Prefabricated esthetic coated stainless steel crown - primary tooth Ⓑ   E

Medicare Statute 1862A(12)

⊘ **D2940** Protective restoration Ⓑ   E

Medicare Statute 1862A(12)

D2941 Interim therapeutic restoration – primary dentition Ⓑ   E

▶ New   ↻ Revised   ✔ Reinstated   ~~deleted~~ Deleted   ⊘ Not covered or valid by Medicare

⊛ Special coverage instructions   ✱ Carrier discretion   Ⓑ Bill local carrier   Ⓑ Bill DME MAC

D2949 Restorative foundation for an indirect restoration ⓑ E

⊘ **D2950** Core build-up, including any pins when required ⓑ E

Medicare Statute 1862A(12)

⊘ **D2951** Pin retention-per tooth, in addition to restoration ⓑ E

Medicare Statute 1862A(12)

⊘ **D2952** Post and core in addition to crown, indirectly fabricated ⓑ E

Medicare Statute 1862A(12)

⊘ **D2953** Each additional indirectly fabricated post - same tooth ⓑ E

Medicare Statute 1862A(12)

⊘ **D2954** Prefabricated post and core in addition to crown ⓑ E

Medicare Statute 1862A(12)

⊘ **D2955** Post removal ⓑ E

Medicare Statute 1862A(12)

⊘ **D2957** Each additional prefabricated post - same tooth ⓑ E

Medicare Statute 1862A(12)

⊘ **D2960** Labial veneer (laminate)-chairside ⓑ E

Medicare Statute 1862A(12)

⊘ **D2961** Labial veneer (resin laminate)-laboratory ⓑ E

Medicare Statute 1862A(12)

⊘ **D2962** Labial veneer (porcelain laminate)-laboratory ⓑ E

Medicare Statute 1862A(12)

✲ **D2970** Temporary crown (fractured tooth) ⓑ E

IOM: 100-02, 15, 150; 100-02, 16, 140

⊘ **D2971** Additional procedures to construct new crown under existing partial denture framework ⓑ E

Medicare Statute 1862A(12)

↺⊘ **D2975** Coping ⓑ E

Medicare Statute 1862A(12)

⊘ **D2980** Crown repair, necessitated by restorative material failure ⓑ E

Medicare Statute 1862A(12)

D2981 Inlay repair necessitated by restorative material failure ⓑ E

D2982 Onlay repair necessitated by restorative material failure ⓑ E

D2983 Veneer repair necessitated by restorative material failure ⓑ E

Other Restorative Services

D2990 Resin infiltration of incipient smooth surface lesions ⓑ E

✲ **D2999** Unspecified restorative procedure, by report ⓑ S

Endodontics
Pulp Capping

⊘ **D3110** Pulp cap-direct (excluding final restoration) ⓑ E

Medicare Statute 1862A(12)

⊘ **D3120** Pulp cap-indirect (excluding final restoration) ⓑ E

Medicare Statute 1862A(12)

Pulpotomy

⊘ **D3220** Therapeutic pulpotomy (excluding final restoration) removal of pulp coronal to the dentinocemental junction and application of medicament ⓑ E

Medicare Statute 1862A(12)

⊘ **D3221** Pulpal debridement, primary and permanent teeth ⓑ E

Medicare Statute 1862A(12)

⊘ **D3222** Partial pulpotomy for apexogenesis-permanent tooth with incomplete root development ⓑ E

Medicare Statute 1862A(12)

Endodontic Therapy on Primary Teeth

⊘ **D3230** Pulpal therapy (resorbable filling)-anterior, primary tooth (excluding final restoration) ⓑ E

Medicare Statute 1862A(12)

⊘ **D3240** Pulpal therapy (resorbable filling)-posterior, primary tooth (excluding final restoration) ⓑ E

Medicare Statute 1862A(12)

Endodontic Therapy (Including Treatment Plan, Clinical Procedures and Follow-Up Care)

⊘ **D3310** Endodontic therapy, anterior tooth (excluding final restoration) ⓑ E

Medicare Statute 1862A(12)

⊘ **D3320** Endodontic therapy bicuspid tooth (excluding final restoration) ⓑ E

Medicare Statute 1862A(12)

⊘ **D3330** Endodontic therapy molar (excluding final restoration) ⑧   E

Medicare Statute 1862A(12)

⊘ **D3331** Treatment of root canal obstruction; non-surgical access ⑧   E

Medicare Statute 1862A(12)

⊘ **D3332** Incomplete endodontic therapy; inoperable, unrestorable or fractured tooth ⑧   E

Medicare Statute 1862A(12)

⊘ **D3333** Internal root repair of perforation defects ⑧   E

Medicare Statute 1862A(12)

Endodontic Retreatment

⊘ **D3346** Retreatment of previous root canal therapy-anterior ⑧   E

Medicare Statute 1862A(12)

⊘ **D3347** Retreatment of previous root canal therapy-bicuspid ⑧   E

Medicare Statute 1862A(12)

⊘ **D3348** Retreatment of previous root canal therapy-molar ⑧   E

Medicare Statute 1862A(12)

Apexification/Recalcification

↻ ⊘ **D3351** Apexification/recalcification-initial visit (apical closure/calcific repair of perforations, root resorption, etc.) ⑧   E

Medicare Statute 1862A(12)

⊘ **D3352** Apexification/recalcification-interim medication replacement (apical closure/calcific repair of perforations, root resorption, pulp space disinfection, etc.) ⑧   E

Medicare Statute 1862A(12)

⊘ **D3353** Apexification/recalcification-final visit (includes completed root canal therapy-apical closure/calcific repair of perforations, root resorption, etc.) ⑧   E

Medicare Statute 1862A(12)

Pulpal Regeneration

D3355 Pulpal regeneration - initial visit ⑧   E

D3356 Pulpal regeneration - interim medication replacement ⑧   E

D3357 Pulpal regeneration - completion of treatment ⑧   E

Apicoectomy/Periradicular Services

⊘ **D3410** Apicoectomy/periradicular surgery-anterior ⑧   E

Medicare Statute 1862A(12)

⊘ **D3421** Apicoectomy-bicuspid (first root) ⑧   E

Medicare Statute 1862A(12)

⊘ **D3425** Apicoectomy-molar (first root) ⑧   E

Medicare Statute 1862A(12)

⊘ **D3426** Apicoectomy (each additional root) ⑧   E

Medicare Statute 1862A(12)

D3427 Periradicular surgery without apicoectomy ⑧   E

D3428 Bone graft in conjunction with periradicular surgery – per tooth, single site ⑧   E

D3429 Bone graft in conjunction with periradicular surgery – each additional contiguous tooth in the same surgical site ⑧   E

⊘ **D3430** Retrograde filling-per root ⑧   E

Medicare Statute 1862A(12)

D3431 Bologic materials to aid in soft and osseous tissue regeneration in conjunction with periradicular surgery ⑧   E

D3432 Guided tissue regeneration, resorbable barrier, per site, in conjunction with periradicular surgery ⑧   E

⊘ **D3450** Root amputation-per root ⑧   E

Medicare Statute 1862A(12)

✸ **D3460** Endodontic endosseous implant ⑧   S

IOM: 100-02, 15, 150; 100-02, 16, 140

⊘ **D3470** Intentional replantation (including necessary splinting) ⑧   E

Medicare Statute 1862A(12)

Other Endodontic Procedures

⊘ **D3910** Surgical procedure for isolation of tooth with rubber dam ⑧   E

Medicare Statute 1862A(12)

⊘ **D3920** Hemisection (including any root removal), not including root canal therapy ⑧   E

Medicare Statute 1862A(12)

▶ New	↻ Revised	✔ Reinstated	deleted Deleted	⊘ Not covered or valid by Medicare
✸ Special coverage instructions		✳ Carrier discretion	⑧ Bill local carrier	⑧ Bill DME MAC

⊘ **D3950** Canal preparation and fitting of preformed dowel or post Ⓑ   E

Medicare Statute 1862A(12)

⊛ **D3999** Unspecified endodontic procedure, by report Ⓑ   S

IOM: 100-02, 15, 150; 100-02, 16, 140

Periodontics

Surgical Services (Including Usual Postoperative Care)

⊘ **D4210** Gingivectomy or gingivoplasty - four or more contiguous teeth or tooth bounded spaces per quadrant Ⓑ   E

Cross Reference CPT 41820

⊘ **D4211** Gingivectomy or gingivoplasty - one to three contiguous teeth or tooth bounded spaces per quadrant Ⓑ   E

Cross Reference CPT

D4212 Gingivectomy or gingivoplasty to allow access for restorative procedure, per tooth Ⓑ   E

⊘ **D4230** Anatomical crown exposure - four or more contiguous teeth per quadrant Ⓑ   E

Medicare Statute 1862A(12)

⊘ **D4231** Anatomical crown exposure - one to three teeth per quadrant Ⓑ   E

Medicare Statute 1862A(12)

⊘ **D4240** Gingival flap procedure, including root planing - four or more contiguous teeth or tooth bounded spaces per quadrant Ⓑ   E

Medicare Statute 1862A(12)

⊘ **D4241** Gingival flap procedure, including root planing - one to three contiguous teeth or tooth bounded spaces per quadrant Ⓑ   E

Medicare Statute 1862A(12)

⊘ **D4245** Apically positioned flap Ⓑ   E

Medicare Statute 1862A(12)

↻ ⊘ **D4249** Clinical crown lengthening-hard tissue Ⓑ   E

Medicare Statute 1862A(12)

↻ ⊛ **D4260** Osseous surgery (including elevation of a full thickness flap and closure) - four or more contiguous teeth or tooth bounded spaces per quadrant Ⓑ   S

IOM: 100-2, 15, 150; 100-02, 16, 140

↻ ⊘ **D4261** Osseous surgery (including elevation of a full thickness flap and closure) - one to three contiguous teeth or tooth bounded spaces per quadrant Ⓑ   E

Medicare Statute 1862A(12)

⊛ **D4263** Bone replacement graft - first site in quadrant Ⓑ   S

IOM: 100-02, 15, 150; 100-02, 16, 140; 100-03, 4, 260.6

⊛ **D4264** Bone replacement graft - each additional site in quadrant Ⓑ   S

IOM: 100-02, 15, 150; 100-2, 16, 140; 100-3, 4, 260.6

⊘ **D4265** Biologic materials to aid in soft and osseous tissue regeneration Ⓑ   E

Medicare Statute 1862A(12)

⊘ **D4266** Guided tissue regeneration - resorbable barrier, per site Ⓑ   E

Medicare Statute 1862A(12)

⊘ **D4267** Guided tissue regeneration - nonresorbable barrier, per site, (includes membrane removal) Ⓑ   E

Medicare Statute 1862A(12)

⊛ **D4268** Surgical revision procedure, per tooth Ⓑ   S

IOM: 100-02; 15, 150; 100-02, 16, 140

⊛ **D4270** Pedicle soft tissue graft procedure Ⓑ   S

IOM: 100-02, 15, 150; 100-02, 16, 140

⊛ **D4273** Subepithelial connective tissue graft procedures, per tooth Ⓑ   S

IOM:100-02, 15, 150; 100-02, 16, 140; 100-03, 4, 260.6

⊘ **D4274** Distal or proximal wedge procedure (when not performed in conjuction with surgical procedures in the same anatomical area) Ⓑ   E

Medicare Statute 1862A(12)

⊘ **D4275** Soft tissue allograft Ⓑ   E

Medicare Statute 1862A(12)

⊘ **D4276** Combined connective tissue and double pedicle graft, per tooth Ⓑ   E

Medicare Statute 1862A(12)

D4277 Free soft tissue graft procedure (including donor site surgery), first tooth or edentulous tooth position in graft Ⓑ   E

D4278 Free soft tissue graft procedure (including donor site surgery), each additional contiguous tooth or edentulous tooth position in same graft site Ⓑ   E

Non-Surgical Periodontal Services

⊘ **D4320** Provisional splinting-intracoronal ⓑ — E
Medicare Statute 1862A(12)

⊘ **D4321** Provisional splinting-extracoronal ⓑ — E
Medicare Statute 1862A(12)

⊘ **D4341** Periodontal scaling and root planing - four or more teeth per quadrant ⓑ — E
Medicare Statute 1862A(12)

⊘ **D4342** Periodontal scaling and root planing - one to three teeth, per quadrant ⓑ — E
Medicare Statute 1862A(12)

✲ **D4355** Full mouth debridement to enable comprehensive evaluation and diagnosis ⓑ — S
IOM: 100-02, 15, 150; 100-02, 16, 140

✲ **D4381** Localized delivery of antimicrobial agents via a controlled release vehicle into diseased crevicular tissue, per tooth ⓑ — S
IOM: 100-02, 15, 150; 100-02, 16, 140

Other Periodontal Services

⊘ **D4910** Periodontal maintenance ⓑ — E
Medicare Statute 1862A(12)

⊘ **D4920** Unscheduled dressing change (by someone other than treating dentist or their staff) ⓑ — E
Medicare Statute 1862A(12)

D4921 Gingival irrigation – per quadrant ⓑ — E

⊘ **D4999** Unspecified periodontal procedure, by report ⓑ — E
Medicare Statute 1862A(12)

Prosthodontics (removable)

Complete Dentures (Including Routine Post-Delivery Care)

⊘ **D5110** Complete denture – maxillary ⓑ — E
Medicare Statute 1862A(12)

⊘ **D5120** Complete denture – mandibular ⓑ — E
Medicare Statute 1862A(12)

⊘ **D5130** Immediate denture – maxillary ⓑ — E
Medicare Statute 1862A(12)

⊘ **D5140** Immediate denture – mandibular ⓑ — E
Medicare Statute 1862A(12)

Partial Dentures (Including Routine Post-Delivery Care)

⊘ **D5211** Upper partial-resin base (including any conventional clasps, rests and teeth) ⓑ — E
Medicare Statute 1862A(12)

⊘ **D5212** Lower partial-resin base (including any conventional clasps, rests and teeth) ⓑ — E
Medicare Statute 1862A(12)

⊘ **D5213** Maxillary partial denture - cast metal framework with resin denture bases (including any conventional clasps, rests and teeth) ⓑ — E
Medicare Statute 1862A(12)

⊘ **D5214** Mandibular partial denture - cast metal framework with resin denture bases (including any conventional clasps, rests and teeth) ⓑ — E
Medicare Statute 1862A(12)

⊘ **D5225** Maxillary partial denture - flexible base (including any clasps, rests and teeth) ⓑ — E
Medicare Statute 1862A(12)

⊘ **D5226** Mandibular partial denture - flexible base (including any clasps, rests and teeth) ⓑ — E
Medicare Statute 1862A(12)

⊘ **D5281** Removable unilateral partial denture-one piece cast metal (including clasps and teeth) ⓑ — E
Medicare Statute 1862A(12)

Adjustment to Dentures

⊘ **D5410** Adjust complete denture – maxillary ⓑ — E
Medicare Statute 1862A(12)

⊘ **D5411** Adjust complete denture – mandibular ⓑ — E
Medicare Statute 1862A(12)

⊘ **D5421** Adjust partial denture – maxillary ⓑ — E
Medicare Statute 1862A(12)

⊘ **D5422** Adjust partial denture – mandibular ⓑ — E
Medicare Statute 1862A(12)

▶ New   ↻ Revised   ✔ Reinstated   ~~deleted~~ Deleted   ⊘ Not covered or valid by Medicare
✲ Special coverage instructions   ✳ Carrier discretion   ⓑ Bill local carrier   ⓓ Bill DME MAC

Repairs to Complete Dentures

⊘ **D5510** Repair broken complete denture base Ⓑ   E
Medicare Statute 1862A(12)

⊘ **D5520** Replace missing or broken teeth-complete denture (each tooth) Ⓑ   E
Medicare Statute 1862A(12)

Repairs to Partial Dentures

⊘ **D5610** Repair resin denture base Ⓑ   E
Medicare Statute 1862A(12)

⊘ **D5620** Repair cast framework Ⓑ   E
Medicare Statute 1862A(12)

⊘ **D5630** Repair or replace broken clasp Ⓑ   E
Medicare Statute 1862A(12)

⊘ **D5640** Replace broken teeth-per tooth Ⓑ   E
Medicare Statute 1862A(12)

⊘ **D5650** Add tooth to existing partial denture Ⓑ   E
Medicare Statute 1862A(12)

⊘ **D5660** Add clasp to existing partial denture Ⓑ   E
Medicare Statute 1862A(12)

⊘ **D5670** Replace all teeth and acrylic on cast metal framework (maxillary) Ⓑ   E
Medicare Statute 1862A(12)

⊘ **D5671** Replace all teeth and acrylic on cast metal framework (mandibular) Ⓑ   E
Medicare Statute 1862A(12)

Denture Rebase Procedures

⊘ **D5710** Rebase complete maxillary denture Ⓑ   E
Medicare Statute 1862A(12)

⊘ **D5711** Rebase complete mandibular denture Ⓑ   E
Medicare Statute 1862A(12)

⊘ **D5720** Rebase maxillary partial denture Ⓑ   E
Medicare Statute 1862A(12)

⊘ **D5721** Rebase mandibular partial denture Ⓑ   E
Medicare Statute 1862A(12)

Denture Reline Procedures

⊘ **D5730** Reline complete maxillary denture (chairside) Ⓑ   E
Medicare Statute 1862A(12)

⊘ **D5731** Reline lower complete mandibular denture (chairside) Ⓑ   E
Medicare Statute 1862A(12)

⊘ **D5740** Reline maxillary partial denture (chairside) Ⓑ   E
Medicare Statute 1862A(12)

⊘ **D5741** Reline mandibular partial denture (chairside) Ⓑ   E
Medicare Statute 1862A(12)

⊘ **D5750** Reline complete maxillary denture (laboratory) Ⓑ   E
Medicare Statute 1862A(12)

⊘ **D5751** Reline complete mandibular denture (laboratory) Ⓑ   E
Medicare Statute 1862A(12)

⊘ **D5760** Reline maxillary partial denture (laboratory) Ⓑ   E
Medicare Statute 1862A(12)

⊘ **D5761** Reline mandibular partial denture (laboratory) Ⓑ   E
Medicare Statute 1862A(12)

Interim Prosthesis

⊘ **D5810** Interim complete denture (maxillary) Ⓑ   E
Medicare Statute 1862A(12)

⊘ **D5811** Interim complete denture (mandibular) Ⓑ   E
Medicare Statute 1862A(12)

⊘ **D5820** Interim partial denture (maxillary) Ⓑ   E
Medicare Statute 1862A(12)

⊘ **D5821** Interim partial denture (mandibular) Ⓑ   E
Medicare Statute 1862A(12)

⊘ **D5850** Tissue conditioning, maxillary Ⓑ   E
Medicare Statute 1862A(12)

⊘ **D5851** Tissue conditioning, mandibular Ⓑ   E
Medicare Statute 1862A(12)

⊘ **D5862** Precision attachment, by report Ⓑ   E
Medicare Statute 1862A(12)

D5863 Overdenture – complete maxillary Ⓑ   E

PQRS   **Qp** Quantity Physician Appendix A   **Qh** Quantity Hospital Appendix B   ♀ Female only
♂ Male only   **A** Age   ♿ DMEPOS   A2-Z3 ASC Payment Indicator   A-Y ASC Status Indicator   Coding Clinic

DENTAL PROCEDURES   D5510 – D5863

157

D5864 Overdenture – partial maxillary Ⓑ   E

D5865 Overdenture – complete mandibular Ⓑ   E

D5866 Overdenture – partial mandibular Ⓑ   E

⊘ **D5867** Replacement of replaceable part of semi-precision or precision attachment (male or female component) Ⓑ   E

Medicare Statute 1862A(12)

⊘ **D5875** Modification of removable prosthesis following implant surgery Ⓑ   E

Medicare Statute 1862A(12)

⊘ **D5899** Unspecified removable prosthodontic procedure, by report Ⓑ   E

Medicare Statute 1862A(12)

Maxillofacial Prosthetics

✹ **D5911** Facial moulage (sectional) Ⓑ   S

IOM: 100-02, 15, 150; 100-02, 16, 140

✹ **D5912** Facial moulage (complete) Ⓑ   S

IOM: 100-02, 15, 150

⊘ **D5913** Nasal prosthesis Ⓑ   E

Cross Reference CPT 21087

⊘ **D5914** Auricular prosthesis Ⓑ   E

Cross Reference CPT 21086

⊘ **D5915** Orbital prosthesis Ⓑ   E

Cross Reference CPT L8611

⊘ **D5916** Ocular prosthesis Ⓑ   E

Cross Reference CPT, V2623, V2629

⊘ **D5919** Facial prosthesis Ⓑ   E

Cross Reference CPT 21088

⊘ **D5922** Nasal septal prosthesis Ⓑ   E

Cross Reference CPT 30220

⊘ **D5923** Ocular prosthesis, interim Ⓑ   E

Cross Reference CPT 92330

⊘ **D5924** Cranial prosthesis Ⓑ   E

Cross Reference CPT 62143

⊘ **D5925** Facial augmentation implant prosthesis Ⓑ   E

Cross Reference CPT 21208

⊘ **D5926** Nasal prosthesis, replacement Ⓑ   E

Cross Reference CPT 21087

⊘ **D5927** Auricular prosthesis, replacement Ⓑ   E

Cross Reference CPT 21086

⊘ **D5928** Orbital prosthesis, replacement Ⓑ   E

Cross Reference CPT 67550

⊘ **D5929** Facial prosthesis, replacement Ⓑ   E

Cross Reference CPT 21088

⊘ **D5931** Obturator prosthesis, surgical Ⓑ   E

Cross Reference CPT 21079

⊘ **D5932** Obturator prosthesis, definitive Ⓑ   E

Cross Reference CPT 21080

⊘ **D5933** Obturator prosthesis, modification Ⓑ   E

Cross Reference CPT 21080

⊘ **D5934** Mandibular resection prosthesis with guide flange Ⓑ   E

Cross Reference CPT 21081

⊘ **D5935** Mandibular resection prosthesis without guide flange Ⓑ   E

Cross Reference CPT 21081

⊘ **D5936** Obturator/prosthesis, interim Ⓑ   E

Cross Reference CPT 21079

⊘ **D5937** Trismus appliance (not for tm treatment) Ⓑ   E

IOM: 100-02, 15, 150

✹ **D5951** Feeding aid Ⓑ   E

IOM: 100-02, 15, 150; 100-02, 16, 140

⊘ **D5952** Speech aid prosthesis, pediatric Ⓑ **A**   E

Cross Reference CPT 21084

⊘ **D5953** Speech aid prosthesis, adult Ⓑ **A**   E

Cross Reference CPT 21084

⊘ **D5954** Palatal augmentation prosthesis Ⓑ   E

Cross Reference CPT 21082

⊘ **D5955** Palatal lift prosthesis, definitive Ⓑ   E

Cross Reference CPT 21083

⊘ **D5958** Palatal lift prosthesis, interim Ⓑ   E

Cross Reference CPT 21083

⊘ **D5959** Palatal lift prosthesis, modification Ⓑ   E

Cross Reference CPT 21083

⊘ **D5960** Speech aid prosthesis, modification Ⓑ   E

Cross Reference CPT 21084

⊘ **D5982** Surgical stent Ⓑ   E

Cross Reference CPT 21085

Carriers

✹ **D5983** Radiation carrier Ⓑ   S

IOM: 100-02, 15, 150; 100-02, 16, 140

✹ **D5984** Radiation shield Ⓑ   S

IOM: 100-02, 15, 150; 100-02, 16, 140

▶ **New**   ⟳ **Revised**   ✔ **Reinstated**   ~~deleted~~ **Deleted**   ⊘ **Not covered or valid by Medicare**

✹ **Special coverage instructions**   ✳ **Carrier discretion**   Ⓑ **Bill local carrier**   Ⓓ **Bill DME MAC**

⊘ **D5985** Radiation cone locator ⓑ   S
IOM: 100-02, 15, 150; 100-02, 16, 140

⃠ **D5986** Fluoride gel carrier ⓑ   E
Medicare Statute 1862A(12)

⊘ **D5987** Commissure splint ⓑ   S
IOM: 100-02, 15, 150; 100-02, 16, 140

⃠ **D5988** Surgical splint ⓑ   E
Cross Reference CPT

⃠ **D5991** Vesicobullous disease medicament carrier ⓑ   E
Medicare Statute 1862A(12)

⃠ **D5992** Adjust maxillofacial prosthetic appliance, by report ⓑ   E

⃠ **D5993** Maintenance and cleaning of a maxillofacial prosthesis (extra or intraoral) other than required adjustments, by report ⓑ   E

D5994 Periodontal medicament carrier with peripheral seal – laboratory processed ⓑ   E

⃠ **D5999** Unspecified maxillofacial prosthesis, by report ⓑ   E
Cross Reference CPT

Implant Services

D6010-D6199: FPD 5 fixed partial denture

Surgical Services

⃠ **D6010** Surgical placement of implant body: endosteal implant ⓑ   E
Cross Reference CPT 21248

D6011 Second stage implant surgery ⓑ   E

⃠ **D6012** Surgical placement of interim implant body for transitional prosthesis: endosteal implant ⓑ   E
Medicare Statute 1862A(12)

D6013 Surgical placement of mini implant ⓑ   E

⃠ **D6040** Surgical placement: eposteal implant ⓑ   E
Cross Reference CPT 21245

⃠ **D6050** Surgical placement: transosteal implant ⓑ   E
Cross Reference CPT 21244

D6051 Interim abutment - includes placement and removal ⓑ   E

D6052 Semi-precision attachment abutment ⓑ   E

~~D6053 Implant/abutment supported removable denture for completely edentulous arch~~ ✖

~~D6054 Implant/abutment supported removable denture for partially edentulous arch~~ ✖

Implant Supported Prosthetics

⃠ **D6055** Connecting bar — implant supported or abutment supported ⓑ   E
IOM: 100-02, 15, 150

⃠ **D6056** Prefabricated abutment - includes modification and placement ⓑ   E
IOM: 100-02, 15, 150

⃠ **D6057** Custom fabricated abutment - includes placement ⓑ   E
IOM: 100-02, 15, 150

↩⃠ **D6058** Abutment supported porcelain/ceramic crown ⓑ   E
IOM: 100-02, 15, 150

↩⃠ **D6059** Abutment supported porcelain fused to metal crown (high noble metal) ⓑ   E
IOM: 100-02, 15, 150

↩⃠ **D6060** Abutment supported porcelain fused to metal crown (predominantly base metal) ⓑ   E
IOM: 100-02, 15, 150

↩⃠ **D6061** Abutment supported porcelain fused to metal crown (noble metal) ⓑ   E
IOM: 100-02, 15, 150

↩⃠ **D6062** Abutment supported cast metal crown (high noble metal) ⓑ   E
IOM: 100-02, 15, 150

↩⃠ **D6063** Abutment supported cast metal crown (predominantly base metal) ⓑ   E
IOM: 100-02, 15, 150

↩⃠ **D6064** Abutment supported cast metal crown (noble metal) ⓑ   E
IOM: 100-02, 15, 150

↩⃠ **D6065** Implant supported porcelain/ceramic crown ⓑ   E
IOM: 100-02, 15, 150

↩⃠ **D6066** Implant supported porcelain fused to metal crown (titanium, titanium alloy, high noble metal) ⓑ   E
IOM: 100-02, 15, 150

↩⃠ **D6067** Implant supported metal crown (titanium, titanium alloy, high noble metal) ⓑ   E
IOM: 100-02, 15, 150

DENTAL PROCEDURES   D5985 – D6067

↻ ⊘ **D6068** Abutment supported retainer for porcelain/ceramic FPD ⑧   E

IOM: 100-02, 15, 150

↻ ⊘ **D6069** Abutment supported retainer for porcelain fused to metal FPD (high noble metal) ⑧   E

IOM: 100-02, 15, 150

↻ ⊘ **D6070** Abutment supported retainer for porcelain fused to metal FPD (predominantly base metal) ⑧   E

IOM: 100-02, 15, 150

↻ ⊘ **D6071** Abutment supported retainer for porcelain fused to metal FPD (noble metal) ⑧   E

IOM: 100-02, 15, 150

↻ ⊘ **D6072** Abutment supported retainer for cast metal FPD (high noble metal) ⑧   E

IOM: 100-02, 15, 150

↻ ⊘ **D6073** Abutment supported retainer for cast metal FPD (predominantly base metal) ⑧   E

IOM: 100-02, 15, 150

↻ ⊘ **D6074** Abutment supported retainer for cast metal FPD (noble metal) ⑧   E

IOM: 100-02, 15, 150

↻ ⊘ **D6075** Implant supported retainer for ceramic FPD ⑧   E

IOM: 100-02, 15, 150

↻ ⊘ **D6076** Implant supported retainer for porcelain fused to metal FPD (titanium, titanium alloy, or high noble metal) ⑧   E

IOM: 100-02, 15, 150

↻ ⊘ **D6077** Implant supported retainer for cast metal FPD (titanium, titanium alloy, or high noble metal) ⑧   E

IOM: 100-02, 15, 150

~~D6078~~ ~~Implant/abutment supported fixed denture for completely edentulous arch~~   ✖

~~D6079~~ ~~Implant/abutment supported fixed denture for partially edentulous arch~~   ✖

Other Implant Services

⊘ **D6080** Implant maintenance procedures when prostheses are removed and reinserted, including cleansing of prostheses and abutments ⑧   E

IOM: 100-02, 15, 150

⊘ **D6090** Repair implant supported prosthesis by report ⑧   E

Cross Reference CPT 21299

⊘ **D6091** Replacement of semi-precision or precision attachment (male or female component) of implant/abutment supported prosthesis, per attachment ⑧   E

Medicare Statute 1862A(12)

↻ ⊘ **D6092** Re-cement or re-bond implant/abutment supported crown ⑧   E

Medicare Statute 1862A(12)

↻ ⊘ **D6093** Re-cement or re-bond implant/abutment supported fixed partial denture ⑧   E

Medicare Statute 1862A(12)

↻ ⊘ **D6094** Abutment supported crown - (titanium) ⑧   E

Medicare Statute 1862A(12)

⊘ **D6095** Repair implant abutment, by report ⑧   E

Cross Reference CPT 21299

⊘ **D6100** Implant removal, by report ⑧   E

Cross Reference CPT 21299

↻ **D6101** Debridement of a peri-implant defect or defects surrounding a single implant, and surface cleaning of exposed implant surfaces, including flap entry and closure ⑧   E

↻ **D6102** Debridement and osseous contouring of a peri-implant defect or defects surrounding a single implant and includes surface cleaning of the exposed implant surfaces and flap entry and closure ⑧   E

↻ **D6103** Bone graft for repair of peri-implant defect – does not include flap entry and closure. Placement of a barrier membrane or biologic materials to aid in osseous regeneration are reported separately ⑧   E

D6104 Bone graft at time of implant placement ⑧   E

▶ **D6110** Implant /abutment supported removable denture for edentulous arch – maxillary   E

▶ **D6111** Implant /abutment supported removable denture for edentulous arch – mandibular   E

▶ **D6112** Implant /abutment supported removable denture for partially edentulous arch – maxillary   E

▶ **New**   ↻ **Revised**   ✔ **Reinstated**   ~~deleted~~ **Deleted**   ⊘ **Not covered or valid by Medicare**

⊙ **Special coverage instructions**   ✳ **Carrier discretion**   ⑧ **Bill local carrier**   ⑧ **Bill DME MAC**

D6068 – D6112 DENTAL PROCEDURES

▶ **D6113** Implant /abutment supported removable denture for partially edentulous arch – mandibular   E

▶ **D6114** Implant /abutment supported fixed denture for edentulous arch – maxillary   E

▶ **D6115** Implant /abutment supported fixed denture for edentulous arch – mandibular   E

▶ **D6116** Implant /abutment supported fixed denture for partially edentulous arch – maxillary   E

▶ **D6117** Implant /abutment supported fixed denture for partially edentulous arch – mandibular   E

⊘ **D6190** Radiographic/surgical implant index, by report Ⓑ   E

Medicare Statute 1862A(12)

↻ ⊘ **D6194** Abutment supported retainer crown for FPD - (titanium) Ⓑ   E

Medicare Statute 1862A(12)

⊘ **D6199** Unspecified implant procedure, by report Ⓑ   E

Cross Reference CPT 21299

Prosthodontics, fixed

Fixed Partial Denture Pontics

⊘ **D6205** Pontic - indirect resin based composite Ⓑ   E

Medicare Statute 1862A(12)

⊘ **D6210** Pontic-cast high noble metal Ⓑ   E

Medicare Statute 1862A(12)

⊘ **D6211** Pontic-cast predominantly base metal Ⓑ   E

Medicare Statute 1862A(12)

⊘ **D6212** Pontic-cast noble metal Ⓑ   E

Medicare Statute 1862A(12)

⊘ **D6214** Pontic – titanium Ⓑ   E

Medicare Statute 1862A(12)

⊘ **D6240** Pontic-porcelain fused to high noble metal Ⓑ   E

Medicare Statute 1862A(12)

⊘ **D6241** Pontic-porcelain fused to predominantly base metal Ⓑ   E

Medicare Statute 1862A(12)

⊘ **D6242** Pontic-porcelain fused to noble metal Ⓑ   E

Medicare Statute 1862A(12)
IOM: 100-02, 15, 150

⊘ **D6245** Pontic - porcelain/ceramic Ⓑ   E

IOM: 100-02, 15, 150

⊘ **D6250** Pontic-resin with high noble metal Ⓑ   E

Medicare Statute 1862A(12)

⊘ **D6251** Pontic-resin with predominantly base metal Ⓑ   E

Medicare Statute 1862A(12)

⊘ **D6252** Pontic-resin with noble metal Ⓑ   E

Medicare Statute 1862A(12)

⊘ **D6253** Provisional pontic Ⓑ   E

Medicare Statute 1862A(12)

Fixed Partial Denture Retainers – Inlays/Onlays

⊘ **D6545** Retainer-cast metal for resin bonded fixed prosthesis Ⓑ   E

Medicare Statute 1862A(12)

⊘ **D6548** Retainer - porcelain/ceramic for resin bonded fixed prosthesis Ⓑ   E

IOM: 100-02, 15, 150

▶ **D6549** Resin retainer – for resin bonded fixed prosthesis   E

⊘ **D6600** Inlay-porcelain/ceramic, two surfaces Ⓑ   E

IOM: 100-02, 15, 150

⊘ **D6601** Inlay - porcelain/ceramic, three or more surfaces Ⓑ   E

IOM: 100-02, 15, 150

⊘ **D6602** Inlay - cast high noble metal, two surfaces Ⓑ   E

IOM: 100-02, 15, 150

⊘ **D6603** Inlay - cast high noble metal, three or more surfaces Ⓑ   E

IOM: 100-02, 15, 150

⊘ **D6604** Inlay - cast predominantly base metal, two surfaces Ⓑ   E

IOM: 100-02, 15, 150

⊘ **D6605** Inlay - cast predominantly base metal, three or more surfaces Ⓑ   E

IOM: 100-02, 15, 150

⊘ **D6606** Inlay - cast noble metal, two surfaces Ⓑ   E

IOM: 100-02, 15, 150

⊘ **D6607** Inlay - cast noble metal, three or more surfaces Ⓑ   E

IOM: 100-02, 15, 150

PQRS   **Qp** Quantity Physician Appendix A   **Qh** Quantity Hospital Appendix B   ♀ Female only   ♂ Male only   **A** Age   ♿ DMEPOS   A2-Z3 ASC Payment Indicator   A-Y ASC Status Indicator   Coding Clinic

DENTAL PROCEDURES D6113 – D6607

161

⊘ **D6608**   Onlay - porcelain/ceramic, two surfaces Ⓑ   E
IOM: 100-02, 15, 150

⊘ **D6609**   Onlay - porcelain/ceramic, three or more surfaces Ⓑ   E
IOM: 100-02, 15, 150

⊘ **D6610**   Onlay - cast high noble metal, two surfaces Ⓑ   E
IOM: 100-02, 15, 150

⊘ **D6611**   Onlay - cast high noble metal, three or more surfaces Ⓑ   E
IOM: 100-02, 15, 150

⊘ **D6612**   Onlay - cast predominantly base metal, two surfaces Ⓑ   E
IOM: 100-02, 15, 150

⊘ **D6613**   Onlay - cast predominantly base metal, three or more surfaces Ⓑ   E
IOM: 100-02, 15, 150

⊘ **D6614**   Onlay - cast noble metal, two surfaces Ⓑ   E
IOM: 100-02, 15, 150

⊘ **D6615**   Onlay - cast noble metal, three or more surfaces Ⓑ   E
IOM: 100-02, 15, 150

⊘ **D6624**   Inlay – titanium Ⓑ   E
Medicare Statute 1862A(12)

⊘ **D6634**   Onlay – titanium Ⓑ   E
Medicare Statute 1862A(12)

Fixed Partial Denture Retainers – Crowns

⊘ **D6710**   Crown - indirect resin based composite Ⓑ   E
Medicare Statute 1862A(12)

⊘ **D6720**   Crown-resin with high noble metal Ⓑ   E
Medicare Statute 1862A(12)

⊘ **D6721**   Crown-resin with predominantly base metal Ⓑ   E
Medicare Statute 1862A(12)

⊘ **D6722**   Crown-resin with noble metal Ⓑ   E
Medicare Statute 1862A(12)

⊘ **D6740**   Crown - porcelain/ceramic Ⓑ   E
IOM: 100-02, 15, 150

⊘ **D6750**   Crown-porcelain fused to high noble metal Ⓑ   E
Medicare Statute 1862A(12)

⊘ **D6751**   Crown-porcelain fused to predominantly base metal Ⓑ   E
Medicare Statute 1862A(12)

⊘ **D6752**   Crown-porcelain fused to noble metal Ⓑ   E
Medicare Statute 1862A(12)

⊘ **D6780**   Crown-3/4 cast high noble metal Ⓑ   E
Medicare Statute 1862A(12)

⊘ **D6781**   Crown - 3/4 cast predominantly based metal Ⓑ   E
IOM: 100-02, 15, 150

⊘ **D6782**   Crown - 3/4 cast noble metal Ⓑ   E
IOM: 100-02, 15, 150

⊘ **D6783**   Crown - 3/4 porcelain/ceramic Ⓑ   E
IOM: 100-02, 15, 150

⊘ **D6790**   Crown-full cast high noble metal Ⓑ   E
Medicare Statute 1862A(12)

⊘ **D6791**   Crown-full cast predominantly base metal Ⓑ   E
Medicare Statute 1862A(12)

⊘ **D6792**   Crown-full cast noble metal Ⓑ   E
Medicare Statute 1862A(12)

⊘ **D6793**   Provisional retainer crown Ⓑ   E
Medicare Statute 1862A(12)

⊘ **D6794**   Crown - titanium Ⓑ   E
Medicare Statute 1862A(12)

Other Fixed Partial Denture Services

✷ **D6920**   Connector bar Ⓑ   S
IOM: 100-02, 15, 150; 100-02, 16, 140; 100-03, 4, 260.6

↻ ⊘ **D6930**   Re-cement or re-bond fixed partial denture Ⓑ   E
Medicare Statute 1862A(12)

⊘ **D6940**   Stress breaker Ⓑ   E
Medicare Statute 1862A(12)

⊘ **D6950**   Precision attachment Ⓑ   E
Medicare Statute 1862A(12)

~~D6975~~   ~~Coping~~   ✖

⊘ **D6980**   Bridge repair necessitated by restorative material failure Ⓑ   E
Medicare Statute 1862A(12)

⊘ **D6985**   Pediatric partial denture, fixed Ⓑ **A**   E
Medicare Statute 1862A(12)

▶ **New**   ↻ **Revised**   ✔ **Reinstated**   ~~deleted~~ **Deleted**   ⊘ **Not covered or valid by Medicare**
✷ **Special coverage instructions**   ✲ **Carrier discretion**   Ⓑ **Bill local carrier**   Ⓑ **Bill DME MAC**

⊘ **D6999** Unspecified fixed prosthodontic procedure, by report ⓑ   E

Medicare Statute 1862A(12)

Oral and Maxillofacial Surgery

Extractions (Includes Local Anesthesia, Suturing, If Needed, and Routine Postoperative Care)

✳ **D7111** Extraction, coronal remnants - deciduous tooth ⓑ   S

IOM: 100-02, 16, 140

🅟 ✳ **D7140** Extraction, erupted tooth or exposed root (elevation and/or forceps removal) ⓑ   S

IOM: 100-02, 16, 140

Surgical Extractions (Includes Local Anesthesia, Suturing, If Needed, and Routine Postoperative Care)

🅟 ✳ **D7210** Surgical removal of erupted tooth requiring removal of bone and/or section of tooth, and elevation of mucoperiosteal flap ⓑ   S

IOM: 100-02, 15, 150; 100-02, 16, 140

✳ **D7220** Removal of impacted tooth-soft tissue ⓑ   S

IOM: 100-02, 15, 150; 100-02, 16, 140

✳ **D7230** Removal of impacted tooth-partially bony ⓑ   S

IOM: 100-02, 15, 150; 100-02, 16, 140

✳ **D7240** Removal of impacted tooth-completely bony ⓑ   S

IOM: 100-02, 15, 150; 100-02, 16, 140

✳ **D7241** Removal of impacted tooth-completely bony, with unusual surgical complications ⓑ   S

IOM: 100-02, 15, 150; 100-02, 16, 140

✳ **D7250** Surgical removal of residual tooth roots (cutting procedure) ⓑ   S

IOM: 100-02, 15, 150; 100-02, 16, 140

⊘ **D7251** Coronectomy — intentional partial tooth removal ⓑ   E

Other Surgical Procedures

✳ **D7260** Oral antral fistula closure ⓑ   S

IOM: 100-02, 15, 150; 100-02, 16, 140

✳ **D7261** Primary closure of a sinus perforation ⓑ   S

IOM: 100-02, 16, 140

⊘ **D7270** Tooth reimplantation and/or stabilization of accidentally evulsed or displaced tooth ⓑ   E

Medicare Statute 1862A(12)

⊘ **D7272** Tooth transplantation (includes reimplantation from one site to another and splinting and/or stabilization) ⓑ   E

Medicare Statute 1862A(12)

⊘ **D7280** Surgical access of an unerupted tooth ⓑ   E

Medicare Statute 1862A(12)

⊘ **D7282** Mobilization of erupted or malpositioned tooth to aid eruption ⓑ   E

Medicare Statute 1862A(12)

✳ **D7283** Placement of device to facilitate eruption of impacted tooth ⓑ   B

↻⊘ **D7285** Incisional biopsy of oral tissue - hard (bone, tooth) ⓑ   E

Cross Reference CPT 20220, 20225, 20240, 20245

↻⊘ **D7286** Incisional biopsy of oral tissue – soft ⓑ   E

Cross Reference CPT 40808

⊘ **D7287** Exfoliative cytological sample collection ⓑ   E

✳ **D7288** Brush biopsy - transepithelial sample collection ⓑ   B

⊘ **D7290** Surgical repositioning of teeth ⓑ   E

Medicare Statute 1862A(12)

✳ **D7291** Transseptal fiberotomy/supra crestal fiberotomy, by report ⓑ   S

IOM: 100-02, 15, 150; 100-02, 16, 140

↻⊘ **D7292** Surgical placement of temporary anchorage device [screw retained plate] requiring flap; includes device removal ⓑ   E

Medicare Statute 1862A(12)

↻⊘ **D7293** Surgical placement of temporary anchorage device requiring flap; includes device removal ⓑ   E

Medicare Statute 1862A(12)

↻⊘ **D7294** Surgical placement of temporary anchorage device without flap; includes device removal ⓑ   E

Medicare Statute 1862A(12)

⊘ **D7295** Harvest of bone for use in autogenous grafting procedure ⓑ   E

Alveoloplasty – Surgical Preparation of Ridge

⊘ **D7310** Alveoloplasty in conjunction with extractions - four or more teeth or tooth spaces, per quadrant Ⓑ　　E

Cross Reference CPT 41874

⊘ **D7311** Alveoloplasty in conjunction with extractions - one to three teeth or tooth spaces, per quadrant Ⓑ　　E

Medicare Statute 1862A(12)

⊘ **D7320** Alveoloplasty not in conjunction with extractions - four or more teeth or tooth spaces, per quadrant Ⓑ　　E

Cross Reference CPT 41870

✹ **D7321** Alveoloplasty not in conjunction with extractions - one to three teeth or tooth spaces, per quadrant Ⓑ　　B

Vestibuloplasty

⊘ **D7340** Vestibuloplasty-ridge extension (second epithelialization) Ⓑ　　E

Cross Reference CPT 40840, 40842, 40843, 40844

⊘ **D7350** Vestibuloplasty-ridge extension (including soft tissue grafts, muscle re-attachments, revision of soft tissue attachment, and management of hypertrophied and hyperplastic tissue) Ⓑ　　E

Cross Reference CPT 40845

Surgical Excision of Soft Tissue Lesions

⊘ **D7410** Excision of benign lesion up to 1.25 cm Ⓑ　　E

Cross Reference CPT

⊘ **D7411** Excision of benign lesion greater than 1.25 cm Ⓑ　　E

⊘ **D7412** Excision of benign lesion, complicated Ⓑ　　E

⊘ **D7413** Excision of malignant lesion up to 1.25 cm Ⓑ　　E

⊘ **D7414** Excision of malignant lesion greater than 1.25 cm Ⓑ　　E

⊘ **D7415** Excision of malignant lesion, complicated Ⓑ　　E

Surgical Excision of Intra-Osseous Lesions

⊘ **D7440** Excision of malignant tumor-lesion diameter up to 1.25 cm Ⓑ　　E

Cross Reference CPT

⊘ **D7441** Excision of malignant tumor-lesion diameter greater than 1.25 cm Ⓑ　　E

Cross Reference CPT

⊘ **D7450** Removal of benign odontogenic cyst or tumor-lesion diameter up to 1.25 cm Ⓑ　　E

Cross Reference CPT

⊘ **D7451** Removal of benign odontogenic cyst or tumor-lesion diameter greater than 1.25 cm Ⓑ　　E

Cross Reference CPT

⊘ **D7460** Removal of benign nonodontogenic cyst or tumor-lesion diameter up to 1.25 cm Ⓑ　　E

Cross Reference CPT

⊘ **D7461** Removal of benign nonodontogenic cyst or tumor-lesion diameter greater than 1.25 cm　　E

Cross Reference CPT

⊘ **D7465** Destruction of lesion(s) by physical or chemical methods, by report Ⓑ　　E

Cross Reference CPT 41850

Excision of Bone Tissue

⊘ **D7471** Removal of lateral exostosis (maxilla or mandible) Ⓑ　　E

Cross Reference CPT 21031, 21032

⊘ **D7472** Removal of torus palatinus Ⓑ　　E

⊘ **D7473** Removal of torus mandibularis Ⓑ　　E

⊘ **D7485** Surgical reduction of osseous tuberosity Ⓑ　　E

⊘ **D7490** Radical resection of maxilla or mandible Ⓑ　　E

Cross Reference CPT 21095

Surgical Incision

⊘ **D7510** Incision and drainage of abscess-intraoral soft tissue Ⓑ　　E

Cross Reference CPT 41800

✹ **D7511** Incision and drainage of abscess - intraoral soft tissue-complicated (includes drainage of multiple fascial spaces) Ⓑ　　B

⊘ **D7520** Incision and drainage of abscess-extraoral soft tissue Ⓑ　　E

Cross Reference CPT 41800

✹ **D7521** Incision and drainage of abscess - extraoral soft tissue - complicated (includes drainage of multiple fascial spaces) Ⓑ　　B

▶ **New**　ↄ **Revised**　✔ **Reinstated**　~~deleted~~ **Deleted**　⊘ **Not covered or valid by Medicare**

✹ **Special coverage instructions**　✳ **Carrier discretion**　Ⓑ **Bill local carrier**　Ⓓ **Bill DME MAC**

⊘ **D7530** Removal of foreign body from mucosa, skin, or subcutaneous alveolar tissue ⓑ   E

Cross Reference CPT 41805, 41828

⊘ **D7540** Removal of reaction-producing foreign bodies-musculoskeletal system ⓑ   E

Cross Reference CPT 20520, 41800, 41806

⊘ **D7550** Partial ostectomy/sequestrectomy for removal of non-vital bone ⓑ   E

Cross Reference CPT 20999

⊘ **D7560** Maxillary sinusotomy for removal of tooth fragment or foreign body ⓑ   E

Cross Reference CPT 31020

Treatment of Fractures – Simple

⊘ **D7610** Maxilla-open reduction (teeth immobilized if present) ⓑ   E

Cross Reference CPT

⊘ **D7620** Maxilla-closed reduction (teeth immobilized if present) ⓑ   E

Cross Reference CPT

⊘ **D7630** Mandible-open reduction (teeth immobilized if present) ⓑ   E

Cross Reference CPT

⊘ **D7640** Mandible-closed reduction (teeth immobilized if present) ⓑ   E

Cross Reference CPT

⊘ **D7650** Malar and/or zygomatic arch-open reduction ⓑ   E

Cross Reference CPT

⊘ **D7660** Malar and/or zygomatic arch-closed reduction ⓑ   E

Cross Reference CPT

⊘ **D7670** Alveolus - closed reduction, may include stabilization of teeth ⓑ   E

Cross Reference CPT

⊘ **D7671** Alveolus - open reduction, may include stabilization of teeth ⓑ   E

⊘ **D7680** Facial bones-complicated reduction with fixation and multiple surgical approaches ⓑ   E

Cross Reference CPT

Treatment of Fractures – Compound

⊘ **D7710** Maxilla-open reduction ⓑ   E

Cross Reference CPT 21346

⊘ **D7720** Maxilla-closed reduction ⓑ   E

Cross Reference CPT 21345

⊘ **D7730** Mandible-open reduction ⓑ   E

Cross Reference CPT 21461, 21462

⊘ **D7740** Mandible-closed reduction ⓑ   E

Cross Reference CPT 21455

⊘ **D7750** Malar and/or zygomatic arch-open reduction ⓑ   E

Cross Reference CPT 21360, 21365

⊘ **D7760** Malar and/or zygomatic arch-closed reduction ⓑ   E

Cross Reference CPT 21355

⊘ **D7770** Alveolus - open reduction stabilization of teeth ⓑ   E

Cross Reference CPT 21422

⊘ **D7771** Alveolus, closed reduction stabilization of teeth ⓑ   E

⊘ **D7780** Facial bones-complicated reduction with fixation and multiple surgical approaches ⓑ   E

Cross Reference CPT 21433, 21435

Reduction of Dislocation and Management of Other Temporomandibular Joint Dysfunction

⊘ **D7810** Open reduction of dislocation ⓑ   E

Cross Reference CPT 21490

⊘ **D7820** Closed reduction of dislocation ⓑ   E

Cross Reference CPT 21480

⊘ **D7830** Manipulation under anesthesia ⓑ   E

Cross Reference CPT 00190

⊘ **D7840** Condylectomy ⓑ   E

Cross Reference CPT 21050

⊘ **D7850** Surgical discectomy; with/without implant ⓑ   E

Cross Reference CPT 21060

⊘ **D7852** Disc repair ⓑ   E

Cross Reference CPT 21299

⊘ **D7854** Synovectomy ⓑ   E

Cross Reference CPT 21299

⊘ **D7856** Myotomy ⓑ   E

Cross Reference CPT 21299

⊘ **D7858** Joint reconstruction ⓑ   E

Cross Reference CPT 21242, 21243

⊘ **D7860** Arthrotomy ⓑ   E

IOM: 100-02, 15, 150; 100-02, 16, 140

⊘ **D7865** Arthroplasty ⓑ   E

Cross Reference CPT 21240

ⓟ PQRS	Qp Quantity Physician Appendix A	Qh Quantity Hospital Appendix B	♀ Female only	
♂ Male only	A Age	♿ DMEPOS	A2-Z3 ASC Payment Indicator	A-Y ASC Status Indicator Coding Clinic

⊘ **D7870** Arthrocentesis ⓑ E

Cross Reference CPT 21060

⊘ **D7871** Non-arthroscopic lysis and lavage ⓑ E

Medicare Statute 1862A(12)

⊘ **D7872** Arthroscopy-diagnosis, with or without biopsy ⓑ E

Cross Reference CPT 29800

⊘ **D7873** Arthroscopy-surgical: lavage and lysis of adhesions ⓑ E

Cross Reference CPT 29804

⊘ **D7874** Arthroscopy-surgical: disc repositioning and stabilization ⓑ E

Cross Reference CPT 29804

⊘ **D7875** Arthroscopy-surgical: synovectomy ⓑ E

Cross Reference CPT 29804

⊘ **D7876** Arthroscopy-surgical: discectomy ⓑ E

Cross Reference CPT 29804

⊘ **D7877** Arthroscopy-surgical: debridement ⓑ E

Cross Reference CPT 29804

⊘ **D7880** Occlusal orthotic appliance ⓑ E

Cross Reference CPT 21499

⊘ **D7899** Unspecified TMD therapy, by report ⓑ E

Cross Reference CPT 21499

Repair of Traumatic Wounds

⊘ **D7910** Suture of recent small wounds up to 5 cm ⓑ E

Cross Reference CPT 12011, 12013

Complicated Suturing (Reconstruction Requiring Delicate Handling of Tissue and Wide Undermining for Meticulous Closure)

⊘ **D7911** Complicated suture-up to 5 cm ⓑ E

Cross Reference CPT 12051, 12052

⊘ **D7912** Complicated suture-greater than 5 cm ⓑ E

Cross Reference CPT 13132

Other Repair Procedures

⊘ **D7920** Skin graft (identify defect covered, location, and type of graft) ⓑ E

Cross Reference CPT

D7921 Collection and application of autologous blood concentrate product ⓑ E

✿ **D7940** Osteoplasty-for orthognathic deformities ⓑ S

IOM: 100-02, 15, 150; 100-02, 16, 140

⊘ **D7941** Osteotomy - mandibular rami ⓑ E

Cross Reference CPT 21193, 21195, 21196

⊘ **D7943** Osteotomy - mandibular rami with bone graft; includes obtaining the graft ⓑ E

Cross Reference CPT 21194

⊘ **D7944** Osteotomy-segmented or subapical ⓑ E

Cross Reference CPT 21198, 21206

⊘ **D7945** Osteotomy-body of mandible ⓑ E

Cross Reference CPT 21193, 21194, 21195, 21196

⊘ **D7946** Lefort I (maxilla-total) ⓑ E

Cross Reference CPT 21147

⊘ **D7947** Lefort I (maxilla-segmented) ⓑ E

Cross Reference CPT 21145, 21146

⊘ **D7948** Lefort II or lefort III (osteoplasty of facial bones for midface hypoplasia or retrusion)-without bone graft ⓑ E

Cross Reference CPT 21150

⊘ **D7949** Lefort II or lefort III-with bone graft ⓑ E

Cross Reference CPT

⊘ **D7950** Osseous, osteoperiosteal, or cartilage graft of the mandible or maxilla - autogenous or nonautogenous, by report ⓑ E

Cross Reference CPT 21247

⊘ **D7951** Sinus augmentation with bone or bone substitutes ⓑ E

Medicare Statute 1862A(12)

D7952 Sinus augmentation via a vertical approach ⓑ E

⊘ **D7953** Bone replacement graft for ridge preservation - per site ⓑ E

Medicare Statute 1862A(12)

⊘ **D7955** Repair of maxillofacial soft and/or hard tissue defect ⓑ E

Cross Reference CPT 21299

▶ New   ↻ Revised   ✔ Reinstated   ~~deleted~~ Deleted   ⊘ Not covered or valid by Medicare
✿ Special coverage instructions   ✳ Carrier discretion   ⓑ Bill local carrier   ⓓ Bill DME MAC

⊘ **D7960** Frenulectomy also known as frenectomy or frenotomy-separate procedure not incidental to another procedure ⑧   E

Cross Reference CPT 40819, 41010, 41115

⊘ **D7963** Frenuloplasty ⑧   E

Medicare Statute 1862A(12)

⊘ **D7970** Excision of hyperplastic tissue-per arch ⑧   E

Cross Reference CPT

⊘ **D7971** Excision of pericoronal gingival ⑧   E

Cross Reference CPT 41821

⊘ **D7972** Surgical reduction of fibrous tuberosity ⑧   E

⊘ **D7980** Sialolithotomy ⑧   E

Cross Reference CPT 42330, 42335, 42340

⊘ **D7981** Excision of salivary gland, by report ⑧   E

Cross Reference CPT 42408

⊘ **D7982** Sialodochoplasty ⑧   E

Cross Reference CPT 42500

⊘ **D7983** Closure of salivary fistula ⑧   E

Cross Reference CPT 42600

⊘ **D7990** Emergency tracheotomy ⑧   E

Cross Reference CPT 21070

⊘ **D7991** Coronoidectomy ⑧   E

Cross Reference CPT 21070

⊘ **D7995** Synthetic graft-mandible or facial bones, by report ⑧   E

Cross Reference CPT 21299

⊘ **D7996** Implant-mandible for augmentation purposes (excluding alveolar ridge), by report ⑧   E

Cross Reference CPT 21299

⊘ **D7997** Appliance removal (not by dentist who placed appliance), includes removal of archbar ⑧   E

Medicare Statute 1862A(12)

⊘ **D7998** Intraoral placement of a fixation device not in conjunction with a fracture ⑧   E

Medicare Statute 1862A(12)

⊘ **D7999** Unspecified oral surgery procedure, by report ⑧   E

Cross Reference CPT 21299

Orthodontics

Limited Orthodontic Treatment

⊘ **D8010** Limited orthodontic treatment of the primary dentition ⑧   E

Medicare Statute 1862A(12)

⊘ **D8020** Limited orthodontic treatment of the transitional dentition ⑧   E

Medicare Statute 1862A(12)

⊘ **D8030** Limited orthodontic treatment of the adolescent dentition ⑧ **A**   E

Medicare Statute 1862A(12)

⊘ **D8040** Limited orthodontic treatment of the adult dentition ⑧ **A**   E

Medicare Statute 1862A(12)

Interceptive Orthodontic Treatment

⊘ **D8050** Interceptive orthodontic treatment of the primary dentition ⑧   E

Medicare Statute 1862A(12)

⊘ **D8060** Interceptive orthodontic treatment of the transitional dentition ⑧   E

Medicare Statute 1862A(12)

Comprehensive Orthodontic Treatment

⊘ **D8070** Comprehensive orthodontic treatment of the transitional dentition ⑧   E

Medicare Statute 1862A(12)

⊘ **D8080** Comprehensive orthodontic treatment of the adolescent dentition ⑧ **A**   E

Medicare Statute 1862A(12)

⊘ **D8090** Comprehensive orthodontic treatment of the adult dentition ⑧ **A**   E

Medicare Statute 1862A(12)

Minor Treatment to Control Harmful Habits

⊘ **D8210** Removable appliance therapy ⑧   E

Medicare Statute 1862A(12)

⊘ **D8220** Fixed appliance therapy ⑧   E

Medicare Statute 1862A(12)

Other Orthodontic Services

↩ ⊘ **D8660** Pre-orthodontic examination to monitor growth and development ⑧   E

Medicare Statute 1862A(12)

ᴾᑫᴿˢ PQRS	**Qp** Quantity Physician Appendix A	**Qh** Quantity Hospital Appendix B	♀ Female only
♂ Male only	**A** Age	♿ DMEPOS	A2-Z3 ASC Payment Indicator A-Y ASC Status Indicator *Coding Clinic*

↻ ⊘ **D8670** Periodic orthodontic treatment visit Ⓑ   E

Medicare Statute 1862A(12)

⊘ **D8680** Orthodontic retention (removal of appliances, construction and placement of retainer(s)) Ⓑ   E

Medicare Statute 1862A(12)

⊘ **D8690** Orthodontic treatment (alternative billing to a contract fee) Ⓑ   E

Medicare Statute 1862A(12)

⊘ **D8691** Repair of orthodontic appliance Ⓑ   E

Medicare Statute 1862A(12)

⊘ **D8692** Replacement of lost or broken retainer Ⓑ   E

Medicare Statute 1862A(12)

↻ ⊘ **D8693** Re-cement or re-bond of fixed retainer Ⓑ   E

Medicare Statute 1862A(12)

D8694 Repair of fixed retainers, includes reattachment Ⓑ   E

⊘ **D8999** Unspecified orthodontic procedure, by report Ⓑ   E

Medicare Statute 1862A(12)

Adjunctive General Services

Unclassified Treatment

✿ **D9110** Palliative (emergency) treatment of dental pain-minor procedures Ⓑ   N

IOM: 100-02, 15, 150; 100-02, 16, 140

⊘ **D9120** Fixed partial denture sectioning Ⓑ   E

Medicare Statute 1862A(12)

Anesthesia

⊘ **D9210** Local anesthesia not in conjunction with operative or surgical procedures Ⓑ   E

Cross Reference CPT 90784

⊘ **D9211** Regional block anesthesia Ⓑ   E

Cross Reference CPT 01995

⊘ **D9212** Trigeminal division block anesthesia Ⓑ   E

Cross Reference CPT 64400

⊘ **D9215** Local anesthesia in conjunction with operative or surgical procedures Ⓑ   E

Cross Reference CPT 90784

▶ **D9219** Evaluation for deep sedation or general anesthesia   E

⊘ **D9220** Deep sedation/general anesthesia-first 30 minutes Ⓑ   E

Cross Reference CPT

↻ ⊘ **D9221** Deep sedation/general anesthesia-each additional 15 minutes Ⓑ   E

IOM: 100-02, 15, 150; 100-02, 16, 140

✿ **D9230** Inhalation of nitrous oxide/analgesia, anxiolysis Ⓑ   N

IOM: 100-02, 15, 150; 100-02, 16, 140

↻ ⊘ **D9241** Intravenous moderate (conscious) sedation/analgesia - first 30 minutes Ⓑ   E

Cross Reference CPT 90784

↻ ⊘ **D9242** Intravenous moderate (conscious) sedation/ analgesia - each additional 15 minutes Ⓑ   E

Cross Reference CPT 90784

↻ ✿ **D9248** Non-intravenous moderate (conscious) sedation Ⓑ   N

Professional Consultation

⊘ **D9310** Consultation - diagnostic service provided by dentist or physician other than requesting dentist or physician Ⓑ   E

Cross Reference CPT

Professional Visits

⊘ **D9410** House/extended care facility call Ⓑ   E

Cross Reference CPT

⊘ **D9420** Hospital or ambulatory surgical center call Ⓑ   E

Cross Reference CPT

⊘ **D9430** Office visit for observation (during regularly scheduled hours) no other services performed Ⓑ   E

Cross Reference CPT

⊘ **D9440** Office visit-after regularly scheduled hours Ⓑ   E

Cross Reference CPT 99050

⊘ **D9450** Case presentation, detailed and extensive treatment planning Ⓑ   E

▶ **New**   ↻ **Revised**   ✔ **Reinstated**   ~~deleted~~ **Deleted**   ⊘ **Not covered or valid by Medicare**

✿ **Special coverage instructions**   ✳ **Carrier discretion**   Ⓛ **Bill local carrier**   Ⓑ **Bill DME MAC**

Drugs

⊘ **D9610** Therapeutic parenteral drug, single administration ⑧   E

⊘ **D9612** Therapeutic parenteral drugs, two or more administrations, different medications ⑧   E

Medicare Statute 1862A(12)

✪ **D9630** Other drugs and/or medicaments, by report ⑧   S

IOM: 100-02, 15, 150; 100-02, 16, 140

Miscellaneous Services

⊘ **D9910** Application of desensitizing medicament ⑧   E

Medicare Statute 1862A(12)

⊘ **D9911** Application of desensitizing resin for cervical and/or root surface, per tooth ⑧   E

Medicare Statute 1862A(12)

⊘ **D9920** Behavior management, by report ⑧   E

Medicare Statute 1862A(12)

✪ **D9930** Treatment of complications (postsurgical) - unusual circumstances, by report ⑧   S

IOM: 100-02, 15, 150; 100-02, 16, 140

▶ **D9931** Cleaning and inspection of removable appliance   E

✪ **D9940** Occlusal guards, by report ⑧   S

IOM: 100-02, 15, 150; 100-02, 16, 140

⊘ **D9941** Fabrication of athletic mouthguard ⑧   E

Medicare Statute 1862A(12)

Cross Reference CPT 21089

⊘ **D9942** Repair and/or reline of occlusal guard ⑧   E

Medicare Statute 1862A(12)

✪ **D9950** Occlusion analysis-mounted case ⑧   S

IOM: 100-02, 15, 150; 100-02, 16, 140

✪ **D9951** Occlusal adjustment-limited ⑧   S

IOM: 100-02, 15, 150; 100-02, 16, 140

✪ **D9952** Occlusal adjustment-complete ⑧   S

IOM: 100-02, 15, 150; 100-02, 16, 140

⊘ **D9970** Enamel microabrasion ⑧   E

Medicare Statute 1862A(12)

⊘ **D9971** Odontoplasty 1 - 2 teeth; includes removal of enamel projections ⑨   E

Medicare Statute 1862A(12)

⊘ **D9972** External bleaching - per arch - performed in office ⑧   E

Medicare Statute 1862A(12)

⊘ **D9973** External bleaching - per tooth ⑧   E

Medicare Statute 1862A(12) ⑧

⊘ **D9974** Internal bleaching - per tooth ⑧   E

Medicare Statute 1862A(12)

D9975 External bleaching for home application, per arch ⑧   E

D9985 Sales tax ⑧   E

Non-Clinical Procedures

▶ **D9986** Missed appointment   E

▶ **D9987** Cancelled appointment   E

⊘ **D9999** Unspecified adjunctive procedure, by report ⑧   E

Cross Reference CPT 21499

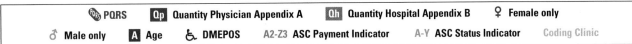

🅟 PQRS   🆀ᵖ **Quantity Physician Appendix A**   🆀ʰ **Quantity Hospital Appendix B**   ♀ **Female only**

♂ **Male only**   🅰 **Age**   ♿ **DMEPOS**   A2-Z3 **ASC Payment Indicator**   A-Y **ASC Status Indicator**   *Coding Clinic*

DURABLE MEDICAL EQUIPMENT (E0100-E1841)

Canes

⊕ **E0100**   Cane, includes canes of all materials, adjustable or fixed, with tip ⑧ **Qp** **Qh** ♿   Y

IOM: 100-02, 15, 110.1; 100-03, 4, 280.1; 100-03, 4, 280.2

DMEPOS Modifier(s): NU, RR, UE

⊕ **E0105**   Cane, quad or three prong, includes canes of all materials, adjustable or fixed, with tips ⑧ **Qp** **Qh** ♿   Y

IOM: 100-02, 15, 110.1; 100-03, 4, 280.1; 100-03, 4, 280.2

DMEPOS Modifier(s): NU, RR, UE

Crutches

⊕ **E0110**   Crutches, forearm, includes crutches of various materials, adjustable or fixed, pair, complete with tips and handgrips ⑧ **Qp** **Qh** ♿   Y

Crutches are covered when prescribed for a patient who is normally ambulatory but suffers from a condition that impairs ambulation. Provides minimal to moderate weight support while ambulating.

IOM: 100-02, 15, 110.1; 100-03, 4, 280.1

DMEPOS Modifier(s): NU, RR, UE

⊕ **E0111**   Crutch forearm, includes crutches of various materials, adjustable or fixed, each, with tips and handgrips ⑧ **Qp** **Qh** ♿   Y

IOM: 100-02, 15, 110.1; 100-03, 4, 280.1

DMEPOS Modifier(s): NU, RR, UE

⊕ **E0112**   Crutches, underarm, wood, adjustable or fixed, pair, with pads, tips, and handgrips ⑧ **Qp** **Qh** ♿   Y

IOM: 100-02, 15, 110.1; 100-03, 4, 280.1

DMEPOS Modifier(s): NU, RR, UE

⊕ **E0113**   Crutch underarm, wood, adjustable or fixed, each, with pad, tip, and handgrip ⑧ **Qp** **Qh** ♿   Y

IOM: 100-02, 15, 110.1; 100-03, 4, 280.1

DMEPOS Modifier(s): NU, RR, UE

⊕ **E0114**   Crutches, underarm, other than wood, adjustable or fixed, pair, with pads, tips and handgrips ⑧ **Qp** **Qh** ♿   Y

IOM: 100-02, 15, 110.1; 100-03, 4, 280.1

DMEPOS Modifier(s): NU, RR, UE

⊕ **E0116**   Crutch, underarm, other than wood, adjustable or fixed, with pad, tip, handgrip, with or without shock absorber, each ⑧ **Qp** **Qh** ♿   Y

IOM: 100-02, 15, 110.1; 100-03, 4, 280.1

DMEPOS Modifier(s): NU, RR, UE

↻ ⊕ **E0117**   Crutch, underarm, articulating, spring assisted, each ⑧ **Qp** **Qh** ♿   Y

IOM: 100-02, 15, 110.1

DMEPOS Modifier(s): RR

✳ **E0118**   Crutch substitute, lower leg platform, with or without wheels, each ⑧ **Qp** **Qh**   E

Walkers

⊕ **E0130**   Walker, rigid (pickup), adjustable or fixed height ⑧ **Qp** **Qh** ♿   Y

Standard walker criteria for payment: Individual has a mobility limitation that significantly impairs ability to participate in mobility-related activities of daily living that cannot be adequately or safely addressed by a cane. The patient is able to use the walker safely; the functional mobility deficit can be resolved with use of a standard walker.

IOM: 100-02, 15, 110.1; 100-03, 4, 280.1

DMEPOS Modifier(s): NU, RR, UE

⊕ **E0135**   Walker, folding (pickup), adjustable or fixed height ⑧ **Qp** **Qh** ♿   Y

IOM: 100-02, 15, 110.1; 100-03, 4, 280.1

DMEPOS Modifier(s): NU, RR, UE

⊕ **E0140**   Walker, with trunk support, adjustable or fixed height, any type ⑧ **Qp** **Qh** ♿   Y

IOM: 100-02, 15, 110.1; 100-03, 4, 280.1

DMEPOS Modifier(s): NU, RR, UE

⊕ **E0141**   Walker, rigid, wheeled, adjustable or fixed height ⑧ **Qp** **Qh** ♿   Y

IOM: 100-02, 15, 110.1; 100-03, 4, 280.1

DMEPOS Modifier(s): NU, RR, UE

⊕ **E0143**   Walker, folding, wheeled, adjustable or fixed height ⑧ **Qp** **Qh** ♿   Y

IOM: 100-02, 15, 110.1; 100-03, 4, 280.1

DMEPOS Modifier(s): NU, RR, UE

↻ ⊕ **E0144**   Walker, enclosed, four sided framed, rigid or folding, wheeled, with posterior seat ⑧ **Qp** **Qh** ♿   Y

IOM: 100-02, 15, 110.1; 100-03, 4, 280.1

DMEPOS Modifier(s): RR

▶ **New**   ↻ **Revised**   ✔ **Reinstated**   ~~deleted~~ **Deleted**   ⊘ **Not covered or valid by Medicare**
⊕ **Special coverage instructions**   ✳ **Carrier discretion**   ⑧ **Bill local carrier**   ⑧ **Bill DME MAC**

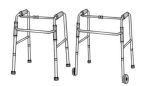

Figure 11 Walkers.

⚙ **E0147** Walker, heavy duty, multiple braking system, variable wheel resistance Ⓑ Qp Qh ♿ Y

Heavy-duty walker is labeled as capable of supporting more than 300 pounds

IOM: 100-02, 15, 110.1; 100-03, 4, 280.1

DMEPOS Modifier(s): NU, RR, UE

✳ **E0148** Walker, heavy duty, without wheels, rigid or folding, any type, each Ⓑ Qp Qh ♿ Y

Heavy-duty walker is labeled as capable of supporting more than 300 pounds

DMEPOS Modifier(s): NU, RR, UE

✳ **E0149** Walker, heavy duty, wheeled, rigid or folding, any type Ⓑ Qp Qh ♿ Y

Heavy-duty walker is labeled as capable of supporting more than 300 pounds

DMEPOS Modifier(s): NU, RR, UE

✳ **E0153** Platform attachment, forearm crutch, each Ⓑ Qp Qh ♿ Y

DMEPOS Modifier(s): NU, RR, UE

✳ **E0154** Platform attachment, walker, each Ⓑ Qp Qh ♿ Y

DMEPOS Modifier(s): NU, RR, UE

✳ **E0155** Wheel attachment, rigid pick-up walker, per pair Ⓑ Qp Qh ♿ Y

DMEPOS Modifier(s): NU, RR, UE

Attachments

✳ **E0156** Seat attachment, walker Ⓑ Qp Qh ♿ Y

DMEPOS Modifier(s): NU, RR, UE

✳ **E0157** Crutch attachment, walker, each Ⓑ Qp Qh ♿ Y

DMEPOS Modifier(s): NU, RR, UE

✳ **E0158** Leg extensions for walker, per set of four (4) Ⓑ Qp Qh ♿ Y

Leg extensions are considered medically necessary DME for patients 6 feet tall or more

DMEPOS Modifier(s): NU, RR, UE

✳ **E0159** Brake attachment for wheeled walker, replacement, each Ⓑ Qp Qh ♿ Y

DMEPOS Modifier(s): NU, RR, UE

Commodes

⚙ **E0160** Sitz type bath or equipment, portable, used with or without commode Ⓑ Qp Qh ♿ Y

IOM: 100-03, 4, 280.1

DMEPOS Modifier(s): NU, RR, UE

⚙ **E0161** Sitz type bath or equipment, portable, used with or without commode, with faucet attachment/ s Ⓑ Qp Qh ♿ Y

IOM: 100-03, 4, 280.1

DMEPOS Modifier(s): NU, RR, UE

⚙ **E0162** Sitz bath chair Ⓑ Qp Qh ♿ Y

IOM: 100-03, 4, 280.1

DMEPOS Modifier(s): NU, RR, UE

⚙ **E0163** Commode chair, mobile or stationary, with fixed arms Ⓑ Qp Qh ♿ Y

IOM: 100-02, 15, 110.1; 100-03, 4, 280.1

DMEPOS Modifier(s): NU, RR, UE

⚙ **E0165** Commode chair, mobile or stationary, with detachable arms Ⓑ Qp Qh ♿ Y

IOM: 100-02, 15, 110.1; 100-03, 4, 280.1

DMEPOS Modifier(s): RR

⚙ **E0167** Pail or pan for use with commode chair, replacement only Ⓑ Qp Qh ♿ Y

IOM: 100-03, 4, 280.1

DMEPOS Modifier(s): NU, RR, UE

✳ **E0168** Commode chair, extra wide and/ or heavy duty, stationary or mobile, with or without arms, any type, each Ⓑ Qp Qh ♿ Y

Extra-wide or heavy duty commode chair is labeled as capable of supporting more than 300 pounds

DMEPOS Modifier(s): NU, RR, UE

✳ **E0170** Commode chair with integrated seat lift mechanism, electric, any type Ⓑ Qp Qh ♿ Y

DMEPOS Modifier(s): RR

✳ **E0171** Commode chair with integrated seat lift mechanism, non-electric, any type Ⓑ Qp Qh ♿ Y

DMEPOS Modifier(s): RR

⊘ **E0172** Seat lift mechanism placed over or on top of toilet, any type Qp Qh Ⓑ E

Medicare Statute 1861 SSA

✳ **E0175** Foot rest, for use with commode chair, each Ⓑ Qp Qh ♿ Y

DMEPOS Modifier(s): NU, RR, UE

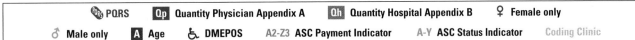

ⓅQRS PQRS	Qp Quantity Physician Appendix A	Qh Quantity Hospital Appendix B	♀ Female only
♂ Male only	Ⓐ Age	♿ DMEPOS	A2-Z3 ASC Payment Indicator	A-Y ASC Status Indicator	Coding Clinic

Decubitus Care Equipment

⊛ **E0181** Powered pressure reducing mattress overlay/pad, alternating, with pump, includes heavy duty Ⓑ 〔Qp〕〔Qh〕 ♿   Y

Requires the provider to determine medical necessity compliance. To demonstrate the requirements in the medical policy were met, attach -KX.

IOM: 100-03, 4, 280.1; 100-08, 5, 5.2.3

DMEPOS Modifier(s): RR

⊛ **E0182** Pump for alternating pressure pad, for replacement only Ⓑ 〔Qp〕〔Qh〕 ♿   Y

IOM: 100-03, 4, 280.1; 100-08, 5, 5.2.3

DMEPOS Modifier(s): RR

⊛ **E0184** Dry pressure mattress Ⓑ 〔Qp〕〔Qh〕 ♿   Y

IOM: 100-03, 4, 280.1; 100-08, 5, 5.2.3

DMEPOS Modifier(s): NU, RR, UE

⊛ **E0185** Gel or gel-like pressure pad for mattress, standard mattress length and width Ⓑ 〔Qp〕〔Qh〕 ♿   Y

IOM: 100-03, 4, 280.1; 100-08, 5, 5.2.3

DMEPOS Modifier(s): NU, RR, UE

⊛ **E0186** Air pressure mattress Ⓑ 〔Qp〕〔Qh〕 ♿   Y

IOM: 100-03, 4, 280.1

DMEPOS Modifier(s): RR

⊛ **E0187** Water pressure mattress Ⓑ 〔Qp〕〔Qh〕 ♿   Y

IOM: 100-03, 4, 280.1

DMEPOS Modifier(s): RR

⊛ **E0188** Synthetic sheepskin pad Ⓑ 〔Qp〕〔Qh〕 ♿   Y

IOM: 100-03, 4, 280.1; 100-08, 5, 5.2.3

DMEPOS Modifier(s): NU, RR, UE

⊛ **E0189** Lambswool sheepskin pad, any size Ⓑ 〔Qp〕〔Qh〕 ♿   Y

IOM: 100-03, 4, 280.1; 100-08, 5, 5.2.3

DMEPOS Modifier(s): NU, RR, UE

⊛ **E0190** Positioning cushion/pillow/wedge, any shape or size, includes all components and accessories Ⓑ 〔Qp〕〔Qh〕   E

IOM: 100-02, 15, 110.1

✳ **E0191** Heel or elbow protector, each Ⓑ 〔Qp〕〔Qh〕 ♿   Y

DMEPOS Modifier(s): NU, RR, UE

✳ **E0193** Powered air flotation bed (low air loss therapy) Ⓑ 〔Qp〕〔Qh〕 ♿   Y

DMEPOS Modifier(s): RR

⊛ **E0194** Air fluidized bed Ⓑ 〔Qp〕〔Qh〕 ♿   Y

IOM: 100-03, 4, 280.1

DMEPOS Modifier(s): RR

⊛ **E0196** Gel pressure mattress Ⓑ 〔Qp〕〔Qh〕 ♿   Y

IOM: 100-03, 4, 280.1

DMEPOS Modifier(s): RR

⊛ **E0197** Air pressure pad for mattress, standard mattress length and width Ⓑ 〔Qp〕〔Qh〕 ♿   Y

IOM: 100-03, 4, 280.1

DMEPOS Modifier(s): NU, RR, UE

↻ ⊛ **E0198** Water pressure pad for mattress, standard mattress length and width Ⓑ 〔Qp〕〔Qh〕 ♿   Y

IOM: 100-03, 4, 280.1

DMEPOS Modifier(s): RR

⊛ **E0199** Dry pressure pad for mattress, standard mattress length and width Ⓑ 〔Qp〕〔Qh〕 ♿   Y

IOM: 100-03, 4, 280.1

DMEPOS Modifier(s): NU, RR, UE

Heat/Cold Application

⊛ **E0200** Heat lamp, without stand (table model), includes bulb, or infrared element Ⓑ 〔Qp〕〔Qh〕 ♿   Y

Covered when medical review determines patient's medical condition is one for which application of heat by heat lamp is therapeutically effective

IOM: 100-02, 15, 110.1; 100-03, 4, 280.1

DMEPOS Modifier(s): NU, RR, UE

✳ **E0202** Phototherapy (bilirubin) light with photometer Ⓑ 〔Qp〕〔Qh〕 ♿   Y

DMEPOS Modifier(s): RR

⊘ **E0203** Therapeutic lightbox, minimum 10,000 lux, table top model Ⓑ 〔Qp〕〔Qh〕   E

IOM: 100-03, 4, 280.1

⊛ **E0205** Heat lamp, with stand, includes bulb, or infrared element Ⓑ 〔Qp〕〔Qh〕 ♿   Y

IOM: 100-02, 15, 110.1; 100-03, 4, 280.1

DMEPOS Modifier(s): NU, RR, UE

▶ New   ↻ Revised   ✔ Reinstated   ~~deleted~~ Deleted   ⊘ Not covered or valid by Medicare
⊛ Special coverage instructions   ✳ Carrier discretion   Ⓑ Bill local carrier   Ⓓ Bill DME MAC

✳ **E0210** Electric heat pad, standard ⑧ Qp Qh ♿   Y

Flexible device containing electric resistive elements producing heat; has fabric cover to prevent burns; with or without timing devices for automatic shut-off

IOM: 100-03, 4, 280.1

DMEPOS Modifier(s): NU, RR, UE

✳ **E0215** Electric heat pad, moist ⑧ Qp Qh ♿   Y

Flexible device containing electric resistive elements producing heat. Must have component that will absorb and retain liquid (water)

IOM: 100-03, 4, 280.1

DMEPOS Modifier(s): NU, RR, UE

✳ **E0217** Water circulating heat pad with pump ⑧ Qp Qh ♿   Y

Consists of flexible pad containing series of channels through which water is circulated by means of electrical pumping mechanism and heated in external reservoir

IOM: 100-03, 4, 280.1

DMEPOS Modifier(s): NU, RR, UE

✳ **E0218** Water circulating cold pad with pump ⑧ Qp Qh   Y

IOM: 100-03, 4, 280.1

✳ **E0221** Infrared heating pad system ⑧ Qp Qh   Y

✳ **E0225** Hydrocollator unit, includes pads ⑧ Qp Qh ♿   Y

IOM: 100-02, 15, 230; 100-03, 4, 280.1

DMEPOS Modifier(s): NU, RR, UE

⊘ **E0231** Non-contact wound warming device (temperature control unit, AC adapter and power cord) for use with warming card and wound cover ⑧ Qp Qh   E

IOM: 100-02, 16, 20

⊘ **E0232** Warming card for use with the non-contact wound warming device and non-contact wound warming wound cover ⑧ Qp Qh   E

IOM: 100-02, 16, 20

✳ **E0235** Paraffin bath unit, portable (see medical supply code A4265 for paraffin) ⑧ Qp Qh ♿   Y

Ordered by physician and patient's condition expected to be relieved by long term use of modality

IOM: 100-02, 15, 230; 100-03, 4, 280.1

DMEPOS Modifier(s): RR

✳ **E0236** Pump for water circulating pad ⑧ Qp Qh ♿   Y

IOM: 100-03, 4, 280.1

DMEPOS Modifier(s): RR

✳ **E0239** Hydrocollator unit, portable ⑧ Qp Qh ♿   Y

IOM: 100-02, 15, 230; 100-03, 4, 280.1

DMEPOS Modifier(s): NU, RR, UE

Bath and Toilet Aids

⊘ **E0240** Bath/shower chair, with or without wheels, any size ⑧ Qp Qh   E

IOM: 100-03, 4, 280.1

⊘ **E0241** Bath tub wall rail, each ⑧ Qp Qh   E

IOM: 100-02, 15, 110.1; 100-03, 4, 280.1

⊘ **E0242** Bath tub rail, floor base ⑧ Qp Qh   E

IOM: 100-02, 15, 110.1; 100-03, 4, 280.1

⊘ **E0243** Toilet rail, each ⑧ Qp Qh   E

IOM: 100-02, 15, 110.1; 100-03, 4, 280.1

⊘ **E0244** Raised toilet seat ⑧ Qp Qh   E

IOM: 100-03, 4, 280.1

⊘ **E0245** Tub stool or bench ⑧ Qp Qh   E

IOM: 100-03, 4, 280.1

✳ **E0246** Transfer tub rail attachment ⑧ Qp Qh   E

✳ **E0247** Transfer bench for tub or toilet with or without commode opening ⑧ Qp Qh   E

IOM: 100-03, 4, 280.1

✳ **E0248** Transfer bench, heavy duty, for tub or toilet with or without commode opening ⑧ Qp Qh   E

Heavy duty transfer bench is labeled as capable of supporting more than 300 pounds

IOM: 100-03, 4, 280.1

✻ **E0249** Pad for water circulating heat unit, for replacement only Ⓑ Qp Qh ♿ Y

Describes durable replacement pad used with water circulating heat pump system

IOM: 100-03, 4, 280.1

DMEPOS Modifier(s): NU, RR, UE

Hospital Beds and Accessories

◌ **E0250** Hospital bed, fixed height, with any type side rails, with mattress Ⓑ Qp Qh ♿ Y

IOM: 100-02, 15, 110.1; 100-03, 4, 280.7

DMEPOS Modifier(s): RR

◌ **E0251** Hospital bed, fixed height, with any type side rails, without mattress Ⓑ Qp Qh ♿ Y

IOM:100-02, 15, 110.1; 100-03, 4, 280.7

DMEPOS Modifier(s): RR

◌ **E0255** Hospital bed, variable height, hi-lo, with any type side rails, with mattress Ⓑ Qp Qh ♿ Y

IOM: 100-02, 15, 110.1; 100-03, 4, 280.7

DMEPOS Modifier(s): RR

◌ **E0256** Hospital bed, variable height, hi-lo, with any type side rails, without mattress Ⓑ Qp Qh ♿ Y

IOM: 100-02, 15, 110.1; 100-03, 4, 280.7

DMEPOS Modifier(s): RR

◌ **E0260** Hospital bed, semi-electric (head and foot adjustment), with any type side rails, with mattress Ⓑ Qp Qh ♿ Y

IOM: 100-02, 15, 110.1; 100-03, 4, 280.7

DMEPOS Modifier(s): RR

◌ **E0261** Hospital bed, semi-electric (head and foot adjustment), with any type side rails, without mattress Ⓑ Qp Qh ♿ Y

IOM: 100-02, 15, 110.1; 100-03, 4, 280.7

DMEPOS Modifier(s): RR

◌ **E0265** Hospital bed, total electric (head, foot and height adjustments), with any type side rails, with mattress Ⓑ Qp Qh ♿ Y

IOM: 100-02, 15, 110.1; 100-03, 4, 280.7

DMEPOS Modifier(s): RR

◌ **E0266** Hospital bed, total electric (head, foot and height adjustments), with any type side rails, without mattress Ⓑ Qp Qh ♿ Y

IOM: 100-02, 15, 110.1; 100-03, 4, 280.7

DMEPOS Modifier(s): RR

⃠ **E0270** Hospital bed, institutional type includes: oscillating, circulating and Stryker frame, with mattress Ⓑ Qp Qh E

IOM: 100-03, 4, 280.1

◌ **E0271** Mattress, innerspring Ⓑ Qp Qh ♿ Y

IOM: 100-03, 4, 280.1; 100-03, 4, 280.7

DMEPOS Modifier(s): NU, RR, UE

◌ **E0272** Mattress, foam rubber Ⓑ Qp Qh ♿ Y

IOM: 100-03, 4, 280.1; 100-03, 4, 280.7

DMEPOS Modifier(s): NU, RR, UE

⃠ **E0273** Bed board Ⓑ Qp Qh E

IOM: 100-03, 4, 280.1

⃠ **E0274** Over-bed table Ⓑ Qp Qh E

IOM: 100-03, 4, 280.1

◌ **E0275** Bed pan, standard, metal or plastic Ⓑ Qp Qh ♿ Y

IOM: 100-03, 4, 280.1

DMEPOS Modifier(s): NU, RR, UE

◌ **E0276** Bed pan, fracture, metal or plastic Ⓑ Qp Qh ♿ Y

IOM: 100-03, 4, 280.1

DMEPOS Modifier(s): NU, RR, UE

◌ **E0277** Powered pressure-reducing air mattress Ⓑ Qp Qh ♿ Y

IOM: 100-03, 4, 280.1

DMEPOS Modifier(s): RR

✻ **E0280** Bed cradle, any type Ⓑ Qp Qh ♿ Y

DMEPOS Modifier(s): NU, RR, UE

◌ **E0290** Hospital bed, fixed height, without side rails, with mattress Ⓑ Qp Qh ♿ Y

IOM: 100-02, 15, 110.1; 100-03, 4, 280.7

DMEPOS Modifier(s): RR

◌ **E0291** Hospital bed, fixed height, without side rails, without mattress Ⓑ Qp Qh ♿ Y

IOM: 100-02, 15, 110.1; 100-03, 4, 280.7

DMEPOS Modifier(s): RR

◌ **E0292** Hospital bed, variable height, hi-lo, without side rails, with mattress Ⓑ Qp Qh ♿ Y

IOM: 100-02, 15, 110.1; 100-03, 4, 280.7

DMEPOS Modifier(s): RR

▶ New ⤾ Revised ✔ Reinstated ~~deleted~~ Deleted ⃠ Not covered or valid by Medicare
◌ Special coverage instructions ✻ Carrier discretion Ⓑ Bill local carrier Ⓑ Bill DME MAC

○ **E0293** Hospital bed, variable height, hi-lo, without side rails, without mattress ⑧ Qp Qh   Y

IOM: 100-02, 15, 110.1; 100-03, 4, 280.7

DMEPOS Modifier(s): RR

○ **E0294** Hospital bed, semi-electric (head and foot adjustment), without side rails, with mattress ⑧ Qp Qh &   Y

IOM: 100-02, 15, 110.1; 100-03, 4, 280.7

DMEPOS Modifier(s): RR

○ **E0295** Hospital bed, semi-electric (head and foot adjustment), without side rails, without mattress ⑧ Qp Qh &   Y

IOM: 100-02, 15, 110.1; 100-03, 4, 280.7

DMEPOS Modifier(s): RR

○ **E0296** Hospital bed, total electric (head, foot and height adjustments). Without side rails, with mattress ⑧ Qp Qh &   Y

IOM: 100-02, 15, 110.1; 100-03, 4, 280.7

DMEPOS Modifier(s): RR

○ **E0297** Hospital bed, total electric (head, foot and height adjustments), without side rails, without mattress ⑧ Qp Qh &   Y

IOM: 100-02, 15, 110.1; 100-03, 4, 280.7

DMEPOS Modifier(s): RR

↺ ✳ **E0300** Pediatric crib, hospital grade, fully enclosed, with or without top enclosure ⑧ Qp Qh A &   Y

DMEPOS Modifier(s): RR

○ **E0301** Hospital bed, heavy duty, extra wide, with weight capacity greater than 350 pounds, but less than or equal to 600 pounds, with any type side rails, without mattress ⑧ Qp Qh &   Y

IOM: 100-03, 4, 280.7

DMEPOS Modifier(s): RR

○ **E0302** Hospital bed, extra heavy duty, extra wide, with weight capacity greater than 600 pounds, with any type side rails, without mattress ⑧ Qp Qh &   Y

IOM: 100-03, 4, 280.7

DMEPOS Modifier(s): RR

○ **E0303** Hospital bed, heavy duty, extra wide, with weight capacity greater than 350 pounds, but less than or equal to 600 pounds, with any type side rails, with mattress ⑧ Qp Qh &   Y

IOM: 100-03, 4, 280.7

DMEPOS Modifier(s): RR

○ **E0304** Hospital bed, extra heavy duty, extra wide, with weight capacity greater than 600 pounds, with any type side rails, with mattress ⑧ Qp Qh &   Y

IOM: 100-03, 4, 280.7

DMEPOS Modifier(s): RR

○ **E0305** Bed side rails, half length ⑧ Qh &   Y

IOM: 100-03, 4, 280.7

DMEPOS Modifier(s): RR

○ **E0310** Bed side rails, full length ⑧ Qp Qh &   Y

IOM: 100-03, 4, 280.7

DMEPOS Modifier(s): NU, RR, UE

⊘ **E0315** Bed accessory: board, table, or support device, any type ⑧ Qp Qh   E

IOM: 100-03, 4, 280.1

✳ **E0316** Safety enclosure frame/canopy for use with hospital bed, any type ⑧ Qp Qh &   Y

DMEPOS Modifier(s): RR

○ **E0325** Urinal; male, jug-type, any material ⑧ ♂ Qp Qh &   Y

IOM: 100-03, 4, 280.1

DMEPOS Modifier(s): NU, RR, UE

○ **E0326** Urinal; female, jug-type, any material ⑧ ♀ Qp Qh &   Y

IOM: 100-03, 4, 280.1

DMEPOS Modifier(s): NU, RR, UE

✳ **E0328** Hospital bed, pediatric, manual, 360 degree side enclosures, top of headboard, footboard and side rails up to 24 inches above the spring, includes mattress ⑧ Qp Qh A   Y

✳ **E0329** Hospital bed, pediatric, electric or semi-electric, 360 degree side enclosures, top of headboard, footboard and side rails up to 24 inches above the spring, includes mattress ⑧ Qp Qh A   Y

✳ **E0350** Control unit for electronic bowel irrigation/evacuation system ⑧ Qp Qh   E

Pulsed Irrigation Enhanced Evacuation (PIEE) is pulsed irrigation of severely impacted fecal material and may be necessary for patients who have not responded to traditional bowel program.

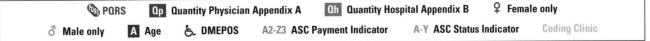

PQRS   Qp **Quantity Physician Appendix A**   Qh **Quantity Hospital Appendix B**   ♀ **Female only**

♂ **Male only**   A **Age**   & **DMEPOS**   A2-Z3 **ASC Payment Indicator**   A-Y **ASC Status Indicator**   Coding Clinic

✳ **E0352** Disposable pack (water reservoir bag, speculum, valving mechanism and collection bag/box) for use with the electronic bowel irrigation/evacuation system Ⓑ **Qp** **Qh**   E

Therapy kit includes 1 B-Valve circuit, 2 containment bags, 1 lubricating jelly, 1 bed pad, 1 tray liner-waste disposable bag, and 2 hose clamps

✳ **E0370** Air pressure elevator for heel Ⓑ **Qp** **Qh**   E

✳ **E0371** Non powered advanced pressure reducing overlay for mattress, standard mattress length and width Ⓑ **Qp** **Qh** ♿   Y

Patient has at least one large Stage III or Stage IV pressure sore (greater than 2 × 2 cm.) on trunk, with only two turning surfaces on which to lie

DMEPOS Modifier(s): RR

✳ **E0372** Powered air overlay for mattress, standard mattress length and width Ⓑ **Qp** **Qh** ♿   Y

DMEPOS Modifier(s): RR

✳ **E0373** Non powered advanced pressure reducing mattress Ⓑ **Qp** **Qh** ♿   Y

DMEPOS Modifier(s): RR

Oxygen and Related Respiratory Equipment

⊛ **E0424** Stationary compressed gaseous oxygen system, rental; includes container, contents, regulator, flowmeter, humidifier, nebulizer, cannula or mask, and tubing Ⓑ **Qp** **Qh** ♿   Y

IOM: 100-03, 4, 280.1; 100-04, 20, 30.6

DMEPOS Modifier(s): RR

⊛ **E0425** Stationary compressed gas system, purchase; includes regulator, flowmeter, humidifier, nebulizer, cannula or mask, and tubing Ⓑ **Qp** **Qh**   E

IOM: 100-03, 4, 280.1; 100-04, 20, 30.6

⊛ **E0430** Portable gaseous oxygen system, purchase; includes regulator, flowmeter, humidifier, cannula or mask, and tubing Ⓑ **Qp** **Qh**   E

IOM: 100-03, 4, 280.1; 100-04, 20, 30.6

⊛ **E0431** Portable gaseous oxygen system, rental; includes portable container, regulator, flowmeter, humidifier, cannula or mask, and tubing Ⓑ **Qp** **Qh** ♿   Y

IOM: 100-03, 4, 280.1; 100-04, 20, 30.6

DMEPOS Modifier(s): RR

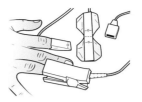

Figure 12 Oximeter device.

✳ **E0433** Portable liquid oxygen system, rental; home liquefier used to fill portable liquid oxygen containers, includes portable containers, regulator, flowmeter, humidifier, cannula or mask and tubing, with or without supply reservoir and contents gauge Ⓑ **Qh** ♿   Y

DMEPOS Modifier(s): RR

⊛ **E0434** Portable liquid oxygen system, rental; includes portable container, supply reservoir, humidifier, flowmeter, refill adaptor, contents gauge, cannula or mask, and tubing Ⓑ **Qp** **Qh** ♿   Y

Fee schedule payments for stationary oxygen system rentals are all-inclusive and represent monthly allowance for beneficiary. Non-Medicare payers may rent device to beneficiaries, or arrange for purchase of device

IOM: 100-03, 4, 280.1; 100-04, 20, 30.6

DMEPOS Modifier(s): RR

⊛ **E0435** Portable liquid oxygen system, purchase; includes portable container, supply reservoir, flowmeter, humidifier, contents gauge, cannula or mask, tubing and refill adaptor Ⓑ **Qp** **Qh**   E

IOM: 100-03, 4, 280.1; 100-04, 20, 30.6

⊛ **E0439** Stationary liquid oxygen system, rental; includes container, contents, regulator, flowmeter, humidifier, nebulizer, cannula or mask, & tubing Ⓑ **Qp** **Qh** ♿   Y

This allowance includes payment for equipment, contents, and accessories furnished during rental month

IOM: 100-03, 4, 280.1; 100-04, 20, 30.6

DMEPOS Modifier(s): RR

⊛ **E0440** Stationary liquid oxygen system, purchase; includes use of reservoir, contents indicator, regulator, flowmeter, humidifier, nebulizer, cannula or mask, and tubing Ⓑ **Qp** **Qh**   E

IOM: 100-03, 4, 280.1; 100-04, 20, 30.6

✳ **E0441** Stationary oxygen contents, gaseous, 1 month's supply = 1 unit Ⓑ **Qp** **Qh** ♿   Y

IOM: 100-03, 4, 280.1; 100-04, 20, 30.6

▶ **New**   ⤺ **Revised**   ✔ **Reinstated**   ~~deleted~~ **Deleted**   ⊘ **Not covered or valid by Medicare**
⊛ **Special coverage instructions**   ✳ **Carrier discretion**   Ⓑ **Bill local carrier**   Ⓖ **Bill DME MAC**

✳ **E0442** Stationary oxygen contents, liquid, 1 month's supply = 1 unit Ⓑ Qp Qh ♿   Y

IOM: 100-03, 4, 280.1; 100-04, 20, 30.6

✳ **E0443** Portable oxygen contents, gaseous, 1 month's supply = 1 unit Ⓑ Qp Qh ♿   Y

IOM: 100-03, 4, 280.1; 100-04, 20, 30.6

✳ **E0444** Portable oxygen contents, liquid, 1 month's supply = 1 unit Ⓑ Qp Qh ♿   Y

IOM: 100-03, 4, 280.1; 100-04, 20, 30.6

✳ **E0445** Oximeter device for measuring blood oxygen levels non-invasively Ⓑ Qp Qh   N

⊘ **E0446** Topical oxygen delivery system, not otherwise specified, includes all supplies and accessories Ⓑ Qp Qh   E

⊛ **E0450** Volume control ventilator, without pressure support mode, may include pressure control mode, used with invasive interface (e.g., tracheostomy tube) Ⓑ Qp Qh ♿   Y

Patient confined to wheelchair during day may receive reimbursement for 2 ventilators. One ventilator is mounted to wheelchair and second used while in bed

IOM: 100-03, 4, 280.1

DMEPOS Modifier(s): RR

⊛ **E0455** Oxygen tent, excluding croup or pediatric tents Ⓑ Qp Qh   Y

IOM: 100-03, 4, 280.1; 100-04, 20, 30.6

⊘ **E0457** Chest shell (cuirass) Ⓑ Qp Qh ♿   E

DMEPOS Modifier(s): NU, RR, UE

⊘ **E0459** Chest wrap Ⓑ Qp Qh ♿   E

DMEPOS Modifier(s): RR

⊛ **E0460** Negative pressure ventilator; portable or stationary Ⓑ Qp Qh ♿   Y

Noninvasive device, generates airflow into lungs by creating negative pressure around chest by means of interface

IOM: 100-03, 4, 240.2

DMEPOS Modifier(s): RR

⊛ **E0461** Volume control ventilator, without pressure support mode, may include pressure control mode, used with non-invasive interface (e.g. mask) Ⓑ Qp Qh ♿   Y

IOM: 100-03, 4, 240.2

DMEPOS Modifier(s): RR

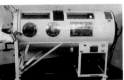
Figure 13 Pressure ventilator.

✳ **E0462** Rocking bed with or without side rails Ⓑ Qp Qh ♿   Y

DMEPOS Modifier(s): RR

✳ **E0463** Pressure support ventilator with volume control mode, may include pressure control mode, used with invasive interface (e.g., tracheostomy tube) Ⓑ Qp Qh ♿   Y

DMEPOS Modifier(s): RR

✳ **E0464** Pressure support ventilator with volume control mode, may include pressure control mode, used with non-invasive interface (e.g., mask) Ⓑ Qp Qh ♿   Y

DMEPOS Modifier(s): RR

⊛ **E0470** Respiratory assist device, bi-level pressure capability, without backup rate feature, used with noninvasive interface, e.g., nasal or facial mask (intermittent assist device with continuous positive airway pressure device) Ⓑ Qp Qh ♿   Y

IOM: 100-03, 4, 240.2

DMEPOS Modifier(s): RR

⊛ **E0471** Respiratory assist device, bi-level pressure capability, with back-up rate feature, used with noninvasive interface, e.g., nasal or facial mask (intermittent assist device with continuous positive airway pressure device) Ⓑ Qp Qh ♿   Y

IOM: 100-03, 4, 240.2

DMEPOS Modifier(s): RR

⊛ **E0472** Respiratory assist device, bi-level pressure capability, with backup rate feature, used with invasive interface, e.g., tracheostomy tube (intermittent assist device with continuous positive airway pressure device) Ⓑ Qp Qh ♿   Y

IOM: 100-03, 4, 240.2

DMEPOS Modifier(s): RR

⊛ **E0480** Percussor, electric or pneumatic, home model Ⓑ Qp Qh ♿   Y

IOM: 100-03, 4, 240.2

DMEPOS Modifier(s): RR

⊘ **E0481** Intrapulmonary percussive ventilation system and related accessories Ⓑ Qp Qh   E

IOM: 100-03, 4, 240.2

* **E0482** Cough stimulating device, alternating positive and negative airway pressure ⑧ Qp Qh ᕦ Y

DMEPOS Modifier(s): RR

* **E0483** High frequency chest wall oscillation air-pulse generator system, (includes hoses and vest), each ⑧ Qp Qh ᕦ Y

DMEPOS Modifier(s): RR

* **E0484** Oscillatory positive expiratory pressure device, non-electric, any type, each ⑧ Qp Qh ᕦ Y

DMEPOS Modifier(s): NU, RR, UE

* **E0485** Oral device/appliance used to reduce upper airway collapsibility, adjustable or non-adjustable, prefabricated, includes fitting and adjustment ⑧ Qp Qh ᕦ Y

DMEPOS Modifier(s): NU, RR, UE

* **E0486** Oral device/appliance used to reduce upper airway collapsibility, adjustable or non-adjustable, custom fabricated, includes fitting and adjustment ⑧ Qp Qh ᕦ Y

DMEPOS Modifier(s): NU, RR, UE

⊛ **E0487** Spirometer, electronic, includes all accessories ⑧ Qp Qh N

IPPB Machines

⊛ **E0500** IPPB machine, all types, with built-in nebulization; manual or automatic valves; internal or external power source ⑧ Qp Qh ᕦ Y

Bill DME MAC

IOM: 100-03, 4, 240.2

DMEPOS Modifier(s): RR

Humidifiers/Nebulizers/Compressors for Use with Oxygen IPPB Equipment

⊛ **E0550** Humidifier, durable for extensive supplemental humidification during IPPB treatments or oxygen delivery ⑧ Qp Qh ᕦ Y

IOM: 100-03, 4, 240.2

DMEPOS Modifier(s): RR

⊛ **E0555** Humidifier, durable, glass or autoclavable plastic bottle type, for use with regulator or flowmeter ⑧ Qp Qh Y

IOM: 100-03, 4, 280.1; 100-04, 20, 30.6

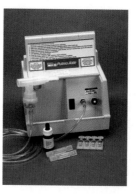

Figure 14 Nebulizer.

⊛ **E0560** Humidifier, durable for supplemental humidification during IPPB treatment or oxygen delivery ⑧ Qp Qh ᕦ Y

IOM: 100-03, 4, 280.1

DMEPOS Modifier(s): NU, RR, UE

* **E0561** Humidifier, non-heated, used with positive airway pressure device ⑧ Qp Qh ᕦ Y

DMEPOS Modifier(s): NU, RR, UE

* **E0562** Humidifier, heated, used with positive airway pressure device ⑧ Qp Qh ᕦ Y

DMEPOS Modifier(s): NU, RR, UE

* **E0565** Compressor, air power source for equipment which is not self-contained or cylinder driven ⑧ Qp Qh ᕦ Y

DMEPOS Modifier(s): RR

⊛ **E0570** Nebulizer, with compressor ⑧ Qp Qh ᕦ Y

IOM: 100-03, 4, 240.2; 100-03, 4, 280.1

DMEPOS Modifier(s): RR

* **E0572** Aerosol compressor, adjustable pressure, light duty for intermittent use ⑧ Qp Qh ᕦ Y

DMEPOS Modifier(s): RR

* **E0574** Ultrasonic/electronic aerosol generator with small volume nebulizer ⑧ Qp Qh ᕦ Y

DMEPOS Modifier(s): RR

⊛ **E0575** Nebulizer, ultrasonic, large volume ⑧ Qp Qh ᕦ Y

IOM: 100-03, 4, 240.2

DMEPOS Modifier(s): RR

⊛ **E0580** Nebulizer, durable, glass or autoclavable plastic, bottle type, for use with regulator or flowmeter ⑧ Qp Qh ᕦ Y

IOM: 100-03, 4, 240.2; 100-03, 4, 280.1

DMEPOS Modifier(s): NU, RR, UE

▶ **New**   ⟳ **Revised**   ✔ **Reinstated**   ~~deleted~~ **Deleted**   ⊘ **Not covered or valid by Medicare**

⊛ **Special coverage instructions**   * **Carrier discretion**   ⑧ **Bill local carrier**   ⑧ **Bill DME MAC**

⊛ **E0585** Nebulizer, with compressor and heater Ⓑ Qp Qh ♿ Y

IOM: 100-03, 4, 240.2; 100-03, 4, 280.1

DMEPOS Modifier(s): RR

Suction Pump/Room Vaporizers

⊛ **E0600** Respiratory suction pump, home model, portable or stationary, electric Ⓑ Qp Qh ♿ Y

IOM: 100-03, 4, 240.2

DMEPOS Modifier(s): RR

⊛ **E0601** Continuous positive airway pressure (CPAP) device Ⓑ Qp Qh ♿ Y

IOM: 100-03, 4, 240.4

DMEPOS Modifier(s): RR

✳ **E0602** Breast pump, manual, any type Ⓑ Qp Qh ♀ ♿ Y

Bill either manual breast pump or breast pump kit

DMEPOS Modifier(s): NU, RR, UE

✳ **E0603** Breast pump, electric (AC and/or DC), any type Ⓑ Qp Qh ♀ N

✳ **E0604** Breast pump, hospital grade, electric (AC and/or DC), any type Ⓑ Qp Qh ♀ A

⊛ **E0605** Vaporizer, room type Qp Qh ♿ Y

IOM: 100-03, 4, 240.2

DMEPOS Modifier(s): NU, RR, UE

⊛ **E0606** Postural drainage board Ⓑ Qp Qh ♿ Y

IOM: 100-03, 4, 240.2

DMEPOS Modifier(s): RR

Monitoring Equipment

⊛ **E0607** Home blood glucose monitor Ⓑ Qp Qh ♿ Y

Document recipient or caregiver is competent to monitor equipment and that device is designed for home rather than clinical use

IOM: 100-03, 4, 280.1; 100-03, 1, 40.2

DMEPOS Modifier(s): NU, RR, UE

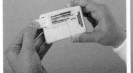 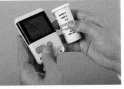

Figure 15 Glucose monitor.

Pacemaker Monitor

⊛ **E0610** Pacemaker monitor, self-contained, (checks battery depletion, includes audible and visible check systems) Ⓑ Qp Qh ♿ Y

IOM: 100-03, 1, 20.8

DMEPOS Modifier(s): NU, RR, UE

⊛ **E0615** Pacemaker monitor, self-contained, checks battery depletion and other pacemaker components, includes digital/visible check systems Ⓑ Qp Qh ♿ Y

IOM: 100-03, 1, 20.8

DMEPOS Modifier(s): NU, RR, UE

✳ **E0616** Implantable cardiac event recorder with memory, activator and programmer Ⓑ Qp Qh N1 N

Assign when two 30-day pre-symptom external loop recordings fail to establish a definitive diagnosis. Bill to local carrier.

✳ **E0617** External defibrillator with integrated electrocardiogram analysis Ⓑ Qp Qh ♿ Y

DMEPOS Modifier(s): RR, KF

✳ **E0618** Apnea monitor, without recording feature Ⓑ Qp Qh ♿ Y

DMEPOS Modifier(s): RR

✳ **E0619** Apnea monitor, with recording feature Ⓑ Qp Qh ♿ Y

DMEPOS Modifier(s): RR

↻ ✳ **E0620** Skin piercing device for collection of capillary blood, laser, each Ⓑ Qp Qh ♿ Y

DMEPOS Modifier(s): RR

Patient Lifts

⊛ **E0621** Sling or seat, patient lift, canvas or nylon Ⓑ Qp Qh ♿ Y

IOM: 100-03, 4, 240.2, 280.4

DMEPOS Modifier(s): NU, RR, UE

⊘ **E0625** Patient lift, bathroom or toilet, not otherwise classified Ⓑ Qp Qh E

IOM: 100-03, 4, 240.2

⊛ **E0627** Seat lift mechanism incorporated into a combination lift-chair mechanism Ⓑ Qp Qh ♿   Y

IOM: 100-03, 4, 280.4; 100-04, 4, 20

Cross Reference Q0080

DMEPOS Modifier(s): NU, RR, UE

⊛ **E0628** Separate seat lift mechanism for use with patient owned furniture - electric Ⓑ Qp Qh ♿   Y

IOM: 100-03, 4, 280.4; 100-04, 4, 20

Cross Reference Q0078

DMEPOS Modifier(s): NU, RR, UE

⊛ **E0629** Separate seat lift mechanism for use with patient owned furniture - non-electric Ⓑ Qp Qh ♿   Y

IOM: 100-04, 4, 20

Cross Reference Q0079

DMEPOS Modifier(s): NU, RR, UE

⊛ **E0630** Patient lift, hydraulic or mechanical, includes any seat, sling, strap(s) or pad(s) Ⓑ Qp Qh ♿   Y

IOM: 100-03, 4, 240.2

DMEPOS Modifier(s): RR

⊛ **E0635** Patient lift, electric, with seat or sling Ⓑ Qp Qh ♿   Y

IOM: 100-03, 4, 240.2

DMEPOS Modifier(s): RR

✳ **E0636** Multipositional patient support system, with integrated lift, patient accessible controls Ⓑ Qp Qh ♿   Y

DMEPOS Modifier(s): RR

⊘ **E0637** Combination sit to stand frame/table system, any size including pediatric, with seat lift feature, with or without wheels Ⓑ Qp Qh   E

IOM: 100-03, 4, 240.2

⊘ **E0638** Standing frame/table system, one position (e.g. upright, supine or prone stander), any size including pediatric, with or without wheels Ⓑ Qp Qh   E

IOM: 100-03, 4, 240.2

✳ **E0639** Patient lift, moveable from room to room with disassembly and reassembly, includes all components/accessories Ⓑ Qp Qh   E

✳ **E0640** Patient lift, fixed system, includes all components/accessories Ⓑ Qp Qh   E

⊘ **E0641** Standing frame/table system, multi-position (e.g. three-way stander), any size including pediatric, with or without wheels Ⓑ Qp Qh   E

IOM: 100-03, 4, 240.2

⊘ **E0642** Standing frame/table system, mobile (dynamic stander), any size including pediatric Ⓑ Qp Qh   E

IOM: 100-03, 4, 240.2

Pneumatic Compressor and Appliances

⊛ **E0650** Pneumatic compressor, non-segmental home model Ⓑ Qp Qh ♿   Y

Lymphedema pumps are classified as segmented or nonsegmented, depending on whether distinct segments of devices can be inflated sequentially

IOM: 100-03, 4, 280.6

DMEPOS Modifier(s): NU, RR, UE

⊛ **E0651** Pneumatic compressor, segmental home model without calibrated gradient pressure Ⓑ Qp Qh ♿   Y

IOM: 100-03, 4, 280.6

DMEPOS Modifier(s): NU, RR, UE

⊛ **E0652** Pneumatic compressor, segmental home model with calibrated gradient pressure Ⓑ Qp Qh ♿   Y

IOM: 100-03, 4, 280.6

DMEPOS Modifier(s): NU, RR, UE

⊛ **E0655** Non-segmental pneumatic appliance for use with pneumatic compressor, half arm Ⓑ Qp Qh ♿   Y

IOM: 100-03, 4, 280.6

DMEPOS Modifier(s): NU, RR, UE

↻ ⊛ **E0656** Segmental pneumatic appliance for use with pneumatic compressor, trunk Ⓑ Qp Qh ♿   Y

DMEPOS Modifier(s): RR

↻ ⊛ **E0657** Segmental pneumatic appliance for use with pneumatic compressor, chest Ⓑ Qp Qh ♿   Y

DMEPOS Modifier(s): RR

⊛ **E0660** Non-segmental pneumatic appliance for use with pneumatic compressor, full leg Ⓑ Qp Qh ♿   Y

IOM: 100-03, 4, 280.6

DMEPOS Modifier(s): NU, RR, UE

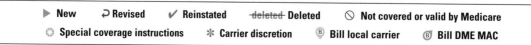

▶ New　　↻ Revised　　✔ Reinstated　　~~deleted~~ Deleted　　⊘ Not covered or valid by Medicare
⊛ Special coverage instructions　　✳ Carrier discretion　　Ⓑ Bill local carrier　　Ⓑ Bill DME MAC

⊛ **E0665** Non-segmental pneumatic appliance for use with pneumatic compressor, full arm ⓑ Qp Qh ♿   Y

IOM: 100-03, 4, 280.6

DMEPOS Modifier(s): NU, RR, UE

⊛ **E0666** Non-segmental pneumatic appliance for use with pneumatic compressor, half leg ⓑ Qp Qh ♿   Y

IOM: 100-03, 4, 280.6

DMEPOS Modifier(s): NU, RR, UE

⊛ **E0667** Segmental pneumatic appliance for use with pneumatic compressor, full leg ⓑ Qp Qh ♿   Y

IOM: 100-03, 4, 280.6

DMEPOS Modifier(s): NU, RR, UE

⊛ **E0668** Segmental pneumatic appliance for use with pneumatic compressor, full arm ⓑ Qp Qh ♿   Y

IOM: 100-03, 4, 280.6

DMEPOS Modifier(s): NU, RR, UE

⊛ **E0669** Segmental pneumatic appliance for use with pneumatic compressor, half leg ⓑ Qp Qh ♿   Y

IOM: 100-03, 4, 280.6

DMEPOS Modifier(s): NU, RR, UE

⊛ **E0670** Segmental pneumatic appliance for use with pneumatic compressor, integrated, 2 full legs and trunk ⓑ Qp Qh ♿   Y

IOM 100-03, 4, 280.6

DMEPOS Modifier(s): NU, RR, UE

⊛ **E0671** Segmental gradient pressure pneumatic appliance, full leg ⓑ Qp Qh ♿   Y

IOM: 100-03, 4, 280.6

DMEPOS Modifier(s): NU, RR, UE

⊛ **E0672** Segmental gradient pressure pneumatic appliance, full arm ⓑ Qp Qh ♿   Y

IOM: 100-03, 4, 280.6

DMEPOS Modifier(s): NU, RR, UE

⊛ **E0673** Segmental gradient pressure pneumatic appliance, half leg ⓑ Qp Qh ♿   Y

IOM: 100-03, 4, 280.6

DMEPOS Modifier(s): NU, RR, UE

✳ **E0675** Pneumatic compression device, high pressure, rapid inflation/deflation cycle, for arterial insufficiency (unilateral or bilateral system) ⓑ Qp Qh ♿   Y

DMEPOS Modifier(s): RR

✳ **E0676** Intermittent limb compression device (includes all accessories), not otherwise specified ⓑ Qp Qh   Y

Ultraviolet Cabinet

✳ **E0691** Ultraviolet light therapy system, includes bulbs/lamps, timer and eye protection; treatment area 2 square feet or less ⓑ Qp Qh ♿   Y

DMEPOS Modifier(s): NU, RR, UE

✳ **E0692** Ultraviolet light therapy system panel, includes bulbs/lamps, timer and eye protection, 4 foot panel ⓑ Qp Qh ♿   Y

DMEPOS Modifier(s): NU, RR, UE

✳ **E0693** Ultraviolet light therapy system panel, includes bulbs/lamps, timer and eye protection, 6 foot panel ⓑ Qp Qh ♿   Y

DMEPOS Modifier(s): NU, RR, UE

✳ **E0694** Ultraviolet multidirectional light therapy system in 6 foot cabinet, includes bulbs/lamps, timer and eye protection ⓑ Qp Qh ♿   Y

DMEPOS Modifier(s): NU, RR, UE

Safety Equipment

✳ **E0700** Safety equipment, device or accessory, any type ⓑ Qp Qh   E

⊛ **E0705** Transfer device, any type, each ⓑ Qp Qh ♿   B

DMEPOS Modifier(s): NU, RR, UE

Restraints

✳ **E0710** Restraints, any type (body, chest, wrist or ankle) ⓑ Qp Qh   E

Transcutaneous and/or Neuromuscular Electrical Nerve Stimulators (TENS)

⊛ **E0720** Transcutaneous electrical nerve stimulation (TENS) device, two lead, localized stimulation ⓑ Qp Qh ♿   Y

A Certificate of Medical Necessity (CMN) is not needed for a TENS rental, but is needed purchase.

IOM: 100-03, 2, 160.2; 100-03, 4, 280.1

DMEPOS Modifier(s): NU

⊛ **E0730** Transcutaneous electrical nerve stimulation (TENS) device, four or more leads, for multiple nerve stimulation ⓑ Qp Qh ♿   Y

IOM: 100-03, 2, 160.2; 100-03, 4, 280.1

DMEPOS Modifier(s): NU

PQRS PQRS	Qp Quantity Physician Appendix A	Qh Quantity Hospital Appendix B	♀ Female only
♂ Male only	A Age ♿ DMEPOS	A2-Z3 ASC Payment Indicator	A-Y ASC Status Indicator Coding Clinic

⊛ **E0731** Form fitting conductive garment for delivery of TENS or NMES (with conductive fibers separated from the patient's skin by layers of fabric) Ⓑ **Qp** **Qh** ♿   Y

IOM: 100-03, 2, 160.13

DMEPOS Modifier(s): NU

↻ ⊛ **E0740** Incontinence treatment system, pelvic floor stimulator, monitor, sensor and/or trainer Ⓑ **Qp** **Qh** ♿   Y

IOM: 100-03, 4, 230.8

DMEPOS Modifier(s): RR

✳ **E0744** Neuromuscular stimulator for scoliosis Ⓑ **Qp** **Qh** ♿   Y

DMEPOS Modifier(s): RR

⊛ **E0745** Neuromuscular stimulator, electronic shock unit Ⓑ **Qp** **Qh** ♿   Y

IOM: 100-03, 2, 160.12

DMEPOS Modifier(s): RR

⊛ **E0746** Electromyography (EMG), biofeedback device Ⓑ **Qp** **Qh**   N

IOM: 100-03, 1, 30.1

⊛ **E0747** Osteogenesis stimulator, electrical, non-invasive, other than spinal applications Ⓑ **Qp** **Qh** ♿   Y

Devices are composed of two basic parts: Coils that wrap around cast and pulse generator that produces electric current

DMEPOS Modifier(s): NU, KF, RR, UE

⊛ **E0748** Osteogenesis stimulator, electrical, non-invasive, spinal applications Ⓑ **Qp** **Qh** ♿   Y

Device should be applied within 30 days as adjunct to spinal fusion surgery

DMEPOS Modifier(s): NU, KF, RR, UE

⊛ **E0749** Osteogenesis stimulator, electrical, surgically implanted Ⓑ **Qp** **Qh** ♿   N1   N

DMEPOS Modifier(s): RR, KF

✳ **E0755** Electronic salivary reflex stimulator (intra-oral/non-invasive) Ⓑ **Qp** **Qh**   E

✳ **E0760** Osteogenesis stimulator, low intensity ultrasound, non-invasive Ⓑ **Qp** **Qh** ♿   Y

Ultrasonic osteogenesis stimulator may not be used concurrently with other noninvasive stimulators

DMEPOS Modifier(s): NU, KF, RR, UE

⊛ **E0761** Non-thermal pulsed high frequency radiowaves, high peak power electromagnetic energy treatment device Ⓑ **Qp** **Qh**   E

↻ ✳ **E0762** Transcutaneous electrical joint stimulation device system, includes all accessories Ⓑ **Qp** **Qh** ♿   B

DMEPOS Modifier(s): RR

↻ ⊛ **E0764** Functional neuromuscular stimulator, transcutaneous stimulation of sequential muscle groups of ambulation with computer control, used for walking by spinal cord injured, entire system, after completion of training program Ⓑ **Qp** **Qh** ♿   Y

IOM: 100-03, 2, 160.12

DMEPOS Modifier(s): RR, KF

✳ **E0765** FDA approved nerve stimulator, with replaceable batteries, for treatment of nausea and vomiting Ⓑ **Qp** **Qh** ♿   Y

DMEPOS Modifier(s): NU, RR, UE

✳ **E0766** Electrical stimulation device used for cancer treatment, includes all accessories, any type Ⓑ **Qp** **Qh**   Y

⊛ **E0769** Electrical stimulation or electromagnetic wound treatment device, not otherwise classified Ⓑ **Qp** **Qh**   B

IOM: 100-04, 32, 11.1

⊛ **E0770** Functional electrical stimulator, transcutaneous stimulation of nerve and/or muscle groups, any type, complete system, not otherwise specified Ⓑ **Qp** **Qh**   Y

Infusion Supplies

✳ **E0776** IV pole Ⓑ **Qp** **Qh** ♿   Y

PEN: On Fee Schedule,

DMEPOS Modifier(s): BA, KE, NU, RR, UE

✳ **E0779** Ambulatory infusion pump, mechanical, reusable, for infusion 8 hours or greater Ⓑ **Qp** **Qh** ♿   Y

Requires prior authorization and copy of invoice

DMEPOS Modifier(s): RR

This is a capped rental infusion pump modifier. The correct monthly modifier (-KH, -KI, -KJ) is used to indicate which month the rental is for (i.e. -KH, month 1; -KI, months 2 and 3; -KJ, months 4 through 13).

▶ **New**   ↻ **Revised**   ✔ **Reinstated**   ~~deleted~~ **Deleted**   ⊘ **Not covered or valid by Medicare**
⊛ **Special coverage instructions**   ✳ **Carrier discretion**   Ⓑ **Bill local carrier**   Ⓓ **Bill DME MAC**

✻ **E0780** Ambulatory infusion pump, mechanical, reusable, for infusion less than 8 hours Ⓑ Qp Qh ♿   Y

Requires prior authorization and copy of invoice

DMEPOS Modifier(s): NU

⊛ **E0781** Ambulatory infusion pump, single or multiple channels, electric or battery operated with administrative equipment, worn by patient Ⓑ Ⓓ Qp Qh ♿   Y

Billable to both the local carrier (Ⓑ) and the DME MAC (Ⓓ). This item may be billed to the DME MAC whenever the infusion is initiated in the physician's office but the patient does not return during the same business day.

IOM: 100-03, 1, 50.3

DMEPOS Modifier(s): RR

⊛ **E0782** Infusion pump, implantable, non-programmable (includes all components, e.g., pump, catheter, connectors, etc.) Ⓑ Qp Qh ♿ N1 N

IOM: 100-03, 1, 50.3

DMEPOS Modifier(s): NU, KF, RR, UE

⊛ **E0783** Infusion pump system, implantable, programmable (includes all components, e.g., pump, catheter, connectors, etc.) Ⓑ Qp Qh ♿ N1 N

IOM: 100-03, 1, 50.3

DMEPOS Modifier(s): NU, KF, RR, UE

⊛ **E0784** External ambulatory infusion pump, insulin Ⓑ Qp Qh ♿   Y

IOM: 100-03, 4, 280.14

DMEPOS Modifier(s): RR

⊛ **E0785** Implantable intraspinal (epidural/ intrathecal) catheter used with implantable infusion pump, replacement Ⓑ Qp Qh ♿ N1 N

IOM: 100-03, 1, 50.3

DMEPOS Modifier(s): KF

⊛ **E0786** Implantable programmable infusion pump, replacement (excludes implantable intraspinal catheter) Ⓑ Qp Qh ♿ N1 N

IOM: 100-03, 1, 50.3

DMEPOS Modifier(s): NU, KF, RR, UE

⊛ **E0791** Parenteral infusion pump, stationary, single or multi-channel Ⓑ Qp Qh ♿   Y

IOM: 100-02, 15, 120; 100-03, 3, 180.2; 100-04, 20, 100.2.2

DMEPOS Modifier(s): RR

Traction Equipment: All Types and Cervical

⊛ **E0830** Ambulatory traction device, all types, each Ⓑ Qp Qh   N

IOM: 100-03, 4, 280.1

DMEPOS Modifier(s): NU

⊛ **E0840** Traction frame, attached to headboard, cervical traction Ⓑ Qp Qh ♿   Y

IOM: 100-03, 4, 280.1

DMEPOS Modifier(s): NU, RR, UE

↺ ✻ **E0849** Traction equipment, cervical, free-standing stand/frame, pneumatic, applying traction force to other than mandible Ⓑ Qp Qh ♿   Y

DMEPOS Modifier(s): RR

⊛ **E0850** Traction stand, free standing, cervical traction Ⓑ Qp Qh ♿   Y

IOM: 100-03, 4, 280.1

DMEPOS Modifier(s): NU, RR, UE

↺ ✻ **E0855** Cervical traction equipment not requiring additional stand or frame Ⓑ Qp Qh ♿   Y

DMEPOS Modifier(s): RR

↺ ✻ **E0856** Cervical traction device, with inflatable air bladder(s) Ⓑ Qp Qh ♿   Y

DMEPOS Modifier(s): RR

Traction: Overdoor

⊛ **E0860** Traction equipment, overdoor, cervical Ⓑ Qp Qh   Y

IOM: 100-03, 4, 280.1

DMEPOS Modifier(s): NU, RR, UE

Traction: Extremity

⊛ **E0870** Traction frame, attached to footboard, extremity traction, (e.g., Buck's) Ⓑ Qp Qh ♿   Y

IOM: 100-03, 4, 280.1

DMEPOS Modifier(s): NU, RR, UE

⊛ **E0880** Traction stand, free standing, extremity traction, (e.g., Buck's) Ⓑ Qp Qh ♿ Y

IOM: 100-03, 4, 280.1

DMEPOS Modifier(s): NU, RR, UE

Traction: Pelvic

⊛ **E0890** Traction frame, attached to footboard, pelvic traction Ⓑ Qp Qh ♿ Y

IOM: 100-03, 4, 280.1

DMEPOS Modifier(s): NU, RR, UE

⊛ **E0900** Traction stand, free standing, pelvic traction, (e.g., Buck's) Ⓑ Qp Qh ♿ Y

IOM: 100-03, 4, 280.1

DMEPOS Modifier(s): NU, RR, UE

Trapeze Equipment, Fracture Frame, and Other Orthopedic Devices

⊛ **E0910** Trapeze bars, A/K/A patient helper, attached to bed, with grab bar Ⓑ Qp Qh ♿ Y

IOM: 100-03, 4, 280.1

DMEPOS Modifier(s): RR

⊛ **E0911** Trapeze bar, heavy duty, for patient weight capacity greater than 250 pounds, attached to bed, with grab bar Ⓑ Qp Qh ♿ Y

IOM: 100-03, 4, 280.1

DMEPOS Modifier(s): RR

⊛ **E0912** Trapeze bar, heavy duty, for patient weight capacity greater than 250 pounds, free standing, complete with grab bar Ⓑ Qp Qh ♿ Y

IOM: 100-03, 4, 280.1

DMEPOS Modifier(s): RR

⊛ **E0920** Fracture frame, attached to bed, includes weights Ⓑ Qp Qh ♿ Y

IOM: 100-03, 4, 280.1

DMEPOS Modifier(s): RR

⊛ **E0930** Fracture frame, free standing, includes weights Ⓑ Qp Qh ♿ Y

IOM: 100-03, 4, 280.1

DMEPOS Modifier(s): RR

⊛ **E0935** Continuous passive motion exercise device for use on knee only Ⓑ Qp Qh ♿ Y

To qualify for coverage, use of device must commence within two days following surgery

IOM: 100-03, 4, 280.1

DMEPOS Modifier(s): RR

⊘ **E0936** Continuous passive motion exercise device for use other than knee Ⓑ Qp Qh E

⊛ **E0940** Trapeze bar, free standing, complete with grab bar Ⓑ Qp Qh ♿ Y

IOM: 100-03, 4, 280.1

DMEPOS Modifier(s): RR

⊛ **E0941** Gravity assisted traction device, any type Ⓑ Qp Qh ♿ Y

IOM: 100-03, 4, 280.1

DMEPOS Modifier(s): RR

✳ **E0942** Cervical head harness/halter Ⓑ Qp Qh ♿ Y

DMEPOS Modifier(s): NU, RR, UE

✳ **E0944** Pelvic belt/harness/boot Ⓑ Qp Qh ♿ Y

DMEPOS Modifier(s): NU, RR, UE

✳ **E0945** Extremity belt/harness Ⓑ Qp Qh ♿ Y

DMEPOS Modifier(s): NU, RR, UE

⊛ **E0946** Fracture, frame, dual with cross bars, attached to bed, (e.g. Balken, 4 poster) Ⓑ Qp Qh ♿ Y

IOM: 100-03, 4, 280.1

DMEPOS Modifier(s): RR

⊛ **E0947** Fracture frame, attachments for complex pelvic traction Ⓑ Qp Qh ♿ Y

IOM: 100-03, 4, 280.1

DMEPOS Modifier(s): NU, RR, UE

⊛ **E0948** Fracture frame, attachments for complex cervical traction Ⓑ Qp Qh ♿ Y

IOM: 100-03, 4, 280.1

DMEPOS Modifier(s): NU, RR, UE

Wheelchair Accessories

⊛ **E0950** Wheelchair accessory, tray, each Ⓑ Qp Qh ♿ Y

IOM: 100-03, 4, 280.1

DMEPOS Modifier(s): NU, KE, RR

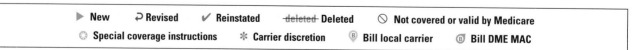

▶ New ↻ Revised ✔ Reinstated ~~deleted~~ Deleted ⊘ Not covered or valid by Medicare
⊛ Special coverage instructions ✳ Carrier discretion Ⓑ Bill local carrier Ⓒ Bill DME MAC

✳ **E0951** Heel loop/holder, any type, with or without ankle strap, each Ⓑ Qp Qh ♿   Y

DMEPOS Modifier(s): NU, KE, RR

✿ **E0952** Toe loop/holder, any type, each Ⓑ Qp Qh ♿   Y

IOM: 100-03, 4, 280.1

DMEPOS Modifier(s): NU, KE, RR

✳ **E0955** Wheelchair accessory, headrest, cushioned, any type, including fixed mounting hardware, each Ⓑ Qp Qh ♿   Y

DMEPOS Modifier(s): NU, KE, RR

✳ **E0956** Wheelchair accessory, lateral trunk or hip support, any type, including fixed mounting hardware, each Ⓑ Qp Qh ♿   Y

DMEPOS Modifier(s): NU, KE, RR

✳ **E0957** Wheelchair accessory, medial thigh support, any type, including fixed mounting hardware, each Ⓑ Qp Qh ♿   Y

DMEPOS Modifier(s): NU, KE, RR

✿ **E0958** Manual wheelchair accessory, one-arm drive attachment, each Ⓑ Qp Qh ♿   Y

IOM: 100-03, 4, 280.1

DMEPOS Modifier(s): RR

✳ **E0959** Manual wheelchair accessory, adapter for amputee, each Qp Qh ♿   B

IOM: 100-03, 4, 280.1

DMEPOS Modifier(s): NU, RR, UE

✳ **E0960** Wheelchair accessory, shoulder harness/straps or chest strap, including any type mounting hardware Ⓑ Qp Qh ♿   Y

DMEPOS Modifier(s): NU, KE, RR

✳ **E0961** Manual wheelchair accessory, wheel lock brake extension (handle), each Ⓑ Qp Qh ♿   B

IOM: 100-03, 4, 280.1

DMEPOS Modifier(s): NU, RR, UE

✳ **E0966** Manual wheelchair accessory, headrest extension, each Ⓑ Qp Qh ♿   B

IOM: 100-03, 4, 280.1

DMEPOS Modifier(s): NU, RR, UE

✿ **E0967** Manual wheelchair accessory, hand rim with projections, any type, each Ⓑ Qp Qh ♿   Y

IOM: 100-03, 4, 280.1

DMEPOS Modifier(s): NU, RR, UE

✿ **E0968** Commode seat, wheelchair Ⓑ Qp Qh ♿   Y

IOM: 100-03, 4, 280.1

DMEPOS Modifier(s): RR

✿ **E0969** Narrowing device, wheelchair Ⓑ ♿   Y

IOM: 100-03, 4, 280.1

DMEPOS Modifier(s): NU, RR, UE

⊘ **E0970** No.2 footplates, except for elevating leg rest Ⓑ Qp Qh   E

IOM: 100-03, 4, 280.1

Cross Reference CPT K0037, K0042

✳ **E0971** Manual wheelchair accessory, anti-tipping device, each Ⓑ Qp Qh ♿   B

IOM: 100-03, 4, 280.1

Cross Reference CPT K0021

DMEPOS Modifier(s): NU, RR, UE

✿ **E0973** Wheelchair accessory, adjustable height, detachable armrest, complete assembly, each Ⓑ Qp Qh ♿   B

IOM: 100-03, 4, 280.1

DMEPOS Modifier(s): NU, KE, RR

✿ **E0974** Manual wheelchair accessory, anti-rollback device, each Ⓑ Qp Qh ♿   B

IOM: 100-03, 4, 280.1

DMEPOS Modifier(s): NU, RR, UE

✳ **E0978** Wheelchair accessory, positioning belt/safety belt/pelvic strap, each Ⓑ Qp Qh ♿   B

DMEPOS Modifier(s): NU, KE, RR

✳ **E0980** Safety vest, wheelchair Ⓑ ♿   Y

DMEPOS Modifier(s): NU, RR, UE

✳ **E0981** Wheelchair accessory, seat upholstery, replacement only, each Ⓑ Qp Qh ♿   Y

DMEPOS Modifier(s): NU, KE, RR

✳ **E0982** Wheelchair accessory, back upholstery, replacement only, each Ⓑ Qp Qh ♿   Y

DMEPOS Modifier(s): NU, KE, RR

✳ **E0983** Manual wheelchair accessory, power add-on to convert manual wheelchair to motorized wheelchair, joystick control Ⓑ Qp Qh ♿   Y

DMEPOS Modifier(s): RR

↻ ✳ **E0984** Manual wheelchair accessory, power add-on to convert manual wheelchair to motorized wheelchair, tiller control Ⓑ Qp Qh ♿   Y

DMEPOS Modifier(s): RR

✳ **E0985** Wheelchair accessory, seat lift mechanism Ⓑ Qp Qh ♿   Y

DMEPOS Modifier(s): NU, RR, UE

↻ ✳ **E0986** Manual wheelchair accessory, push-rim activated power assist system Ⓑ Qp Qh ♿   Y

DMEPOS Modifier(s): RR

✳ **E0988** Manual wheelchair accessory, lever-activated, wheel drive, pair Ⓑ Qp Qh ♿   Y

DMEPOS Modifier(s): PR

✳ **E0990** Wheelchair accessory, elevating leg rest, complete assembly, each Ⓑ Qp Qh ♿   B

IOM: 100-03, 4, 280.1

DMEPOS Modifier(s): NU, KE, RR, UE

✳ **E0992** Manual wheelchair accessory, solid seat insert Ⓑ Qp Qh ♿   B

DMEPOS Modifier(s): NU, RR, UE

◎ **E0994** Arm rest, each Ⓑ Qp Qh ♿   Y

IOM: 100-03, 4, 280.1

DMEPOS Modifier(s): NU, RR, UE

✳ **E0995** Wheelchair accessory, calf rest/pad, each Ⓑ Qp Qh ♿   B

IOM: 100-03, 4, 280.1

DMEPOS Modifier(s): NU, KE, RR, UE

↻ ✳ **E1002** Wheelchair accessory, power seating system, tilt only Ⓑ Qp Qh ♿   Y

DMEPOS Modifier(s): RR, KE

↻ ✳ **E1003** Wheelchair accessory, power seating system, recline only, without shear reduction Ⓑ Qp Qh ♿   Y

DMEPOS Modifier(s): RR, KE

↻ ✳ **E1004** Wheelchair accessory, power seating system, recline only, with mechanical shear reduction Ⓑ Qp Qh ♿   Y

DMEPOS Modifier(s): RR, KE

↻ ✳ **E1005** Wheelchair accessory, power seating system, recline only, with power shear reduction Ⓑ Qp Qh ♿   Y

DMEPOS Modifier(s): RR, KE

↻ ✳ **E1006** Wheelchair accessory, power seating system, combination tilt and recline, without shear reduction Ⓑ Qp Qh ♿   Y

DMEPOS Modifier(s): RR, KE

↻ ✳ **E1007** Wheelchair accessory, power seating system, combination tilt and recline, with mechanical shear reduction Ⓑ Qp Qh ♿   Y

DMEPOS Modifier(s): RR, KE

↻ ✳ **E1008** Wheelchair accessory, power seating system, combination tilt and recline, with power shear reduction Ⓑ Qp Qh ♿   Y

DMEPOS Modifier(s): RR, KE

✳ **E1009** Wheelchair accessory, addition to power seating system, mechanically linked leg elevation system, including pushrod and leg rest, each Ⓑ Qp Qh ♿   Y

DMEPOS Modifier(s): NU, RR, UE

↻ ✳ **E1010** Wheelchair accessory, addition to power seating system, power leg elevation system, including leg rest, pair Ⓑ Qp Qh ♿   Y

DMEPOS Modifier(s): RR, KE

◎ **E1011** Modification to pediatric size wheelchair, width adjustment package (not to be dispensed with initial chair) Qp Qh Ⓐ ♿   Y

IOM: 100-03, 4, 280.1

DMEPOS Modifier(s): NU, RR, UE

↻ ◎ **E1014** Reclining back, addition to pediatric size wheelchair Ⓑ Qp Qh Ⓐ ♿   Y

IOM: 100-03, 4, 280.1

DMEPOS Modifier(s): RR

◎ **E1015** Shock absorber for manual wheelchair, each Ⓑ Qp Qh ♿   Y

IOM: 100-03, 4, 280.1

DMEPOS Modifier(s): NU, RR, UE

◎ **E1016** Shock absorber for power wheelchair, each Ⓑ Qp Qh ♿   Y

IOM: 100-03, 4, 280.1

DMEPOS Modifier(s): NU, KE, RR, UE

◎ **E1017** Heavy duty shock absorber for heavy duty or extra heavy duty manual wheelchair, each Ⓑ Qp Qh ♿   Y

IOM: 100-03, 4, 280.1

DMEPOS Modifier(s): NU, RR, UE

◎ **E1018** Heavy duty shock absorber for heavy duty or extra heavy duty power wheelchair, each Ⓑ Qp Qh ♿   Y

IOM: 100-03, 4, 280.1

DMEPOS Modifier(s): NU, RR, UE

▶ New   ↻ Revised   ✔ Reinstated   ~~deleted~~ Deleted   ⊘ Not covered or valid by Medicare

◎ Special coverage instructions   ✳ Carrier discretion   Ⓑ Bill local carrier   Ⓑ Bill DME MAC

⚙ **E1020** Residual limb support system for wheelchair, any type ⑧ **Qp** **Qh** ♿   Y

IOM: 100-03, 3, 280.3

DMEPOS Modifier(s): NU, KE, RR, UE

✳ **E1028** Wheelchair accessory, manual swing-away, retractable or removable mounting hardware for joystick, other control interface or positioning accessory ⑧ **Qp** **Qh** ♿   Y

DMEPOS Modifier(s): NU, KE, RR, UE

↻ ✳ **E1029** Wheelchair accessory, ventilator tray, fixed ⑧ **Qp** **Qh** ♿   Y

DMEPOS Modifier(s): RR, KE

↻ ✳ **E1030** Wheelchair accessory, ventilator tray, gimbaled ⑧ **Qp** **Qh** ♿   Y

DMEPOS Modifier(s): RR, KE

Rollabout Chair and Transfer System

⚙ **E1031** Rollabout chair, any and all types with castors 5" or greater ⑧ **Qp** **Qh** ♿   Y

IOM: 100-03, 4, 280.1

DMEPOS Modifier(s): RR

✳ **E1035** Multi-positional patient transfer system, with integrated seat, operated by care giver, patient weight capacity up to and including 300 lbs ⑧ **Qp** **Qh** ♿   Y

IOM: 100-02, 15, 110

DMEPOS Modifier(s): RR

✳ **E1036** Multi-positional patient transfer system, extra-wide, with integrated seat, operated by caregiver, patient weight capacity greater than 300 lbs ⑧ **Qh** ♿   Y

DMEPOS Modifier(s): RR

⚙ **E1037** Transport chair, pediatric size ⑧ **Qp** **Qh** **A** ♿   Y

IOM: 100-03, 4, 280.1

DMEPOS Modifier(s): RR

⚙ **E1038** Transport chair, adult size, patient weight capacity up to and including 300 pounds ⑧ **Qp** **Qh** **A** ♿   Y

IOM: 100-03, 4, 280.1

DMEPOS Modifier(s): RR

✳ **E1039** Transport chair, adult size, heavy duty, patient weight capacity greater than 300 pounds ⑧ **Qp** **Qh** **A** ♿   Y

DMEPOS Modifier(s): RR

Wheelchair: Fully Reclining

⚙ **E1050** Fully-reclining wheelchair, fixed full length arms, swing away detachable elevating leg rests ⑧ **Qp** **Qh** ♿   Y

IOM: 100-03, 4, 280.1

DMEPOS Modifier(s): RR

⚙ **E1060** Fully-reclining wheelchair, detachable arms, desk or full length, swing away detachable elevating legrests ⑧ **Qp** **Qh** ♿   Y

IOM: 100-03, 4, 280.1

DMEPOS Modifier(s): RR

⚙ **E1070** Fully-reclining wheelchair, detachable arms (desk or full length) swing away detachable footrests ⑧ **Qp** **Qh** ♿   Y

IOM: 100-03, 4, 280.1

DMEPOS Modifier(s): RR

⚙ **E1083** Hemi-wheelchair, fixed full length arms, swing away detachable elevating leg rest ⑧ **Qp** **Qh** ♿   Y

IOM: 100-03, 4, 280.1

DMEPOS Modifier(s): RR

⚙ **E1084** Hemi-wheelchair, detachable arms desk or full length arms, swing away detachable elevating leg rests ⑧ **Qp** **Qh** ♿   Y

IOM: 100-03, 4, 280.1

DMEPOS Modifier(s): RR

⊘ **E1085** Hemi-wheelchair, fixed full length arms, swing away detachable foot rests ⑧ **Qp** **Qh**   E

IOM: 100-03, 4, 280.1

Cross Reference CPT K0002

⊘ **E1086** Hemi-wheelchair, detachable arms desk or full length, swing away detachable footrests ⑧ **Qp** **Qh**   E

IOM: 100-03, 4, 280.1

Cross Reference CPT K0002

⚙ **E1087** High strength lightweight wheelchair, fixed full length arms, swing away detachable elevating leg rests ⑧ **Qp** **Qh** ♿   Y

IOM: 100-03, 4, 280.1

DMEPOS Modifier(s): RR

⚙ **E1088** High strength lightweight wheelchair, detachable arms desk or full length, swing away detachable elevating leg rests ⑧ **Qp** **Qh** ♿   Y

IOM: 100-03, 4, 280.1

DMEPOS Modifier(s): RR

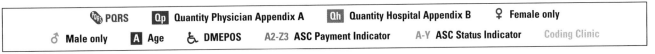
DURABLE MEDICAL EQUIPMENT   E1020 — E1088

⊘ **E1089** High strength lightweight wheelchair, fixed length arms, swing away detachable footrest Ⓑ `Qp` `Qh`   E

IOM: 100-03, 4, 280.1

Cross Reference CPT K0004

⊘ **E1090** High strength lightweight wheelchair, detachable arms desk or full length, swing away detachable foot rests Ⓑ `Qp` `Qh`   E

IOM: 100-03, 4, 280.1

Cross Reference CPT K0004

✪ **E1092** Wide heavy duty wheelchair, detachable arms (desk or full length) swing away detachable elevating leg rests Ⓑ `Qp` `Qh` ♿   Y

IOM: 100-03, 4, 280.1

DMEPOS Modifier(s): RR

✪ **E1093** Wide heavy duty wheelchair, detachable arms (desk or full length arms), swing away detachable foot rests Ⓑ `Qp` `Qh` ♿   Y

IOM: 100-03, 4, 280.1

DMEPOS Modifier(s): RR

Wheelchair: Semi-reclining

✪ **E1100** Semi-reclining wheelchair, fixed full length arms, swing away detachable elevating leg rests Ⓑ `Qp` `Qh` ♿   Y

IOM: 100-03, 4, 280.1

DMEPOS Modifier(s): RR

✪ **E1110** Semi-reclining wheelchair, detachable arms (desk or full length), elevating leg rest Ⓑ `Qp` `Qh` ♿   Y

IOM: 100-03, 4, 280.1

DMEPOS Modifier(s): RR

Wheelchair: Standard

⊘ **E1130** Standard wheelchair, fixed full length arms, fixed or swing away detachable footrests Ⓑ `Qp` `Qh`   E

IOM: 100-03, 4, 280.1

Cross Reference CPT K0001

⊘ **E1140** Wheelchair, detachable arms, desk or full length, swing away detachable footrests Ⓑ `Qp` `Qh`   E

IOM: 100-03, 4, 280.1

Cross Reference CPT K0001

✪ **E1150** Wheelchair, detachable arms, desk or full length, swing away detachable elevating legrests Ⓑ `Qp` `Qh` ♿   Y

IOM: 100-03, 4, 280.1

DMEPOS Modifier(s): RR

✪ **E1160** Wheelchair, fixed full length arms, swing away detachable elevating legrests Ⓑ `Qp` `Qh` ♿   Y

IOM: 100-03, 4, 280.1

DMEPOS Modifier(s): RR

↻ ✳ **E1161** Manual adult size wheelchair, includes tilt in space Ⓑ `Qp` `Qh` `A` ♿   Y

DMEPOS Modifier(s): RR

Wheelchair: Amputee

✪ **E1170** Amputee wheelchair, fixed full length arms, swing away detachable elevating legrests Ⓑ `Qp` `Qh` ♿   Y

IOM: 100-03, 4, 280.1

DMEPOS Modifier(s): RR

✪ **E1171** Amputee wheelchair, fixed full length arms, without footrests or legrest Ⓑ `Qp` `Qh` ♿   Y

IOM: 100-03, 4, 280.1

DMEPOS Modifier(s): RR

✪ **E1172** Amputee wheelchair, detachable arms (desk or full length) without footrests or legrest Ⓑ `Qp` `Qh` ♿   Y

IOM: 100-03, 4, 280.1

DMEPOS Modifier(s): RR

✪ **E1180** Amputee wheelchair, detachable arms (desk or full length) swing away detachable footrests Ⓑ `Qp` `Qh` ♿   Y

IOM: 100-03, 4, 280.1

DMEPOS Modifier(s): RR

✪ **E1190** Amputee wheelchair, detachable arms (desk or full length), swing away detachable legrests Ⓑ `Qp` `Qh` ♿   Y

IOM: 100-03, 4, 280.1

DMEPOS Modifier(s): RR

✪ **E1195** Heavy duty wheelchair, fixed full length arms, swing away detachable elevating legrests Ⓑ `Qp` `Qh` ♿   Y

IOM: 100-03, 4, 280.1

DMEPOS Modifier(s): RR

▶ **New**   ↻ **Revised**   ✔ **Reinstated**   ~~deleted~~ **Deleted**   ⊘ **Not covered or valid by Medicare**

✪ **Special coverage instructions**   ✳ **Carrier discretion**   Ⓑ **Bill local carrier**   Ⓓ **Bill DME MAC**

⊛ **E1200** Amputee wheelchair, fixed full length arms, swing away detachable footrest ⓑ Qp Qh ♿ Y

IOM: 100-03, 4, 280.1

DMEPOS Modifier(s): RR

Wheelchair: Special Size

⊛ **E1220** Wheelchair; specially sized or constructed, (indicate brand name, model number, if any) and justification ⓑ Qp Qh Y

IOM: 100-03, 4, 280.3

⊛ **E1221** Wheelchair with fixed arm, footrests ⓑ Qp Qh ♿ Y

IOM: 100-03, 4, 280.3

DMEPOS Modifier(s): RR

⊛ **E1222** Wheelchair with fixed arm, elevating legrests ⓑ Qp Qh ♿ Y

IOM: 100-03, 4, 280.3

DMEPOS Modifier(s): RR

⊛ **E1223** Wheelchair with detachable arms, footrests ⓑ Qp Qh ♿ Y

IOM: 100-03, 4, 280.3

DMEPOS Modifier(s): RR

⊛ **E1224** Wheelchair with detachable arms, elevating legrests ⓑ Qp Qh ♿ Y

IOM: 100-03, 4, 280.3

DMEPOS Modifier(s): RR

⊛ **E1225** Wheelchair accessory, manual semi-reclining back, (recline greater than 15 degrees, but less than 80 degrees), each ⓑ Qp Qh ♿ Y

IOM: 100-03, 4, 280.3

DMEPOS Modifier(s): RR

⊛ **E1226** Wheelchair accessory, manual fully reclining back, (recline greater than 80 degrees), each ⓑ Qp ♿ B

IOM: 100-03, 4, 280.1

DMEPOS Modifier(s): NU, RR, UE

⊛ **E1227** Special height arms for wheelchair ⓑ ♿ Y

IOM: 100-03, 4, 280.3

DMEPOS Modifier(s): NU, RR, UE

⊛ **E1228** Special back height for wheelchair ⓑ Qp ♿ Y

IOM: 100-03, 4, 280.3

DMEPOS Modifier(s): RR

✳ **E1229** Wheelchair, pediatric size, not otherwise specified ⓑ Qp Qh A Y

⊛ **E1230** Power operated vehicle (three or four wheel non-highway), specify brand name and model number ⓑ Qp Qh ♿ Y

Patient is unable to operate manual wheelchair; patient capable of safely operating controls for scooter; patient can transfer safely in and out of scooter

IOM: 100-08, 5, 5.2.3

DMEPOS Modifier(s): NU, RR, UE

⊛ **E1231** Wheelchair, pediatric size, tilt-in-space, rigid, adjustable, with seating system ⓑ Qp Qh A ♿ Y

IOM: 100-03, 4, 280.1

DMEPOS Modifier(s): NU, RR, UE

↻ ⊛ **E1232** Wheelchair, pediatric size, tilt-in-space, folding, adjustable, with seating system ⓑ Qp Qh A ♿ Y

IOM: 100-03, 4, 280.1

DMEPOS Modifier(s): RR

↻ ⊛ **E1233** Wheelchair, pediatric size, tilt-in-space, rigid, adjustable, without seating system ⓑ Qp Qh A ♿ Y

IOM: 100-03, 4, 280.1

DMEPOS Modifier(s): RR

↻ ⊛ **E1234** Wheelchair, pediatric size, tilt-in-space, folding, adjustable, without seating system ⓑ Qp Qh A ♿ Y

IOM: 100-03, 4, 280.1

DMEPOS Modifier(s): RR

↻ ⊛ **E1235** Wheelchair, pediatric size, rigid, adjustable, with seating system ⓑ Qp Qh A ♿ Y

IOM: 100-03, 4, 280.1

DMEPOS Modifier(s): RR

↻ ⊛ **E1236** Wheelchair, pediatric size, folding, adjustable, with seating system ⓑ Qp Qh A ♿ Y

IOM: 100-03, 4, 280.1

DMEPOS Modifier(s): RR

↻ ⊛ **E1237** Wheelchair, pediatric size, rigid, adjustable, without seating system ⓑ Qp Qh A ♿ Y

IOM: 100-03, 4, 280.1

DMEPOS Modifier(s): RR

↻ ⊛ **E1238** Wheelchair, pediatric size, folding, adjustable, without seating system ⓑ Qp Qh A ♿ Y

IOM: 100-03, 4, 280.1

DMEPOS Modifier(s): RR

✳ **E1239**   Power wheelchair, pediatric size, not otherwise specified Ⓑ **Qp** **Qh** **A**   Y

Wheelchair: Lightweight

⊘ **E1240**   Lightweight wheelchair, detachable arms, (desk or full length) swing away detachable, elevating leg rests Ⓑ **Qp** **Qh** ♿   Y

IOM: 100-03, 4, 280.1

DMEPOS Modifier(s): RR

⊘ **E1250**   Lightweight wheelchair, fixed full length arms, swing away detachable footrest Ⓑ **Qp** **Qh**   E

IOM: 100-03, 4, 280.1

Cross Reference CPT K0003

⊘ **E1260**   Lightweight wheelchair, detachable arms (desk or full length) swing away detachable footrest Ⓑ **Qp** **Qh**   E

IOM: 100-03, 4, 280.1

Cross Reference CPT K0003

⊘ **E1270**   Lightweight wheelchair, fixed full length arms, swing away detachable elevating legrests Ⓑ **Qp** **Qh** ♿   Y

IOM: 100-03, 4, 280.1

DMEPOS Modifier(s): RR

Wheelchair: Heavy Duty

⊘ **E1280**   Heavy duty wheelchair, detachable arms (desk or full length), elevating legrests Ⓑ **Qp** **Qh** ♿   Y

IOM: 100-03, 4, 280.1

DMEPOS Modifier(s): RR

⊘ **E1285**   Heavy duty wheelchair, fixed full length arms, swing away detachable footrest Ⓑ **Qp** **Qh**   E

IOM: 100-03, 4, 280.1

Cross Reference CPT K0006

⊘ **E1290**   Heavy duty wheelchair, detachable arms (desk or full length) swing away detachable footrest Ⓑ **Qp** **Qh**   E

IOM: 100-03, 4, 280.1

Cross Reference CPT K0006

⊘ **E1295**   Heavy duty wheelchair, fixed full length arms, elevating legrest Ⓑ **Qp** **Qh** ♿   Y

IOM: 100-03, 4, 280.1

DMEPOS Modifier(s): RR

⊘ **E1296**   Special wheelchair seat height from floor Ⓑ ♿   Y

IOM: 100-03, 4, 280.3

DMEPOS Modifier(s): NU, RR, UE

⊘ **E1297**   Special wheelchair seat depth, by upholstery Ⓑ ♿   Y

IOM: 100-03, 4, 280.3

DMEPOS Modifier(s): NU, RR, UE

⊘ **E1298**   Special wheelchair seat depth and/or width, by construction Ⓑ ♿   Y

IOM: 100-03, 4, 280.3

DMEPOS Modifier(s): NU, RR, UE

Whirlpool Equipment

⊘ **E1300**   Whirlpool, portable (overtub type) Ⓑ **Qp** **Qh**   E

IOM: 100-03, 4, 280.1

⊘ **E1310**   Whirlpool, non-portable (built-in type) Ⓑ **Qp** **Qh** ♿   Y

IOM: 100-03, 4, 280.1

DMEPOS Modifier(s): NU, RR, UE

Additional Oxygen Related Equipment

✳ **E1352**   Oxygen accessory, flow regulator capable of positive inspiratory pressure Ⓑ **Qp** **Qh**   Y

⊘ **E1353**   Regulator Ⓑ **Qp** **Qh** ♿   Y

IOM: 100-03, 4, 240.2

✳ **E1354**   Oxygen accessory, wheeled cart for portable cylinder or portable concentrator, any type, replacement only, each Ⓑ **Qp** **Qh**   Y

⊘ **E1355**   Stand/rack Ⓑ **Qp** **Qh** ♿   Y

IOM: 100-03, 4, 240.2

✳ **E1356**   Oxygen accessory, battery pack/cartridge for portable concentrator, any type, replacement only, each Ⓑ **Qp** **Qh**   Y

✳ **E1357**   Oxygen accessory, battery charger for portable concentrator, any type, replacement only, each Ⓑ **Qp** **Qh**   Y

↻⊘ **E1358**   Oxygen accessory, DC power adapter for portable concentrator, any type, replacement only, each Ⓑ **Qp** **Qh**   Y

⊘ **E1372**   Immersion external heater for nebulizer Ⓑ **Qp** **Qh** ♿   Y

IOM: 100-03, 4, 240.2

DMEPOS Modifier(s): NU, RR, UE

▶ New   ↻ Revised   ✔ Reinstated   ~~deleted~~ Deleted   ⊘ Not covered or valid by Medicare   ⊛ Special coverage instructions   ✳ Carrier discretion   Ⓑ Bill local carrier   Ⓑ Bill DME MAC

E1390 Oxygen concentrator, single delivery port, capable of delivering 85 percent or greater oxygen concentration at the prescribed flow rate Ⓑ Qp Qh ♿   Y

IOM: 100-03, 4, 240.2

DMEPOS Modifier(s): RR

E1391 Oxygen concentrator, dual delivery port, capable of delivering 85 percent or greater oxygen concentration at the prescribed flow rate, each Ⓑ Qp Qh ♿   Y

IOM: 100-03, 4, 240.2

DMEPOS Modifier(s): RR

E1392 Portable oxygen concentrator, rental Ⓑ Qp Qh ♿   Y

IOM: 100-03, 4, 240.2

DMEPOS Modifier(s): RR

✳ E1399 Durable medical equipment, miscellaneous Ⓑ   Y

Local carrier (Ⓑ) if used with implanted DME.

Example: Therapeutic exercise putty; rubber exercise tubing; anti-vibration gloves

On DMEPOS fee schedule as a payable replacement for miscellaneous implanted or non-implanted items.

E1405 Oxygen and water vapor enriching system with heated delivery Ⓑ Qp Qh ♿   Y

IOM: 100-03, 4, 240.2

DMEPOS Modifier(s): RR

E1406 Oxygen and water vapor enriching system without heated delivery Ⓑ Qp Qh ♿   Y

IOM: 100-03, 4, 240.2

DMEPOS Modifier(s): RR

Artificial Kidney Machines and Accessories

E1500 Centrifuge, for dialysis Ⓑ Qp Qh   A

E1510 Kidney, dialysate delivery syst. kidney machine, pump recirculating, air removal syst. flowrate meter, power off, heater and temperature control with alarm, I.V. poles, pressure gauge, concentrate container Ⓑ Qp Qh   A

E1520 Heparin infusion pump for hemodialysis Ⓑ Qp Qh   A

E1530 Air bubble detector for hemodialysis, each, replacement Ⓑ Qp Qh   A

E1540 Pressure alarm for hemodialysis, each, replacement Ⓑ Qp Qh   A

E1550 Bath conductivity meter for hemodialysis, each Ⓑ Qp Qh   A

E1560 Blood leak detector for hemodialysis, each, replacement Ⓑ Qp Qh   A

E1570 Adjustable chair, for ESRD patients Ⓑ Qp Qh   A

E1575 Transducer protectors/fluid barriers for hemodialysis, any size, per 10 Ⓑ Qp Qh   A

E1580 Unipuncture control system for hemodialysis Ⓑ Qp Qh   A

E1590 Hemodialysis machine Ⓑ Qp Qh   A

E1592 Automatic intermittent peritoneal dialysis system Ⓑ Qp Qh   A

E1594 Cycler dialysis machine for peritoneal dialysis Ⓑ Qp Qh   A

E1600 Delivery and/or installation charges for hemodialysis equipment Ⓑ Qp Qh   A

E1610 Reverse osmosis water purification system, for hemodialysis Ⓑ Qp Qh   A

IOM: 100-03, 4, 230.7

E1615 Deionizer water purification system, for hemodialysis Ⓑ Qp Qh   A

IOM: 100-03, 4, 230.7

E1620 Blood pump for hemodialysis replacement Ⓑ Qp Qh   A

E1625 Water softening system, for hemodialysis Ⓑ Qp Qh   A

IOM: 100-03, 4, 230.7

✳ E1630 Reciprocating peritoneal dialysis system Ⓑ Qp Qh   A

E1632 Wearable artificial kidney, each Ⓑ Qp Qh   A

E1634 Peritoneal dialysis clamps, each Ⓑ Qp Qh   B

IOM: 100-04, 8, 60.4.2; 100-04, 8, 90.1; 100-04, 18, 80; 100-04, 18, 90

E1635 Compact (portable) travel hemodialyzer system Ⓑ Qp Qh   A

E1636 Sorbent cartridges, for hemodialysis, per 10 Ⓑ Qp Qh   A

E1637 Hemostats, each Ⓑ Qp Qh   A

E1639 Scale, each Ⓑ Qp Qh   A

E1699 Dialysis equipment, not otherwise specified Ⓑ   A

Jaw Motion Rehabilitation System and Accessories

✳ E1700 Jaw motion rehabilitation system Ⓑ Qp Qh ♿   Y

Must be prescribed by physician

DMEPOS Modifier(s): RR

PQRS	Qp Quantity Physician Appendix A	Qh Quantity Hospital Appendix B	♀ Female only
♂ Male only	A Age	♿ DMEPOS	A2-Z3 ASC Payment Indicator	A-Y ASC Status Indicator	Coding Clinic

DURABLE MEDICAL EQUIPMENT   E1390 — E1700

191

✳ **E1701** Replacement cushions for jaw motion rehabilitation system, pkg. of 6 ⑧ Qp Qh ♿   Y

✳ **E1702** Replacement measuring scales for jaw motion rehabilitation system, pkg. of 200 ⑧ Qp Qh ♿   Y

Other Orthopedic Devices

✳ **E1800** Dynamic adjustable elbow extension/ flexion device, includes soft interface material ⑧ Qp Qh ♿   Y
DMEPOS Modifier(s): RR

✳ **E1801** Static progressive stretch elbow device, extension and/or flexion, with or without range of motion adjustment, includes all components and accessories ⑧ Qp Qh ♿   Y
DMEPOS Modifier(s): RR

✳ **E1802** Dynamic adjustable forearm pronation/ supination device, includes soft interface material ⑧ Qp Qh ♿   Y
DMEPOS Modifier(s): RR

✳ **E1805** Dynamic adjustable wrist extension/ flexion device, includes soft interface material ⑧ Qp Qh ♿   Y
DMEPOS Modifier(s): RR

✳ **E1806** Static progressive stretch wrist device, flexion and/or extension, with or without range of motion adjustment, includes all components and accessories ⑧ Qp Qh ♿   Y
DMEPOS Modifier(s): RR

✳ **E1810** Dynamic adjustable knee extension/ flexion device, includes soft interface material ⑧ Qp Qh ♿   Y
DMEPOS Modifier(s): RR

✳ **E1811** Static progressive stretch knee device, extension and/or flexion, with or without range of motion adjustment, includes all components and accessories ⑧ Qp Qh ♿   Y
DMEPOS Modifier(s): RR

✳ **E1812** Dynamic knee, extension/ flexion device with active resistance control ⑧ Qp Qh ♿   Y
DMEPOS Modifier(s): RR

✳ **E1815** Dynamic adjustable ankle extension/ flexion device, includes soft interface material ⑧ Qp Qh ♿   Y
DMEPOS Modifier(s): RR

✳ **E1816** Static progressive stretch ankle device, flexion and/or extension, with or without range of motion adjustment, includes all components and accessories ⑧ Qp Qh ♿   Y
DMEPOS Modifier(s): RR

✳ **E1818** Static progressive stretch forearm pronation/supination device with or without range of motion adjustment, includes all components and accessories ⑧ Qp Qh ♿   Y
DMEPOS Modifier(s): RR

✳ **E1820** Replacement soft interface material, dynamic adjustable extension/flexion device ⑧ Qp Qh ♿   Y
DMEPOS Modifier(s): NU, RR, UE

✳ **E1821** Replacement soft interface material/cuffs for bi-directional static progressive stretch device ⑧ Qp Qh ♿   Y
DMEPOS Modifier(s): NU, RR, UE

✳ **E1825** Dynamic adjustable finger extension/ flexion device, includes soft interface material ⑧ Qp Qh ♿   Y
DMEPOS Modifier(s): RR

✳ **E1830** Dynamic adjustable toe extension/ flexion device, includes soft interface material ⑧ Qp Qh ♿   Y
DMEPOS Modifier(s): RR

✳ **E1831** Static progressive stretch toe device, extension and/or flexion, with or without range of motion adjustment, includes all components and accessories ⑧ Qp Qh ♿   Y
DMEPOS Modifier(s): RR

✳ **E1840** Dynamic adjustable shoulder flexion/ abduction/rotation device, includes soft interface material ⑧ Qp Qh ♿   Y
DMEPOS Modifier(s): RR

✳ **E1841** Static progressive stretch shoulder device, with or without range of motion adjustment, includes all components and accessories ⑧ Qp Qh ♿   Y
DMEPOS Modifier(s): RR

MISCELLANEOUS (E1902-E2120)

✳ **E1902** Communication board, non-electronic augmentative or alternative communication device Qp Qh   Y

▶ New   ↻ Revised   ✔ Reinstated   ~~deleted~~ Deleted   ⊘ Not covered or valid by Medicare
⊛ Special coverage instructions   ✳ Carrier discretion   Ⓑ Bill local carrier   ⑧ Bill DME MAC

✳ **E2000**   Gastric suction pump, home model, portable or stationary, electric ⓆⓅ Ⓠⓗ ♿   Y

DMEPOS Modifier(s): RR

⊙ **E2100**   Blood glucose monitor with integrated voice synthesizer ⓆⓅ Ⓠⓗ ♿   Y

IOM: 100-03, 4, 230.16

DMEPOS Modifier(s): NU, RR, UE

⊙ **E2101**   Blood glucose monitor with integrated lancing/blood sample ⓆⓅ Ⓠⓗ ♿   Y

IOM: 100-03, 4, 230.16

DMEPOS Modifier(s): NU, RR, UE

✳ **E2120**   Pulse generator system for tympanic treatment of inner ear endolymphatic fluid ⓆⓅ Ⓠⓗ ♿   Y

DMEPOS Modifier(s): RR

Wheelchair Assessories

✳ **E2201**   Manual wheelchair accessory, nonstandard seat frame, width greater than or equal to 20 inches and less than 24 inches Ⓑ ⓆⓅ Ⓠⓗ ♿   Y

DMEPOS Modifier(s): NU, RR, UE

✳ **E2202**   Manual wheelchair accessory, nonstandard seat frame width, 24-27 inches Ⓑ ⓆⓅ Ⓠⓗ ♿   Y

DMEPOS Modifier(s): NU, RR, UE

✳ **E2203**   Manual wheelchair accessory, nonstandard seat frame depth, 20 to less than 22 inches Ⓑ ⓆⓅ Ⓠⓗ ♿   Y

DMEPOS Modifier(s): NU, RR, UE

✳ **E2204**   Manual wheelchair accessory, nonstandard seat frame depth, 22 to 25 inches Ⓑ ⓆⓅ Ⓠⓗ ♿   Y

DMEPOS Modifier(s): NU, RR, UE

✳ **E2205**   Manual wheelchair accessory, handrim without projections (includes ergonomic or contoured), any type, replacement only, each Ⓑ ⓆⓅ Ⓠⓗ ♿   Y

DMEPOS Modifier(s): NU, RR, UE

✳ **E2206**   Manual wheelchair accessory, wheel lock assembly, complete, each Ⓑ ⓆⓅ Ⓠⓗ ♿   Y

DMEPOS Modifier(s): NU, RR, UE

✳ **E2207**   Wheelchair accessory, crutch and cane holder, each Ⓑ ⓆⓅ Ⓠⓗ ♿   Y

DMEPOS Modifier(s): NU, RR, UE

✳ **E2208**   Wheelchair accessory, cylinder tank carrier, each Ⓑ ⓆⓅ Ⓠⓗ ♿   Y

DMEPOS Modifier(s): NU, KE, RR, UE

✳ **E2209**   Accessory arm trough, with or without hand support, each Ⓑ ⓆⓅ Ⓠⓗ ♿   Y

DMEPOS Modifier(s): NU, KE, RR, UE

✳ **E2210**   Wheelchair accessory, bearings, any type, replacement only, each Ⓑ ⓆⓅ Ⓠⓗ ♿   Y

DMEPOS Modifier(s): NU, KE, RR, UE

✳ **E2211**   Manual wheelchair accessory, pneumatic propulsion tire, any size, each Ⓑ ⓆⓅ Ⓠⓗ ♿   Y

DMEPOS Modifier(s): NU, RR, UE

✳ **E2212**   Manual wheelchair accessory, tube for pneumatic propulsion tire, any size, each Ⓑ ⓆⓅ Ⓠⓗ ♿   Y

DMEPOS Modifier(s): NU, RR, UE

✳ **E2213**   Manual wheelchair accessory, insert for pneumatic propulsion tire (removable), any type, any size, each Ⓑ ⓆⓅ Ⓠⓗ ♿   Y

DMEPOS Modifier(s): NU, RR, UE

✳ **E2214**   Manual wheelchair accessory, pneumatic caster tire, any size, each Ⓑ ⓆⓅ Ⓠⓗ ♿   Y

DMEPOS Modifier(s): NU, RR, UE

✳ **E2215**   Manual wheelchair accessory, tube for pneumatic caster tire, any size, each Ⓑ ⓆⓅ Ⓠⓗ ♿   Y

DMEPOS Modifier(s): NU, RR, UE

✳ **E2216**   Manual wheelchair accessory, foam filled propulsion tire, any size, each Ⓑ ⓆⓅ Ⓠⓗ ♿   Y

DMEPOS Modifier(s): NU, RR, UE

✳ **E2217**   Manual wheelchair accessory, foam filled caster tire, any size, each Ⓑ ⓆⓅ Ⓠⓗ ♿   Y

DMEPOS Modifier(s): NU, RR, UE

✳ **E2218**   Manual wheelchair accessory, foam propulsion tire, any size, each Ⓑ ⓆⓅ Ⓠⓗ ♿   Y

DMEPOS Modifier(s): NU, RR, UE

✳ **E2219**   Manual wheelchair accessory, foam caster tire, any size, each Ⓑ ⓆⓅ Ⓠⓗ ♿   Y

DMEPOS Modifier(s): NU, RR, UE

✳ **E2220**   Manual wheelchair accessory, solid (rubber/plastic) propulsion tire, any size, each Ⓑ ⓆⓅ Ⓠⓗ ♿   Y

DMEPOS Modifier(s): NU, RR, UE

✳ **E2221**   Manual wheelchair accessory, solid (rubber/plastic) caster tire (removable), any size, each Ⓑ ⓆⓅ Ⓠⓗ ♿   Y

DMEPOS Modifier(s): NU, RR, UE

ⓅⓆⓇⓈ PQRS	ⓆⓅ Quantity Physician Appendix A	Ⓠⓗ Quantity Hospital Appendix B	♀ Female only
♂ **Male only**	Ⓐ **Age**	♿ **DMEPOS**	A2-Z3 **ASC Payment Indicator**	A-Y **ASC Status Indicator**	*Coding Clinic*

✳ **E2222** Manual wheelchair accessory, solid (rubber/plastic) caster tire with integrated wheel, any size, each Ⓑ Qp Qh ♿   Y

DMEPOS Modifier(s): NU, RR, UE

✳ **E2224** Manual wheelchair accessory, propulsion wheel excludes tire, any size, each Ⓑ Qp Qh ♿   Y

DMEPOS Modifier(s): NU, RR, UE

✳ **E2225** Manual wheelchair accessory, caster wheel excludes tire, any size, replacement only, each Ⓑ Qp Qh ♿   Y

DMEPOS Modifier(s): NU, RR, UE

✳ **E2226** Manual wheelchair accessory, caster fork, any size, replacement only, each Ⓑ Qp Qh ♿   Y

DMEPOS Modifier(s): NU, RR, UE

↺✳ **E2227** Manual wheelchair accessory, gear reduction drive wheel, each Ⓑ Qp Qh ♿   Y

DMEPOS Modifier(s): RR

✳ **E2228** Manual wheelchair accessory, wheel braking system and lock, complete, each Ⓑ Qp Qh ♿   Y

DMEPOS Modifier(s): NU, RR, UE

↺✳ **E2230** Manual wheelchair accessory, manual standing system Ⓑ   Y

✳ **E2231** Manual wheelchair accessory, solid seat support base (replaces sling seat), includes any type mounting hardware Ⓑ Qp Qh ♿   Y

DMEPOS Modifier(s): NU, RR, UE

✳ **E2291** Back, planar, for pediatric size wheelchair including fixed attaching hardware Ⓑ Qp Qh A   Y

✳ **E2292** Seat, planar, for pediatric size wheelchair including fixed attaching hardware Ⓑ Qp Qh A   Y

✳ **E2293** Back, contoured, for pediatric size wheelchair including fixed attaching hardware Ⓑ Qp Qh A   Y

✳ **E2294** Seat, contoured, for pediatric size wheelchair including fixed attaching hardware Ⓑ Qp Qh A   Y

✳ **E2295** Manual wheelchair accessory, for pediatric size wheelchair, dynamic seating frame, allows coordinated movement of multiple positioning features Ⓑ Qp Qh A   Y

✳ **E2300** Wheelchair accessory, power seat elevation system, any type Ⓑ Qp Qh   Y

✳ **E2301** Wheelchair accessory, power standing system, any type Ⓑ Qp Qh   Y

↺✳ **E2310** Power wheelchair accessory, electronic connection between wheelchair controller and one power seating system motor, including all related electronics, indicator feature, mechanical function selection switch, and fixed mounting hardware Ⓑ Qp Qh ♿   Y

DMEPOS Modifier(s): RR, KE

↺✳ **E2311** Power wheelchair accessory, electronic connection between wheelchair controller and two or more power seating system motors, including all related electronics, indicator feature, mechanical function selection switch, and fixed mounting hardware Ⓑ Qp Qh ♿   Y

DMEPOS Modifier(s): RR, KE

↺✳ **E2312** Power wheelchair accessory, hand or chin control interface, mini-proportional remote joystick, proportional, including fixed mounting hardware Ⓑ Qp Qh ♿   Y

DMEPOS Modifier(s): RR, KC

↺✳ **E2313** Power wheelchair accessory, harness for upgrade to expandable controller, including all fasteners, connectors and mounting hardware, each Ⓑ Qp Qh ♿   Y

DMEPOS Modifier(s): RR

↺✳ **E2321** Power wheelchair accessory, hand control interface, remote joystick, nonproportional, including all related electronics, mechanical stop switch, and fixed mounting hardware Ⓑ Qp Qh ♿   Y

DMEPOS Modifier(s): RR, KC, KE

↺✳ **E2322** Power wheelchair accessory, hand control interface, multiple mechanical switches, nonproportional, including all related electronics, mechanical stop switch, and fixed mounting hardware Ⓑ Qp Qh ♿   Y

DMEPOS Modifier(s): RR, KC, KE

✳ **E2323** Power wheelchair accessory, specialty joystick handle for hand control interface, prefabricated Ⓑ Qp Qh ♿   Y

DMEPOS Modifier(s): KE, NU, RR, UE

✳ **E2324** Power wheelchair accessory, chin cup for chin control interface Ⓑ Qp Qh ♿   Y

DMEPOS Modifier(s): KE, NU, RR, UE

▶ New   ↺ Revised   ✔ Reinstated   ~~deleted~~ Deleted   ⊘ Not covered or valid by Medicare

✪ Special coverage instructions   ✳ Carrier discretion   Ⓑ Bill local carrier   Ⓑ Bill DME MAC

↺ ✳ **E2325** Power wheelchair accessory, sip and puff interface, nonproportional, including all related electronics, mechanical stop switch, and manual swingaway mounting hardware ⑧ Qp Qh ♿   Y

   DMEPOS Modifier(s): RR, KE

↺ ✳ **E2326** Power wheelchair accessory, breath tube kit for sip and puff interface ⑧ Qp Qh ♿   Y

   DMEPOS Modifier(s): RR, KE

↺ ✳ **E2327** Power wheelchair accessory, head control interface, mechanical, proportional, including all related electronics, mechanical direction change switch, and fixed mounting hardware ⑧ Qp Qh ♿   Y

   DMEPOS Modifier(s): RR, KC, KE

↺ ✳ **E2328** Power wheelchair accessory, head control or extremity control interface, electronic, proportional, including all related electronics and fixed mounting hardware ⑧ Qp Qh ♿   Y

   DMEPOS Modifier(s): RR, KE

↺ ✳ **E2329** Power wheelchair accessory, head control interface, contact switch mechanism, nonproportional, including all related electronics, mechanical stop switch, mechanical direction change switch, head array, and fixed mounting hardware ⑧ Qp Qh ♿   Y

   DMEPOS Modifier(s): RR, KE

↺ ✳ **E2330** Power wheelchair accessory, head control interface, proximity switch mechanism, nonproportional, including all related electronics, mechanical stop switch, mechanical direction change switch, head array, and fixed mounting hardware ⑧ Qp Qh ♿   Y

   DMEPOS Modifier(s): RR, KE

✳ **E2331** Power wheelchair accessory, attendant control, proportional, including all related electronics and fixed mounting hardware ⑧ Qp Qh   Y

✳ **E2340** Power wheelchair accessory, nonstandard seat frame width, 20-23 inches Qp Qh ♿   Y

   DMEPOS Modifier(s): NU, RR, UE

✳ **E2341** Power wheelchair accessory, nonstandard seat frame width, 24-27 inches ⑧ Qp Qh ♿   Y

   DMEPOS Modifier(s): NU, RR, UE

✳ **E2342** Power wheelchair accessory, nonstandard seat frame depth, 20 or 21 inches ⑧ Qp Qh ♿   Y

   DMEPOS Modifier(s): NU, RR, UE

✳ **E2343** Power wheelchair accessory, nonstandard seat frame depth, 22-25 inches ⑧ Qp Qh ♿   Y

   DMEPOS Modifier(s): NU, RR, UE

↺ ✳ **E2351** Power wheelchair accessory, electronic interface to operate speech generating device using power wheelchair control interface ⑧ Qp Qh ♿   Y

   DMEPOS Modifier(s): RR, KE

✳ **E2358** Power wheelchair accessory, Group 34 non-sealed lead acid battery, each ⑧ Qp Qh ♿   Y

✳ **E2359** Power wheelchair accessory, Group 34 sealed lead acid battery, each (e.g., gel cell, absorbed glassmat) ⑧ Qp Qh ♿   Y

   DMEPOS Modifier(s): NU, PR, UE

✳ **E2360** Power wheelchair accessory, 22 NF non-sealed lead acid battery, each ⑧ ♿   Y

   DMEPOS Modifier(s): KE, NU, RR, UE

✳ **E2361** Power wheelchair accessory, 22NF sealed lead acid battery, each, (e.g. gel cell, absorbed glassmat) ⑧ Qp Qh ♿   Y

   DMEPOS Modifier(s): KE, NU, RR, UE

✳ **E2362** Power wheelchair accessory, group 24 non-sealed lead acid battery, each ⑧ ♿   Y

   DMEPOS Modifier(s): NU, RR, UE

✳ **E2363** Power wheelchair accessory, group 24 sealed lead acid battery, each (e.g. gel cell, absorbed glassmat) ⑧ Qp Qh ♿   Y

   DMEPOS Modifier(s): KE, NU, RR, UE

✳ **E2364** Power wheelchair accessory, U-1 non-sealed lead acid battery, each ⑧ ♿   Y

   DMEPOS Modifier(s): NU, RR, UE

✳ **E2365** Power wheelchair accessory, U-1 sealed lead acid battery, each (e.g. gel cell, absorbed glassmat) ⑧ Qp Qh ♿   Y

   DMEPOS Modifier(s): KE, NU, RR, UE

✳ **E2366** Power wheelchair accessory, battery charger, single mode, for use with only one battery type, sealed or non-sealed, each ⑧ Qp Qh ♿   Y

   DMEPOS Modifier(s): KE, NU, RR, UE

⒫ PQRS	Qp Quantity Physician Appendix A	Qh Quantity Hospital Appendix B	♀ Female only
♂ Male only	A Age	♿ DMEPOS	A2-Z3 ASC Payment Indicator	A-Y ASC Status Indicator	Coding Clinic

* **E2367** Power wheelchair accessory, battery charger, dual mode, for use with either battery type, sealed or non-sealed, each Ⓑ Qp Qh ♿   Y

DMEPOS Modifier(s): KE, NU, RR, UE

* **E2368** Power wheelchair component, drive wheel motor, replacement only Ⓑ Qp Qh ♿   Y

DMEPOS Modifier(s): KE, NU, RR, UE

* **E2369** Power wheelchair component, drive wheel gear box, replacement only Ⓑ Qp Qh ♿   Y

DMEPOS Modifier(s): KE, NU, RR, UE

* **E2370** Power wheelchair component, integrated drive wheel motor and gear box combination, replacement only Ⓑ Qp Qh ♿   Y

DMEPOS Modifier(s): KE, NU, RR, UE

* **E2371** Power wheelchair accessory, group 27 sealed lead acid battery, (e.g. gel cell, absorbed glass mat), each Ⓑ Qp Qh ♿   Y

DMEPOS Modifier(s): KE, NU, RR, UE

* **E2372** Power wheelchair accessory, group 27 non-sealed lead acid battery, each Ⓑ ♿   Y

DMEPOS Modifier(s): NU, RR, UE

⟳* **E2373** Power wheelchair accessory, hand or chin control interface, compact remote joystick, proportional, including fixed mounting hardware Ⓑ Qp Qh ♿   Y

DMEPOS Modifier(s): RR, KC, KE

⟳◎ **E2374** Power wheelchair accessory, hand or chin control interface, standard remote joystick (not including controller), proportional, including all related electronics and fixed mounting hardware, replacement only Ⓑ Qp Qh ♿   Y

DMEPOS Modifier(s): RR, KE

◎ **E2375** Power wheelchair accessory, non-expandable controller, including all related electronics and mounting hardware, replacement only Ⓑ Qp Qh ♿   Y

DMEPOS Modifier(s): KE, NU, RR, UE

⟳◎ **E2376** Power wheelchair accessory, expandable controller, including all related electronics and mounting hardware, replacement only Ⓑ Qp Qh ♿   Y

DMEPOS Modifier(s): RR, KE

⟳◎ **E2377** Power wheelchair accessory, expandable controller, including all related electronics and mounting hardware, upgrade provided at initial issue Ⓑ Qp Qh ♿   Y

DMEPOS Modifier(s): RR, KE

⟳* **E2378** Power wheelchair component, actuator, replacement only Ⓑ Qp Qh ♿   Y

DMEPOS Modifier(s): NU, RR, UE

◎ **E2381** Power wheelchair accessory, pneumatic drive wheel tire, any size, replacement only, each Ⓑ Qp Qh ♿   Y

DMEPOS Modifier(s): KE, NU, RR, UE

◎ **E2382** Power wheelchair accessory, tube for pneumatic drive wheel tire, any size, replacement only, each Ⓑ Qp Qh ♿   Y

DMEPOS Modifier(s): KE, NU, RR, UE

◎ **E2383** Power wheelchair accessory, insert for pneumatic drive wheel tire (removable), any type, any size, replacement only, each Ⓑ Qp Qh ♿   Y

DMEPOS Modifier(s): KE, NU, RR, UE

◎ **E2384** Power wheelchair accessory, pneumatic caster tire, any size, replacement only, each Ⓑ Qp Qh ♿   Y

DMEPOS Modifier(s): KE, NU, RR, UE

◎ **E2385** Power wheelchair accessory, tube for pneumatic caster tire, any size, replacement only, each Ⓑ Qp Qh ♿   Y

DMEPOS Modifier(s): KE, NU, RR, UE

◎ **E2386** Power wheelchair accessory, foam filled drive wheel tire, any size, replacement only, each Ⓑ Qp Qh ♿   Y

DMEPOS Modifier(s): KE, NU, RR, UE

◎ **E2387** Power wheelchair accessory, foam filled caster tire, any size, replacement only, each Ⓑ Qp Qh ♿   Y

DMEPOS Modifier(s): KE, NU, RR, UE

◎ **E2388** Power wheelchair accessory, foam drive wheel tire, any size, replacement only, each Ⓑ Qp Qh ♿   Y

DMEPOS Modifier(s): KE, NU, RR, UE

◎ **E2389** Power wheelchair accessory, foam caster tire, any size, replacement only, each Ⓑ Qp Qh ♿   Y

DMEPOS Modifier(s): KE, NU, RR, UE

◎ **E2390** Power wheelchair accessory, solid (rubber/plastic) drive wheel tire, any size, replacement only, each Ⓑ Qp Qh ♿   Y

DMEPOS Modifier(s): KE, NU, RR, UE

▶ New   ⟳ Revised   ✔ Reinstated   ~~deleted~~ Deleted   ⃠ Not covered or valid by Medicare
◎ Special coverage instructions   * Carrier discretion   Ⓑ Bill local carrier   Ⓑ Bill DME MAC

⊛ **E2391** Power wheelchair accessory, solid (rubber/plastic) caster tire (removable), any size, replacement only, each ⑥ Qp Qh ⤓   Y

    DMEPOS Modifier(s): KE, NU, RR, UE

⊛ **E2392** Power wheelchair accessory, solid (rubber/plastic) caster tire with integrated wheel, any size, replacement only, each ⑥ Qp Qh ⤓   Y

    DMEPOS Modifier(s): KE, NU, RR, UE

⊛ **E2394** Power wheelchair accessory, drive wheel excludes tire, any size, replacement only, each ⑥ Qp Qh ⤓   Y

    DMEPOS Modifier(s): KE, NU, RR, UE

⊛ **E2395** Power wheelchair accessory, caster wheel excludes tire, any size, replacement only, each ⑥ Qp Qh ⤓   Y

    DMEPOS Modifier(s): KE, NU, RR, UE

⊛ **E2396** Power wheelchair accessory, caster fork, any size, replacement only, each ⑥ Qp Qh ⤓   Y

    DMEPOS Modifier(s): KE, NU, RR, UE

✳ **E2397** Power wheelchair accessory, lithium-based battery, each ⑥ Qp Qh ⤓   Y

    DMEPOS Modifier(s): NU, RR, UE

Negative Pressure

✳ **E2402** Negative pressure wound therapy electrical pump, stationary or portable ⑥ Qp Qh ⤓   Y

    Document at least every 30 calendar days the quantitative wound characteristics, including wound surface area (length, width and depth)

    Medicare coverage up to a maximum of 15 dressing kits (A6550) per wound per month unless documentation states that the wound size requires more than one dressing kit for each dressing change.

    DMEPOS Modifier(s): RR

Speech Device

↻⊛ **E2500** Speech generating device, digitized speech, using pre-recorded messages, less than or equal to 8 minutes recording time ⑥ Qp Qh ⤓   Y

    IOM: 100-03, 1, 50.1

    DMEPOS Modifier(s): RR

↻⊛ **E2502** Speech generating device, digitized speech, using pre-recorded messages, greater than 8 minutes but less than or equal to 20 minutes recording time ⑥ Qp Qh ⤓   Y

    IOM: 100-03, 1, 50.1

    DMEPOS Modifier(s): RR

↻⊛ **E2504** Speech generating device, digitized speech, using pre-recorded messages, greater than 20 minutes but less than or equal to 40 minutes recording time ⑥ Qp Qh ⤓   Y

    IOM: 100-03, 1, 50.1

    DMEPOS Modifier(s): RR

↻⊛ **E2506** Speech generating device, digitized speech, using pre-recorded messages, greater than 40 minutes recording time ⑥ Qp Qh ⤓   Y

    IOM: 100-03, 1, 50.1

    DMEPOS Modifier(s): RR

↻⊛ **E2508** Speech generating device, synthesized speech, requiring message formulation by spelling and access by physical contact with the device ⑥ Qp Qh ⤓   Y

    IOM: 100-03, 1, 50.1

    DMEPOS Modifier(s): RR

↻⊛ **E2510** Speech generating device, synthesized speech, permitting multiple methods of message formulation and multiple methods of device access ⑥ Qp Qh ⤓   Y

    IOM: 100-03, 1, 50.1

    DMEPOS Modifier(s): RR

⊛ **E2511** Speech generating software program, for personal computer or personal digital assistant ⑥ Qp Qh ⤓   Y

    IOM: 100-03, 1, 50.1

    DMEPOS Modifier(s): NU, RR, UE

⊛ **E2512** Accessory for speech generating device, mounting system ⑥ Qp Qh ⤓   Y

    IOM: 100-03, 1, 50.1

    DMEPOS Modifier(s): NU, RR, UE

↻⊛ **E2599** Accessory for speech generating device, not otherwise classified ⑥   Y

    IOM: 100-03, 1, 50.1

Wheelchair, Cushion and Protection

✳ **E2601** General use wheelchair seat cushion, width less than 22 inches, any depth ⑥ Qp Qh ⤓   Y

    DMEPOS Modifier(s): NU, KE, RR, UE

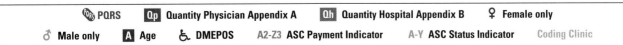

℗ᴏʀˢ PQRS	Qp Quantity Physician Appendix A	Qh Quantity Hospital Appendix B	♀ Female only
♂ Male only	A Age	⤓ DMEPOS	A2-Z3 ASC Payment Indicator	A-Y ASC Status Indicator	Coding Clinic

197

MISCELLANEOUS   E2391 — E2601

* **E2602** General use wheelchair seat cushion, width 22 inches or greater, any depth Ⓑ Qp Qh ♿   Y

  DMEPOS Modifier(s): NU, KE, RR, UE

* **E2603** Skin protection wheelchair seat cushion, width less than 22 inches, any depth Ⓑ Qp Qh ♿   Y

  DMEPOS Modifier(s): NU, KE, RR, UE

* **E2604** Skin protection wheelchair seat cushion, width 22 inches or greater, any depth Ⓑ Qp Qh ♿   Y

  DMEPOS Modifier(s): NU, KE, RR, UE

* **E2605** Positioning wheelchair seat cushion, width less than 22 inches, any depth Ⓑ Qp Qh ♿   Y

* **E2606** Positioning wheelchair seat cushion, width 22 inches or greater, any depth Ⓑ Qp Qh ♿   Y

  DMEPOS Modifier(s): NU, KE, RR, UE

* **E2607** Skin protection and positioning wheelchair seat cushion, width less than 22 inches, any depth Ⓑ Qp Qh ♿   Y

  DMEPOS Modifier(s): NU, KE, RR, UE

* **E2608** Skin protection and positioning wheelchair seat cushion, width 22 inches or greater, any depth Ⓑ Qp Qh ♿   Y

  DMEPOS Modifier(s): NU, KE, RR, UE

* **E2609** Custom fabricated wheelchair seat cushion, any size Ⓑ Qp Qh   Y

* **E2610** Wheelchair seat cushion, powered Ⓑ   B

* **E2611** General use wheelchair back cushion, width less than 22 inches, any height, including any type mounting hardware Ⓑ Qp Qh ♿   Y

  DMEPOS Modifier(s): NU, KE, RR, UE

* **E2612** General use wheelchair back cushion, width 22 inches or greater, any height, including any type mounting hardware Ⓑ Qp Qh ♿   Y

  DMEPOS Modifier(s): NU, KE, RR, UE

* **E2613** Positioning wheelchair back cushion, posterior, width less than 22 inches, any height, including any type mounting hardware Ⓑ Qp Qh ♿   Y

  DMEPOS Modifier(s): NU, KE, RR, UE

* **E2614** Positioning wheelchair back cushion, posterior, width 22 inches or greater, any height, including any type mounting hardware Ⓑ Qp Qh ♿   Y

  DMEPOS Modifier(s): NU, KE, RR, UE

* **E2615** Positioning wheelchair back cushion, posterior-lateral, width less than 22 inches, any height, including any type mounting hardware Ⓑ Qp Qh ♿   Y

  DMEPOS Modifier(s): NU, KE, RR, UE

* **E2616** Positioning wheelchair back cushion, posterior-lateral, width 22 inches or greater, any height, including any type mounting hardware Ⓑ Qp Qh ♿   Y

  DMEPOS Modifier(s): NU, KE, RR, UE

* **E2617** Custom fabricated wheelchair back cushion, any size, including any type mounting hardware Ⓑ Qp Qh   Y

* **E2619** Replacement cover for wheelchair seat cushion or back cushion, each Ⓑ Qp Qh ♿   Y

  DMEPOS Modifier(s): NU, KE, RR, UE

* **E2620** Positioning wheelchair back cushion, planar back with lateral supports, width less than 22 inches, any height, including any type mounting hardware Ⓑ Qp Qh ♿   Y

  DMEPOS Modifier(s): NU, KE, RR, UE

* **E2621** Positioning wheelchair back cushion, planar back with lateral supports, width 22 inches or greater, any height, including any type mounting hardware Ⓑ Qp Qh ♿   Y

  DMEPOS Modifier(s): NU, KE, RR, UE

SKIN PROTECTION, WHEELCHAIR (E2622-E2625)

* **E2622** Skin protection wheelchair seat cushion, adjustable, width less than 22 inches, any depth Qp Qh ♿   Y

  DMEPOS Modifier(s): NU, KE, RR, UE

* **E2623** Skin protection wheelchair seat cushion, adjustable, width 22 inches or greater, any depth Qp Qh ♿   Y

  DMEPOS Modifier(s): NU, KE, RR, UE

* **E2624** Skin protection and positioning wheelchair seat cushion, adjustable, width less than 22 inches, any depth Qp Qh ♿   Y

  DMEPOS Modifier(s): NU, KE, RR, UE

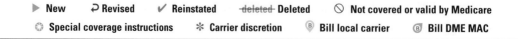

▶ New ↻ Revised ✔ Reinstated ~~deleted~~ Deleted ⊘ Not covered or valid by Medicare
⊛ Special coverage instructions ✳ Carrier discretion Ⓑ Bill local carrier Ⓑ Bill DME MAC

❋ **E2625** Skin protection and positioning wheelchair seat cushion, adjustable, width 22 inches or greater, any depth Qp Qh ♿   Y

DMEPOS Modifier(s): NU, KE, RR, UE

ARM SUPPORT (E2626-E2633)

❋ **E2626** Wheelchair accessory, shoulder elbow, mobile arm support attached to wheelchair, balanced, adjustable Qp Qh ♿   Y

DMEPOS Modifier(s): NU, RR, UE

❋ **E2627** Wheelchair accessory, shoulder elbow, mobile arm support attached to wheelchair, balanced, adjustable rancho type Qp Qh ♿   Y

DMEPOS Modifier(s): NU, RR, UE

❋ **E2628** Wheelchair accessory, shoulder elbow, mobile arm support attached to wheelchair, balanced, reclining Qp Qh ♿   Y

DMEPOS Modifier(s): NU, RR, UE

❋ **E2629** Wheelchair accessory, shoulder elbow, mobile arm support attached to wheelchair, balanced, friction arm support (friction dampening to proximal and distal joints) Qp Qh ♿   Y

DMEPOS Modifier(s): NU, RR, UE

❋ **E2630** Wheelchair accessory, shoulder elbow, mobile arm support, monosuspension arm and hand support, overhead elbow forearm hand sling support, yoke type suspension support Qp Qh ♿   Y

DMEPOS Modifier(s): NU, RR, UE

❋ **E2631** Wheelchair accessory, addition to mobile arm support, elevating proximal arm Qp Qh ♿   Y

DMEPOS Modifier(s): NU, RR, UE

❋ **E2632** Wheelchair accessory, addition to mobile arm support, offset or lateral rocker arm with elastic balance control Qp Qh ♿   Y

DMEPOS Modifier(s): NU, RR, UE

❋ **E2633** Wheelchair accessory, addition to mobile arm support, supinator Qp Qh ♿   Y

DMEPOS Modifier(s): NU, RR, UE

GAIT TRAINER (E8000-E8002)

⊘ **E8000** Gait trainer, pediatric size, posterior support, includes all accessories and components Ⓑ A   E

⊘ **E8001** Gait trainer, pediatric size, upright support, includes all accessories and components Ⓑ A   E

⊘ **E8002** Gait trainer, pediatric size, anterior support, includes all accessories and components Ⓑ A   E

| 🅿️ PQRS | Qp Quantity Physician Appendix A | Qh Quantity Hospital Appendix B | ♀ Female only |
| ♂ Male only | A Age | ♿ DMEPOS | A2-Z3 ASC Payment Indicator | A-Y ASC Status Indicator | Coding Clinic |

199

GAIT TRAINER   E2625 — E8002

TEMPORARY PROCEDURES/PROFESSIONAL SERVICES (G0000-G9999)

NOTE: Series "G", "K", and "Q" in the Level II coding are reserved for CMS assignment. "G", "K", and "Q" codes are temporary national codes for items or services requiring uniform national coding between one year's update and the next. Sometimes "temporary" codes remain for more than one update. If "G", "K", and "Q" codes are not converted to permanent codes in Level I or Level II series in the following update, they will remain active until converted in following years or until CMS notifies contractors to delete them. All active "G", "K", and "Q" codes at the time of update will be included on the update file for contractors. In addition, deleted codes are retained on the file for informational purposes, with a deleted indicator, for four years.

Administration, Vaccine

✳ **G0008** Administration of influenza virus vaccine Ⓑ 〔Qp〕〔Qh〕   S

Coinsurance and deductible do not apply. If provided, report significant, separately identifiable E/M for medically necessary services (V04.81)

✳ **G0009** Administration of pneumococcal vaccine Ⓑ 〔Qp〕〔Qh〕   S

Reported once in a lifetime based on risk; Medicare covers cost of vaccine and administration (V03.82)

Copayment, coinsurance, and deductible waived. (https://www.cms.gov/MLNProducts/downloads/MPS_QuickReferenceChart_1.pdf)

✳ **G0010** Administration of hepatitis B vaccine Ⓑ 〔Qp〕〔Qh〕   S

Report for other than OPPs. Coinsurance and deductible apply; Medicare covers both cost of vaccine and administration (V05.3)

Copayment/coinsurance and deductible are waived. (https://www.cms.gov/MLNProducts/downloads/MPS_QuickReferenceChart_1.pdf)

Semen Analysis

✳ **G0027** Semen analysis; presence and/or motility of sperm excluding Huhner Ⓑ 〔Qp〕〔Qh〕 ♀   N

Laboratory Certification: Hematology

Screening, Cervical

⊛ ◎ **G0101** Cervical or vaginal cancer screening; pelvic and clinical breast examination Ⓑ 〔Qp〕〔Qh〕 ♀   V

Covered once every two years and annually if high risk for cervical/vaginal cancer, or if childbearing age patient has had an abnormal Pap smear in preceding three years. High risk diagnosis, V15.89

Coding Clinic: 2002, Q4, P8

Screening, Prostate

◎ **G0102** Prostate cancer screening; digital rectal examination Ⓑ 〔Qp〕〔Qh〕 ♀   N

Covered annually by Medicare (V76.44). Not separately payable with an E/M code (99201-99499).

IOM: 100-02, 6, 10; 100-04, 4, 240

IOM: 100-04, 18, 50.1

◎ **G0103** Prostate cancer screening; prostate specific antigen test (PSA) Ⓑ 〔Qp〕〔Qh〕 ♀   Z3 N

Covered annually by Medicare (V76.44)

IOM: 100-02, 6, 10; 100-04, 4, 240

IOM: 100-04, 18, 50

Laboratory Certification: Routine chemistry

Screening, Colorectal

◎ **G0104** Colorectal cancer screening; flexible sigmoidoscopy Ⓑ 〔Qp〕〔Qh〕   P3 S

Covered once every 48 months for beneficiaries age 50+

Co-insurance waived under Section 4104.

Coding Clinic: 2011, Q2, P4

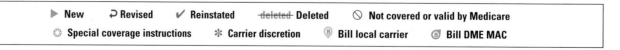

▶ **New**   ↻ **Revised**   ✔ **Reinstated**   ~~deleted~~ **Deleted**   ⊘ **Not covered or valid by Medicare**
⊛ **Special coverage instructions**   ✳ **Carrier discretion**   Ⓑ **Bill local carrier**   Ⓓ **Bill DME MAC**

(PQRS) ⊘ **G0105** Colorectal cancer screening; colonoscopy on individual at high risk Ⓑ Qp Qh A2 T

Screening colonoscopy covered once every 24 months for high risk for developing colorectal cancer. May use modifier 53 if appropriate (physician fee schedule)

Co-insurance waived under Section 4104.

Coding Clinic: 2011, Q2, P4

(PQRS) ⊘ **G0106** Colorectal cancer screening; alternative to G0104, screening sigmoidoscopy, barium enema Ⓑ Qp Qh S

Barium enema (not high risk) (alternative to G0104). Covered once every 4 years for beneficiaries age 50+. Use modifier 26 for professional component only.

Coding Clinic: 2011, Q2, P4

Training Services, Diabetes

(PQRS) ✳ **G0108** Diabetes outpatient self-management training services, individual, per 30 minutes Ⓑ A

Report for beneficiaries diagnosed with diabetes.

Effective January 2011, DSMT will be included in the list of reimbursable Medicare telehealth services.

✳ **G0109** Diabetes outpatient self-management training services, group session (2 or more) per 30 minutes Ⓑ A

Report for beneficiaries diagnosed with diabetes.

Effective January 2011, DSMT will be included in the list of reimbursable Medicare telehealth services.

Screening, Glaucoma

✳ **G0117** Glaucoma screening for high risk patients furnished by an optometrist or ophthalmologist Ⓑ Qp Qh S

Covered once per year (full 11 months between screenings). Bundled with all other ophthalmic services provided on same day. Diagnosis code V80.1

✳ **G0118** Glaucoma screening for high risk patient furnished under the direct supervision of an optometrist or ophthalmologist Ⓑ Qp Qh S

Covered once per year (full 11 months between screenings). Diagnosis code V80.1

Screening, Colorectal, Other

(PQRS) ⊘ **G0120** Colorectal cancer screening; alternative to G0105, screening colonoscopy, barium enema. Qp Qh S

Barium enema for patients with a high risk of developing colorectal. Covered once every 2 years. Used as an alternative to G0105. Use modifier 26 for professional component only

(PQRS) ⊘ **G0121** Colorectal cancer screening; colonoscopy on individual not meeting criteria for high risk Ⓑ Qp Qh A2 T

Screening colonoscopy for patients that are not high risk. Covered once every 10 years, but not within 48 months of a G0104. For non-Medicare patients report 45378.

Co-insurance waived under Section 4104.

⊘ **G0122** Colorectal cancer screening; barium enema Ⓑ E

Medicare: this service is denied as noncovered, because it fails to meet the requirements of the benefit. The beneficiary is liable for payment.

Screening, Cytopathology

⊘ **G0123** Screening cytopathology, cervical or vaginal (any reporting system), collected in preservative fluid, automated thin layer preparation, screening by cytotechnologist under physician supervision Ⓑ Qp Qh ♀ N

Use G0123 or G0143 or G0144 or G0145 or G0147 or G0148 or P3000 for Pap smears NOT requiring physician interpretation (technical component)

IOM: 100-03, 3, 190.2; 100-04, 18, 30

Laboratory Certification: Cytology

| (PQRS) PQRS | Qp Quantity Physician Appendix A | Qh Quantity Hospital Appendix B | ♀ Female only |
| ♂ Male only | A Age | ♿ DMEPOS | A2-Z3 ASC Payment Indicator | A-Y ASC Status Indicator | Coding Clinic |

201

TEMPORARY PROCEDURES/PROFESSIONAL SERVICES   G0105 – G0123

⊘ **G0124** Screening cytopathology, cervical or vaginal (any reporting system), collected in preservative fluid, automated thin layer preparation, requiring interpretation by physician Ⓑ **Qp** **Qh** ♀   B

Report professional component for Pap smears requiring physician interpretation

IOM: 100-03, 3, 190.2; 100-04, 18, 30

Laboratory Certification: Cytology

Trimming, Nail

⮌ ⊘ **G0127** Trimming of dystrophic nails, any number Ⓑ **Qp** **Qh**   P3 Q1

Must be used with a modifier (Q7, Q8, or Q9) to show that the foot care service is needed because the beneficiary has a systemic disease. Limit 1 unit of service

IOM: 100-02, 15, 290

Service, Nursing and OT

⊘ **G0128** Direct (face-to-face with patient) skilled nursing services of a registered nurse provided in a comprehensive outpatient rehabilitation facility, each 10 minutes beyond the first 5 minutes Ⓑ **Qp** **Qh**   B

A separate nursing service that is clearly identifiable in the Plan of Treatment and not part of other services. Documentation must support this service. Examples include: Insertion of a urinary catheter, intramuscular injections, bowel disimpaction, nursing assessment, and education. Restricted coverage by Medicare.

Medicare Statute 1833(a)

✳ **G0129** Occupational therapy services requiring the skills of a qualified occupational therapist, furnished as a component of a partial hospitalization treatment program, per session (45 minutes or more) Ⓑ **Qh**   P

Study, SEXA

⊘ **G0130** Single energy x-ray absorptiometry (SEXA) bone density study, one or more sites; appendicular skeleton (peripheral) (eg, radius, wrist, heel) Ⓑ **Qp** **Qh**   S

Covered every 24 months (more frequently if medically necessary). Use modifier 26 for professional component only

Preventive service; no deductible

IOM: 100-03, 2, 150.3; 100-04, 13, 140.1

Screening, Cytopathology, Other

✳ **G0141** Screening cytopathology smears, cervical or vaginal, performed by automated system, with manual rescreening, requiring interpretation by physician Ⓑ **Qp** **Qh** ♀   B

Co-insurance, copay, and deductible waived

Report professional component for Pap smears requiring physician interpretation. Refer to diagnosis of V15.89, V76.2, V76.47, or V76.49 to report appropriate risk level

Laboratory Certification: Cytology

✳ **G0143** Screening cytopathology, cervical or vaginal (any reporting system), collected in preservative fluid, automated thin layer preparation, with manual screening and rescreening by cytotechnologist under physician supervision Ⓑ **Qp** **Qh** ♀   N

Co-insurance, copay, and deductible waived

Laboratory Certification: Cytology

✳ **G0144** Screening cytopathology, cervical or vaginal (any reporting system), collected in preservative fluid, automated thin layer preparation, with screening by automated system, under physician supervision Ⓑ **Qp** **Qh** ♀   N

Co-insurance, copay, and deductible waived

Laboratory Certification: Cytology

▶ **New**   ⮌ **Revised**   ✔ **Reinstated**   ~~deleted~~ **Deleted**   ⊘ **Not covered or valid by Medicare**
⊘ **Special coverage instructions**   ✳ **Carrier discretion**   Ⓑ **Bill local carrier**   Ⓑ **Bill DME MAC**

✳ **G0145** Screening cytopathology, cervical or vaginal (any reporting system), collected in preservative fluid, automated thin layer preparation, with screening by automated system and manual rescreening under physician supervision ⑧ **Qp** **Qh** ♀   N

Co-insurance, copay, and deductible waived

Laboratory Certification: Cytology

✳ **G0147** Screening cytopathology smears, cervical or vaginal; performed by automated system under physician supervision ⑧ **Qp** **Qh** ♀   N

Co-insurance, copay, and deductible waived

Laboratory Certification: Cytology

✳ **G0148** Screening cytopathology smears, cervical or vaginal; performed by automated system with manual rescreening ⑧ **Qp** **Qh** ♀   N

Co-insurance, copay, and deductible waived

Laboratory Certification: Cytology

Services, Allied Health

✳ **G0151** Services performed by a qualified physical therapist in the home health or hospice setting, each 15 minutes ⑧   B

✳ **G0152** Services performed by a qualified occupational therapist in the home health or hospice setting, each 15 minutes ⑧   B

✳ **G0153** Services performed by a qualified speech-language pathologist in the home health or hospice setting, each 15 minutes ⑧   B

✳ **G0154** Direct skilled nursing services of a licensed nurse (LPN or RN) in the home health or hospice setting, each 15 minutes ⑧   B

✳ **G0155** Services of clinical social worker in home health or hospice settings, each 15 minutes ⑧   B

✳ **G0156** Services of home health/health aide in home health or hospice settings, each 15 minutes ⑧   B

✳ **G0157** Services performed by a qualified physical therapist assistant in the home health or hospice setting, each 15 minutes ⑧   B

✳ **G0158** Services performed by a qualified occupational therapist assistant in the home health or hospice setting, each 15 minutes ⑧   B

✳ **G0159** Services performed by a qualified physical therapist, in the home health setting, in the establishment or delivery of a safe and effective physical therapy maintenance program, each 15 minutes ⑧   B

✳ **G0160** Services performed by a qualified occupational therapist, in the home health setting, in the establishment or delivery of a safe and effective occupational therapy maintenance program, each 15 minutes ⑧   B

✳ **G0161** Services performed by a qualified speech-language pathologist, in the home health setting, in the establishment or delivery of a safe and effective speech-language pathology maintenance program, each 15 minutes ⑧   B

✳ **G0162** Skilled services by a registered nurse (RN) for management and evaluation of the plan of care; each 15 minutes (the patient's underlying condition or complication requires an RN to ensure that essential non-skilled care achieves its purpose in the home health or hospice setting) ⑧   B

Transmittal No. 824 (CR7182)

✳ **G0163** Skilled services of a licensed nurse (LPN or RN) for the observation and assessment of the patient's condition, each 15 minutes (the of change in the patient's condition requires skilled nursing personnel to identify and evaluate the patient's need for possible modification of treatment in the home health or hospice setting) ⑧   B

Transmittal No. 824 (CR7182)

✳ **G0164** Skilled services of a licensed nurse (LPN or RN), in the training and/or education of a patient or family member, in the home health or hospice setting, each 15 minutes ⑧   B

Transmittal No. 824 (CR7182)

◎ **G0166** External counterpulsation, per treatment session ⑧ **Qp** **Qh**   Q1

IOM: 100-03, 1, 20.20

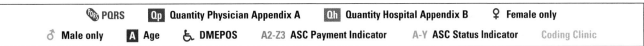

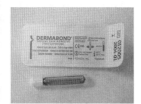

Figure 16 Tissue adhesive.

Wound Closure

✳ **G0168** Wound closure utilizing tissue adhesive(s) only ⑧ **Qp** **Qh**   B

Report for wound closure with only tissue adhesive. If a practitioner utilizes tissue adhesive in addition to staples or sutures to close a wound, HCPCS code G0168 is not separately reportable, but is included in the tissue repair.

The only closure material used for a simple repair, coverage based on payer.

Coding Clinic: 2005, Q1, P5; 2001, Q4, P12; Q3, P13

~~G0173~~   ~~Linear accelerator based stereotactic radiosurgery, complete course of therapy in one session~~   ✖

Team Conference

✳ **G0175** Scheduled interdisciplinary team conference (minimum of three exclusive of patient care nursing staff) with patient present ⑧ **Qp** **Qh**   V

Therapy, Activity

OPPS not separately payable

⊘ **G0176** Activity therapy, such as music, dance, art or play therapies not for recreation, related to the care and treatment of patient's disabling mental health problems, per session (45 minutes or more) ⑧ **Qh**   P

Paid in partial hospitalization

⊘ **G0177** Training and educational services related to the care and treatment of patient's disabling mental health problems per session (45 minutes or more) ⑧ **Qp** **Qh**   N

Paid in partial hospitalization

Physician Services

✳ **G0179** Physician re-certification for Medicare-covered home health services under a home health plan of care (patient not present), including contacts with home health agency and review of reports of patient status required by physicians to affirm the initial implementation of the plan of care that meets patient's needs, per re-certification period ⑧ **Qp** **Qh**   M

The recertification code is used after a patient has received services for at least 60 days (or one certification period) when the physician signs the certification after the initial certification period.

✳ **G0180** Physician certification for Medicare-covered home health services under a home health plan of care (patient not present), including contacts with home health agency and review of reports of patient status required by physicians to affirm the initial implementation of the plan of care that meets patient's needs, per certification period ⑧ **Qp** **Qh**   M

This code can be billed only when the patient has not received Medicare covered home health services for at least 60 days.

✳ **G0181** Physician supervision of a patient receiving Medicare-covered services provided by a participating home health agency (patient not present) requiring complex and multidisciplinary care modalities involving regular physician development and/or revision of care plans, review of subsequent reports of patient status, review of laboratory and other studies, communication (including telephone calls) with other health care professionals involved in the patient's care, integration of new information into the medical treatment plan and/or adjustment of medical therapy, within a calendar month, 30 minutes or more ⑧ **Qp** **Qh**   M

▶ **New**   ↻ **Revised**   ✔ **Reinstated**   ~~deleted~~ **Deleted**   ⊘ **Not covered or valid by Medicare**
⊕ **Special coverage instructions**   ✳ **Carrier discretion**   ⑧ **Bill local carrier**   ⑧ **Bill DME MAC**

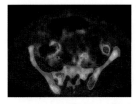

Figure 17 PET scan.

⊛ **G0182** Physician supervision of a patient under a Medicare-approved hospice (patient not present) requiring complex and multidisciplinary care modalities involving regular physician development and/or revision of care plans, review of subsequent reports of patient status, review of laboratory and other studies, communication (including telephone calls) with other health care professionals involved in the patient's care, integration of new information into the medical treatment plan and/or adjustment of medical therapy, within a calendar month, 30 minutes or more ⑧ **Qp** **Qh**   M

Destruction

⊛ **G0186** Destruction of localized lesion of choroid (for example, choroidal neovascularization); photocoagulation, feeder vessel technique (one or more sessions) ⑧ **Qp** **Qh**   R2 T

Mammography

⊛ **G0202** Screening mammography, producing direct digital image, bilateral, all views ⑧ **Qp** **Qh**   A

Screening mammogram reported based on technique, such as 76082, 76083, 76092, or G0202. Requires coinsurance, but no deductible. Diagnosis codes, V76.11 (high risk) or V76.12 (low risk). Use modifier 26 for professional component only

⊅⊛ **G0204** Diagnostic mammography, producing direct 2-D digital image, bilateral, all views ⑧ **Qp** **Qh**   A

Use modifier 26 for professional component only

Coding Clinic: 2013, Q3, P7

⊅⊛ **G0206** Diagnostic mammography, producing direct 2-D digital image, unilateral, all views ⑧ **Qp** **Qh**   A

Use modifier 26 for professional component only

Coding Clinic: 2013, Q3, P7; 2010, Q4, P5

Imaging, PET

⊘ **G0219** PET imaging whole body; melanoma for non-covered indications ⑧   E

Example: Assessing regional lymph nodes in melanoma. Medicare non-covered.

IOM: 100-03, 4, 220.6

Coding Clinic: 2007, Q1, P6

⊘ **G0235** PET imaging, any site, not otherwise specified ⑧ **Qp** **Qh**   E

Example: Prostate cancer diagnosis and initial staging. Medicare non-covered.

IOM: 100-03, 4, 220.6

Coding Clinic: 2007, Q1, P6

Therapeutic Procedures

⊛ **G0237** Therapeutic procedures to increase strength or endurance of respiratory muscles, face to face, one on one, each 15 minutes (includes monitoring) ⑧   Q1

⊛ **G0238** Therapeutic procedures to improve respiratory function, other than described by G0237, one on one, face to face, per 15 minutes (includes monitoring) ⑧   Q1

⊛ **G0239** Therapeutic procedures to improve respiratory function or increase strength or endurance of respiratory muscles, two or more individuals (includes monitoring) ⑧ **Qp** **Qh**   Q1

PQRS   **Qp** Quantity Physician Appendix A   **Qh** Quantity Hospital Appendix B   ♀ **Female only**

♂ **Male only**   **A** **Age**   🦽 **DMEPOS**   A2-Z3 **ASC Payment Indicator**   A-Y **ASC Status Indicator**   *Coding Clinic*

Physician Service, Diabetic

⚙ **G0245** Initial physician evaluation and management of a diabetic patient with diabetic sensory neuropathy resulting in a loss of protective sensation (LOPS) which must include (1) the diagnosis of LOPS, (2) a patient history, (3) a physical examination that consist of at least the following elements: (A) visual inspection of the forefoot, hindfoot and toe web spaces, (B) evaluation of a protective sensation, (C) evaluation of foot structure and biomechanics, (D) evaluation of vascular status and skin integrity, and (E) evaluation and recommendation of footwear, and (4) patient education Ⓑ **Qp** **Qh**   V

Report one of the following diagnosis codes in conjunction with this code: 250.60, 250.61, 250.62, 250.63, or 357.2

IOM: 100-03, 1, 70.2.1

⚙ **G0246** Follow-up physician evaluation and management of a diabetic patient with diabetic sensory neuropathy resulting in a loss of protective sensation (LOPS) to include at least the following: (1) a patient history, (2) a physical examination that includes: (A) visual inspection of the forefoot, hindfoot and toe web spaces, (B) evaluation of protective sensation, (C) evaluation of foot structure and biomechanics, (D) evaluation of vascular status and skin integrity, and (E) evaluation and recommendation of footwear, and (3) patient education Ⓑ **Qp** **Qh**   V

IOM: 100-03, 1, 70.2.1; 100-02, 15, 290

Foot Care

↻ ⚙ **G0247** Routine foot care by a physician of a diabetic patient with diabetic sensory neuropathy resulting in a loss of protective sensation (LOPS) to include, the local care of superficial wounds (i.e. superficial to muscle and fascia) and at least the following if present: (1) local care of superficial wounds, (2) debridement of corns and calluses, and (3) trimming and debridement of nails Ⓑ **Qp** **Qh**   P2 Q1

IOM: 100-03, 1, 70.2.1

Demonstration, INR

⚙ **G0248** Demonstration, prior to initiation, of home INR monitoring for patient with either mechanical heart valve(s), chronic atrial fibrillation, or venous thromboembolism who meets Medicare coverage criteria, under the direction of a physician; includes: face-to-face demonstration of use and care of the INR monitor, obtaining at least one blood sample, provision of instructions for reporting home INR test results, and documentation of patient's ability to perform testing and report results Ⓑ **Qp** **Qh**   V

⚙ **G0249** Provision of test materials and equipment for home INR monitoring of patient with either mechanical heart valve(s), chronic atrial fibrillation, or venous thromboembolism who meets Medicare coverage criteria; includes provision of materials for use in the home and reporting of test results to physician; testing not occurring more frequently than once a week; testing materials, billing units of service include 4 tests Ⓑ **Qp** **Qh**   V

⚙ **G0250** Physician review, interpretation, and patient management of home INR testing for patient with either mechanical heart valve(s), chronic atrial fibrillation, or venous thromboembolism who meets Medicare coverage criteria; testing not occurring more frequently than once a week; billing units of service include 4 tests Ⓑ **Qp** **Qh**   M

G0251 ~~Linear accelerator based stereotactic radiosurgery, delivery including collimator changes and custom plugging, fractionated treatment, all lesions, per session, maximum five sessions per course of treatment~~ ✱

▶ **New**   ↻ **Revised**   ✔ **Reinstated**   ~~deleted~~ **Deleted**   ⊘ **Not covered or valid by Medicare**
⚙ **Special coverage instructions**   ✱ **Carrier discretion**   Ⓑ **Bill local carrier**   Ⓑ **Bill DME MAC**

Imaging, PET

⊘ **G0252** PET imaging, full and partial-ring PET scanners only, for initial diagnosis of breast cancer and/or surgical planning for breast cancer (e.g. initial staging of axillary lymph nodes) Ⓑ   E

IOM: 100-03, 4, 220.6

Coding Clinic: 2007, Q1, P6

SNCT

⊘ **G0255** Current perception threshold/sensory nerve conduction test (SNCT), per limb, any nerve Ⓑ   E

IOM: 100-03, 2, 160.23

Dialysis, Emergency

✪ **G0257** Unscheduled or emergency dialysis treatment for an ESRD patient in a hospital outpatient department that is not certified as an ESRD facility Ⓑ **Qh**   S

Coding Clinic: 2003, Q1, P9

Injection, Arthrography

✪ **G0259** Injection procedure for sacroiliac joint; arthrography Ⓑ **Qp** **Qh**   N1 N

Replaces 27096 for reporting injections for Medicare beneficiaries

Used by Part A only (facility), not priced by Part B Medicare.

✪ **G0260** Injection procedure for sacroiliac joint; provision of anesthetic, steroid and/or other therapeutic agent, with or without arthrography Ⓑ **Qp** **Qh**   A2 T

ASCs report when a therapeutic sacroiliac joint injection is administered in ASC

Removal, Cerumen

✳ **G0268** Removal of impacted cerumen (one or both ears) by physician on same date of service as audiologic function testing Ⓑ **Qp** **Qh**   N1 N

Report only when a physician, not an audiologist, performs the procedure.

Use with DX 380.4 when performed by physician.

Coding Clinic: 2003, Q1, P12

Placement, Occlusive Device

✪ **G0269** Placement of occlusive device into either a venous or arterial access site, post surgical or interventional procedure (e.g. angioseal plug, vascular plug) Ⓑ   N1 N

Report for replacement of vasoseal. Hospitals may report the closure device as a supply with C1760. Bundled status on Physician Fee Schedule.

Coding Clinic: 2011, Q3, P4; 2010, Q4, P6

Therapy, Nutrition

🅟 ✳ **G0270** Medical nutrition therapy; reassessment and subsequent intervention(s) following second referral in same year for change in diagnosis, medical condition or treatment regimen (including additional hours needed for renal disease), individual, face to face with the patient, each 15 minutes Ⓑ   A

Requires physician referral for beneficiaries with diabetes or renal disease. Services must be provided by dietitian/nutritionist. Co-insurance and deductible waived.

🅟 ✳ **G0271** Medical nutrition therapy, reassessment and subsequent intervention(s) following second referral in same year for change in diagnosis, medical condition, or treatment regimen (including additional hours needed for renal disease), group (2 or more individuals), each 30 minutes Ⓑ   A

Requires physician referral for beneficiaries with diabetes or renal disease. Services must be provided by dietitian/nutritionist. Co-insurance and deductible waived.

Blinded Procedure

▶ ✪ **G0276** Blinded procedure for lumbar stenosis, percutaneous image-guided lumbar decompression (PILD) or placebo-control, performed in an approved coverage with evidence development (CED) clinical trial   T

Therapy, Hyperbaric Oxygen

▶ ✪ **G0277** Hyperbaric oxygen under pressure, full body chamber, per 30 minute interval   S

IOM: 100-03, 1, 20.29

🅟 PQRS	**Qp** Quantity Physician Appendix A	**Qh** Quantity Hospital Appendix B	♀ Female only
♂ Male only	**A** Age	♿ DMEPOS	A2-Z3 ASC Payment Indicator	A-Y ASC Status Indicator	Coding Clinic

Angiography

 * **G0278** Iliac and/or femoral artery angiography, non-selective, bilateral or ipsilateral to catheter insertion, performed at the same time as cardiac catheterization and/or coronary angiography, includes positioning or placement of the catheter in the distal aorta or ipsilateral femoral or iliac artery, injection of dye, production of permanent images, and radiologic supervision and interpretation (list separately in addition to primary procedure) ⑧ **Qp** **Qh**   N

Medicare specific code not reported for iliac injection used as a guiding shot for a closure device

Coding Clinic: 2011, Q3, P4; 2006, Q4, P7

Diagnostic

▶ * **G0279** Diagnostic digital breast tomosynthesis, unilateral or bilateral (list separately in addition to G0204 or G0206)   A

Stimulation, Electrical

* **G0281** Electrical stimulation, (unattended), to one or more areas, for chronic stage III and stage IV pressure ulcers, arterial ulcers, diabetic ulcers, and venous stasis ulcers not demonstrating measurable signs of healing after 30 days of conventional care, as part of a therapy plan of care **Qp** **Qh**   A

Reported by encounter/areas and not by site. Therapists report G0281 and G0283 rather than 97014

⊘ **G0282** Electrical stimulation, (unattended), to one or more areas, for wound care other than described in G0281 ⑧   E

IOM: 100-03, 4, 270.1

* **G0283** Electrical stimulation (unattended), to one or more areas for indication(s) other than wound care, as part of a therapy plan of care ⑧ **Qp** **Qh**   A

Reported by encounter/areas and not by site. Therapists report G0281 and G0283 rather than 97014

Angiography, Arthroscopy

* **G0288** Reconstruction, computed tomographic angiography of aorta for surgical planning for vascular surgery ⑧ **Qp** **Qh**   N1 N

* **G0289** Arthroscopy, knee, surgical, for removal of loose body, foreign body, debridement/shaving of articular cartilage (chondroplasty) at the time of other surgical knee arthroscopy in a different compartment of the same knee ⑧ **Qp** **Qh**   N1 N

Add-on code reported with knee arthroscopy code for major procedure performed—reported once per extra compartment

"The code may be reported twice (or with a unit of two) if the physician performs these procedures in two compartments, in addition to the compartment where the main procedure was performed." (http://www.ama-assn.org/resources/doc/cpt/orthopaedics.pdf)

Procedure, Non-Covered

⊛ **G0293** Noncovered surgical procedure(s) using conscious sedation, regional, general or spinal anesthesia in a Medicare qualifying clinical trial, per day ⑧ **Qp** **Qh**   Q1

⊛ **G0294** Noncovered procedure(s) using either no anesthesia or local anesthesia only, in a Medicare qualifying clinical trial, per day ⑧ **Qp** **Qh**   Q1

Therapy, Electromagnetic

⊘ **G0295** Electromagnetic therapy, to one or more areas, for wound care other than described in G0329 or for other uses ⑧   E

IOM: 100-03, 4, 270.1

Services, Pulmonary Surgery

* **G0302** Pre-operative pulmonary surgery services for preparation for LVRS, complete course of services, to include a minimum of 16 days of services ⑧ **Qp** **Qh**   S

* **G0303** Pre-operative pulmonary surgery services for preparation for LVRS, 10 to 15 days of services ⑧ **Qp** **Qh**   S

* **G0304** Pre-operative pulmonary surgery services for preparation for LVRS, 1 to 9 days of services ⑧ **Qp** **Qh**   S

* **G0305** Post-discharge pulmonary surgery services after LVRS, minimum of 6 days of services ⑧ **Qp** **Qh**   S

▶ **New**	⤾ **Revised**	✔ **Reinstated**	~~deleted~~ **Deleted**	⊘ **Not covered or valid by Medicare**
⊛ **Special coverage instructions**		* **Carrier discretion**	⑧ **Bill local carrier**	⑧ **Bill DME MAC**

Laboratory

✳ **G0306** Complete CBC, automated (HgB, HCT, RBC, WBC, without platelet count) and automated WBC differential count ⓑ Qp Qh   N

Laboratory Certification: Hematology

✳ **G0307** Complete CBC, automated (HgB, HCT, RBC, WBC; without platelet count) ⓑ Qp Qh   N

Laboratory Certification: Hematology

◌ **G0328** Colorectal cancer screening; fecal occult blood test, immunoassay, 1-3 simultaneous ⓑ Qp Qh   N

Co-insurance and deductible waived

Reported for Medicare patients 50+; one FOBT per year, with either G0107 (guaiac-based) or G0328 (immunoassay-based)

Laboratory Certification: Routine Chemistry, Hematology

Coding Clinic: 2012, Q2, P9

Therapy, Electromagnetic

✳ **G0329** Electromagnetic therapy, to one or more areas for chronic stage III and stage IV pressure ulcers, arterial ulcers, and diabetic ulcers and venous stasis ulcers not demonstrating measurable signs of healing after 30 days of conventional care as part of a therapy plan of care ⓑ Qp Qh   A

Fee, Pharmacy

◌ **G0333** Pharmacy dispensing fee for inhalation drug(s); initial 30-day supply as a beneficiary ⓑ Qp Qh   M

Medicare will reimburse an initial dispensing fee to a pharmacy for initial 30-day period of inhalation drugs furnished through DME

US machine

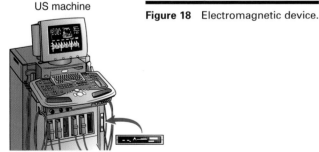

Electromagnetic device

Figure 18 Electromagnetic device.

Hospice

✳ **G0337** Hospice evaluation and counseling services, pre-election ⓑ Qp Qh   B

Radiosurgery, Robotic

✳ **G0339** Image-guided robotic linear accelerator-based stereotactic radiosurgery, complete course of therapy in one session or first session of fractionated treatment ⓑ Qp Qh   B

✳ **G0340** Image-guided robotic linear accelerator-based stereotactic radiosurgery, delivery including collimator changes and custom plugging, fractionated treatment, all lesions, per session, second through fifth sessions, maximum five sessions per course of treatment ⓑ Qp Qh   B

Islet Cell

◌ **G0341** Percutaneous islet cell transplant, includes portal vein catheterization and infusion ⓑ Qp Qh   C

IOM: 100-03, 4, 260.3; 100-04, 32, 70

◌ **G0342** Laparoscopy for islet cell transplant, includes portal vein catheterization and infusion ⓑ Qp Qh   C

IOM: 100-03, 4, 260.3

◌ **G0343** Laparotomy for islet cell transplant, includes portal vein catheterization and infusion ⓑ Qp Qh   C

IOM: 100-03, 4, 260.3

Aspiration, Bone Marrow

⤺ ✳ **G0364** Bone marrow aspiration performed with bone marrow biopsy through the same incision on the same date of service ⓑ Qp Qh   P3 N

For Medicare patients, reported rather than 38220

Coding Clinic: 2012, Q3, P7-8

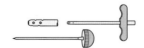

Figure 19 Bone aspiration needles.

| ⓆRS PQRS | Qp Quantity Physician Appendix A | Qh Quantity Hospital Appendix B | ♀ Female only |
| ♂ Male only | A Age | ♿ DMEPOS | A2-Z3 ASC Payment Indicator | A-Y ASC Status Indicator | Coding Clinic |

Mapping, Vessel

✳ **G0365** Vessel mapping of vessels for hemodialysis access (services for preoperative vessel mapping prior to creation of hemodialysis access using an autogenous hemodialysis conduit, including arterial inflow and venous outflow) Ⓑ **Qp** **Qh**   **P2** **S**

Includes evaluation of the relevant arterial and venous vessels. Use modifier 26 for professional component only

⚙ **G0372** Physician service required to establish and document the need for a power mobility device Ⓑ **Qp** **Qh**   **M**

Providers should bill the E/M code and G0372 on the same claim.

Services, Observation and ED

⚙ **G0378** Hospital observation service, per hour Ⓑ   **N**

Report all related services in addition to G0378. Report units of hours spent in observation (rounded to the nearest hour). Hospitals report the ED or clinic visit with a CPT code or, if applicable, G0379 (direct admit to observation) and G0378 (hospital observation services, per hour)

Coding Clinic: 2007, Q1, P10; 2006, Q3, P7-8

⚙ **G0379** Direct admission of patient for hospital observation care Ⓑ **Qh**   **Q3**

Report all related services in addition to G0379. Report units of hours spent in observation (rounded to the nearest hour). Hospitals report the ED or clinic visit with a CPT code or, if applicable, G0379 (direct admit to observation) and G0378 (hospital observation services, per hour)

Coding Clinic: 2007, Q1, P7

✳ **G0380** Level 1 hospital emergency department visit provided in a type B emergency department; (the ED must meet at least one of the following requirements: (1) it is licensed by the state in which it is located under applicable state law as an emergency room or emergency department; (2) it is held out to the public (by name, posted signs, advertising, or other means) as a place that provides care for emergency medical conditions on an urgent basis without requiring a previously scheduled appointment; or (3) during the calendar year immediately preceding the calendar year in which a determination under 42 CFR 489.24 is being made, based on a representative sample of patient visits that occurred during that calendar year, it provides at least one-third of all of its outpatient visits for the treatment of emergency medical conditions on an urgent basis without requiring a previously scheduled appointment) Ⓑ **Qh**   **V**

Coding Clinic: 2009, Q1, P4; 2007, Q2, P1

✳ **G0381** Level 2 hospital emergency department visit provided in a type B emergency department; (the ED must meet at least one of the following requirements: (1) it is licensed by the state in which it is located under applicable state law as an emergency room or emergency department; (2) it is held out to the public (by name, posted signs, advertising, or other means) as a place that provides care for emergency medical conditions on an urgent basis without requiring a previously scheduled appointment; or (3) during the calendar year immediately preceding the calendar year in which a determination under 42 CFR 489.24 is being made, based on a representative sample of patient visits that occurred during that calendar year, it provides at least one-third of all of its outpatient visits for the treatment of emergency medical conditions on an urgent basis without requiring a previously scheduled appointment) Ⓑ **Qh**   **V**

Coding Clinic: 2009, Q1, P4; 2007, Q2, P1

▶ New	↻ Revised	✔ Reinstated	~~deleted~~ Deleted	⊘ Not covered or valid by Medicare
⚙ Special coverage instructions		✳ Carrier discretion	Ⓑ Bill local carrier	Ⓑ Bill DME MAC

* **G0382** Level 3 hospital emergency department visit provided in a type B emergency department; (the ED must meet at least one of the following requirements: (1) it is licensed by the state in which it is located under applicable state law as an emergency room or emergency department; (2) it is held out to the public (by name, posted signs, advertising, or other means) as a place that provides care for emergency medical conditions on an urgent basis without requiring a previously scheduled appointment; or (3) during the calendar year immediately preceding the calendar year in which a determination under 42 CFR 489.24 is being made, based on a representative sample of patient visits that occurred during that calendar year, it provides at least one-third of all of its outpatient visits for the treatment of emergency medical conditions on an urgent basis without requiring a previously scheduled appointment) Ⓑ **Qh**   V

Coding Clinic: 2009, Q1, P4; 2007, Q2, P1

* **G0383** Level 4 hospital emergency department visit provided in a type B emergency department; (the ED must meet at least one of the following requirements: (1) it is licensed by the state in which it is located under applicable state law as an emergency room or emergency department; (2) it is held out to the public (by name, posted signs, advertising, or other means) as a place that provides care for emergency medical conditions on an urgent basis without requiring a previously scheduled appointment; or (3) during the calendar year immediately preceding the calendar year in which a determination under 42 CFR 489.24 is being made, based on a representative sample of patient visits that occurred during that calendar year, it provides at least one-third of all of its outpatient visits for the treatment of emergency medical conditions on an urgent basis without requiring a previously scheduled appointment) Ⓑ **Qh**   V

Coding Clinic: 2009, Q1, P4; 2007, Q2, P1

* **G0384** Level 5 hospital emergency department visit provided in a type B emergency department; (the ED must meet at least one of the following requirements: (1) it is licensed by the state in which it is located under applicable state law as an emergency room or emergency department; (2) it is held out to the public (by name, posted signs, advertising, or other means) as a place that provides care for emergency medical conditions on an urgent basis without requiring a previously scheduled appointment; or (3) during the calendar year immediately preceding the calendar year in which a determination under 42 CFR § 489.24 is being made, based on a representative sample of patient visits that occurred during that calendar year, it provides at least one-third of all of its outpatient visits for the treatment of emergency medical conditions on an urgent basis without requiring a previously scheduled appointment) Ⓑ **Qh**   Q3

Coding Clinic: 2009, Q1, P4; 2007, Q2, P1

Ultrasound, AAA

○ **G0389** Ultrasound B-scan and/or real time with image documentation; for abdominal aortic aneurysm (AAA) screening Ⓑ **Qp** **Qh**   S

Use modifier 26 for professional component only

Eligible beneficiaries must receive a referral for an AAA ultrasound screening as a result of an IPPE (initial preventative physical examination). This is a once in a lifetime benefit per eligible beneficiary. (http://www.cms.gov/MLNProducts/downloads/MPS_QuickReferenceChart_1.pdf)

Team, Trauma Response

○ **G0390** Trauma response team associated with hospital critical care service Ⓑ **Qh**   S

Coding Clinic: 2007, Q2, P5

Assessment/Intervention

* **G0396** Alcohol and/or substance (other than tobacco) abuse structured assessment (e.g., audit, DAST), and brief intervention 15 to 30 minutes ⑧ **Qp** **Qh**   S

   Bill instead of 99408 and 99409

* **G0397** Alcohol and/or substance (other than tobacco) abuse structured assessment (e.g., audit, DAST), and intervention, greater than 30 minutes ⑧ **Qp** **Qh**   S

   Bill instead of 99408 and 99409

Home Sleep Study Test

* **G0398** Home sleep study test (HST) with type II portable monitor, unattended; minimum of 7 channels: EEG, EOG, EMG, ECG/heart rate, airflow, respiratory effort and oxygen saturation ⑧ **Qp** **Qh**   S

* **G0399** Home sleep test (HST) with type III portable monitor, unattended; minimum of 4 channels: 2 respiratory movement/airflow, 1 ECG/heart rate and 1 oxygen saturation ⑧ **Qp** **Qh**   S

* **G0400** Home sleep test (HST) with type IV portable monitor, unattended; minimum of 3 channels ⑧ **Qp** **Qh**   S

Examination, Initial Medicare

⊛ * **G0402** Initial preventive physical examination; face-to-face visit, services limited to new beneficiary during the first 12 months of Medicare enrollment ⑧ **Qp** **Qh**   V

   Depending on circumstances, 99201-99215 may be assigned with modifier 25 to report an E/M service as a significant, separately identifiable service in addition to the Initial Preventive Physical Examination (IPPE), G0402.

   Copayment and coinsurance waived, deductible waived.

   Coding Clinic: 2009, Q4, P8

Electrocardiogram

* **G0403** Electrocardiogram, routine ECG with 12 leads; performed as a screening for the initial preventive physical examination with interpretation and report ⑧ **Qp** **Qh**   M

   Optional service may be ordered or performed at discretion of physician. Once in a life-time screening, stemming from a referral from Initial Preventive Physical Examination (IPPE). Both deductible and co-payment apply.

* **G0404** Electrocardiogram, routine ECG with 12 leads; tracing only, without interpretation and report, performed as a screening for the initial preventive physical examination ⑧ **Qp** **Qh**   S

* **G0405** Electrocardiogram, routine ECG with 12 leads; interpretation and report only, performed as a screening for the initial preventive physical examination ⑧ **Qp** **Qh**   B

Telehealth

* **G0406** Follow-up inpatient consultation, limited, physicians typically spend 15 minutes communicating with the patient via telehealth ⑧ **Qp**   B

   These telehealth modifers are required when billing for telehealth services with codes G0406-G0408 and G0425-G0427:

   • GT, via interactive audio and video telecommunications system

   • GQ, via asynchronous telecommunications system

* **G0407** Follow-up inpatient consultation, intermediate, physicians typically spend 25 minutes communicating with the patient via telehealth ⑧ **Qp**   B

* **G0408** Follow-up inpatient consultation, complex, physicians typically spend 35 minutes communicating with the patient via telehealth ⑧ **Qp**   B

Services, Social, Psychological

* **G0409** Social work and psychological services, directly relating to and/or furthering the patient's rehabilitation goals, each 15 minutes, face-to-face; individual (services provided by a CORF-qualified social worker or psychologist in a CORF) ⑧   B

▶ **New**   ↻ **Revised**   ✔ **Reinstated**   ~~deleted~~ **Deleted**   ⊘ **Not covered or valid by Medicare**
⑨ **Special coverage instructions**   ✳ **Carrier discretion**   ⑧ **Bill local carrier**   ⑨ **Bill DME MAC**

❋ **G0410** Group psychotherapy other than of a multiple-family group, in a partial hospitalization setting, approximately 45 to 50 minutes ⓑ   P

Coding Clinic: 2009, Q4, P9, 10

❋ **G0411** Interactive group psychotherapy, in a partial hospitalization setting, approximately 45 to 50 minutes ⓑ   P

Coding Clinic: 2009, Q4, P9, 10

Treatment, Bone

❋ **G0412** Open treatment of iliac spine(s), tuberosity avulsion, or iliac wing fracture(s), unilateral or bilateral for pelvic bone fracture patterns which do not disrupt the pelvic ring includes internal fixation, when performed ⓑ **Qp** **Qh**   C

❋ **G0413** Percutaneous skeletal fixation of posterior pelvic bone fracture and/or dislocation, for fracture patterns which disrupt the pelvic ring, unilateral or bilateral, (includes ilium, sacroiliac joint and/or sacrum) ⓑ **Qp** **Qh**   T

❋ **G0414** Open treatment of anterior pelvic bone fracture and/or dislocation for fracture patterns which disrupt the pelvic ring, unilateral or bilateral, includes internal fixation when performed (includes pubic symphysis and/or superior/inferior rami) ⓑ **Qp** **Qh**   C

❋ **G0415** Open treatment of posterior pelvic bone fracture and/or dislocation, for fracture patterns which disrupt the pelvic ring, unilateral or bilateral, includes internal fixation, when performed (includes ilium, sacroiliac joint and/or sacrum) ⓑ **Qp** **Qh**   C

Pathology, Surgical

⤶❋ **G0416** Surgical pathology, gross and microscopic examinations for prostate needle biopsy, any method ⓑ **Qp** **Qh** ♂   S

This testing requires a facility to have either a CLIA certificate of registration (certificate type code 9), a CLIA certificate of compliance (certificate type code 1), or a CLIA certificate of accreditation (certificate type code 3). A facility without a valid, current, CLIA certificate, with a current CLIA certificate of waiver (certificate type code 2) or with a current CLIA certificate for provider-performed microscopy procedures (certificate type code 4), must not be permitted to be paid for these tests. This code has a -TC, -26 (physician), or gobal component.

Laboratory Certification: Histopathology

Coding Clinic: 2013, Q2, P6

~~G0417   Surgical pathology, gross and microscopic examination for prostate needle biopsy, any method, 21-40 specimens~~   ✖

~~G0418   Surgical pathology, gross and microscopic examination, for prostate needle biopsy, any method, 41-60 specimens~~   ✖

~~G0419   Surgical pathology, gross and microscopic examination for prostate needle biopsy, any method, .60 specimens~~   ✖

Educational Services, Rehabilitation, Telehealth, and Miscellaneous

❋ **G0420** Face-to-face educational services related to the care of chronic kidney disease; individual, per session, per one hour ⓑ **Qp** **Qh**   A

CKD is kidney damage of 3 months or longer, regardless of the cause of kidney damage. Sessions billed in increments of one hour (if session is less than 1 hour, it must last at least 31 minutes to be billable. Sessions less than one hour and longer than 31 minutes is billable as one session. No more than 6 sessions of KDE services in a beneficiary's lifetime

* **G0421** Face-to-face educational services related to the care of chronic kidney disease; group, per session, per one hour ⑧   A

Group setting: 2 to 20, report codes G0420 and G0421 with diagnosis code 585.4.

* **G0422** Intensive cardiac rehabilitation; with or without continuous ECG monitoring with exercise, per session ⑧   S

Includes the same service as 93798 but at a greater frequency; may be reported with as many as six hourly sessions on a single date of service. Includes medical nutrition services to reduce cardiac disease risk factors.

* **G0423** Intensive cardiac rehabilitation; with or without continuous ECG monitoring; without exercise, per session ⑧   S

Includes the same service as 93797 but at a greater frequency; may be reported with as many as six hourly sessions on a single date of service. Includes medical nutrition services to reduce cardiac disease risk factors.

* **G0424** Pulmonary rehabilitation, including exercise (includes monitoring), one hour, per session, up to two sessions per day ⑧ **Qp** **Qh**   Q1

Includes therapeutic services and all related monitoring services to inprove respiratory function. Do not report with G0237, G0238, or G0239.

* **G0425** Telehealth consultation, emergency department or initial inpatient, typically 30 minutes communicating with the patient via telehealth ⑧ **Qp**   B

Problem Focused: Problem focused history and examination, with straightforward medical decision making complexity. Typically 30 minutes communicating with patient via telehealth

* **G0426** Initial inpatient telehealth consultation, emergency department or initial inpatient, typically 50 minutes communicating with the patient via telehealth ⑧ **Qp**   B

Detailed: Detailed history and examination, with moderate medical decision making complexity. Typically 50 minutes communicating with patient via telehealth

* **G0427** Initial inpatient telehealth consultation, emergency department or initial inpatient, typically 70 minutes or more communicating with the patient via telehealth ⑧ **Qp**   B

Comprehensive: Comprehensive history and examination, with high medical decision making complexity. Typically 70 minutes or more communicating with patient via telehealth.

⊘ **G0428** Collagen meniscus implant procedure for filling meniscal defects (e.g., cmi, collagen scaffold, menaflex) ⑧   E

* **G0429** Dermal filler injection(s) for the treatment of facial lipodystrophy syndrome (LDS) (e.g., as a result of highly active antiretroviral therapy) ⑧ **Qp** **Qh**   B

Designated for dermal fillers Sculptra® and Radiesse (Medicare). (https://www.cms.gov/ContractorLearningResources/downloads/JA6953.pdf)

Coding Clinic: 2010, Q3, P8

* **G0431** Drug screen, qualitative; multiple drug classes by high complexity test method (e.g., immunoassay, enzyme assay), per patient encounter ⑧ **Qp** **Qh**   N

http://www.cms.hhs.gov/mlnmattersarticles/downloads/se1001.pdf.

Laboratory Certification: Toxicology

* **G0432** Infectious agent antibody detection by enzyme immunoassay (EIA) technique, HIV-1 and/or HIV-2, screening ⑧ **Qp** **Qh**   N

Laboratory Certification: Virology, General immunology

Coding Clinic: 2010, Q2, P10

* **G0433** Infectious agent antibody detection by enzyme-linked immunosorbent assay (ELISA) technique, HIV-1 and/or HIV-2, screening ⑧ **Qp** **Qh**   N

Laboratory Certification: Virology, General immunology

Coding Clinic: 2010, Q2, P10

* **G0434** Drug screen, other than chromatographic; any number of drug classes, by CLIA waived test or moderate complexity test, per patient encounter ⑧ **Qp** **Qh**   N

Laboratory Certification: Toxicology

Coding Clinic: 2012, Q2, P9

▶ **New**   ↻ **Revised**   ✔ **Reinstated**   deleted **Deleted**   ⊘ **Not covered or valid by Medicare**
⊛ **Special coverage instructions**   * **Carrier discretion**   ⑧ **Bill local carrier**   ⑦ **Bill DME MAC**

* **G0435** Infectious agent antibody detection by rapid antibody test, HIV-1 and/or HIV-2, screening ⓑ Qp Qh   N

Coding Clinic: 2010, Q2, P10

* **G0436** Smoking and tobacco cessation counseling visit for the asymptomatic patient; intermediate, greater than 3 minutes, up to 10 minutes ⓑ Qp Qh   S

Coding Clinic: 2011, Q1, P5

* **G0437** Smoking and tobacco cessation counseling visit for the asymptomatic patient; intensive, greater than 10 minutes ⓑ Qp Qh   S

Coding Clinic: 2011, Q1, P5

* **G0438** Annual wellness visit; includes a personalized prevention plan of service (pps), initial visit ⓑ Qp Qh   A

* **G0439** Annual wellness visit, includes a personalized prevention plan of service (pps), subsequent visit ⓑ Qp Qh   A

* **G0442** Annual alcohol misuse screening, 15 minutes ⓑ Qp Qh   S

Coding Clinic: 2012, Q1, P7

* **G0443** Brief face-to-face behavioral counseling for alcohol misuse, 15 minutes ⓑ Qp Qh   S

Coding Clinic: 2012, Q1, P7

* **G0444** Annual depression screening, 15 minutes ⓑ Qp Qh   S

* **G0445** High intensity behavioral counseling to prevent sexually transmitted infection; face-to-face, individual, includes: education, skills training and guidance on how to change sexual behavior; performed semi-annually, 30 minutes ⓑ Qp Qh   S

* **G0446** Annual, face-to-face intensive behavioral therapy for cardiovascular disease, individual, 15 minutes ⓑ   S

Coding Clinic: 2012, Q2, P8

* **G0447** Face-to-face behavioral counseling for obesity, 15 minutes ⓑ   S

Coding Clinic: 2012, Q1, P8

↻ * **G0448** Insertion or replacement of a permanent pacing cardioverter-defibrillator system with transvenous lead(s), single or dual chamber with insertion of pacing electrode, cardiac venous system, for left ventricular pacing ⓑ Qp Qh   J8 B

* **G0451** Development testing, with interpretation and report, per standardized instrument form   Q3

* **G0452** Molecular pathology procedure; physician interpretation and report ⓑ Qp Qh   B

* **G0453** Continuous intraoperative neurophysiology monitoring, from outside the operating room (remote or nearby), per patient, (attention directed exclusively to one patient) each 15 minutes (list in addition to primary procedure) ⓑ   N1 N

* **G0454** Physician documentation of face-to-face visit for durable medical equipment determination performed by nurse practitioner, physician assistant or clinical nurse specialist ⓑ Qp Qh   B

* **G0455** Preparation with instillation of fecal microbiota by any method, including assessment of donor specimen ⓑ Qp Qh   Q1

Coding Clinic: 2013, Q3, P8

~~G0456~~ ~~Negative pressure wound therapy, (e.g., vacuum assisted drainage collection) using a mechanically powered device, not durable medical equipment, including provision of cartridge and dressing(s), topical application(s), wound assessment, and instructions for ongoing care, per session; total wounds(s) surface area less than or equal to 50 square centimeters~~ ✖

~~G0457~~ ~~Negative pressure wound therapy, (e.g., vacuum assisted drainage collection) using a mechanically powered device, not durable medical equipment, including provision of cartridge and dressing(s), topical application(s), wound assessment, and instructions for ongoing care, per session; total wounds(s) surface area greater than 50 square centimeters~~ ✖

* **G0458** Low dose rate (LDR) prostate brachytherapy services, composite rate ⓑ Qp Qh   G2 B

* **G0459** Inpatient telehealth pharmacologic management, including prescription, use, and review of medication with no more than minimal medical psychotherapy ⓑ Qp Qh   B

* **G0460** Autologous platelet rich plasma for chronic wounds/ulcers, incuding phlebotomy, centrifugation, and all other preparatory procedures, administration and dressings, per treatment ⓑ Qp Qh   T

~~G0461~~ ~~Immunohistochemistry or immunocytochemistry, per specimen; first single or multiplex antibody stain~~ ✖

PQRS Qp Quantity Physician Appendix A Qh Quantity Hospital Appendix B ♀ Female only

♂ Male only A Age DMEPOS A2-Z3 ASC Payment Indicator A-Y ASC Status Indicator Coding Clinic

~~G0462~~ ~~Immunohistochemistry or~~ ✖
~~immunocytochemistry, per specimen;~~
~~each additional single or multiplex~~
~~antibody stain (list separately in~~
~~addition to code for primary procedure)~~

✳ **G0463** Hospital outpatient clinic visit for
assessment and management of a
patient Ⓑ **Qp** **Qh** Q3

▶ ✳ **G0464** Colorectal cancer screening; stool-based
DNA and fecal occult hemoglobin (e.g.,
KRAS, NDRG4 and BMP3) **N1** **N**

*Laboratory Certification: General
immunology, Routine chemistry, Clinical
cytogenetics*

▶ ✳ **G0466** Federally qualified health center
(FQHC) visit, new patient; a medically-
necessary, face-to-face encounter (one-
on-one) between a new patient and
a FQHC practitioner during which
time one or more FQHC services
are rendered and includes a typical
bundle of Medicare-covered services
that would be furnished per diem to a
patient receiving a FQHC visit **A**

▶ ✳ **G0467** Federally qualified health center
(FQHC) visit, established patient;
a medically-necessary, face-to-face
encounter (one-on-one) between
an established patient and a FQHC
practitioner during which time one
or more FQHC services are rendered
and includes a typical bundle of
Medicare-covered services that would
be furnished per diem to a patient
receiving a FQHC visit **A**

▶ ✳ **G0468** Federally qualified health center
(FQHC) visit, IPPE or AWV; a FQHC
visit that includes an initial preventive
physical examination (IPPE) or annual
wellness visit (AWV) and includes a
typical bundle of Medicare-covered
services that would be furnished per
diem to a patient receiving an IPPE or
AWV **A**

▶ ✳ **G0469** Federally qualified health center
(FQHC) visit, mental health, new
patient; a medically-necessary, face-
to-face mental health encounter (one-
on-one) between a new patient and
a FQHC practitioner during which
time one or more FQHC services
are rendered and includes a typical
bundle of Medicare-covered services
that would be furnished per diem to
a patient receiving a mental health
visit **A**

▶ ✳ **G0470** Federally qualified health center
(FQHC) visit, mental health, established
patient; a medically-necessary, face-to-
face mental health encounter (one-on-
one) between an established patient
and a FQHC practitioner during which
time one or more FQHC services
are rendered and includes a typical
bundle of Medicare-covered services
that would be furnished per diem to
a patient receiving a mental health
visit **A**

▶ ✳ **G0471** Collection of venous blood by
venipuncture or urine sample by
catheterization from an individual in
a skilled nursing facility (SNF) or by a
laboratory on behalf of a home health
agency (HHA) **A**

▶ ◎ **G0472** Hepatitis C antibody screening, for
individual at high risk and other
covered indication(s) **N1** **N**

Medicare Statute 1861SSA

▶ ✳ **G0473** Face-to-face behavioral counseling for
obesity, group (2-10), 30 minutes **S**

~~G0908~~ ~~Most recent hemoglobin (HGB) level~~ ✖
~~>12.0 g/dl~~

~~G0909~~ ~~Hemoglobin level measurement not~~ ✖
~~documented, reason not given~~

~~G0910~~ ~~Most recent hemoglobin level~~ ✖
~~<= 12.0 g/dl~~

Ⓟ ✳ **G0913** Improvement in visual function
achieved within 90 days following
cataract surgery Ⓑ **M**

Ⓟ ✳ **G0914** Patient care survey was not completed
by patient Ⓑ **M**

Ⓟ ✳ **G0915** Improvement in visual function not
achieved within 90 days following
cataract surgery Ⓑ **M**

Ⓟ ✳ **G0916** Satisfaction with care achieved within
90 days following cataract
surgery Ⓑ **M**

Ⓟ ✳ **G0917** Patient satisfaction survey was not
completed by patient Ⓑ **M**

Ⓟ ✳ **G0918** Satisfaction with care not achieved
within 90 days following cataract
surgery Ⓑ **M**

~~G0919~~ ~~Influenza immunization ordered or~~ ✖
~~recommended (to be given at alternate~~
~~location or alternate provider); vaccine~~
~~not available at time of visit~~

~~G0920~~ ~~Type, anatomic location, and activity~~ ✖
~~all documented~~

~~G0921~~ ~~Documentation of patient reason(s)~~ ✖
~~for not being able to assess (e.g.,~~
~~patient refuses endoscopic and/or~~
~~radiologic assessment)~~

▶ New	↻ Revised	✔ Reinstated	~~deleted~~ Deleted	◯ Not covered or valid by Medicare
◎ Special coverage instructions		✳ Carrier discretion	Ⓑ Bill local carrier	Ⓑ Bill DME MAC

~~G0922~~ ~~No documentation of disease type,~~ ✖
~~anatomic location, and activity, reason~~
~~not given~~

Tositumomab

❋ **G3001** Administration and supply of
tositumomab, 450 mg Ⓑ **Qp** **Qh** S

The therapeutic regimen consists of
a dosimetric step of tositumomab
infusion followed 7–14 days later by
a therapeutic step of iodine I-131
tositumomab infusion.

Guidance

▶ ⊘ **G6001** Ultrasonic guidance for placement of
radiation therapy fields B

▶ ❋ **G6002** Stereoscopic X-ray guidance for
localization of target volume for the
delivery of radiation therapy B

Treatment, Radiation

▶ ❋ **G6003** Radiation treatment delivery, single
treatment area, single port or parallel
opposed ports, simple blocks or no
blocks: up to 5mev B

▶ ❋ **G6004** Radiation treatment delivery, single
treatment area, single port or parallel
opposed ports, simple blocks or no
blocks: 6-10mev B

▶ ❋ **G6005** Radiation treatment delivery, single
treatment area, single port or parallel
opposed ports, simple blocks or no
blocks: 11-19mev B

▶ ❋ **G6006** Radiation treatment delivery, single
treatment area, single port or parallel
opposed ports, simple blocks or no
blocks: 20mev or greater B

▶ ❋ **G6007** Radiation treatment delivery, 2 separate
treatment areas, 3 or more ports on a
single treatment area, use of multiple
blocks: up to 5mev B

▶ ❋ **G6008** Radiation treatment delivery, 2 separate
treatment areas, 3 or more ports on a
single treatment area, use of multiple
blocks: 6-10mev B

▶ ❋ **G6009** Radiation treatment delivery, 2 separate
treatment areas, 3 or more ports on a
single treatment area, use of multiple
blocks: 11-19mev B

▶ ❋ **G6010** Radiation treatment delivery, 2 separate
treatment areas, 3 or more ports on a
single treatment area, use of multiple
blocks: 20 mev or greater B

▶ ❋ **G6011** Radiation treatment delivery, 3 or
more separate treatment areas, custom
blocking, tangential ports, wedges,
rotational beam, compensators,
electron beam; up to 5mev B

▶ ❋ **G6012** Radiation treatment delivery, 3 or
more separate treatment areas, custom
blocking, tangential ports, wedges,
rotational beam, compensators,
electron beam; 6-10mev B

▶ ❋ **G6013** Radiation treatment delivery, 3 or
more separate treatment areas, custom
blocking, tangential ports, wedges,
rotational beam, compensators,
electron beam; 11-19mev B

▶ ❋ **G6014** Radiation treatment delivery, 3 or
more separate treatment areas, custom
blocking, tangential ports, wedges,
rotational beam, compensators,
electron beam; 20mev or greater B

▶ ❋ **G6015** Intensity modulated treatment
delivery, single or multiple fields/arcs,
via narrow spatially and temporally
modulated beams, binary, dynamic
MLC, per treatment session B

▶ ❋ **G6016** Compensator-based beam modulation
treatment delivery of inverse planned
treatment using 3 or more high
resolution (milled or cast) compensator,
convergent beam modulated fields, per
treatment session B

▶ ❋ **G6017** Intra-fraction localization and tracking
of target or patient motion during
delivery of radiation therapy (eg,
3D positional tracking, gating, 3D
surface tracking), each fraction of
treatment B

Intestinal

▶ ❋ **G6018** Ileoscopy, through stoma; with
transendoscopic stent placement
(includes predilation) B

▶ ❋ **G6019** Colonoscopy through stoma; with
ablation of tumor(s), polyp(s), or other
lesion(s) not amenable to removal by
hot biopsy forceps, bipolar cautery or
snare technique B

▶ ❋ **G6020** Colonoscopy through stoma; with
transendoscopic stent placement
(includes predilation) B

▶ ❋ **G6021** Unlisted procedure, intestine B

▶ ❋ **G6022** Sigmoidoscopy, flexible; with ablation
of tumor(s), polyp(s), or other lesions(s)
not amenable to removal by hot biopsy
forceps, bipolar cautery or snare
technique B

ⓅQRS PQRS	**Qp** Quantity Physician Appendix A	**Qh** Quantity Hospital Appendix B	♀ Female only
♂ Male only	**A** Age	♿ DMEPOS A2-Z3 ASC Payment Indicator	A-Y ASC Status Indicator Coding Clinic

▶ ✳ **G6023**   Sigmoidoscopy, flexible; with transendoscopic stent placement (includes predilation)   B

▶ ✳ **G6024**   Colonoscopy, flexible; proximal to splenic flexure; with ablation of tumor(s), polyp(s), or other lesion(s) not amenable to removal by hot biopsy forceps, bipolar cautery or snare technique   B

▶ ✳ **G6025**   Colonoscopy, flexible, proximal to splenic flexure; with transendoscopic stent placement (includes predilation)   B

▶ ✳ **G6027**   Anoscopy, high resolution (HRA) (with magnification and chemical agent enhancement); diagnostic, including collection of specimen(s) by brushing or washing when performed   B

▶ ✳ **G6028**   Anoscopy, high resolution (HRA) (with magnification and chemical agent enhancement); with biopsy(ies)   B

Drugs

▶ ✳ **G6030**   Amitriptyline   N
Laboratory Certification: Toxicology

▶ ✳ **G6031**   Benzodiazepines   N
Laboratory Certification: Toxicology

▶ ✳ **G6032**   Desipramine   N
Laboratory Certification: Toxicology

▶ ✳ **G6034**   Doxepin   N
Laboratory Certification: Toxicology

▶ ✳ **G6035**   Gold   N
Laboratory Certification: Toxicology

▶ ✳ **G6036**   Assay of imipramine   N
Laboratory Certification: Toxicology

▶ ✳ **G6037**   Nortriptyline   N
Laboratory Certification: Toxicology

▶ ✳ **G6038**   Salicylate   N
Laboratory Certification: Toxicology

▶ ✳ **G6039**   Acetaminophen   N
Laboratory Certification: Toxicology

▶ ✳ **G6040**   Alcohol (ethanol); any specimen except breath   N
Laboratory Certification: Toxicology

▶ ✳ **G6041**   Alkaloids, urine, quantitative   N
Laboratory Certification: Toxicology

▶ ✳ **G6042**   Amphetamine or methamphetamine   N
Laboratory Certification: Toxicology

▶ ✳ **G6043**   Barbiturates, not elsewhere specified   N
Laboratory Certification: Toxicology

▶ ✳ **G6044**   Cocaine or metabolite   N
Laboratory Certification: Toxicology

▶ ✳ **G6045**   Dihydrocodeinone   N
Laboratory Certification: Toxicology

▶ ✳ **G6046**   Dihydromorphinone   N
Laboratory Certification: Toxicology

▶ ✳ **G6047**   Dihydrotestosterone   N
Laboratory Certification: Toxicology

▶ ✳ **G6048**   Dimethadione   N
Laboratory Certification: Toxicology

▶ ✳ **G6049**   Epiandrosterone   N
Laboratory Certification: Toxicology

▶ ✳ **G6050**   Ethchlorvynol   N
Laboratory Certification: Toxicology

▶ ✳ **G6051**   Flurazepam   N
Laboratory Certification: Toxicology

▶ ✳ **G6052**   Meprobamate   N
Laboratory Certification: Toxicology

▶ ✳ **G6053**   Methadone   N
Laboratory Certification: Toxicology

▶ ✳ **G6054**   Methsuximide   N
Laboratory Certification: Toxicology

▶ ✳ **G6055**   Nicotine   N
Laboratory Certification: Toxicology

▶ ✳ **G6056**   Opiate(s), drug and metabolites, each procedure   N
Laboratory Certification: Toxicology

▶ ✳ **G6057**   Phenothiazine   N
Laboratory Certification: Toxicology

▶ ✳ **G6058**   Drug confirmation, each procedure   N
Laboratory Certification: Toxicology

Documentation

~~G8126~~   ~~Patient with a diagnosis of major depression documented as being treated with antidepressant medication during the entire 84 day (12 week) acute treatment phase~~   ✖

~~G8127~~   ~~Patient with a diagnosis of major depression not documented as being treated with antidepressant medication during the entire 84 day (12 week) acute treatment phase~~   ✖

▶ New	↻ Revised	✔ Reinstated	~~deleted~~ Deleted	⊘ Not covered or valid by Medicare
✷ Special coverage instructions		✳ Carrier discretion	Ⓑ Bill local carrier	Ⓑ Bill DME MAC

~~G8128~~ ~~Clinician documented that patient was not an eligible candidate for antidepressant medication during the entire 12 week acute treatment phase measure~~ ✖

* **G8395** Left ventricular ejection fraction (LVEF) > = 40% or documentation as normal or mildly depressed left ventricular systolic function Ⓑ   M

* **G8396** Left ventricular ejection fraction (LVEF) not performed or documented Ⓑ   M

(PQRS) * **G8397** Dilated macular or fundus exam performed, including documentation of the presence or absence of macular edema and level of severity of retinopathy Ⓑ   M

(PQRS) * **G8398** Dilated macular or fundus exam not performed Ⓑ   M

(PQRS) * **G8399** Patient with central dual-energy x-ray absorptiometry (DXA) results documented or ordered or pharmacologic therapy (other than minerals/vitamins) for osteoporosis prescribed) Ⓑ   M

(PQRS) * **G8400** Patient with central dual-energy x-ray absorptiometry (DXA) results not documented or not ordered or pharmacologic therapy (other than minerals/vitamins) for osteoporosis not prescribed, reason not given Ⓑ   M

(PQRS) * **G8401** Clinician documented that patient was not an eligible candidate for screening or therapy for osteoporosis for women measure Ⓑ ♀   M

(PQRS) * **G8404** Lower extremity neurological exam performed and documented Ⓑ   M

(PQRS) * **G8405** Lower extremity neurological exam not performed Ⓑ   M

~~G8406~~ ~~Clinician documented that patient was not an eligible candidate for lower extremity neurological exam measure~~ ✖

(PQRS) * **G8410** Footwear evaluation performed and documented Ⓑ   M

(PQRS) * **G8415** Footwear evaluation was not performed Ⓑ   M

(PQRS) * **G8416** Clinician documented that patient was not an eligible candidate for footwear evaluation measure Ⓑ   M

(PQRS) * **G8417** BMI is documented above normal parameters and a follow-up plan is documented Ⓑ   M

(PQRS) * **G8418** BMI is documented below normal parameters and a follow-up plan is documented Ⓑ   M

(PQRS) * **G8419** BMI is documented outside normal parameters, no follow-up plan documented, no reason given Ⓑ   M

(PQRS) * **G8420** BMI is documented within normal parameters and no follow-up plan is required Ⓑ   M

(PQRS) * **G8421** BMI not documented and no reason is given Ⓑ   M

(PQRS) * **G8422** BMI not documented, documentation the patient is not eligible for BMI calculation Ⓑ   M

(PQRS) * **G8427** Eligible professional attests to documenting in the medical record they obtained, updated, or reviewed the patient's current medications Ⓑ   M

(PQRS) * **G8428** Current list of medications not documented as obtained, updated, or reviewed by the eligible professional, reason not given Ⓑ   M

(PQRS) * **G8430** Eligible professional attests to documenting in the medical record the patient is not eligible for a current list of medications being obtained, updated, or reviewed by the eligible professional Ⓑ   M

(PQRS) * **G8431** Screening for clinical depression is documented as being positive and a follow-up plan is documented Ⓑ   M

(PQRS) * **G8432** Clinical depression screening not documented, reason not given Ⓑ   M

(PQRS) * **G8433** Screening for clinical depression not documented, documentation stating the patient is not eligible Ⓑ   M

(PQRS) * **G8442** Pain assessment not documented as being performed, documentation the patient is not eligible for a pain assessment using a standardized tool Ⓑ   M

(PQRS) * **G8450** Beta-blocker therapy prescribed Ⓑ   M

(PQRS) * **G8451** Beta-blocker therapy for LVEF <40% not prescribed for reasons documented by the clinician (e.g., low blood pressure, fluid overload, asthma, patients recently treated with an intravenous positive inotropic agent, allergy, intolerance, other medical reasons, patient declined, other patient reasons or other reasons attributable to the healthcare system) Ⓑ   M

(PQRS) * **G8452** Beta-blocker therapy not prescribed Ⓑ   M

* **G8458** Clinician documented that patient is not an eligible candidate for genotype testing; patient not receiving antiviral treatment for hepatitis C Ⓑ   M

(PQRS) PQRS	Qp Quantity Physician Appendix A	Qh Quantity Hospital Appendix B	♀ Female only
♂ Male only	A Age	DMEPOS	A2-Z3 ASC Payment Indicator A-Y ASC Status Indicator Coding Clinic

* **G8460** Clinician documented that patient is not an eligible candidate for quantitative RNA testing at week 12; patient not receiving antiviral treatment for hepatitis C Ⓑ   M

Ⓟ ⮌ * **G8461** Patient receiving antiviral treatment for hepatitis C during the measurement period Ⓑ   M

~~G8464~~ ~~Clinician documented that prostate cancer patient is not an eligible candidate for adjuvant hormonal therapy; low or intermediate risk of recurrence or risk of recurrence not determined~~ ✖

Ⓟ * **G8465** High risk of recurrence of prostate cancer Ⓑ ♂   M

Ⓟ * **G8473** Angiotensin converting enzyme (ACE) inhibitor or angiotensin receptor blocker (ARB) therapy prescribed Ⓑ   M

Ⓟ ⮌ * **G8474** Angiotensin converting enzyme (ACE) inhibitor or angiotensin receptor blocker (ARB) therapy not prescribed for reasons documented by the clinician (eg, allergy, intolerance, pregnancy, renal failure due to ACE inhibitor, diseases of the aortic or mitral valve, other medical reasons) or (eg, patient declined, other patient reasons) or (eg, lack of drug availability, other reasons attributable to the health care system) Ⓑ   M

Ⓟ * **G8475** Angiotensin converting enzyme (ACE) inhibitor or angiotensin receptor blocker (ARB) therapy not prescribed, reason not given Ⓑ   M

Ⓟ ⮌ * **G8476** Most recent blood pressure has a systolic measurement of <140 mmHg and a diastolic measurement of <90 mmHg Ⓑ   M

Ⓟ ⮌ * **G8477** Most recent blood pressure has a systolic measurement of > =140 mmHg and/or a diastolic measurement of > =90 mmHg Ⓑ   M

Ⓟ * **G8478** Blood pressure measurement not performed or documented, reason not given Ⓑ   M

Ⓟ * **G8482** Influenza immunization administered or previously received Ⓑ   M

Ⓟ ⮌ * **G8483** Influenza immunization was not administered for reasons documented by clinician (e.g., patient allergy or other medical reasons, patient declined or other patient reasons, vacine not available or other system reasons) Ⓑ   M

Ⓟ ⮌ * **G8484** Influenza immunization was not administered, reason not given Ⓑ   M

* **G8485** I intend to report the diabetes mellitus (DM) measures group Ⓑ   M

* **G8486** I intend to report the preventive care measures group Ⓑ   M

* **G8487** I intend to report the chronic kidney disease (CKD) measures group Ⓑ   M

* **G8489** I intend to report the coronary artery disease (CAD) measures group Ⓑ   M

* **G8490** I intend to report the rheumatoid arthritis (RA) measures group Ⓑ   M

* **G8491** I intend to report the HIV/AIDS measures group Ⓑ   M

~~G8492~~ ~~I intend to report the perioperative care measures group~~ ✖

~~G8493~~ ~~I intend to report the back pain measures group~~ ✖

* **G8494** All quality actions for the applicable measures in the diabetes mellitus (DM) measures group have been performed for this patient Ⓑ   M

Composite code, do not report with G8485

* **G8495** All quality actions for the applicable measures in the chronic kidney disease (CKD) measures group have been performed for this patient Ⓑ   M

Composite code, do not report with G8487

* **G8496** All quality actions for the applicable measures in the Preventive Care measures group have been performed for this patient Ⓑ   M

Composite code, do not report with G8486

* **G8497** All quality actions for the applicable measures in the Coronary Artery Bypass Graft (CABG) measures group have been performed for this patient Ⓑ   M

Composite code.

* **G8498** All quality actions for the applicable measures in the Coronary Artery Disease (CAD) measures group have been performed for this patient Ⓑ   M

Composite code.

* **G8499** All quality actions for the applicable measures in the Rheumatoid Arthritis (RA) measures group have been performed for this patient Ⓑ   M

Composite code, do not report with G8490

▶ **New**   ⮌ **Revised**   ✔ **Reinstated**   ~~deleted~~ **Deleted**   ⃠ **Not covered or valid by Medicare**

✪ **Special coverage instructions**   ✱ **Carrier discretion**   Ⓑ **Bill local carrier**   Ⓑ **Bill DME MAC**

＊ **G8500** All quality actions for the applicable measures in the HIV/AIDS measures group have been performed for this patient Ⓑ M

Composite code.

~~G8501 All quality actions for the applicable measures in the Perioperative Care measures group have been performed for this patient~~ ✖

~~G8502 All quality actions for the applicable measures in the Back Pain measures group have been performed for this patient~~ ✖

⒫ ＊ **G8506** Patient receiving angiotensin converting enzyme (ACE) inhibitor or angiotensin receptor blocker (ARB) therapy Ⓑ M

⒫ ＊ **G8509** Pain assessment documented as positive using a standardized tool, follow-up plan not documented, reason not given Ⓑ M

⒫ ＊ **G8510** Screening for clinical depression is documented as negative, a follow-up plan is not required Ⓑ M

⒫ ＊ **G8511** Screening for clinical depression documented as positive, follow up plan not documented, reason not given Ⓑ M

⒫ ＊ **G8530** Autogenous AV fistula received M

⒫ ＊ **G8531** Clinician documented that patient was not an eligible candidate for autogenous AV fistula Ⓑ M

⒫ ＊ **G8532** Clinician documented that patient received vascular access other than autogenous AV fistula, reason not given Ⓑ M

⒫ ＊ **G8535** Elder maltreatment screen not documented; documentation that patient not eligible for the elder maltreatment screen Ⓑ Ⓐ M

⒫ ＊ **G8536** No documentation of an elder maltreatment screen, reason not given Ⓑ Ⓐ M

⒫ ＊ **G8539** Functional outcome assessment documented as positive using a standardized tool and a care plan based on identified deficiencies on the date of functional outcome assessment is documented Ⓑ M

⒫ ＊ **G8540** Functional outcome assessment not documented as being performed, documentation the patient is not eligible for a functional outcome assessment using a standardized tool Ⓑ M

⒫ ＊ **G8541** Functional outcome assessment using a standardized tool not documented, reason not given Ⓑ M

⒫ ＊ **G8542** Functional outcome assessment using a standardized tool is documented; no functional deficiencies identified, care plan not required Ⓑ M

⒫ ＊ **G8543** Documentation of a positive functional outcome assessment using a standardized tool; care plan not documented, reason not given Ⓑ M

＊ **G8544** I intend to report the coronary artery bypass graft (CABG) measures group Ⓑ M

＊ **G8545** I intend to report the Hepatitis C measures group Ⓑ M

~~G8547 I intend to report the Ischemic Vascular Disease (IVD) measures group~~ ✖

＊ **G8548** I intend to report the Heart Failure (HF) measures group Ⓑ M

＊ **G8549** All quality actions for the applicable measures in the Hepatitis C measures group have been performed for this patient Ⓑ M

Composite code, do not report with G8545

＊ **G8551** All quality actions for the applicable measures in the Heart Failure (HF) measures group have been performed for this patient Ⓑ M

Composite code.

~~G8552 All quality actions for the applicable measures in the Ischemic Vascular Disease (IVD) measures group have been performed for this patient~~ ✖

＊ **G8559** Patient referred to a physician (preferably a physician with training in disorders of the ear) for an otologic evaluation Ⓑ M

＊ **G8560** Patient has a history of active drainage from the ear within the previous 90 days Ⓑ M

＊ **G8561** Patient is not eligible for the referral for otologic evaluation for patients with a history of active drainage measure Ⓑ M

＊ **G8562** Patient does not have a history of active drainage from the ear within the previous 90 days Ⓑ M

＊ **G8563** Patient not referred to a physician (preferably a physician with training in disorders of the ear) for an otologic evaluation, reason not given Ⓑ M

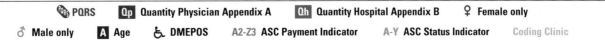

* **G8564** Patient was referred to a physician (preferably a physician with training in disorders of the ear) for an otologic evaluation, reason not specified) Ⓑ M

* **G8565** Verification and documentation of sudden or rapidly progressive hearing loss Ⓑ M

* **G8566** Patient is not eligible for the "referral for otologic evaluation for sudden or rapidly progressive hearing loss" measure Ⓑ M

* **G8567** Patient does not have verification and documentation of sudden or rapidly progressive hearing loss Ⓑ M

* **G8568** Patient was not referred to a physician (preferably a physician with training in disorders of the ear) for an otologic evaluation, reason not given Ⓑ M

PQRS * **G8569** Prolonged postoperative intubation (>24 hrs) required Ⓑ M

PQRS * **G8570** Prolonged postoperative intubation (>24 hrs) not required Ⓑ M

PQRS ↻ * **G8571** Development of deep sternal wound infection/mediastinitis within 30 days postoperatively Ⓑ M

PQRS ↻ * **G8572** No deep sternal wound infection/ mediastinitis Ⓑ M

PQRS * **G8573** Stroke following isolated CABG surgery Ⓑ M

PQRS * **G8574** No stroke following isolated CABG surgery Ⓑ M

PQRS * **G8575** Developed postoperative renal failure or required dialysis Ⓑ M

PQRS * **G8576** No postoperative renal failure/ dialysis not required Ⓑ M

PQRS * **G8577** Re-exploration required due to mediastinal bleeding with or without tamponade, graft occlusion, valve disfunction, or other cardiac reason Ⓑ M

PQRS * **G8578** Re-exploration not required due to mediastinal bleeding with or without tamponade, graft occlusion, valve dysfunction, or other cardiac reason Ⓑ M

~~G8579~~ ~~Antiplatelet medication at discharge~~ ✖

~~G8580~~ ~~Antiplatelet medication contraindicated~~ ✖

~~G8581~~ ~~No antiplatelet medication at discharge~~ ✖

~~G8582~~ ~~Beta-blocker at discharge~~ ✖

~~G8583~~ ~~Beta-blocker contraindicated~~ ✖

~~G8584~~ ~~No beta-blocker at discharge~~ ✖

~~G8585~~ ~~Anti-lipid treatment at discharge~~ ✖

~~G8586~~ ~~Anti-lipid treatment contraindicated~~ ✖

~~G8587~~ ~~No anti-lipid treatment at discharge~~ ✖

~~G8593~~ ~~Lipid profile results documented and reviewed (must include total cholesterol, HDL-C, triglycerides and calculated LDL-C)~~ ✖

~~G8594~~ ~~Lipid profile not performed, reason not given~~ ✖

~~G8595~~ ~~Most recent LDL-C < 100 mg/dl~~ ✖

~~G8597~~ ~~Most recent LDL-C >5 100 mg/dl~~ ✖

PQRS * **G8598** Aspirin or another antithrombotic therapy used Ⓑ M

PQRS * **G8599** Aspirin or another antithrombotic therapy not used, reason not given Ⓑ M

PQRS * **G8600** IV T-PA initiated within three hours (<= 180 minutes) of time last known well Ⓑ M

PQRS * **G8601** IV T-PA not initiated within three hours (<= 180 minutes) of time last known well for reasons documented by clinician Ⓑ M

PQRS * **G8602** IV T-PA not initiated within three hours (<= 180 minutes) of time last known well, reason not given Ⓑ M

PQRS * **G8627** Surgical procedure performed within 30 days following cataract surgery for major complications (e.g. retained nuclear fragments, endophthalmitis, dislocated or wrong power IOL, retinal detachment, or wound dehiscence) Ⓑ M

PQRS * **G8628** Surgical procedure not performed within 30 days following cataract surgery for major complications (e.g. retained nuclear fragments, endophthalmitis, dislocated or wrong power IOL, retinal detachment, or wound dehiscence) Ⓑ M

~~G8629~~ ~~Documentation of order for prophylactic parenteral antibiotic to be given within one hour (if fluoroquinolone or vancomycin, two hours) prior to surgical incision (or start of procedure when no incision is required)~~ ✖

▶ **New** ↻ **Revised** ✔ **Reinstated** ~~deleted~~ **Deleted** ⊘ **Not covered or valid by Medicare**
✺ **Special coverage instructions** ✱ **Carrier discretion** Ⓑ **Bill local carrier** Ⓑ **Bill DME MAC**

~~G8630~~ ~~Documentation that administration~~ ✖
~~of prophylactic parenteral antibiotics~~
~~was initiated within one hour (if~~
~~fluoroquinolone or vancomycin, two~~
~~hours) prior to surgical incision (or~~
~~start of procedure when no incision is~~
~~required), as ordered~~

~~G8631~~ ~~Clinician documented that patient~~ ✖
~~was not an eligible candidate for~~
~~ordering prophylactic parenteral~~
~~antibiotics to be given within one hour~~
~~(if fluoroquinolone or vancomycin, two~~
~~hours) prior to surgical incision (or~~
~~start of procedure when no incision is~~
~~required)~~

~~G8632~~ ~~Prophylactic parenteral antibiotics~~ ✖
~~were not ordered to be given or given~~
~~within one hour (if fluoroquinolone or~~
~~vancomycin, two hours) prior to the~~
~~surgical incision (or start of procedure~~
~~when no incision is required), reason~~
~~not given)~~

(PQRS) ✳ **G8633** Pharmacologic therapy (other than
minierals/vitamins) for osteoporosis
prescribed Ⓑ M

(PQRS) ✳ **G8634** Clinician documented patient not an
eligible candidate to receive
pharmacologic therapy for
osteoporosis Ⓑ M

(PQRS) ✳ **G8635** Pharmacologic therapy for osteoporosis
was not prescribed, reason not
given Ⓑ M

✳ **G8645** I intend to report the asthma measures
group Ⓑ M

✳ **G8646** All quality actions for the applicable
measures in the asthma measures
group have been performed for this
patient Ⓑ M

(PQRS) ✳ **G8647** Risk-adjusted functional status change
residual score for the knee successfully
calculated and the score was equal to
zero (0) or greater than zero
(>0) Ⓑ M

(PQRS) ✳ **G8648** Risk-adjusted functional status change
residual score for the knee successfully
calculated and the score was less than
zero (<0) Ⓑ M

(PQRS) ✳ **G8649** Risk-adjusted functional status change
residual scores for the knee not
measured because the patient did not
complete FOTO'S functional intake on
admission and/or follow up status
survey near discharge, patient not
eligible/not appropriate Ⓑ M

(PQRS) ✳ **G8650** Risk-adjusted functional status change
residual scores for the knee not
measured because the patient did not
complete FOTO'S functional intake on
admission and/or follow up status
survey near discharge, reason not
given Ⓑ M

(PQRS) ✳ **G8651** Risk-adjusted functional status change
residual score for the hip successfully
calculated and the score was equal to
zero (0) or greater than zero
(>0) Ⓑ M

(PQRS) ✳ **G8652** Risk-adjusted functional status change
residual score for the hip successfully
calculated and the score was less than
zero (<0) Ⓑ M

(PQRS) ✳ **G8653** Risk-adjusted functional status change
residual scores for the hip not
measured because the patient did not
complete FOTO'S functional intake on
admission and/or follow up status
survey near discharge, patient not
eligible/not appropriate Ⓑ M

(PQRS) ✳ **G8654** Risk-adjusted functional status change
residual scores for the hip not
measured because the patient did not
complete FOTO'S functional intake on
admission and/or follow up status
survey near discharge, reason not
given Ⓑ M

(PQRS) ✳ **G8655** Risk-adjusted functional status change
residual score for the lower leg, foot or
ankle successfully calculated and the
score was equal to zero (0) or greater
than zero (>0) Ⓑ M

(PQRS) ✳ **G8656** Risk-adjusted functional status change
residual score for the lower leg, foot or
ankle successfully calculated and the
score was less than zero (<0) Ⓑ M

(PQRS) ✳ **G8657** Risk-adjusted functional status change
residual scores for the lower leg, foot or
ankle not measured because the patient
did not complete FOTO'S functional
intake on admission and/or follow up
status survey near discharge, patient
not eligible/not appropriate Ⓑ M

(PQRS) ✳ **G8658** Risk-adjusted functional status change
residual scores for the lower leg, foot or
ankle not measured because the patient
did not complete FOTO'S functional
intake on admission and/or follow up
status survey near discharge, reason
not given Ⓑ M

(PQRS) ✳ **G8659** Risk-adjusted functional status change
residual score for the lumbar spine
successfully calculated and the score
was equal to zero (0) or greater than
zero (>0) Ⓑ M

(PQRS) PQRS	Qp Quantity Physician Appendix A	Qh Quantity Hospital Appendix B	♀ Female only
♂ Male only	A Age	♿ DMEPOS	A2-Z3 ASC Payment Indicator A-Y ASC Status Indicator Coding Clinic

⊕ＰＱＲＳ * **G8660** Risk-adjusted functional status change residual score for the lumbar spine successfully calculated and the score was less than zero (<0) ⓑ　　M

⊕ＰＱＲＳ * **G8661** Risk-adjusted functional status change residual scores for the lumbar spine not measured because the patient did not complete FOTO'S functional intake on admission and/or follow up status survey near discharge, patient not eligible/not appropriate ⓑ　　M

⊕ＰＱＲＳ * **G8662** Risk-adjusted functional status change residual scores for the lumbar spine not measured because the patient did not complete FOTO'S functional intake on admission and/or follow up status survey near discharge, reason not given ⓑ　　M

⊕ＰＱＲＳ * **G8663** Risk-adjusted functional status change residual score for the shoulder successfully calculated and the score was equal to zero (0) or greater than zero (>0) ⓑ　　M

⊕ＰＱＲＳ * **G8664** Risk-adjusted functional status change residual score for the shoulder successfully calculated and the score was less than zero (<0) ⓑ　　M

⊕ＰＱＲＳ * **G8665** Risk-adjusted functional status change residual scores for the shoulder not measured because the patient did not complete FOTO'S functional intake on admission and/or follow up status survey near discharge, patient not eligible/not appropriate ⓑ　　M

⊕ＰＱＲＳ * **G8666** Risk-adjusted functional status change residual scores for the shoulder not measured because the patient did not complete FOTO'S functional intake on admission and/or follow up status survey near discharge, reason not given ⓑ　　M

⊕ＰＱＲＳ * **G8667** Risk-adjusted functional status change residual score for the elbow, wrist or hand successfully calculated and the score was equal to zero (0) or greater than zero (>0) ⓑ　　M

⊕ＰＱＲＳ * **G8668** Risk-adjusted functional status change residual score for the elbow, wrist or hand successfully calculated and the score was less than zero (<0) ⓑ　　M

⊕ＰＱＲＳ * **G8669** Risk-adjusted functional status change residual scores for the elbow, wrist or hand not measured because the patient did not complete FOTO'S functional intake on admission and/or follow up status survey near discharge, patient not eligible/not appropriate ⓑ　　M

⊕ＰＱＲＳ * **G8670** Risk-adjusted functional status change residual scores for the elbow, wrist or hand not measured because the patient did not complete FOTO'S functional intake on admission and/or follow up status survey near discharge, reason not given ⓑ　　M

⊕ＰＱＲＳ * **G8671** Risk-adjusted functional status change residual score for the neck, cranium, mandible, thoracic spine, ribs, or other general orthopedic impairment successfully calculated and the score was equal to zero (0) or greater than zero (>0) ⓑ　　M

⊕ＰＱＲＳ * **G8672** Risk-adjusted functional status change residual score for the neck, cranium, mandible, thoracic spine, ribs, or other general orthopedic impairment successfully calculated and the score was less than zero (<0) ⓑ　　M

⊕ＰＱＲＳ * **G8673** Risk-adjusted functional status change residual scores for the neck, cranium, mandible, thoracic spine, ribs, or other general orthopedic impairment not measured because the patient did not complete FOTO'S functional intake on admission and/or follow up status survey near discharge, patient not eligible/not appropriate ⓑ　　M

⊕ＰＱＲＳ * **G8674** Risk-adjusted functional status change residual scores for the neck, cranium, mandible, thoracic spine, ribs, or other general orthopedic impairment not measured because the patient did not complete FOTO'S functional intake on admission and/or follow up status survey near discharge, reason not given ⓑ　　M

⊕ＰＱＲＳ * **G8682** LVF testing documented as being performed prior to discharge or in the previous 12 months ⓑ　　M

~~G8683~~ ~~LVF testing not performed prior to discharge or in the previous 12 months for a medical or patient documented reason~~ ✖

~~G8685~~ ~~LVF testing not documented as being performed prior to discharge or in the previous 12 months, reason not given~~ ✖

⊕ＰＱＲＳ * **G8694** Left ventriucular ejection fraction (LVEF) <40% ⓑ　　M

⊕ＰＱＲＳ * **G8696** Antithrombotic therapy prescribed at discharge ⓑ　　M

▶ **New**　↺ **Revised**　✔ **Reinstated**　~~deleted~~ **Deleted**　⊘ **Not covered or valid by Medicare**
↻ **Special coverage instructions**　✱ **Carrier discretion**　ⓑ **Bill local carrier**　ⓓ **Bill DME MAC**

⊗ * **G8697** Antithrombotic therapy not prescribed for documented reasons (e.g., patients admitted for performance of elective carotid intervention, patient had stroke during hospital stay, patient expired during inpatient stay, other medical reason(s)); (e.g., patient left against medical advice, other patient reason(s)) Ⓑ M

⊗ * **G8698** Antithrombotic therapy was not prescribed at discharge, reason not given Ⓑ M

~~**G8699** Rehabilitation services (occupational, physical or speech) ordered at or prior to discharge~~ ✖

~~**G8700** Rehabilitation services (occupational, physical or speech) not indicated at or prior to discharge~~ ✖

~~**G8701** Rehabilitation services were not ordered, reason not otherwise specified~~ ✖

~~**G8702** Documentation that prophylactic antibiotics were given within 4 hours prior to surgical incision or intraoperatively~~ ✖

~~**G8703** Documentation that prophylactic antibiotics were neither given within 4 hours prior to surgical incision nor intraoperatively~~ ✖

~~**G8704** 12 lead electrocardiogram (ECG) performed~~ ✖

~~**G8705** Documentation of medical reason(s) for not performing a 12 lead electrocardiogram (ECG)~~ ✖

~~**G8706** Documentation of patient reason(s) for not performing a 12 lead electrocardiogram (ECG)~~ ✖

~~**G8707** 12 lead electrocardiogram (ECG) not performed, reason not given~~ ✖

⊗ * **G8708** Patient not prescribed or dispensed antibiotic Ⓑ M

⊗ * **G8709** Patient prescribed or dispensed antibiotic for documented medical reason(s) (e.g. intestinal infection, pertussis, bacterial infection, Lyme disease, otitis media, acute sinusitis, acute pharyngitis, acute tonsillitis, chronic sinusitis, infection of the pharynx/larynx/tonsils/adenoids, prostatitis, cellulitis, mastoiditis, or bone infections, acute lymphadenitis, impetigo, skin staph infections, pneumonia/gonococcal infections, venereal disease (syphilis, chlamydia, inflammatory diseases (female reproductive organs), infections of the kidney, cystitis or UTI, and acne) Ⓑ M

⊗ * **G8710** Patient prescribed or dispensed antibiotic Ⓑ M

⊗ * **G8711** Prescribed or dispensed antibiotic Ⓑ M

* **G8712** Antibiotic not prescribed or dispensed Ⓑ M

⊗ * **G8713** SPKT/V greater than or equal to 1.2 (single-pool clearance of urea [KT] / volume [V]) Ⓑ M

⊗ * **G8714** Hemodialysis treatment performed exactly three times per week for >90 days Ⓑ M

⊗ * **G8717** SPKT/V less than 1.2 (single-pool clearance of urea [KT] / volume [V]), reason not given Ⓑ M

⊗ * **G8718** Total KT/V greater than or equal to 1.7 per week (total clearance of urea [KT] / volume [V]) Ⓑ M

⊗ ⟳ * **G8720** Total KT/V less than 1.7 per week (total clearance of urea [KT] / volume [V]) Ⓑ M

⊗ * **G8721** PT category (primary tumor), PN category (regional lymph nodes), and histologic grade were documented in pathology report Ⓑ M

⊗ * **G8722** Documentation of medical reason(s) for not including the PT category, the PN category or the histologic grade in the pathology report (e.g., re-excision without residual tumor; non-carcinomasanal canal) Ⓑ M

⊗ * **G8723** Specimen site is other than anatomic location of primary tumor Ⓑ M

⊗ * **G8724** PT category, PN category and histologic grade were not documented in the pathology report, reason not given Ⓑ M

* **G8725** Fasting lipid profile performed (triglycerides, LDL-C, HDL-C and total cholesterol) Ⓑ M

⊗ * **G8726** Clinician has documented reason for not performing fasting lipid profile (e.g., patient declined, other patient reasons) Ⓑ M

⊗ * **G8728** Fasting lipid profile not performed, reason not given Ⓑ M

⊗ * **G8730** Pain assessment documented as positive using a standardized tool and a follow-up plan is documented Ⓑ M

⊗ * **G8731** Pain assessment using a standardized tool is documented as negative, no follow-up plan required Ⓑ M

⊗ * **G8732** No documentation of pain assessment, reason not given Ⓑ M

⊗ **PQRS**   **Qp Quantity Physician Appendix A**   **Qh Quantity Hospital Appendix B**   ♀ **Female only**

♂ **Male only**   **A Age**   ♿ **DMEPOS**   **A2-Z3 ASC Payment Indicator**   **A-Y ASC Status Indicator**   Coding Clinic

TEMPORARY PROCEDURES/PROFESSIONAL SERVICES G8697 — G8732

225

⊕ ✳ **G8733** Elder maltreatment screen documented as positive and a follow-up plan is documented Ⓑ **A**   M

⊕ ✳ **G8734** Elder maltreatment screen documented as negative, no follow-up required Ⓑ **A**   M

⊕ ✳ **G8735** Elder maltreatment screen documented as positive, follow-up plan not documented, reason not given Ⓑ **A**   M

~~G8736~~ ~~Most current LDL C <100 mg/dl~~ ✖

~~G8737~~ ~~Most current LDL C >= 100 mg/dl~~ ✖

~~G8738~~ ~~Left ventricular ejection fraction (LVEF) <40% or documentation of severely or moderately depressed left ventricular systolic function~~ ✖

~~G8739~~ ~~Left ventricular ejection fraction (LVEF) >= 40% or documentation as normal or mildly depressed left ventricular systolic function~~ ✖

~~G8740~~ ~~Left ventricular ejection fraction (LVEF) not performed or assessed, reason not given~~ ✖

⊕ ✳ **G8749** Absence of signs of melanoma (cough, dyspnea, tenderness, localized neurologic signs such as weakness, jaundice or any other sign suggesting systemic spread) or absence of symptoms of melanoma (pain, paresthesia, or any other symptom suggesting the possibility of systemic spread of melanoma) Ⓑ   M

~~G8751~~ ~~Smoking status and exposure to second hand smoke in the home not assessed, reason not given~~ ✖

⊕ ✳ **G8752** Most recent systolic blood pressure <140 mm hg Ⓑ   M

⊕ ✳ **G8753** Most recent systolic blood pressure >= 140 mm hg Ⓑ   M

⊕ ✳ **G8754** Most recent diastolic blood pressure <90 mm hg Ⓑ   M

⊕ ✳ **G8755** Most recent diastolic blood pressure >= 90 mm hg Ⓑ   M

⊕ ✳ **G8756** No documentation of blood pressure measurement, reason not given Ⓑ   M

✳ **G8757** All quality actions for the applicable measures in the chronic obstructive pulmonary disease (COPD) measures group have been performed for this patient Ⓑ   M

✳ **G8758** All quality actions for the applicable measures in the inflammatory bowel disease (IBD) measures group have been performed for this patient Ⓑ   M

✳ **G8759** All quality actions for the applicable measures in the sleep apnea measures group have been performed for this patient Ⓑ   M

✳ **G8761** All quality actions for the applicable measures in the dementia measures group have been performed for this patient Ⓑ   M

✳ **G8762** All quality actions for the applicable measures in the Parkinson's disease measures group have been performed for this patient Ⓑ   M

~~G8763~~ ~~All quality actions for the applicable measures in the hypertension (HTN) measures group have been performed for this patient~~ ✖

~~G8764~~ ~~All quality actions for the applicable measures in the cardiovascular prevention measures group have been performed for this patient~~ ✖

✳ **G8765** All quality actions for the applicable measures in the cataract measures group have been performed for this patient Ⓑ   M

~~G8767~~ ~~Lipid panel results documented and reviewed (must include total cholesterol, HDL C, triglycerides and calculated LDL C)~~ ✖

~~G8768~~ ~~Documentation of medical reason(s) for not performing lipid profile (e.g., patients with palliative goals or for whom treatment of hypertension with standard treatment goals is not clinically appropriate)~~ ✖

~~G8769~~ ~~Lipid profile not performed, reason not given~~ ✖

~~G8770~~ ~~Urine protein test result documented and reviewed~~ ✖

~~G8771~~ ~~Documentation of diagnosis of chronic kidney disease~~ ✖

~~G8772~~ ~~Documentation of medical reason(s) for not performing urine protein test (e.g., patients with palliative goals or for whom treatment of hypertension with standard treatment goals is not clinically appropriate)~~ ✖

~~G8773~~ ~~Urine protein test was not performed, reason not given~~ ✖

~~G8774~~ ~~Serum creatinine test result documented and reviewed~~ ✖

~~G8775~~ ~~Documentation of medical reason(s) for not performing serum creatinine test (e.g., patients with palliative goals or for whom treatment of hypertension with standard treatment goals is not clinically appropriate)~~ ✖

▶ **New**   ↻ **Revised**   ✔ **Reinstated**   ~~deleted~~ **Deleted**   ⊘ **Not covered or valid by Medicare**

⊕ **Special coverage instructions**   ✳ **Carrier discretion**   Ⓢ **Bill local carrier**   Ⓑ **Bill DME MAC**

~~G8776~~ ~~Serum creatinine test not performed,~~ ✖
~~reason not given~~

~~G8777~~ ~~Diabetes screening test performed~~ ✖

~~G8778~~ ~~Documentation of medical reason(s)~~ ✖
~~for not performing diabetes screening~~
~~test (e.g., patients with a diagnosis of~~
~~diabetes, or with palliative goals or~~
~~for whom treatment of hypertension~~
~~with standard treatment goals is not~~
~~clinically appropriate)~~

~~G8779~~ ~~Diabetes screening test not~~ ✖
~~performed, reason not given~~

~~G8780~~ ~~Counseling for diet and physical~~ ✖
~~activity performed~~

~~G8781~~ ~~Documentation of medical reason(s)~~ ✖
~~for patient not receiving counseling~~
~~for diet and physical activity (e.g.,~~
~~patients with palliative goals or for~~
~~whom treatment of hypertension~~
~~with standard treatment goals is not~~
~~clinically appropriate)~~

~~G8782~~ ~~Counseling for diet and physical~~ ✖
~~activity not performed, reason not~~
~~given~~

(PQRS) ✳ **G8783** Normal blood pressure reading
documented, follow-up not
required Ⓑ M

(PQRS) ✳ **G8784** Blood pressure reading not
documented, documentation the
patient is not eligible Ⓑ M

(PQRS) ✳ **G8785** Blood pressure reading not
documented, reason not given Ⓑ M

(PQRS) ✳ **G8797** Specimen site other than anatomic
location of esophagus Ⓑ M

(PQRS) ✳ **G8798** Specimen site other than anatomic
location of prostate Ⓑ M

(PQRS) ✳ **G8806** Performance of trans-abdominal or
trans-vaginal ultrasound Ⓑ M

(PQRS) ✳ **G8807** Trans-abdominal or trans-vaginal
ultrasound not performed for reasons
documented by clinician (e.g., patient
has visited the ED multiple times
within 72 hours, patient has a
documented intrauterine pregnancy
[IUP]) Ⓑ M

(PQRS) ✳ **G8808** Performance of trans-abdominal or
trans-vaginal ultrasound not ordered,
reason not given (e.g., patient has
visited the ED multiple times with no
documentation of a trans-abdominal or
trans-vaginal ultrasound within ED or
from referring eligible
professional) Ⓑ M

(PQRS) ✳ **G8809** Rh-immunoglobulin (RhoGAM)
ordered Ⓑ M

(PQRS) ✳ **G8810** Rh-immunoglobulin (RhoGAM) not
ordered for reasons documented by
clinician (e.g., patient had prior
documented report of RhoGAM within
12 weeks, patient refusal) Ⓑ M

(PQRS) ✳ **G8811** Documentation RH-immunoglobulin
(RhoGAM) was not ordered, reason not
given Ⓑ M

(PQRS) ✳ **G8815** Statin therapy not prescribed for
documented reasons (e.g., medical
intolerance to statin, death of patient
prior to discharge, transfer of care to
another acute care or federal hospital,
hospice admission, left against medical
advice) Ⓑ M

(PQRS) ✳ **G8816** Statin medication prescribed at
discharge Ⓑ M

(PQRS) ✳ **G8817** Statin therapy not prescribed at
discharge, reason not given Ⓑ M

(PQRS) ✳ **G8818** Patient discharge to home no later than
post-operative day #7 Ⓑ M

(PQRS) ✳ **G8825** Patient not discharged to home by postoperative day #7 Ⓑ M

(PQRS) ✳ **G8826** Patient discharge to home no later than
post-operative day #2 following
EVAR Ⓑ M

(PQRS) ✳ **G8833** Patient not discharged to home by postoperative day #2 following EVAR Ⓑ M

(PQRS) ✳ **G8834** Patient discharged to home no later
than post-operative day #2 following
CEA Ⓑ M

(PQRS) ✳ **G8838** Patient not discharged to home by postoperative day #2 following CEA Ⓑ M

✳ **G8839** Sleep apnea symptoms assessed,
including presence or absence of
snoring and daytime sleepiness Ⓑ M

↻✳ **G8840** Documentation of reason(s) for not
documenting an assessment of sleep
symptoms (e.g., patient didn't have
initial daytime sleepiness, patient
visited between initial testing and
initiation of therapy) Ⓑ M

✳ **G8841** Sleep apnea symptoms not assessed,
reason not given Ⓑ M

✳ **G8842** Apnea Hypopnea Index (AHI) or
Respiratory Disturbance Index
(RDI) measured at the time of initial
diagnosis Ⓑ M

↻✳ **G8843** Documentation of reason(s) for not
measuring an Apnea Hypopnea Index
(AHI) or a Respiratory Disturbance
Index (RDI) at the time of initial
diagnosis (e.g., psychiatric disease,
dementia, patient declined, financial,
insurance coverage, test ordered but
not yet completed) Ⓑ M

(PQRS) PQRS	**Qp** Quantity Physician Appendix A	**Qh** Quantity Hospital Appendix B	♀ Female only
♂ Male only	**A** Age	♿ DMEPOS	A2-Z3 ASC Payment Indicator	A-Y ASC Status Indicator	Coding Clinic

* **G8844** Apnea Hypopnea Index (AHI) or Respiratory Disturbance Index (RDI) not measured at the time of initial diagnosis, reason not given Ⓑ   M

* **G8845** Positive airway pressure therapy prescribed Ⓑ   M

* **G8846** Moderate or severe obstructive sleep apnea (Apnea Hypopnea Index (AHI) or Respiratory Disturbance Index (RDI) of 15 or greater) Ⓑ   M

* **G8848** Mild obstructive sleep apnea (Apnea Hypopnea Index (AHI) or Respiratory Disturbance Index (RDI) of less than 15) Ⓑ   M

* **G8849** Documentation of reason(s) for not prescribing positive airway pressure therapy (e.g., patient unable to tolerate, alternative therapies use, patient declined, financial, insurance coverage) Ⓑ   M

* **G8850** Positive airway pressure therapy not prescribed, reason not given Ⓑ   M

* **G8851** Objective measurement of adherence to positive airway pressure therapy, documented Ⓑ   M

* **G8852** Positive airway pressure therapy prescribed Ⓑ   M

* **G8853** Positive airway pressure therapy not prescribed Ⓑ   M

* **G8854** Documentation of reason(s) for not objectively measuring adherence to positive airway pressure therapy (e.g., patient didn't bring data from continuous positive airway pressure [CPAP], therapy was not yet initiated, not available on machine) Ⓑ   M

* **G8855** Objective measurement of adherence to positive airway pressure therapy not performed, reason not given Ⓑ   M

(PQRS) * **G8856** Referral to a physician for an otologic evaluation performed Ⓑ   M

(PQRS) * **G8857** Patient is not eligible for the referral for otologic evaluation measure (e.g., patients who are already under the care of a physician for acute or chronic dizziness) Ⓑ   M

(PQRS) * **G8858** Referral to a physician for an otologic evaluation not performed, reason not given Ⓑ   M

~~G8859~~ ~~Patient receiving corticosteroids greater than or equal to 10 mg/day for 60 or greater consecutive days~~ ✖

~~G8860~~ ~~Patients who have received dose of corticosteroids greater than or equal to 10 mg/day for 60 or greater consecutive days~~ ✖

↺ * **G8861** Within the past 2 years, central dual-energy x-ray absorptiometry (DXA) ordered and documented, review of systems and medication history or pharmacologic therapy (other than minerals/vitamins) for osteoporosis prescribed Ⓑ   M

~~G8862~~ ~~Patients not receiving corticosteroids greater than or equal to 10 mg/day for 60 or greater consecutive days~~ ✖

* **G8863** Patients not assessed for risk of bone loss, reason not given Ⓑ   M

* **G8864** Pneumococcal vaccine administered or previously received Ⓑ   M

* **G8865** Documentation of medical reason(s) for not administering or previously receiving pneumococcal vaccine (e.g., patient allergic reaction, potential adverse drug reaction) Ⓑ   M

* **G8866** Documentation of patient reason(s) for not administering or previously receiving pneumococcal vaccine (e.g., patient refusal) Ⓑ   M

* **G8867** Pneumococcal vaccine not administered or previously received, reason not given Ⓑ   M

* **G8868** Patients receiving a first course of anti-TNF therapy Ⓑ   M

* **G8869** Patient has documented immunity to hepatitis B and is receiving a first course of anti-TNF therapy Ⓑ   M

* **G8870** Hepatitis B vaccine injection administered or previously received and is receiving a first course of anti-TNF therapy Ⓑ   M

* **G8871** Patient not receiving a first course of anti-TNF therapy Ⓑ   M

(PQRS) * **G8872** Excised tissue evaluated by imaging intraoperatively to confirm successful inclusion of targeted lesion Ⓑ   M

(PQRS) * **G8873** Patients with needle localization specimens which are not amenable to intraoperative imaging such as MRI needle wire localization, or targets which are tentatively identified on mammogram or ultrasound which do not contain a biopsy marker but which can be verified on intraoperative inspection or pathology (e.g., needle biopsy site where the biopsy marker is remote from the actual biopsy site) Ⓑ   M

(PQRS) * **G8874** Excised tissue not evaluated by imaging intraoperatively to confirm successful inclusion of targeted lesion Ⓑ   M

(PQRS) * **G8875** Clinician diagnosed breast cancer preoperatively by a minimally invasive biopsy method Ⓑ   M

▶ **New**   ↺ **Revised**   ✔ **Reinstated**   ~~deleted~~ **Deleted**   ⊘ **Not covered or valid by Medicare**
⟳ **Special coverage instructions**   * **Carrier discretion**   Ⓑ **Bill local carrier**   Ⓓ **Bill DME MAC**

⟲* **G8876** Documentation of reason(s) for not performing minimally invasive biopsy to diagnose breast cancer properatively (e.g., lesion too close to skin, implant, chest wall, etc., lesion could not be adequately visualized for needle biopsy, patient condition prevents needle biopsy [weight, breast thickness, etc.], duct excision without imaging abnormality, prophylactic mastectomy, reduction mammoplasty, excisional biopsy performed by another physician) ⓑ M

* **G8877** Clinician did not attempt to achieve the diagnosis of breast cancer preoperatively by a minimally invasive biopsy method, reason not given ⓑ M

* **G8878** Sentinel lymph node biopsy procedure performed ⓑ M

* **G8879** Clinically node negative (T1N0M0 or T2N0M0) invasive breast cancer ⓑ M

* **G8880** Documentation of reason(s) sentinel lymph node biopsy not performed (e.g., reasons could include but not limited to; non-invasive cancer, incidental discovery of breast cancer on prophylactic mastectomy, incidental discovery of breast cancer on reduction mammoplasty, pre-operative biopsy proven lymph node (LN) metastases, inflammatory carcinoma, stage 3 locally advanced cancer, recurrent invasive breast cancer, patient refusal after informed consent) ⓑ M

* **G8881** Stage of breast cancer is greater than T1N0M0 or T2N0M0 ⓑ M

* **G8882** Sentinel lymph node biopsy procedure not performed, reason not given ⓑ M

* **G8883** Biopsy results reviewed, communicated, tracked and documented ⓑ M

* **G8884** Clinician documented reason that patient's biopsy results were not reviewed ⓑ M

* **G8885** Biopsy results not reviewed, communicated, tracked or documented ⓑ M

~~G8886~~ ~~Most recent blood pressure under control~~ ✖

~~G8887~~ ~~Documentation of medical reason(s) for most recent blood pressure not being under control (e.g., patients with palliative goals or for whom treatment of hypertension with standard treatment goals is not clinically appropriate)~~ ✖

~~G8888~~ ~~Most recent blood pressure not under control, results documented and reviewed~~ ✖

~~G8889~~ ~~No documentation of blood pressure measurement, reason not given~~ ✖

~~G8890~~ ~~Most recent LDL-C under control, results documented and reviewed~~ ✖

~~G8891~~ ~~Documentation of medical reason(s) for most recent LDL-C not under control (e.g., patients with palliative goals for whom treatment of hypertension with standard treatment goals is not clinically appropriate)~~ ✖

~~G8892~~ ~~Documentation of medical reason(s) for not performing LDL-C test (e.g., patients with palliative goals or for whom treatment of hypertension with standard treatment goals is not clinically appropriate)~~ ✖

~~G8893~~ ~~Most recent LDL-C not under control, results documented and reviewed~~ ✖

~~G8894~~ ~~LDL-C not performed, reason not given~~ ✖

~~G8895~~ ~~Oral aspirin or other antithrombotic therapy prescribed~~ ✖

~~G8896~~ ~~Documentation of medical reason(s) for not prescribing oral aspirin or other antithrombotic therapy (e.g., patient documented to be low risk or patient with terminal illness or treatment of hypertension with standard treatment goals is not clinically appropriate or for whom risk of aspirin or other antithrombotic therapy exceeds potential benefits such as for individuals whose blood pressure is poorly controlled)~~ ✖

~~G8897~~ ~~Oral aspirin or other antithrombotic therapy was not prescribed, reason not given~~ ✖

* **G8898** I intend to report the chronic obstructive pulmonary disease (COPD) measures group ⓑ M

* **G8899** I intend to report the inflammatory bowel disease (IBD) measures group ⓑ M

* **G8900** I intend to report the sleep apnea measures group ⓑ M

* **G8902** I intend to report the dementia measures group ⓑ M

* **G8903** I intend to report the Parkinson's disease measures group ⓑ M

~~G8904~~ ~~I intend to report the hypertension (HTN) measures group~~ ✖

~~G8905~~ ~~I intend to report the cardiovascular prevention measures group~~ ✖

* **G8906** I intend to report the cataract measures group ⑧ **M**

* **G8907** Patient documented not to have experienced any of the following events: a burn prior to discharge; a fall within the facility; wrong site/side/patient/procedure/implant event; or a hospital transfer or hospital admission upon discharge from the facility ⑧

* **G8908** Patient documented to have received a burn prior to discharge ⑧

* **G8909** Patient documented not to have received a burn prior to discharge ⑧

* **G8910** Patient documented to have experienced a fall within ASC ⑧

* **G8911** Patient documented not to have experienced a fall within ambulatory surgical center ⑧

* **G8912** Patient documented to have experienced a wrong site, wrong side, wrong patient, wrong procedure or wrong implant event ⑧

* **G8913** Patient documented not to have experienced a wrong site, wrong side, wrong patient, wrong procedure or wrong implant event ⑧

* **G8914** Patient documented to have experienced a hospital transfer or hospital admission upon discharge from ASC ⑧

* **G8915** Patient documented not to have experienced a hospital transfer or hospital admission upon discharge from ASC ⑧

* **G8916** Patient with preoperative order for IV antibiotic surgical site infection (SSI) prophylaxis, antibiotic initiated on time ⑧

* **G8917** Patient with preoperative order for IV antibiotic surgical site infection (SSI) prophylaxis, antibiotic not initiated on time ⑧

* **G8918** Patient without preoperative order for IV antibiotic surgical site infection(SSI) prophylaxis ⑧

⊗ * **G8923** Left ventricular ejection fraction (LVEF) <40% or documentation of moderately or severely depressed left ventricular systolic function ⑧ **M**

⊗ ↻ * **G8924** Spirometry test results demonstrate FEV1/FVC <60% and patient has COPD symptoms (e.g., dyspnea, cough/sputum, wheezing) ⑧ **M**

⊗ * **G8925** Spirometry test results demonstrate FEV1/FVC >=60% or patient does not have COPD symptoms ⑧ **M**

⊗ * **G8926** Spirometry test not performed or documented, reason not given ⑧ **M**

⊗ * **G8927** Adjuvant chemotherapy referred, prescribed or previously received for AJCC stage III, colon cancer ⑧ **M**

⊗ * **G8928** Adjuvant chemotherapy not prescribed or previously received, for documented reasons (e.g., medical co-morbidities, diagnosis date more than 5 years prior to the current visit date, patient's cancer has metastasized, medical contraindication/allergy, poor performance status, other medical reasons, patient refusal, other patient reasons, patient is currently enrolled in a clinical trial that precludes prescription of chemotherapy, other system reasons) ⑧ **M**

⊗ * **G8929** Adjuvant chemotherapy not prescribed or previously received, reason not specified ⑧ **M**

~~G8930 Assessment of depression severity at the initial evaluation~~ ✘

~~G8931 Assessment of depression severity not documented, reason not given~~ ✘

~~G8932 Suicide risk assessed at the initial evaluation~~ ✘

~~G8933 Suicide risk not assessed at the initial evaluation, reason not given~~ ✘

⊗ * **G8934** Left ventricular ejection fraction (LVEF) <40% or documentation of moderately or severely depressed left ventricular systolic function ⑧ **M**

⊗ * **G8935** Clinician prescribed angiotensin converting enzyme (ACE) inhibitor or angiotensin receptor blocker (ARB) therapy ⑧ **M**

⊗ ↻ * **G8936** Clinician documented that patient was not an eligible candidate for angiotensin converting enzyme (ACE) inhibitor or angiotensin receptor blocker (ARB) therapy (eg, allergy, intolerance, pregnancy, renal failure due to ace inhibitor, diseases of the aortic or mitral valve, other medical reasons) or (eg, patient declined, other patient reasons) or (eg, lack of drug availability, other reasons attributable to the health care system) ⑧ **M**

▶ **New**   ↻ **Revised**   ✔ **Reinstated**   ~~deleted~~ **Deleted**   ⊘ **Not covered or valid by Medicare**

✿ **Special coverage instructions**   * **Carrier discretion**   ⑧ **Bill local carrier**   ⑧ **Bill DME MAC**

(PQRS) ✳ **G8937** Clinician did not prescribe angiotensin converting enzyme (ACE) inhibitor or angiotensin receptor blocker (ARB) therapy, reason not given Ⓑ   M

(PQRS) ✳ **G8938** BMI is documented as being outside of normal limits, follow-up plan is not documented, documentation the patient is not eligible Ⓑ   M

(PQRS) ✳ **G8939** Pain assessment documented as positive, follow-up plan not documented, documentation the patient is not eligible Ⓑ   M

(PQRS) ✳ **G8940** Screening for clinical depression documented as positive, a follow-up plan not documented, documentation stating the patient is not eligible Ⓑ   M

(PQRS) ✳ **G8941** Elder maltreatment screen documented as positive, follow-up plan not documented, documentation the patient is not eligible Ⓑ 🅰   M

(PQRS) ✳ **G8942** Functional outcomes assessment using a standardized tool is documented within the previous 30 days and care plan, based on identified deficiencies on the date of the functional outcome assessment, is documented Ⓑ   M

~~G8943   LDL-C result not present or not within 12 months prior~~ ✖

(PQRS) ✳ **G8944** AJCC melanoma cancer stage 0 through IIC melanoma Ⓑ   M

(PQRS) ✳ **G8946** Minimally invasive biopsy method attempted but not diagnostic of breast cancer (e.g., high risk lesion of breast such as atypical ductal hyperplasia, lobular neoplasia, atypical lobular hyperplasia, lobular carcinoma in situ, atypical columnar hyperplasica, flat epithelial atypia, radial scar, complex sclerosing lesion, papillary lesion, or any lesion with spindle cells) Ⓑ   M

✳ **G8947** One or more neuropsychiatric symptoms Ⓑ   M

✳ **G8948** No neuropsychiatric symptoms Ⓑ   M

~~G8949   Documentation of patient reason(s) for patient not receiving counseling for diet and physical activity (e.g., patient is not willing to discuss diet or exercise interventions to help control blood pressure, or the patient said he/she refused to make these changes)~~ ✖

(PQRS) ✳ **G8950** Pre-hypertensive or hypertensive blood pressure reading documented, and the indicated follow-up documented Ⓑ   M

(PQRS) ✳ **G8951** Pre-hypertensive or hypertensive blood pressure reading documented, indicated follow-up not documented, documentation the patient is not eligible Ⓑ   M

(PQRS) ✳ **G8952** Pre-hypertensive or hypertensive blood pressure reading documented, indicated follow-up not documented, reason not given Ⓑ   M

✳ **G8953** All quality actions for the applicable measures in the oncology measures group have been performed for this patient Ⓑ   M

(PQRS) ✳ **G8955** Most recent assessment of adequacy of volume management Ⓑ   M

(PQRS) ✳ **G8956** Patient receiving maintenance hemodialysis in an outpatient dialysis facility Ⓑ   M

~~G8957   Patient not receiving maintenance hemodialysis in an outpatient dialysis facility~~ ✖

(PQRS) ✳ **G8958** Assessment of adequacy of volume management not documented, reason not given Ⓑ   M

(PQRS) ✳ **G8959** Clinician treating major depressive disorder communicates to clinician treating comorbid condition Ⓑ   M

(PQRS) ✳ **G8960** Clinician treating major depressive disorder did not communicate to clinician treating comorbid condition, reason not given Ⓑ   M

(PQRS) ✳ **G8961** Cardiac stress imaging test primarily performed on low-risk surgery patient for preoperative evaluation within 30 days preceding this surgery Ⓑ   M

(PQRS) ✳ **G8962** Cardiac stress imaging test performed on patient for any reason including those who did not have low risk surgery or test that was performed more than 30 days preceding low risk surgery Ⓑ   M

(PQRS) ✳ **G8963** Cardiac stress imaging performed primarily for monitoring of asymptomatic patient who had PCI within 2 years Ⓑ   M

(PQRS) ✳ **G8964** Cardiac stress imaging test performed primarily for any other reason than monitoring of asymptomatic patient who had PCI within 2 years (e.g., symptomatic patient, patient greater than 2 years since PCI, initial evaluation, etc.) Ⓑ   M

(PQRS) ✳ **G8965** Cardiac stress imaging test primarily performed on low CHD risk patient for initial detection and risk assessment Ⓑ   M

(PQRS) PQRS	Op Quantity Physician Appendix A	Oh Quantity Hospital Appendix B	♀ Female only
♂ Male only	🅰 Age	♿ DMEPOS	A2-Z3 ASC Payment Indicator	A-Y ASC Status Indicator	Coding Clinic

QRS * **G8966** Cardiac stress imaging test performed on symptomatic or higher than low CHD risk patient or for any reason other than initial detection and risk assessment ⒷM

QRS * **G8967** Warfarin or another oral anticoagulant that is FDA approved prescribed ⒷM

QRS ↻* **G8968** Documentation of medical reason(s) for not prescribing warfarin or another oral anticoagulant that is FDA approved for the prevention of thromboembolism [eg, patients with mitral stenosis or prosthetic heart valves, patients with transient or reversible causes of AF (eg, pneumonia, hyperthyroidism, pregnancy, cardiac surgery), allergy, risk of bleeding, other medical reasons] ⒷM

QRS * **G8969** Documentation of patient reason(s) for not prescribing warfarin or another oral anticoagulant that is FDA approved (e.g., economic, social, and/or religious impediments, noncompliance patient refusal, other patient reasons) ⒷM

QRS * **G8970** No risk factors or one moderate risk factor for thromboembolism ⒷM

QRS * **G8971** Warfarin or another oral anticoagulant that is FDA approved not prescribed, reason not given ⒷM

QRS * **G8972** One or more high risk factors for thromboembolism or more than one moderate risk factor for thromboembolism ⒷM

QRS * **G8973** Most recent hemoglobin (Hgb) level <10 g/dl ⒷM

QRS * **G8974** Hemoglobin level measurement not documented, reason not given ⒷM

QRS * **G8975** Documentation of medical reason(s) for patient having a hemoglobin level <10 g/dl (e.g., patients who have non-renal etiologies of anemia [e.g., sickle cell anemia or other hemoglobinopathies, hypersplenism, primary bone marrow disease, anemia related to chemotherapy for diagnosis of malignancy, postoperative bleeding, active bloodstream or peritoneal infection], other medical reasons) ⒷM

QRS * **G8976** Most recent hemoglobin (Hgb) level >= 10 g/dl ⒷM

* **G8977** I intend to report the oncology measures group ⒷM

* **G8978** Mobility: walking & moving around functional limitation, current status, at therapy episode outset and at reporting intervals ⒷE

* **G8979** Mobility: walking & moving around functional limitation, projected goal status, at therapy episode outset, at reporting intervals, and at discharge or to end reporting ⒷE

* **G8980** Mobility: walking & moving around functional limitation, discharge status, at discharge from therapy or to end reporting ⒷE

* **G8981** Changing & maintaining body position functional limitation, current status, at therapy episode outset and at reporting intervals ⒷE

* **G8982** Changing & maintaining body position functional limitation, projected goal status, at therapy episode outset, at reporting intervals, and at discharge or to end reporting ⒷE

* **G8983** Changing & maintaining body position functional limitation, discharge status, at discharge from therapy or to end reporting ⒷE

* **G8984** Carrying, moving & handling objects functional limitation, current status, at therapy episode outset and at reporting intervals ⒷE

* **G8985** Carrying, moving and handling objects, projected goal status, at therapy episode outset, at reporting intervals, and at discharge or to end reporting ⒷE

* **G8986** Carrying, moving & handling objects functional limitation, discharge status, at discharge from therapy or to end reporting ⒷE

* **G8987** Self-care functional limitation, current status, at therapy episode outset and at reporting intervals ⒷE

* **G8988** Self-care functional limitation, projected goal status, at therapy episode outset, at reporting intervals, and at discharge or to end reporting ⒷE

* **G8989** Self-care functional limitation, discharge status, at discharge from therapy or to end reporting ⒷE

* **G8990** Other physical or occupational therapy primary functional limitation, current status, at therapy episode outset and at reporting intervals ⒷE

▶ **New**   ↻ **Revised**   ✔ **Reinstated**   ~~deleted~~ **Deleted**   ⊘ **Not covered or valid by Medicare**

⊛ **Special coverage instructions**   * **Carrier discretion**   Ⓑ **Bill local carrier**   Ⓑ **Bill DME MAC**

* **G8991** Other physical or occupational therapy primary functional limitation, projected goal status, at therapy episode outset, at reporting intervals, and at discharge or to end reporting ⓑ   E

* **G8992** Other physical or occupational therapy primary functional limitation, discharge status, at discharge from therapy or to end reporting ⓑ   E

* **G8993** Other physical or occupational therapy subsequent functional limitation, current status, at therapy episode outset and at reporting intervals ⓑ   E

* **G8994** Other physical or occupational therapy subsequent functional limitation, projected goal status, at therapy episode outset, at reporting intervals, and at discharge or to end reporting ⓑ   E

* **G8995** Other physical or occupational therapy subsequent functional limitation, discharge status, at discharge from therapy or to end reporting ⓑ   E

* **G8996** Swallowing functional limitation, current status at therapy episode outset and at reporting intervals ⓑ   E

* **G8997** Swallowing functional limitation, projected goal status, at therapy episode outset, at reporting intervals, and at discharge or to end reporting ⓑ   E

* **G8998** Swallowing functional limitation, discharge status, at discharge from therapy or to end reporting ⓑ   E

* **G8999** Motor speech functional limitation, current status at therapy episode outset and at reporting intervals ⓑ   E

⊙ **G9001** Coordinated care fee, initial rate ⓑ   B

⊙ **G9002** Coordinated care fee, maintenance rate ⓑ   B

⊙ **G9003** Coordinated care fee, risk adjusted high, initial ⓑ   B

⊙ **G9004** Coordinated care fee, risk adjusted low, initial ⓑ   B

⊙ **G9005** Coordinated care fee, risk adjusted maintenance ⓑ   B

⊙ **G9006** Coordinated care fee, home monitoring ⓑ   B

⊙ **G9007** Coordinated care fee, scheduled team conference ⓑ   B

⊙ **G9008** Coordinated care fee, physician coordinated care oversight services ⓑ   B

⊙ **G9009** Coordinated care fee, risk adjusted maintenance, level 3 ⓑ   B

⊙ **G9010** Coordinated care fee, risk adjusted maintenance, level 4 ⓑ   B

⊙ **G9011** Coordinated care fee, risk adjusted maintenance, level 5 ⓑ   B

⊙ **G9012** Other specified case management services not elsewhere classified ⓑ   B

⊘ **G9013** ESRD demo basic bundle Level I ⓑ   E

Medicare non-covered.

⊘ **G9014** ESRD demo expanded bundle, including venous access and related services ⓑ   E

Medicare non-covered.

⊘ **G9016** Smoking cessation counseling, individual, in the absence of or in addition to any other evaluation and management service, per session (6-10 minutes) [demo project code only] ⓑ   E

Medicare non-covered.

* **G9017** Amantadine hydrochloride, oral, per 100 mg (for use in a Medicare-approved demonstration project) ⓑ   A

* **G9018** Zanamivir, inhalation powder, administered through inhaler, per 10 mg (for use in a Medicare-approved demonstration project) ⓑ   A

* **G9019** Oseltamivir phosphate, oral, per 75 mg (for use in a Medicare-approved demonstration project) ⓑ   A

* **G9020** Rimantadine hydrochloride, oral, per 100 mg (for use in a Medicare-approved demonstration project) ⓑ   A

* **G9033** Amantadine hydrochloride, oral brand, per 100 mg (for use in a Medicare-approved demonstration project) ⓑ   A

* **G9034** Zanamivir, inhalation powder, administered through inhaler, brand, per 10 mg (for use in a Medicare-approved demonstration project) ⓑ   A

* **G9035** Oseltamivir phosphate, oral, brand, per 75 mg (for use in a Medicare-approved demonstration project) ⓑ   A

* **G9036** Rimantadine hydrochloride, oral, brand, per 100 mg (for use in a Medicare-approved demonstration project) ⓑ   A

TEMPORARY PROCEDURES/PROFESSIONAL SERVICES   G8991 — G9036

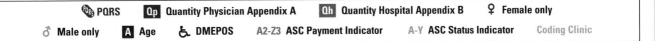

⊘ **G9050** Oncology; primary focus of visit; work-up, evaluation, or staging at the time of cancer diagnosis or recurrence (for use in a Medicare-approved demonstration project) ⑬   E

⊘ **G9051** Oncology; primary focus of visit; treatment decision-making after disease is staged or restaged, discussion of treatment options, supervising/coordinating active cancer directed therapy or managing consequences of cancer directed therapy (for use in a Medicare-approved demonstration project) ⑬   E

⊘ **G9052** Oncology; primary focus of visit; surveillance for disease recurrence for patient who has completed definitive cancer-directed therapy and currently lacks evidence of recurrent disease; cancer directed therapy might be considered in the future (for use in a Medicare-approved demonstration project) ⑬   E

⊘ **G9053** Oncology; primary focus of visit; expectant management of patient with evidence of cancer for whom no cancer directed therapy is being administered or arranged at present; cancer directed therapy might be considered in the future (for use in a Medicare-approved demonstration project) ⑬   E

⊘ **G9054** Oncology; primary focus of visit; supervising, coordinating or managing care of patient with terminal cancer or for whom other medical illness prevents further cancer treatment; includes symptom management, end-of-life care planning, management of palliative therapies (for use in a Medicare-approved demonstration project) ⑬   E

⊘ **G9055** Oncology; primary focus of visit; other, unspecified service not otherwise listed (for use in a Medicare-approved demonstration project ⑬   E

⊘ **G9056** Oncology; practice guidelines; management adheres to guidelines (for use in a Medicare-approved demonstration project) ⑬   E

⊘ **G9057** Oncology; practice guidelines; management differs from guidelines as a result of patient enrollment in an institutional review board approved clinical trial (for use in a Medicare-approved demonstration project) ⑬   E

⊘ **G9058** Oncology; practice guidelines; management differs from guidelines because the treating physician disagrees with guideline recommendations (for use in a Medicare-approved demonstration project) ⑬   E

⊘ **G9059** Oncology; practice guidelines; management differs from guidelines because the patient, after being offered treatment consistent with guidelines, has opted for alternative treatment or management, including no treatment (for use in a Medicare-approved demonstration project) ⑬   E

⊘ **G9060** Oncology; practice guidelines; management differs from guidelines for reason(s) associated with patient comorbid illness or performance status not factored into guidelines (for use in a Medicare-approved demonstration project) ⑬   E

⊘ **G9061** Oncology; practice guidelines; patient's condition not addressed by available guidelines (for use in a Medicare-approved demonstration project) ⑬   E

⊘ **G9062** Oncology; practice guidelines; management differs from guidelines for other reason(s) not listed (for use in a Medicare-approved demonstration project) ⑬   E

∗ **G9063** Oncology; disease status; limited to non-small cell lung cancer; extent of disease initially established as stage I (prior to neo-adjuvant therapy, if any) with no evidence of disease progression, recurrence, or metastases (for use in a Medicare-approved demonstration project) ⑬   M

∗ **G9064** Oncology; disease status; limited to non-small cell lung cancer; extent of disease initially established as stage II (prior to neo-adjuvant therapy, if any) with no evidence of disease progression, recurrence, or metastases (for use in a Medicare-approved demonstration project) ⑬   M

∗ **G9065** Oncology; disease status; limited to non-small cell lung cancer; extent of disease initially established as stage IIIA (prior to neo-adjuvant therapy, if any) with no evidence of disease progression, recurrence, or metastases (for use in a Medicare-approved demonstration project) ⑬   M

▶ **New**   ↻ **Revised**   ✔ **Reinstated**   deleted **Deleted**   ⊘ **Not covered or valid by Medicare**
⟳ **Special coverage instructions**   ∗ **Carrier discretion**   Ⓑ **Bill local carrier**   ⑬ **Bill DME MAC**

✳ **G9066** Oncology; disease status; limited to non-small cell lung cancer; stage IIIB-IV at diagnosis, metastatic, locally recurrent, or progressive (for use in a Medicare-approved demonstration project) Ⓑ M

✳ **G9067** Oncology; disease status; limited to non-small cell lung cancer; extent of disease unknown, staging in progress, or not listed (for use in a Medicare-approved demonstration project) Ⓑ M

✳ **G9068** Oncology; disease status; limited to small cell and combined small cell/non-small cell; extent of disease initially established as limited with no evidence of disease progression, recurrence, or metastases (for use in a Medicare-approved demonstration project) Ⓑ M

✳ **G9069** Oncology; disease status; small cell lung cancer, limited to small cell and combined small cell/non-small cell; extensive stage at diagnosis, metastatic, locally recurrent, or progressive (for use in a Medicare-approved demonstration project) Ⓑ M

✳ **G9070** Oncology; disease status; small cell lung cancer, limited to small cell and combined small cell/non-small cell; extent of disease unknown, staging in progress, or not listed (for use in a Medicare-approved demonstration project) Ⓑ M

✳ **G9071** Oncology; disease status; invasive female breast cancer (does not include ductal carcinoma in situ); adenocarcinoma as predominant cell type; stage I or stage IIA-IIB; or T3, N1, M0; and ER and/or PR positive; with no evidence of disease progression, recurrence, or metastases (for use in a Medicare-approved demonstration project) Ⓑ ♀ M

✳ **G9072** Oncology; disease status; invasive female breast cancer (does not include ductal carcinoma in situ); adenocarcinoma as predominant cell type; stage I, or stage IIA-IIB; or T3, N1, M0; and ER and PR negative; with no evidence of disease progression, recurrence, or metastases (for use in a Medicare-approved demonstration project) Ⓑ ♀ M

✳ **G9073** Oncology; disease status; invasive female breast cancer (does not include ductal carcinoma in situ); adenocarcinoma as predominant cell type; stage IIIA-IIIB; and not T3, N1, M0; and ER and/or PR positive; with no evidence of disease progression, recurrence, or metastases (for use in a Medicare-approved demonstration project) Ⓑ ♀ M

✳ **G9074** Oncology; disease status; invasive female breast cancer (does not include ductal carcinoma in situ); adenocarcinoma as predominant cell type; stage IIIA-IIIB; and not T3, N1, M0; and ER and PR negative; with no evidence of disease progression, recurrence, or metastases (for use in a Medicare-approved demonstration project) Ⓑ ♀ M

✳ **G9075** Oncology; disease status; invasive female breast cancer (does not include ductal carcinoma in situ); adenocarcinoma as predominant cell type; M1 at diagnosis, metastatic, locally recurrent, or progressive (for use in a Medicare-approved demonstration project) Ⓑ ♀ M

✳ **G9077** Oncology; disease status; prostate cancer, limited to adenocarcinoma as predominant cell type; T1-T2c and Gleason 2-7 and PSA < or equal to 20 at diagnosis with no evidence of disease progression, recurrence, or metastases (for use in a Medicare-approved demonstration project) Ⓑ ♂ M

✳ **G9078** Oncology; disease status; prostate cancer, limited to adenocarcinoma as predominant cell type; T2 or T3a Gleason 8-10 or PSA > 20 at diagnosis with no evidence of disease progression, recurrence, or metastases (for use in a Medicare-approved demonstration project) Ⓑ ♂ M

✳ **G9079** Oncology; disease status; prostate cancer, limited to adenocarcinoma as predominant cell type; T3b-T4, any N; any T, N1 at diagnosis with no evidence of disease progression, recurrence, or metastases (for use in a Medicare-approved demonstration project) Ⓑ ♂ M

✳ **G9080** Oncology; disease status; prostate cancer, limited to adenocarcinoma; after initial treatment with rising PSA or failure of PSA decline (for use in a Medicare-approved demonstration project) Ⓑ ♂ M

ⓅQRS PQRS	Ⓠp Quantity Physician Appendix A	Ⓠh Quantity Hospital Appendix B	♀ Female only
♂ Male only	Ⓐ Age	♿ DMEPOS	A2-Z3 ASC Payment Indicator A-Y ASC Status Indicator Coding Clinic

* **G9083** Oncology; disease status; prostate cancer, limited to adenocarcinoma; extent of disease unknown, staging in progress, or not listed (for use in a Medicare-approved demonstration project) ⑧ ♂   M

* **G9084** Oncology; disease status; colon cancer, limited to invasive cancer, adenocarcinoma as predominant cell type; extent of disease initially established as T1-3, N0, M0 with no evidence of disease progression, recurrence, or metastases (for use in a Medicare-approved demonstration project) ⑧   M

* **G9085** Oncology; disease status; colon cancer, limited to invasive cancer, adenocarcinoma as predominant cell type; extent of disease initially established as T4, N0, M0 with no evidence of disease progression, recurrence, or metastases (for use in a Medicare-approved demonstration project) ⑧   M

* **G9086** Oncology; disease status; colon cancer, limited to invasive cancer, adenocarcinoma as predominant cell type; extent of disease initially established as T1-4, N1-2, M0 with no evidence of disease progression, recurrence, or metastases (for use in a Medicare-approved demonstration project) ⑧   M

* **G9087** Oncology; disease status; colon cancer, limited to invasive cancer, adenocarcinoma as predominant cell type; M1 at diagnosis, metastatic, locally recurrent, or progressive with current clinical, radiologic, or biochemical evidence of disease (for use in a Medicare-approved demonstration project) ⑧   M

* **G9088** Oncology; disease status; colon cancer, limited to invasive cancer, adenocarcinoma as predominant cell type; M1 at diagnosis, metastatic, locally recurrent, or progressive without current clinical, radiologic, or biochemical evidence of disease (for use in a Medicare-approved demonstration project) ⑧   M

* **G9089** Oncology; disease status; colon cancer, limited to invasive cancer, adenocarcinoma as predominant cell type; extent of disease unknown, staging in progress, or not listed (for use in a Medicare-approved demonstration project) ⑧   M

* **G9090** Oncology; disease status; rectal cancer, limited to invasive cancer, adenocarcinoma as predominant cell type; extent of disease initially established as T1-2, N0, M0 (prior to neo-adjuvant therapy, if any) with no evidence of disease progression, recurrence, or metastases (for use in a Medicare-approved demonstration project) ⑧   M

* **G9091** Oncology; disease status; rectal cancer, limited to invasive cancer, adenocarcinoma as predominant cell type; extent of disease initially established as T3, N0, M0 (prior to neo-adjuvant therapy, if any) with no evidence of disease progression, recurrence, or metastases (for use in a Medicare-approved demonstration project) ⑧   M

* **G9092** Oncology; disease status; rectal cancer, limited to invasive cancer, adenocarcinoma as predominant cell type; extent of disease initially established as T1-3, N1-2, M0 (prior to neo-adjuvant therapy, if any) with no evidence of disease progression, recurrence or metastases (for use in a Medicare-approved demonstration project) ⑧   M

* **G9093** Oncology; disease status; rectal cancer, limited to invasive cancer, adenocarcinoma as predominant cell type; extent of disease initially established as T4, any N, M0 (prior to neo-adjuvant therapy, if any) with no evidence of disease progression, recurrence, or metastases (for use in a Medicare-approved demonstration project) ⑧   M

* **G9094** Oncology; disease status; rectal cancer, limited to invasive cancer, adenocarcinoma as predominant cell type; M1 at diagnosis, metastatic, locally recurrent, or progressive (for use in a Medicare-approved demonstration project) ⑧   M

* **G9095** Oncology; disease status; rectal cancer, limited to invasive cancer, adenocarcinoma as predominant cell type; extent of disease unknown, staging in progress, or not listed (for use in a Medicare-approved demonstration project) ⑧   M

▶ **New**   ↻ **Revised**   ✔ **Reinstated**   ~~deleted~~ **Deleted**   ⃠ **Not covered or valid by Medicare**

✸ **Special coverage instructions**   ✱ **Carrier discretion**   ⑧ **Bill local carrier**   ⑧ **Bill DME MAC**

✳ **G9096** Oncology; disease status; esophageal cancer, limited to adenocarcinoma or squamous cell carcinoma as predominant cell type; extent of disease initially established as T1-T3, N0-N1 or NX (prior to neo-adjuvant therapy, if any) with no evidence of disease progression, recurrence, or metastases (for use in a Medicare-approved demonstration project) Ⓑ   M

✳ **G9097** Oncology; disease status; esophageal cancer, limited to adenocarcinoma or squamous cell carcinoma as predominant cell type; extent of disease initially established as T4, any N, M0 (prior to neo-adjuvant therapy, if any) with no evidence of disease progression, recurrence, or metastases (for use in a Medicare-approved demonstration project) Ⓑ   M

✳ **G9098** Oncology; disease status; esophageal cancer, limited to adenocarcinoma or squamous cell carcinoma as predominant cell type; M1 at diagnosis, meta-static, locally recurrent, or progressive (for use in a Medicare-approved demonstration project) Ⓑ   M

✳ **G9099** Oncology; disease status; esophageal cancer, limited to adenocarcinoma or squamous cell carcinoma as predominant cell type; extent of disease unknown, staging in progress, or not listed (for use in a Medicare-approved demonstration project) Ⓑ   M

✳ **G9100** Oncology; disease status; gastric cancer, limited to adenocarcinoma as predominant cell type; post R0 resection (with or without neoadjuvant therapy) with no evidence of disease recurrence, progression, or metastases (for use in a Medicare-approved demonstration project) Ⓑ   M

✳ **G9101** Oncology; disease status; gastric cancer, limited to adenocarcinoma as predominant cell type; post R1 or R2 resection (with or without neoadjuvant therapy) with no evidence of disease progression, or metastases (for use in a Medicare-approved demonstration project) Ⓑ   M

✳ **G9102** Oncology; disease status; gastric cancer, limited to adenocarcinoma as predominant cell type; clinical or pathologic M0, unresectable with no evidence of disease progression, or metastases (for use in a Medicare-approved demonstration project) Ⓑ   M

✳ **G9103** Oncology; disease status; gastric cancer, limited to adenocarcinoma as predominant cell type; clinical or pathologic M1 at diagnosis, metastatic, locally recurrent, or progressive (for use in a Medicare-approved demonstration project) Ⓑ   M

✳ **G9104** Oncology; disease status; gastric cancer, limited to adenocarcinoma as predominant cell type; extent of disease unknown, staging in progress, or not listed (for use in a Medicare-approved demonstration project) Ⓑ   M

✳ **G9105** Oncology; disease status; pancreatic cancer, limited to adenocarcinoma as predominant cell type; post R0 resection without evidence of disease progression, recurrence, or metastases (for use in a Medicare-approved demonstration project) Ⓑ   M

✳ **G9106** Oncology; disease status; pancreatic cancer, limited to adenocarcinoma; post R1 or R2 resection with no evidence of disease progression or metastases (for use in a Medicare-approved demonstration project) Ⓑ   M

✳ **G9107** Oncology; disease status; pancreatic cancer, limited to adenocarcinoma; unresectable at diagnosis, M1 at diagnosis, metastatic, locally recurrent, or progressive (for use in a Medicare-approved demonstration project) Ⓑ   M

✳ **G9108** Oncology; disease status; pancreatic cancer, limited to adenocarcinoma; extent of disease unknown, staging in progress, or not listed (for use in a Medicare-approved demonstration project) Ⓑ   M

✳ **G9109** Oncology; disease status; head and neck cancer, limited to cancers of oral cavity, pharynx and larynx with squamous cell as predominant cell type; extent of disease initially established as T1-T2 and N0, M0 (prior to neo-adjuvant therapy, if any) with no evidence of disease progression, recurrence, or metastases (for use in a Medicare-approved demonstration project) Ⓑ   M

✳ **G9110** Oncology; disease status; head and neck cancer, limited to cancers of oral cavity, pharynx, and larynx with squamous cell as predominant cell type; extent of disease initially established as T3-4 and/ or N1-3, M0 (prior to neo-adjuvant therapy, if any) with no evidence of disease progression, recurrence, or metastases (for use in a Medicare-approved demonstration project) Ⓑ   M

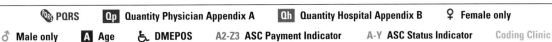

* **G9111** Oncology; disease status; head and neck cancer, limited to cancers of oral cavity, pharynx and larynx with squamous cell as predominant cell type; M1 at diagnosis, metastatic, locally recurrent, or progressive (for use in a Medicare-approved demonstration project) Ⓑ　　　M

* **G9112** Oncology; disease status; head and neck cancer, limited to cancers of oral cavity, pharynx and larynx with squamous cell as predominant cell type; extent of disease unknown, staging in progress, or not listed (for use in a Medicare-approved demonstration project) Ⓑ　　　M

* **G9113** Oncology; disease status; ovarian cancer, limited to epithelial cancer; pathologic stage IA-B (grade 1) without evidence of disease progression, recurrence, or metastases (for use in a Medicare-approved demonstration project) Ⓑ ♀　　　M

* **G9114** Oncology; disease status; ovarian cancer, limited to epithelial cancer; pathologic stage IA-B (grade 2-3); or stage IC (all grades); or stage II; without evidence of disease progression, recurrence, or metastases (for use in a Medicare-approved demonstration project) Ⓑ ♀　　　M

* **G9115** Oncology; disease status; ovarian cancer, limited to epithelial cancer; pathologic stage III-IV; without evidence of progression, recurrence, or metastases (for use in a Medicare-approved demonstration project) Ⓑ ♀　　　M

* **G9116** Oncology; disease status; ovarian cancer, limited to epithelial cancer; evidence of disease progression, or recurrence and/or platinum resistance (for use in a Medicare-approved demonstration project) Ⓑ ♀　　　M

* **G9117** Oncology; disease status; ovarian cancer, limited to epithelial cancer; extent of disease unknown, staging in progress, or not listed (for use in a Medicare-approved demonstration project) Ⓑ ♀　　　M

* **G9123** Oncology; disease status; chronic myelogenous leukemia, limited to Philadelphia chromosome positive and/or BCR-ABL positive; chronic phase not in hematologic, cytogenetic, or molecular remission (for use in a Medicare-approved demonstration project) Ⓑ　　　M

* **G9124** Oncology; disease status; chronic myelogenous leukemia, limited to Philadelphia chromosome positive and/or BCR-ABL positive; accelerated phase not in hematologic cytogenetic, or molecular remission (for use in a Medicare-approved demonstration project) Ⓑ　　　M

* **G9125** Oncology; disease status; chronic myelogenous leukemia, limited to Philadelphia chromosome positive and/or BCR-ABL positive; blast phase not in hematologic, cytogenetic, or molecular remission (for use in a Medicare-approved demonstration project) Ⓑ　　　M

* **G9126** Oncology; disease status; chronic myelogenous leukemia, limited to Philadelphia chromosome positive and/or BCR-ABL positive; in hematologic, cytogenetic, or molecular remission (for use in a Medicare-approved demonstration project) Ⓑ　　　M

G9128 Oncology: disease status; limited to multiple myeloma, systemic disease; smouldering, stage I (for use in a Medicare-approved demonstration project) Ⓑ　　　M

* **G9129** Oncology; disease status; limited to multiple myeloma, systemic disease; stage II or higher (for use in a Medicare-approved demonstration project) Ⓑ　　　M

* **G9130** Oncology; disease status; limited to multiple myeloma, systemic disease; extent of disease unknown, staging in progress, or not listed (for use in a Medicare-approved demonstration project) Ⓑ　　　M

* **G9131** Oncology; disease status; invasive female breast cancer (does not include ductal carcinoma in situ); adenocarcinoma as predominant cell type; extent of disease unknown, staging in progress, or not listed (for use in a Medicare-approved demonstration project) Ⓑ ♀　　　M

* **G9132** Oncology; disease status; prostate cancer, limited to adenocarcinoma; hormone-refractory/androgen-independent (e.g., rising PSA on anti-androgen therapy or post-orchiectomy); clinical metastases (for use in a Medicare-approved demonstration project) Ⓑ ♂　　　M

▶ New　↻ Revised　✔ Reinstated　~~deleted~~ Deleted　⊘ Not covered or valid by Medicare
✪ Special coverage instructions　* Carrier discretion　Ⓛ Bill local carrier　Ⓑ Bill DME MAC

✳ **G9133** Oncology; disease status; prostate cancer, limited to adenocarcinoma; hormone-responsive; clinical metastases or M1 at diagnosis (for use in a Medicare-approved demonstration project) ⑧ ♂   M

✳ **G9134** Oncology; disease status; non-Hodgkin's lymphoma, any cellular classification; stage I, II at diagnosis, not relapsed, not refractory (for use in a Medicare-approved demonstration project) ⑧   M

✳ **G9135** Oncology; disease status; non-Hodgkin's lymphoma, any cellular classification; stage III, IV, not relapsed, not refractory (for use in a Medicare-approved demonstration project) ⑧   M

✳ **G9136** Oncology; disease status; non-Hodgkin's lymphoma, transformed from original cellular diagnosis to a second cellular classification (for use in a Medicare-approved demonstration project) ⑧   M

✳ **G9137** Oncology; disease status; non-Hodgkin's lymphoma, any cellular classification; relapsed/refractory (for use in a Medicare-approved demonstration project) ⑧   M

✳ **G9138** Oncology; disease status; non-Hodgkin's lymphoma, any cellular classification; diagnostic evaluation, stage not determined, evaluation of possible relapse or non-response to therapy, or not listed (for use in a Medicare-approved demonstration project) ⑧   M

✳ **G9139** Oncology; disease status; chronic myelogenous leukemia, limited to Philadelphia chromosome positive and/or BCR-ABL positive; extent of disease unknown, staging in progress, not listed (for use in a Medicare-approved demonstration project) ⑧   M

✳ **G9140** Frontier extended stay clinic demonstration; for a patient stay in a clinic approved for the CMS demonstration project; the following measures should be present: the stay must be equal to or greater than 4 hours; weather or other conditions must prevent transfer or the case falls into a category of monitoring and observation cases that are permitted by the rules of the demonstration; there is a maximum frontier extended stay clinic (FESC) visit of 48 hours, except in the case when weather or other conditions prevent transfer; payment is made on each period up to 4 hours, after the first 4 hours ⑧   A

Influenza A (H1N1) and Warfarin Responsiveness Testing

✳ **G9143** Warfarin responsiveness testing by genetic technique using any method, any number of specimen(s) **Qp** **Qh**   N

This would be a once-in-a-lifetime test unless there is a reason to believe that the patient's personal genetic characteristics would change over time. (https://www.cms.gov/ContractorLearningResources/downloads/JA6715.pdf)

Laboratory Certification: General immunology, hematology

Coding Clinic: 2010, Q2, P10

⊘ **G9147** Outpatient intravenous insulin treatment (OIVIT) either pulsatile or continuous, by any means, guided by the results of measurements for: respiratory quotient; and/or, urine urea nitrogen (UUN); and/or, arterial, venous or capillary glucose; and/or potassium concentration   E

On December 23, 2009, CMS issued a national non-coverage decision on the use of OIVIT. CR 6775.

Not covered on Physician Fee Schedule

Coding Clinic: 2010, Q2, P10

✳ **G9148** National committee for quality assurance - level 1 medical home

✳ **G9149** National committee for quality assurance - level 2 medical home

✳ **G9150** National committee for quality assurance - level 3 medical home

✳ **G9151** MAPCP demonstration - state provided services

✳ **G9152** MAPCP demonstration - community health teams

✳ **G9153** MAPCP demonstration - physician incentive pool

✳ **G9156** Evaluation for wheelchair requiring face to face visit with physician **Qp** **Qh**   M

↻✳ **G9157** Transesophageal doppler measurement of cardiac output (including probe placement, image acquisition, and interpretation per course of treatment) for monitoring purposes **Qp** **Qh**   B

✳ **G9158** Motor speech functional limitation, discharge status, at discharge from therapy or to end reporting   E

✳ **G9159** Spoken language comprehension functional limitation, current status at therapy episode outset and at reporting intervals   E

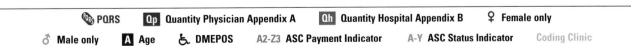

PQRS   **Qp** Quantity Physician Appendix A   **Qh** Quantity Hospital Appendix B   ♀ Female only
♂ Male only   **A** Age   ＆ DMEPOS   A2-Z3 ASC Payment Indicator   A-Y ASC Status Indicator   Coding Clinic

⮌✳ **G9160** Spoken language comprehension functional limitation, projected goal status at therapy episode outset, at reporting intervals, and at discharge or to end reporting E

✳ **G9161** Spoken language comprehension functional limitation, discharge status at discharge from therapy or to end reporting E

✳ **G9162** Spoken language expression functional limitation, current status at therapy episode outset and at reporting intervals E

⮌✳ **G9163** Spoken language expression functional limitation, projected goal status at therapy episode outset, at reporting intervals, and at discharge or to end reporting E

✳ **G9164** Spoken language expression functional limitation, discharge status at discharge from therapy or to end reporting E

✳ **G9165** Attention functional limitation, current status at therapy episode outset and at reporting intervals E

⮌✳ **G9166** Attention functional limitation, projected goal status at therapy episode outset, at reporting intervals, and at discharge or to end reporting E

✳ **G9167** Attention functional limitation, discharge status at discharge from therapy or to end reporting E

✳ **G9168** Memory functional limitation, current status at therapy episode outset and at reporting intervals E

⮌✳ **G9169** Memory functional limitation, projected goal status at therapy episode outset, at reporting intervals, and at discharge or to end reporting E

✳ **G9170** Memory functional limitation, discharge status at discharge from therapy or to end reporting E

✳ **G9171** Voice functional limitation, current status at therapy episode outset and at reporting intervals E

⮌✳ **G9172** Voice functional limitation, projected goal status at therapy episode outset, at reporting intervals, and at discharge or to end reporting E

✳ **G9173** Voice functional limitation, discharge status at discharge from therapy or to end reporting E

✳ **G9174** Other speech language pathology functional limitation, current status at therapy episode outset and at reporting intervals E

⮌✳ **G9175** Other speech language pathology functional limitation, projected goal status at therapy episode outset, at reporting intervals, and at discharge or to end reporting E

✳ **G9176** Other speech language pathology functional limitation, discharge status at discharge from therapy or to end reporting E

⮌✳ **G9186** Motor speech functional limitation, projected goal status at therapy episode outset, at reporting intervals, and at discharge or to end reporting E

✳ **G9187** Bundled payments for care improvement initiative home visit for patient assessment performed by a qualified health care professional for individuals not considered homebound including, but not limited to, assessment of safety, falls, clinical status, fluid status, medication reconciliation/management, patient compliance with orders/plan of care, performance of activities of daily living, appropriateness of care setting; (for use only in the Medicare-approved bundled payments for care improvement initiative); may not be billed for a 30-day period covered by a transitional care management code **Qp** **Qh** E

⊘ ✳ **G9188** Beta-blocker therapy not prescribed, reason not given M

⊘ ✳ **G9189** Beta-blocker therapy prescribed or currently being taken M

⊘ ✳ **G9190** Documentation of medical reason(s) for not prescribing beta-blocker therapy (e.g., allergy, intolerance, other medical reasons) M

⊘ ✳ **G9191** Documentation of patient reason(s) for not prescribing beta-blocker therapy (e.g., patient declined, other patient reasons) M

⊘ ✳ **G9192** Documentation of system reason(s) for not prescribing beta-blocker therapy (e.g., other reasons attributable to the health care system) M

~~G9193~~ ~~Clinician documented that patient with a diagnosis of major depression was not an eligible candidate for antidepressant medication treatment or patient did not have a diagnosis of major depression~~ ✖

~~G9194~~ ~~Patient with a diagnosis of major depression documented as being treated with antidepressant medication during the entire 180 day (6 month) continuation treatment phase~~ ✖

▶ **New** ⮌ **Revised** ✔ **Reinstated** ~~deleted~~ **Deleted** ⊘ **Not covered or valid by Medicare**

⊙ **Special coverage instructions** ✳ **Carrier discretion** Ⓑ **Bill local carrier** Ⓓ **Bill DME MAC**

G9195 ~~Patient with a diagnosis of major depression not documented as being treated with antidepressant medication during the entire 180 day (6 months) continuation treatment phase~~ ✖

(PQRS) ✳ **G9196** Documentation of medical reason(s) for not ordering first or second generation cephalosporin for antimicrobial prophylaxis M

(PQRS) ✳ **G9197** Documentation of order for first or second generation cephalosporin for antimicrobial prophylaxis M

(PQRS) ✳ **G9198** Order for first or second generation cephalosporin for antimicrobial prophylaxis was not documented, reason not given M

G9199 ~~Venous thromboembolism (VTE) prophylaxis not administered the day of or the day after hospital admission for documented reasons (e.g., patient is ambulatory, patient expired during inpatient stay, patient already on warfarin or another anticoagulant, other medical reason(s) or e.g., patient left against medical advice, other patient reason(s))~~ ✖

G9200 ~~Venous thromboembolism (VTE) prophylaxis was not administered the day of or the day after hospital admission, reason not given~~ ✖

G9201 ~~Venous thromboembolism (VTE) prophylaxis administered the day of or the day after hospital admission~~ ✖

G9202 ~~Patients with a positive hepatitis C antibody test~~ ✖

(PQRS) ✳ **G9203** Rna testing for hepatitis C documented as performed within 12 months prior to initiation of antiviral treatment for hepatitis C M

(PQRS) ✳ **G9204** Rna testing for hepatitis C was not documented as performed within 12 months prior to initiation of antiviral treatment for hepatitis C, reason not given M

(PQRS) ✳ **G9205** Patient starting antiviral treatment for hepatitis C during the measurement period M

(PQRS) ✳ **G9206** Patient starting antiviral treatment for hepatitis C during the measurement period M

(PQRS) ✳ **G9207** Hepatitis C genotype testing documented as performed within 12 months prior to initiation of antiviral treatment for hepatitis C M

(PQRS) ✳ **G9208** Hepatitis C genotype testing was not documented as performed within 12 months prior to initiation of antiviral treatment for hepatitis C, reason not given M

(PQRS) ✳ **G9209** Hepatitis C quantitative RNA testing documented as performed between 4-12 weeks after the initiation of antiviral treatment M

(PQRS) ⟳ ✳ **G9210** Hepatitis C quantitative RNA testing not performed between 4-12 weeks after the initiation of antiviral treatment for documented reason(s) (e.g., patients whose treatment was discontinued during the testing period prior to testing, other medical reasons, patient declined, other patient reasons) M

(PQRS) ✳ **G9211** Hepatitis C quantitative RNA testing was not documented as performed between 4-12 weeks after the initiation of antiviral treatment, reason not given M

✳ **G9212** DSM-IVTM criteria for major depressive disorder documented at the initial evaluation M

✳ **G9213** DSM-IV-TR criteria for major depressive disorder not documented at the initial evaluation, reason not otherwise specified M

G9214 ~~CD4+ cell count or CD4+ cell percentage results documented~~ ✖

G9215 ~~CD4+ cell count or percentage not documented as performed, reason not given~~ ✖

G9216 ~~PCP prophylaxis was not prescribed at time of diagnosis of HIV, reason not given~~ ✖

(PQRS) ✳ **G9217** PCP prophylaxis was not prescribed within 3 months of low CD4+ cell count below 200 cells/mm^3, reason not given M

G9218 ~~PCP prophylaxis was not prescribed within 3 months of low CD4+ cell count below 500 cells/mm3 or a CD4 percentage below 15%, reason not given~~ ✖

(PQRS) ✳ **G9219** Pneumocystis jiroveci pneumonia prophylaxis not prescribed within 3 months of low CD4+ cell count below 200 cells/mm^3 for medical reason (i.e., patient's CD4+ cell count above threshold within 3 months after CD4+ cell count below threshold, indicating that the patient's CD4+ levels are within an acceptable range and the patient does not require PCP prophylaxis) M

~~G9220~~ ~~Pneumocystis jiroveci pneumonia~~ ✖
~~prophylaxis not prescribed within~~
~~3 months of low CD4+ cell count below~~
~~500 cells/mm3 or a CD4 percentage~~
~~below 15% for medical reason (i.e.,~~
~~patient's CD4+ cell count above~~
~~threshold within 3 months after CD4+~~
~~cell count below threshold, indicating~~
~~that the patient's CD4+ levels are within~~
~~an acceptable range and the patient~~
~~does not require PCP~~
~~prophylaxis)~~

~~G9221~~ ~~Pneumocystis jiroveci pneumonia~~ ✖
~~prophlaxis prescribed~~

(PQRS) ✳ **G9222** Pneumocystis jiroveci pneumonia
prophylaxis prescribed wthin 3 months
of low CD4+ cell count below
200 cells/mm3   M

(PQRS) ✳ **G9223** Pneumocystis jiroveci pneumonia
prophylaxis prescribed within 3 months
of low CD4+ cell count below 500 cells/
mm^3 or a CD4 percentage below
15%   M

~~G9224~~ ~~Documentation of medical reason for~~ ✖
~~not performing foot exam (e.g., patient~~
~~with bilateral foot/leg~~
~~amputation)~~

(PQRS) ✳ **G9225** Foot exam was not performed, reason
not given   M

(PQRS) ✳ **G9226** Foot examination performed (includes
examination through visual inspection,
sensory exam with monofilament, and
pulse exam - report when all of the
3 components are completed)   M

(PQRS) ✳ **G9227** Functional outcome assessment
documented, care plan not
documented, documentation the
patient is not eligible for a care
plan   M

(PQRS) ✳ **G9228** Chlamydia, gonorrhea and syphilis
screening results documented (report
when results are present for all of the 3
screenings)   M

(PQRS) ✳ **G9229** Chlamydia, gonorrhea, and syphilis not
screened, due to documented reason
(patient refusal is the only allowed
exclusion)   M

(PQRS) ✳ **G9230** Chlamydia, gonorrhea, and syphilis not
screened, reason not given   M

(PQRS) ✳ **G9231** Documentation of end stage renal
disease (ESRD), dialysis, renal
transplant or pregnancy   M

(PQRS) ✳ **G9232** Clinician treating major depressive
disorder did not communicate to
clinician treating comorbid condition
for specified patient reason   M

✳ **G9233** All quality actions for the applicable
measures in the total knee replacement
measures group have been performed
for this patient   M

✳ **G9234** I intend to report the total knee
replacement measures group   M

✳ **G9235** All quality actions for the applicable
measures in the general surgery
measures group have been performed
for this patient   M

✳ **G9236** All quality actions for the applicable
measures in the optimizing patient
exposure to ionizing radiation
measures group have been performed
for this patient   M

✳ **G9237** I intend to report the general surgery
measures group   M

✳ **G9238** I intend to report the optimizing
patient exposure to ionizing radiation
measures group   M

(PQRS) ✳ **G9239** Documentation of reasons for patient
initiating maintenance hemodialysis
with a catheter as the mode of vascular
access (e.g., patient has a maturing
AVF/AVG, time-limited trial of
hemodialysis, patients undergoing
palliative dialysis, other medical
reasons, patient declined AVF/AVG,
other patient reasons, patient followed
by reporting nephrologist for fewer
than 90 days, other system reasons)
  M

(PQRS) ✳ **G9240** Patient whose mode of vascular access
is a catheter at the time maintenance
hemodialysis is initiated   M

(PQRS) ✳ **G9241** Patient whose mode of vascular access
is not a catheter at the time
maintenance hemodialysis is
initiated   M

(PQRS) ↻ ✳ **G9242** Documentation of viral load equal to or
greater than 200 copies/ml or viral load
not performed   M

(PQRS) ✳ **G9243** Documentation of viral load less than
200 copies/ml   M

(PQRS) ✳ **G9244** Antiretroviral therapy not
prescribed   M

(PQRS) ✳ **G9245** Antiretroviral therapy prescribed   M

✳ **G9246** Patient did not have at least one
medical visit in each 6 month period
of the 24 month measurement period,
with a minimum of 60 days between
medical visits   M

✳ **G9247** Patient had at least one medical visit in
each 6 month period of the 24 month
measurement period, with a minimum
of 60 days between medical visits   M

▶ **New**   ↻ **Revised**   ✔ **Reinstated**   ~~deleted~~ **Deleted**   ⃠ **Not covered or valid by Medicare**

✲ **Special coverage instructions**   ✳ **Carrier discretion**   ⑧ **Bill local carrier**   ⑧ **Bill DME MAC**

G9248 ~~Patient did not have a medical visit in the last 6 months~~ ✖

G9249 ~~Patient had a medical visit in the last 6 months~~ ✖

⊛ **G9250** Documentation of patient pain brought to a comfortable level within 48 hours from initial assessment M

⊛ **G9251** Documentation of patient with pain not brought to a comfortable level within 48 hours from initial assessment M

G9252 ~~Adenoma(s) or other neoplasm detected during screening colonoscopy~~ ✖

G9253 ~~Adenoma(s) or other neoplasm not detected during screening colonoscopy~~ ✖

⊛ **G9254** Documentation of patient discharged to home later than post-operative day 2 following CAS M

⊛ **G9255** Documentation of patient discharged to home no later than post operative day 2 following CAS M

⊛ **G9256** Documentation of patient death following CAS M

⊛ **G9257** Documentation of patient stroke following CAS M

⊛ **G9258** Documentation of patient stroke following CEA M

⊛ **G9259** Documentation of patient survival and absence of stroke following CAS M

⊛ **G9260** Documentation of patient death following CEA M

⊛ **G9261** Documentation of patient survival and absence of stroke following CEA M

⊛ **G9262** Documentation of patient death in the hospital following endovascular AAA repair M

⊛ **G9263** Documentation of patient survival in the hospital following endovascular AAA repair M

⊛ **G9264** Documentation of patient receiving maintenance hemodialysis for greater than or equal to 90 days with a catheter for documented reasons (e.g., patient is undergoing palliative dialysis with a catheter, patient approved by a qualified transplant program and scheduled to receive a living donor kidney transplant, other medical reasons, patient declined AVF/AVG, other patient reasons) M

⊛ **G9265** Patient receiving maintenance hemodialysis for greater than or equal to 90 days with a catheter as the mode of vascular access M

⊛ **G9266** Patient receiving maintenance hemodialysis for greater than or equal to 90 days without a catheter as the mode of vascular access M

⊛ **G9267** Documentation of patient with one or more complications or mortality within 30 days M

⊛ **G9268** Documentation of patient with one or more complications within 90 days M

⊛ **G9269** Documentation of patient without one or more complications and without mortality within 30 days M

⊛ **G9270** Documentation of patient without one or more complications within 90 days M

G9271 ~~LDL value < 100~~ ✖

G9272 ~~LDL value >= 100~~ ✖

⊛ **G9273** Blood pressure has a systolic value of < 140 and a diastolic value of < 90 M

⊛ **G9274** Blood pressure has a systolic value of =140 and a diastolic value of = 90 or systolic value < 140 and diastolic value = 90 or systolic value = 140 and diastolic value < 90 M

⊛ **G9275** Documentation that patient is a current non-tobacco user M

⊛ **G9276** Documentation that patient is a current tobacco user M

⮌⊛ **G9277** Documentation that the patient is on daily aspirin or anti-platelet or has documentation of a valid contraindication to aspirin/anti-platelet. Automatic contraindications include anti-coagulant use, allergy, and history of gastrointestinal bleed. Additionally, any reason documented by the physician as a reason for not taking daily aspirin or anti-platelet is acceptable (examples include non-steroidal anti-inflammatory agents, risk for drug interaction, or uncontrolled hypertension defined as > 180 systolic or > 110 diastolic) M

⮌⊛ **G9278** Documentation that the patient is not on daily aspirin or anti-platelet regimen M

⊛ **G9279** Pneumococcal screening performed and documentation of vaccination received prior to discharge M

⊛ **G9280** Pneumococcal vaccination not administered prior to discharge, reason not specified M

⊛ **G9281** Screening performed and documentation that vaccination not indicated/patient refusal M

---

* **G9282** Documentation of medical reason(s) for not reporting the histological type or NSCLC-NOS classification with an explanation (e.g., biopsy taken for other purposes in a patient with a history of non-small cell lung cancer or other documented medical reasons) M

* **G9283** Non small cell lung cancer biopsy and cytology specimen report documents classification into specific histologic type or classified as NSCLC-NOS with an explanation M

* **G9284** Non-small cell lung cancer biopsy and cytology specimen report does not document classification into specific histologic type or classified as NSCLC-NOS with an explanation M

* **G9285** Specimen site other than anatomic location of lung or is not classified as non small cell lung cancer M

* **G9286** Documentation of antibiotic regimen prescribed within 7 days of diagnosis or within 10 days after onset of symptoms M

* **G9287** No antibiotic regimen prescribed within 7 days of diagnosis or within 10 days after onset of symptoms M

* **G9288** Documentation of medical reason(s) for not reporting the histological type or NSCLC-NOS classification with an explanation (e.g., a solitary fibrous tumor in a person with a history of non-small cell carcinoma or other documented medical reasons) M

* **G9289** Non-small cell lung cancer biopsy and cytology specimen report documents classification into specific histologic type or classified as NSCLC-NOS with an explanation M

* **G9290** Non-small cell lung cancer biopsy and cytology specimen report does not document classification into specific histologic type or classified as NSCLC-NOS with an explanation M

* **G9291** Specimen site other than anatomic location of lung, is not classified as non small cell lung cancer or classified as NSCLC-NOS M

* **G9292** Documentation of medical reason(s) for not reporting PT category and a statement on thickness and ulceration and for PT1, mitotic rate (e.g., negative skin biopsies in a patient with a history of melanoma or other documented medical reasons) M

* **G9293** Pathology report does not include the PT category and a statement on thickness and ulceration and for PT1, mitotic rate M

* **G9294** Pathology report includes the PT category and a statement on thickness and ulceration and for PT1, mitotic rate M

* **G9295** Specimen site other than anatomic cutaneous location M

↻ * **G9296** Patients with documented shared decision-making including discussion of conservative (non-surgical) therapy (e.g., NSAIDs, analgesics, weight loss, exercise, injections) prior to the procedure M

↻ * **G9297** Shared decision-making including discussion of conservative (non-surgical) therapy (e.g., NSAIDs, analgesics, weight loss, exercise, injections) prior to the procedure not documented, reason not given M

↻ * **G9298** Patients who are evaluated for venous thromboembolic and cardiovascular risk factors within 30 days prior to the procedure (e.g., history of DVT, PE, MI, arrhythmia and stroke) M

↻ * **G9299** Patients who are not evaluated for venous thromboembolic and cardiovascular risk factors within 30 days prior to the procedure (e.g., history of DVT, PE, MI, arrhythmia and stroke, reason not given) M

* **G9300** Documentation of medical reason(s) for not completely infusing the prophylactic antibiotic prior to the inflation of the proximal tourniquet (e.g., a tourniquet was not used) M

* **G9301** Patients who had the prophylactic antibiotic completely infused prior to the inflation of the proximal tourniquet M

* **G9302** Prophylactic antibiotic not completely infused prior to the inflation of the proximal tourniquet, reason not given M

↻ * **G9303** Operative report does not identify the prosthetic implant specifications including the prosthetic implant manufacturer, the brand name of the prosthetic implant and the size of each prosthetic implant, reason not given M

↻ * **G9304** Operative report identifies the prosthetic implant specifications including the prosthetic implant manufacturer, the brand name of the prosthetic implant and the size of each prosthetic implant M

▶ New   ↻ Revised   ✔ Reinstated   ~~deleted~~ Deleted   ⊘ Not covered or valid by Medicare

⊛ Special coverage instructions   ✳ Carrier discretion   Ⓑ Bill local carrier   Ⓑ Bill DME MAC

* **G9305** Intervention for presence of leak of endoluminal contents through an anastomosis not required   M

* **G9306** Intervention for presence of leak of endoluminal contents through an anastomosis required   M

* **G9307** No return to the operating room for a surgical procedure, for any reason, within 30 days of the principal operative procedure   M

* **G9308** Unplanned return to the operating room for a surgical procedure, for any reason, within 30 days of the principal operative procedure   M

* **G9309** No unplanned hospital readmission within 30 days of principal procedure   M

* **G9310** Unplanned hospital readmission within 30 days of principal procedure   M

* **G9311** No surgical site infection   M

* **G9312** Surgical site infection   M

(PQRS) * **G9313** Amoxicillin, with or without clavulanate, not prescribed as first line antibiotic at the time of diagnosis for documented reason (e.g., cystic fibrosis, immotile cilia disorders, ciliary dyskinesia, immune deficiency, prior history of sinus surgery within the past 12 months, and anatomic abnormalities, such as deviated nasal septum, resistant organisms, allergy to medication, recurrent sinusitis, chronic sinusitis, or other reasons)   M

(PQRS) * **G9314** Amoxicillin, with or without clavulanate, not prescribed as first line antibiotic at the time of diagnosis, reason not given   M

(PQRS) * **G9315** Documentation amoxicillin, with or without clavulanate, prescribed as a first line antibiotic at the time of diagnosis   M

(PQRS) * **G9316** Documentation of patient-specific risk assessment with a risk calculator based on multi-institutional clinical data, the specific risk calculator used, and communication of risk assessment from risk calculator with the patient or family   M

(PQRS) * **G9317** Documentation of patient-specific risk assessment with a risk calculator based on multi-institutional clinical data, the specific risk calculator used, and communication of risk assessment from risk calculator with the patient or family not completed   M

* **G9318** Imaging study named according to standardized nomenclature   M

* **G9319** Imaging study not named according to standardized nomenclature, reason not given   M

* **G9320** Documentation of medical reason(s) for not naming CT studies according to a standardized nomenclature provided (e.g., CT studies performed for radiation treatment planning or image-guided radiation treatment delivery)   M

* **G9321** Count of previous CT (any type of CT) and cardiac nuclear medicine (myocardial perfusion) studies documented in the 12-month period prior to the current study   M

* **G9322** Count of previous CT and cardiac nuclear medicine (myocardial perfusion) studies not documented in the 12-month period prior to the current study, reason not given   M

* **G9323** Documentation of medical reason(s) for not counting previous CT and cardiac nuclear medicine (myocardial perfusion) studies (e.g., CT studies performed for radiation treatment planning or image-guided radiation treatment delivery)   M

* **G9324** All necessary data elements not included, reason not given   M

* **G9325** CT studies not reported to a radiation dose index registry due to medical reasons (e.g., CT studies performed for radiation treatment planning or image-guided radiation treatment delivery)   M

* **G9326** CT studies performed not reported to a radiation dose index registry, reason not given   M

* **G9327** CT studies performed reported to a radiation dose index registry with all necessary data elements   M

* **G9328** DICOM format image data availability not documented in final report due to medical reasons (e.g., CT studies performed for radiation treatment planning or image-guided radiation treatment delivery)   M

↻* **G9329** DICOM format image data available to non-affiliated external healthcare facilities or entities on a secure, media free, reciprocally searchable basis with patient authorization for at least a 12-month period after the study not documented in final report, reason not given   M

↻＊ **G9340** Final report documented that DICOM format image data available to non-affiliated external healthcare facilities or entities on a secure, media free, reciprocally searchable basis with patient authorization for at least a 12-month period after the study   M

↻＊ **G9341** Search conducted for prior patient CT studies completed at non-affiliated external healthcare facilities or entities within the past 12-months and are available through a secure, authorized, media-free, shared archive prior to an imaging study being performed   M

↻＊ **G9342** Search not conducted prior to an imaging study being performed for prior patient CT studies completed at non-affiliated external healthcare facilities or entities within the past 12-months and are available through a secure, authorized, media-free, shared archive, reason not given   M

↻＊ **G9343** Due to medical reasons, search not conducted for DICOM format images for prior patient CT imaging studies completed at non-affiliated external healthcare facilities or entities within the past 12 months that are available through a secure, authorized, media-free, shared archive (e.g., CT studies performed for radiation treatment planning or image-guided radiation treatment delivery)   M

↻＊ **G9344** Due to system reasons search not conducted for DICOM format images for prior patient CT imaging studies completed at non-affiliated external healthcare facilities or entities within the past 12 months that are available through a secure, authorized, media-free, shared archive (e.g., non-affiliated external healthcare facilities or entities does not have archival abilities through a shared archival system)   M

↻＊ **G9345** Follow-up recommendations documented according to recommended guidelines for incidentally detected pulmonary nodules (e.g., follow-up CT imaging studies needed or that no follow-up is needed) based at a minimum on nodule size and patient risk factors   M

↻＊ **G9346** Follow-up recommendations not documented according to recommended guidelines for incidentally detected pulmonary nodules due to medical reasons (e.g., patients with known malignant disease, patients with unexplained fever, CT studies performed for radiation treatment planning or image-guided radiation treatment delivery)   M

↻＊ **G9347** Follow-up recommendations not documented according to recommended guidelines for incidentally detected pulmonary nodules, reason not given   M

(PQRS) ＊ **G9348** CT scan of the paranasal sinuses ordered at the time of diagnosis for documented reasons (e.g., persons with sinusitis symptoms lasting at least 7 to 10 days, antibiotic resistance, immunocompromised, recurrent sinusitis, acute frontal sinusitis, acute sphenoid sinusitis, periorbital cellulitis, or other medical)   M

(PQRS) ＊ **G9349** Documentation of a CT scan of the paranasal sinuses ordered at the time of diagnosis or received within 28 days after date of diagnosis   M

(PQRS) ＊ **G9350** CT scan of the paranasal sinuses not ordered at the time of diagnosis or received within 28 days after date of diagnosis   M

(PQRS) ＊ **G9351** More than one CT scan of the paranasal sinuses ordered or received within 90 days after diagnosis   M

(PQRS) ＊ **G9352** More than one CT scan of the paranasal sinuses ordered or received within 90 days after the date of diagnosis, reason not given   M

(PQRS) ＊ **G9353** More than one CT scan of the paranasal sinuses ordered or received within 90 days after the date of diagnosis for documented reasons (e.g., patients with complications, second CT obtained prior to surgery, other medical reasons)   M

(PQRS) ＊ **G9354** More than one CT scan of the paranasal sinuses not ordered within 90 days after the date of diagnosis   M

(PQRS) ＊ **G9355** Elective delivery or early induction not performed   M

(PQRS) ＊ **G9356** Elective delivery or early induction performed   M

(PQRS) ＊ **G9357** Post-partum screenings, evaluations and education performed   M

(PQRS) ＊ **G9358** Post-partum screenings, evaluations and education not performed   M

(PQRS) ＊ **G9359** Documentation of negative or managed positive TB screen with further evidence that TB is not active   M

(PQRS) ＊ **G9360** No documentation of negative or managed positive TB screen   M

▶ **New**   ↻ **Revised**   ✔ **Reinstated**   ~~deleted~~ **Deleted**   ⊘ **Not covered or valid by Medicare**
⊕ **Special coverage instructions**   ＊ **Carrier discretion**   Ⓑ **Bill local carrier**   Ⓓ **Bill DME MAC**

✳ **G9361** Medical indication for induction (documentation of reason(s) for elective delivery or early induction (e.g., hemorrhage and placental complications, hypertension, preeclampsia and eclampsia, rupture of membranes-premature, prolonged maternal conditions complicating pregnancy/delivery, fetal conditions complicating pregnancy/delivery, malposition and malpresentation of fetus, late pregnancy, prior uterine surgery, or participation in clinical trial))   M

▶ ✳ **G9362** Duration of monitored anesthesia care (MAC) or peripheral nerve block (PNB) without the use of general anesthesia during an applicable procedure 60 minutes or longer, as documented in the anesthesia record   M

▶ ✳ **G9363** Duration of monitored anesthesia care (MAC) or peripheral nerve block (PNB) without the use of general anesthesia during an applicable procedure or general or neuraxial anesthesia less than 60 minutes, as documented in the anesthesia record   M

▶ ✳ **G9364** Sinusitis caused by, or presumed to be caused by, bacterial infection   M

▶ ✳ **G9365** One high-risk medication ordered   M

▶ ✳ **G9366** One high-risk medication not ordered   M

▶ ✳ **G9367** At least two different high-risk medications ordered   M

▶ ✳ **G9368** At least two different high-risk medications not ordered   M

▶ ✳ **G9369** Individual filled at least two prescriptions for any antipsychotic medication and had a PDC of 0.8 or greater   M

▶ ✳ **G9370** Individual who did not fill at least two prescriptions for any antipsychotic medication or did not have a PDC of 0.8 or greater   M

▶ ✳ **G9376** Patient continued to have the retina attached at the 6 months follow up visit (+/- 1 month) following only one surgery   M

▶ ✳ **G9377** Patient did not have the retina attached after 6 months following only one surgery   M

▶ ✳ **G9378** Patient continued to have the retina attached at the 6 months follow up visit (+/- 1 month)   M

▶ ✳ **G9379** Patient did not achieve flat retinas six months post surgery   M

▶ ✳ **G9380** Patient offered assistance with end of life issues during the measurement period   M

▶ ✳ **G9381** Documentation of medical reason(s) for not offering assistance with end of life issues (eg, patient in hospice and in terminal phase) during the measurement period   M

▶ ✳ **G9382** Patient not offered assistance with end of life issues during the measurement period   M

▶ ✳ **G9383** Patient received screening for HCV infection within the 12 month reporting period   M

▶ ✳ **G9384** Documentation of medical reason(s) for not receiving screening for HCV infection within the 12 month reporting period (e.g., decompensated cirrhosis including advanced disease [ie, ascites, esophageal variceal bleeding, hepatic encephalopathy], hepatocellular carcinoma, or waitlist for organ transplant, limited life expectancy, other medical reasons)   M

▶ ✳ **G9385** Documentation of patient reason(s) for not receiving screening for HCV infection within the 12 month reporting period (e.g., patient declined, other patient reasons)   M

▶ ✳ **G9386** Screening for HCV infection not received within the 12 month reporting period, reason not given   M

▶ ✳ **G9389** Unplanned rupture of the posterior capsule requiring vitrectomy   M

▶ ✳ **G9390** No unplanned rupture of the posterior capsule requiring vitrectomy   M

▶ ✳ **G9391** Patient achieves refraction +-1 d for the eye that underwent cataract surgery, measured at the one month follow up visit   M

▶ ✳ **G9392** Patient does not achieve refraction +-1 d for the eye that underwent cataract surgery, measured at the one month follow up visit   M

▶ ✳ **G9393** Patient with an initial PHQ-9 score greater than nine who achieves remission at twelve months as demonstrated by a twelve month (+/- 30 days) phq-9 score of less than five   M

▶ ✳ **G9394** Patient who had a diagnosis of bipolar disorder or personality disorder, death, permanent nursing home resident or receiving hospice or palliative care any time during the measurement or assessment period   M

🄿 PQRS	🅀🄿 Quantity Physician Appendix A	🅀🄷 Quantity Hospital Appendix B	♀ Female only
♂ Male only	🄰 Age	🦽 DMEPOS	A2-Z3 ASC Payment Indicator	A-Y ASC Status Indicator	Coding Clinic

TEMPORARY PROCEDURES/PROFESSIONAL SERVICES   G9361 — G9394

247

▶ ✳ **G9395** Patient with an initial PHQ-9 score greater than nine who did not achieve remission at twelve months as demonstrated by a twelve month (+/- 30 days) phq-9 score greater than or equal to five **M**

▶ ✳ **G9396** Patient with an initial PHQ-9 score greater than nine who was not assessed for remission at twelve months (+/- 30 days) **M**

▶ ✳ **G9399** Documentation in the patient record of a discussion between the physician/clinician and the patient that includes all of the following: treatment choices appropriate to genotype, risks and benefits, evidence of effectiveness, and patient preferences toward the outcome of the treatment **M**

▶ ✳ **G9400** Documentation of medical or patient reason(s) for not discussing treatment options; medical reasons: patient is not a candidate for treatment due to advanced physical or mental health comorbidity (including active substance use); currently receiving antiviral treatment; successful antiviral treatment (with sustained virologic response) prior to reporting period; other documented medical reasons; patient reasons: patient unable or unwilling to participate in the discussion or other patient reasons **M**

▶ ✳ **G9401** No documentation of a discussion in the patient record of a discussion between the physician or other qualified healthcare professional and the patient that includes all of the following: treatment choices appropriate to genotype, risks and benefits, evidence of effectiveness, and patient preferences toward treatment **M**

▶ ✳ **G9402** Patient received follow-up on the date of discharge or within 30 days after discharge **M**

▶ ✳ **G9403** Clinician documented reason patient was not able to complete 30 day follow-up from acute inpatient setting discharge (e.g., patient death prior to follow-up visit, patient non-compliant for visit follow-up) **M**

▶ ✳ **G9404** Patient did not receive follow-up on the date of discharge or within 30 days after discharge **M**

▶ ✳ **G9405** Patient received follow-up within 7 days from discharge **M**

▶ ✳ **G9406** Clinician documented reason patient was not able to complete 7 day follow-up from acute inpatient setting discharge (i.e patient death prior to follow-up visit, patient non-compliance for visit follow-up) **M**

▶ ✳ **G9407** Patient did not receive follow-up on or within 7 days after discharge **M**

▶ ✳ **G9408** Patients with cardiac tamponade and/or pericardiocentesis occurring within 30 days **M**

▶ ✳ **G9409** Patients without cardiac tamponade and/or pericardiocentesis occurring within 30 days **M**

▶ ✳ **G9410** Patient admitted within 180 days, status post CIED implantation, replacement, or revision with an infection requiring device removal or surgical revision **M**

▶ ✳ **G9411** Patient not admitted within 180 days, status post CIED implantation, replacement, or revision with an infection requiring device removal or surgical revision **M**

▶ ✳ **G9412** Patient admitted within 180 days, status post CIED implantation, replacement, or revision with an infection requiring device removal or surgical revision **M**

▶ ✳ **G9413** Patient not admitted within 180 days, status post CIED implantation, replacement, or revision with an infection requiring device removal or surgical revision **M**

▶ ✳ **G9414** Patient had one dose of meningococcal vaccine on or between the patient's 11th and 13th birthdays **M**

▶ ✳ **G9415** Patient did not have one dose of meningococcal vaccine on or between the patient's 11th and 13th birthdays **M**

▶ ✳ **G9416** Patient had one tetanus, diphtheria toxoids and acellular pertussis vaccine (Tdap) or one tetanus, diphtheria toxoids vaccine (Td) on or between the patient's 10th and 13th birthdays or one tetanus and one diptheria vaccine on or between the patient's 10th and 13th birthdays **M**

▶ ✳ **G9417** Patient did not have one tetanus, diphtheria toxoids and acellular pertussis vaccine (Tdap) or one tetanus, diphtheria toxoids vaccine (Td) on or between the patient's 10th and 13th birthdays or one tetanus and one diptheria vaccine on or between the patient's 10th and 13th birthdays **M**

▶ New   ↻ Revised   ✔ Reinstated   ~~deleted~~ Deleted   ⊘ Not covered or valid by Medicare

⊙ Special coverage instructions   ✳ Carrier discretion   Ⓑ Bill local carrier   Ⓑ Bill DME MAC

▶ ✳ **G9418** Primary non-small cell lung cancer biopsy and cytology specimen report documents classification into specific histologic type or classified as NSCLC-NOS with an explanation   M

▶ ✳ **G9419** Documentation of medical reason(s) for not reporting the histological type or NSCLC-NOS classification with an explanation (e.g., biopsy taken for other purposes in a patient with a history of primary non-small cell lung cancer or other documented medical reasons)   M

▶ ✳ **G9420** Specimen site other than anatomic location of lung or is not classified as primary non-small cell lung cancer   M

▶ ✳ **G9421** Primary non-small cell lung cancer biopsy and cytology specimen report does not document classification into specific histologic type or classified as NSCLC-NOS with an explanation   M

▶ ✳ **G9422** Non-small cell lung cancer biopsy and cytology specimen report documents classification into specific histologic type or classified as NSCLC-NOS with an explanation   M

▶ ✳ **G9423** Documentation of medical reason(s) for not reporting the histological type or NSCLC-NOS classification with an explanation (e.g., a solitary fibrous tumor in a person with a history of non-small cell carcinoma or other documented medical reasons)   M

▶ ✳ **G9424** Specimen site other than anatomic location of lung, is not classified as non-small cell lung cancer or classified as NSCLC-NOS   M

▶ ✳ **G9425** Non small cell lung cancer biopsy and cytology specimen report does not document classification into specific histologic type or classified as NSCLC-NOS with an explanation   M

▶ ✳ **G9426** Improvement in median time from ED arrival to initial ED oral or parenteral pain medication administration performed for ED admitted patients   M

▶ ✳ **G9427** Improvement in median time from ED arrival to initial ED oral or parenteral pain medication administration not performed for ED admitted patients   M

▶ ✳ **G9428** Pathology report includes the pT category and a statement on thickness and ulceration and for pT1, mitotic rate   M

▶ ✳ **G9429** Documentation of medical reason(s) for not reporting pT category and a statement on thickness and ulceration and for pT1, mitotic rate (e.g., negative skin biopsies in a patient with a history of melanoma or other documented medical reasons)   M

▶ ✳ **G9430** Specimen site other than anatomic cutaneous location   M

▶ ✳ **G9431** Pathology report does not include the pT category and a statement on thickness and ulceration and for pT1, mitotic rate   M

▶ ✳ **G9432** Asthma well-controlled based on the ACT, C-ACT, ACQ, or ATAQ score and results documented   M

▶ ✳ **G9433** Death, permanent nursing home resident or receiving hospice or palliative care any time during the measurement period   M

▶ ✳ **G9434** Asthma not well-controlled based on the ACT, C-ACT, ACQ, or ATAQ score, or specified asthma control tool not used, reason not given   M

▶ ✳ **G9435** Aspirin prescribed at discharge   M

▶ ✳ **G9436** Aspirin not prescribed for documented reasons (e.g., allergy, medical intolerance, history of bleed)   M

▶ ✳ **G9437** Aspirin not prescribed at discharge   M

▶ ✳ **G9438** P2Y inhibitor prescribed at discharge   M

▶ ✳ **G9439** P2Y inhibitor not prescribed for documented reasons (e.g., allergy, medical intolerance, history of bleed)   M

▶ ✳ **G9440** P2Y inhibitor not prescribed at discharge   M

▶ ✳ **G9441** Statin prescribed at discharge   M

▶ ✳ **G9442** Statin not prescribed for documented reasons (e.g., allergy, medical intolerance)   M

▶ ✳ **G9443** Statin not prescribed at discharge   M

▶ ✳ **G9448** Patients who were born in the years 1945?1965   M

▶ ✳ **G9449** History of receiving blood transfusions prior to 1992   M

▶ ✳ **G9450** History of injection drug use   M

▶ ✳ **G9451** Patient received one-time screening for HCV infection   M

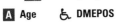 PQRS	Op Quantity Physician Appendix A	Qh Quantity Hospital Appendix B	♀ Female only
♂ Male only A Age & DMEPOS	A2-Z3 ASC Payment Indicator	A-Y ASC Status Indicator	Coding Clinic

▶ ✳ **G9452** Documentation of medical reason(s) for not receiving one-time screening for HCV infection (e.g., decompensated cirrhosis indicating advanced disease [ie, ascites, esophageal variceal bleeding, hepatic encephalopathy], hepatocellular carcinoma, waitlist for organ transplant, limited life expectancy, other medical reasons)   M

▶ ✳ **G9453** Documentation of patient reason(s) for not receiving one-time screening for HCV infection (e.g., patient declined, other patient reasons)   M

▶ ✳ **G9454** One-time screening for HCV infection not received within 12 month reporting period and no documentation of prior screening for HCV infection, reason not given   M

▶ ✳ **G9455** Patient underwent abdominal imaging with ultrasound, contrast enhanced CT or contrast MRI for HCC   M

▶ ✳ **G9456** Documentation of medical or patient reason(s) for not ordering or performing screening for HCC. medical reason: comorbid medical conditions with expected survival < 5 years, hepatic decompensation and not a candidate for liver transplantation, or other medical reasons; patient reasons: patient declined or other patient reasons (e.g., cost of tests, time related to accessing testing equipment)   M

▶ ✳ **G9457** Patient did not undergo abdominal imaging and did not have a documented reason for not undergoing abdominal imaging in the reporting period   M

▶ ✳ **G9458** Patient documented as tobacco user and received tobacco cessation intervention (must include at least one of the following: advice given to quit smoking or tobacco use, counseling on the benefits of quitting smoking or tobacco use, assistance with or referral to external smoking or tobacco cessation support programs, or current enrollment in smoking or tobacco use cessation program) if identified as a tobacco user   M

▶ ✳ **G9459** Currently a tobacco non-user   M

▶ ✳ **G9460** Tobacco assessment or tobacco cessation intervention not performed, reason not otherwise specified   M

▶ ✳ **G9463** I intend to report the sinusitis measures group   M

▶ ✳ **G9464** All quality actions for the applicable measures in the sinusitis measures group have been performed for this patient   M

▶ ✳ **G9465** I intend to report the acute otitis externa (AOE) measures group   M

▶ ✳ **G9466** All quality actions for the applicable measures in the AOE measures group have been performed for this patient   M

▶ ✳ **G9467** Patient who have received or are receiving corticosteroids greater than or equal to 10 mg/day of prednisone equivalents for 60 or greater consecutive days or a single prescription equating to 600mg prednisone or greater for all fills   M

▶ ✳ **G9468** Patient not receiving corticosteroids greater than or equal to 10 mg/day of prednisone equivalents for 60 or greater consecutive days or a single prescription equating to 600mg prednisone or greater for all fills   M

▶ ✳ **G9469** Patients who have received or are receiving corticosteroids greater than or equal to 10 mg/day of prednisone equivalents for 60 or greater consecutive days or a single prescription equating to 600mg prednisone or greater for all fills   M

▶ ✳ **G9470** Patients not receiving corticosteroids greater than or equal to 10 mg/day of prednisone equivalents for 60 or greater consecutive days or a single prescription equating to 600mg prednisone or greater for all fills   M

▶ ✳ **G9471** Within the past 2 years, central dual-energy X-ray absorptiometry (DXA) not ordered or documented   M

▶ ✳ **G9472** Within the past 2 years, central dual-energy X-ray absorptiometry (DXA) not ordered and documented, no review of systems and no medication history or pharmacologic therapy (other than minerals/vitamins) for osteoporosis prescribed   M

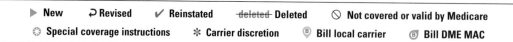

▶ New   ↻ Revised   ✔ Reinstated   deleted Deleted   ⊘ Not covered or valid by Medicare
⊙ Special coverage instructions   ✳ Carrier discretion   ⑧ Bill local carrier   ⑧ Bill DME MAC

BEHAVIORAL HEALTH AND/OR SUBSTANCE ABUSE TREATMENT SERVICES (H0001-H9999)

Used by Medicaid state agencies because no national code exists to meet the reporting needs of these agencies.

⊘ **H0001** Alcohol and/or drug assessment

⊘ **H0002** Behavioral health screening to determine eligibility for admission to treatment program

⊘ **H0003** Alcohol and/or drug screening; laboratory analysis of specimens for presence of alcohol and/or drugs

⊘ **H0004** Behavioral health counseling and therapy, per 15 minutes

⊘ **H0005** Alcohol and/or drug services; group counseling by a clinician

⊘ **H0006** Alcohol and/or drug services; case management

⊘ **H0007** Alcohol and/or drug services; crisis intervention (outpatient)

⊘ **H0008** Alcohol and/or drug services; sub-acute detoxification (hospital inpatient)

⊘ **H0009** Alcohol and/or drug services; acute detoxification (hospital inpatient)

⊘ **H0010** Alcohol and/or drug services; sub-acute detoxification (residential addiction program inpatient)

⊘ **H0011** Alcohol and/or drug services; acute detoxification (residential addiction program inpatient)

⊘ **H0012** Alcohol and/or drug services; sub-acute detoxification (residential addiction program outpatient)

⊘ **H0013** Alcohol and/or drug services; acute detoxification (residential addiction program outpatient)

⊘ **H0014** Alcohol and/or drug services; ambulatory detoxification

⊘ **H0015** Alcohol and/or drug services; intensive outpatient (treatment program that operates at least 3 hours/day and at least 3 days/week and is based on an individualized treatment plan), including assessment, counseling; crisis intervention, and activity therapies or education

⊘ **H0016** Alcohol and/or drug services; medical/somatic (medical intervention in ambulatory setting)

⊘ **H0017** Behavioral health; residential (hospital residential treatment program), without room and board, per diem

⊘ **H0018** Behavioral health; short-term residential (non-hospital residential treatment program), without room and board, per diem

⊘ **H0019** Behavioral health; long-term residential (non-medical, non-acute care in a residential treatment program where stay is typically longer than 30 days), without room and board, per diem

⊘ **H0020** Alcohol and/or drug services; methadone administration and/or service (provision of the drug by a licensed program)

⊘ **H0021** Alcohol and/or drug training service (for staff and personnel not employed by providers)

⊘ **H0022** Alcohol and/or drug intervention service (planned facilitation)

⊘ **H0023** Behavioral health outreach service (planned approach to reach a targeted population)

⊘ **H0024** Behavioral health prevention information dissemination service (one-way direct or non-direct contact with service audiences to affect knowledge and attitude)

⊘ **H0025** Behavioral health prevention education service (delivery of services with target population to affect knowledge, attitude and/or behavior)

⊘ **H0026** Alcohol and/or drug prevention process service, community-based (delivery of services to develop skills of impactors)

⊘ **H0027** Alcohol and/or drug prevention environmental service (broad range of external activities geared toward modifying systems in order to mainstream prevention through policy and law)

⊘ **H0028** Alcohol and/or drug prevention problem identification and referral service (e.g. student assistance and employee assistance programs), does not include assessment

⊘ **H0029** Alcohol and/or drug prevention alternatives service (services for populations that exclude alcohol and other drug use e.g. alcohol-free social events)

⊘ **H0030** Behavioral health hotline service

⊘ **H0031** Mental health assessment, by non-physician

⊘ **H0032** Mental health service plan development by non-physician

⊘ **H0033** Oral medication administration, direct observation

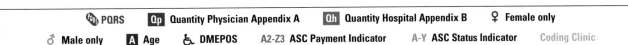

⊘ **H0034** Medication training and support, per 15 minutes

⊘ **H0035** Mental health partial hospitalization, treatment, less than 24 hours

⊘ **H0036** Community psychiatric supportive treatment, face-to-face, per 15 minutes

⊘ **H0037** Community psychiatric supportive treatment program, per diem

⊘ **H0038** Self-help/peer services, per 15 minutes

⊘ **H0039** Assertive community treatment, face-to-face, per 15 minutes

⊘ **H0040** Assertive community treatment program, per diem

⊘ **H0041** Foster care, child, non-therapeutic, per diem **A**

⊘ **H0042** Foster care, child, non-therapeutic, per month **A**

⊘ **H0043** Supported housing, per diem

⊘ **H0044** Supported housing, per month

⊘ **H0045** Respite care services, not in the home, per diem

⊘ **H0046** Mental health services, not otherwise specified

⊘ **H0047** Alcohol and/or other drug abuse services, not otherwise specified

⊘ **H0048** Alcohol and/or other drug testing: collection and handling only, specimens other than blood

⊘ **H0049** Alcohol and/or drug screening

⊘ **H0050** Alcohol and/or drug services, brief intervention, per 15 minutes

⊘ **H1000** Prenatal care, at-risk assessment ♀

⊘ **H1001** Prenatal care, at-risk enhanced service; antepartum management ♀

⊘ **H1002** Prenatal care, at-risk enhanced service; care coordination ♀

⊘ **H1003** Prenatal care, at-risk enhanced service; education ♀

⊘ **H1004** Prenatal care, at-risk enhanced service; follow-up home visit ♀

⊘ **H1005** Prenatal care, at-risk enhanced service package (includes H1001-H1004) ♀

⊘ **H1010** Non-medical family planning education, per session

⊘ **H1011** Family assessment by licensed behavioral health professional for state defined purposes

⊘ **H2000** Comprehensive multidisciplinary evaluation

⊘ **H2001** Rehabilitation program, per 1/2 day

⊘ **H2010** Comprehensive medication services, per 15 minutes

⊘ **H2011** Crisis intervention service, per 15 minutes

⊘ **H2012** Behavioral health day treatment, per hour

⊘ **H2013** Psychiatric health facility service, per diem

⊘ **H2014** Skills training and development, per 15 minutes

⊘ **H2015** Comprehensive community support services, per 15 minutes

⊘ **H2016** Comprehensive community support services, per diem

⊘ **H2017** Psychosocial rehabilitation services, per 15 minutes

⊘ **H2018** Psychosocial rehabilitation services, per diem

⊘ **H2019** Therapeutic behavioral services, per 15 minutes

⊘ **H2020** Therapeutic behavioral services, per diem

⊘ **H2021** Community-based wrap-around services, per 15 minutes

⊘ **H2022** Community-based wrap-around services, per diem

⊘ **H2023** Supported employment, per 15 minutes

⊘ **H2024** Supported employment, per diem

⊘ **H2025** Ongoing support to maintain employment, per 15 minutes

⊘ **H2026** Ongoing support to maintain employment, per diem

⊘ **H2027** Psychoeducational service, per 15 minutes

⊘ **H2028** Sexual offender treatment service, per 15 minutes

⊘ **H2029** Sexual offender treatment service, per diem

⊘ **H2030** Mental health clubhouse services, per 15 minutes

⊘ **H2031** Mental health clubhouse services, per diem

⊘ **H2032** Activity therapy, per 15 minutes

⊘ **H2033** Multisystemic therapy for juveniles, per 15 minutes **A**

⊘ **H2034** Alcohol and/or drug abuse halfway house services, per diem

⊘ **H2035** Alcohol and/or other drug treatment program, per hour

⊘ **H2036** Alcohol and/or other drug treatment program, per diem

⊘ **H2037** Developmental delay prevention activities, dependent child of client, per 15 minutes **A**

▶ **New**   ↻ **Revised**   ✔ **Reinstated**   ~~deleted~~ **Deleted**   ⊘ **Not covered or valid by Medicare**

☼ **Special coverage instructions**   ✳ **Carrier discretion**   ⑧ **Bill local carrier**   ⑧ **Bill DME MAC**

DRUGS OTHER THAN CHEMOTHERAPY
(J0100-J8999)

J0120-J3570: Bill local carrier (Ⓑ) if incident to a physician's service or used in an implanted infusion pump. If other, bill DME MAC (Ⓑ).

↻☼ **J0120** Injection, tetracycline, **up to 250 mg** Ⓑ Ⓑ   K2 K

Other: Achromycin

IOM: 100-02, 15, 50

✱ **J0129** Injection, abatacept, **10 mg** Ⓑ Ⓑ   K2 K

☼ **J0130** Injection, abciximab **10 mg** (Code may be used for Medicare when drug administered under the direct supervision of a physician; not for use when drug is self-administered) Ⓑ Ⓑ **Qp** **Qh**   K2 K

NDC: ReoPro

IOM: 100-02, 15, 50

✱ **J0131** Injection, acetaminophen, **10 mg** Ⓑ Ⓑ **Qp** **Qh**   N1 N

Coding Clinic: 2012, Q1, P9

✱ **J0132** Injection, acetylcysteine, **100 mg** Ⓑ Ⓑ   K2 K

NDC: Acetadote

✱ **J0133** Injection, acyclovir, **5 mg** Ⓑ Ⓑ **Qp** **Qh**   N1 N

✱ **J0135** Injection, adalimumab, **20 mg** Ⓑ Ⓑ **Qp** **Qh**   K2 K

NDC: Humira

IOM: 100-02, 15, 50

~~J0150   Injection, adenosine, for therapeutic use, 6 mg (not to be used to report any adenosine phosphate compounds, instead use A9270)~~ ✖

~~J0151   Injection, adenosine for diagnostic use, 1 mg (not to be used to report any adenosine phosphate compounds, instead use A9270)~~ ✖

▶ ☼ **J0153** Injection, adenosine, 1 mg (not to be used to report any adenosine phosphate compounds)   N1 N

☼ **J0171** Injection, adrenalin, epinephrine, **0.1 mg** Ⓑ Ⓑ   N1 N

IOM: 100-02, 15, 50

Coding Clinic: 2011, Q1, P8

✱ **J0178** Injection, aflibercept, **1 mg** Ⓑ Ⓑ **Qp** **Qh**   K2 K

✱ **J0180** Injection, agalsidase beta, **1 mg** Ⓑ Ⓑ   K2 K

NDC: Fabrazyme

IOM: 100-02, 15, 50

☼ **J0190** Injection, biperiden lactate, **per 5 mg** Ⓑ Ⓑ   E

Other: Akineton

IOM: 100-02, 15, 50

↻☼ **J0200** Injection, alatrofloxacin mesylate, **100 mg**   K2 K

Other: Trovan

IOM: 100-02, 15, 50

↻☼ **J0205** Injection, alglucerase, **per 10 units** Ⓑ Ⓑ   E

Other: Ceredase

IOM: 100-02, 15, 50

☼ **J0207** Injection, amifostine, **500 mg** Ⓑ Ⓑ   K2 K

NDC: Ethyol

IOM: 100-02, 15, 50

☼ **J0210** Injection, methyldopate HCL, **up to 250 mg** Ⓑ Ⓑ **Qp** **Qh**   N1 N

Other: Aldomet

IOM: 100-02, 15, 50

✱ **J0215** Injection, alefacept, **0.5 mg** Ⓑ Ⓑ **Qp** **Qh**   K2 K

NDC: Amevive

✱ **J0220** Injection, alglucosidase alfa, not otherwise specified, **10 mg** Ⓑ Ⓑ **Qp** **Qh**   K2 K

NDC: Myozyme

Other: Lumizyme

Coding Clinic: 2013: Q2, P5; 2012, Q1, P9

✱ **J0221** Injection, alglucosidase alfa, (lumizyme), **10 mg** Ⓑ Ⓑ **Qp** **Qh**   K2 K

Coding Clinic: 2013: Q2, P5

☼ **J0256** Injection, alpha 1 - proteinase inhibitor (human), not otherwise specified, **10 mg** Ⓑ Ⓑ **Qp** **Qh**   K2 K

NDC: Aralast, Aralast NP, Prolastin, Prolastin-C, Zemaira

IOM: 100-02, 15, 50

Coding Clinic: 2012, Q1, P9

☼ **J0257** Injection, alpha 1 proteinase inhibitor (human), (glassia), **10 mg** Ⓑ Ⓑ **Qp** **Qh**   K2 K

IOM: 100-02, 15, 50

Coding Clinic: 2012, Q1, P8

ⓅQRS PQRS	**Qp** Quantity Physician Appendix A	**Qh** Quantity Hospital Appendix B	♀ Female only
♂ **Male only**	**A** Age	♿ **DMEPOS**	A2-Z3 **ASC Payment Indicator**	A-Y **ASC Status Indicator**	Coding Clinic

⊛ **J0270** Injection, alprostadil, **per 1.25 mcg** (Code may be used for Medicare when drug administered under the direct supervision of a physician, not for use when drug is self administered) Ⓑ Ⓑ   B

Other: Caverject, Prostaglandin E1

IOM: 100-02, 15, 50

⊛ **J0275** Alprostadil urethral suppository (Code may be used for Medicare when drug administered under the direct supervision of a physician, not for use when drug is self administered) Ⓑ Ⓑ Qp Qh   B

Other: Muse

IOM: 100-02, 15, 50

＊ **J0278** Injection, amikacin sulfate, **100 mg** Ⓑ Ⓑ Qp Qh   N1 N

Other: Amikin

⊛ **J0280** Injection, aminophylline, **up to 250 mg** Ⓑ Ⓑ Qp Qh   N1 N

IOM: 100-02, 15, 50

⊛ **J0282** Injection, amiodarone hydrochloride, **30 mg** Ⓑ Ⓑ   N1 N

Other: Cordarone

IOM: 100-02, 15, 50

⊛ **J0285** Injection, amphotericin B, **50 mg** Ⓑ Ⓑ   N1 N

Other: ABLC, Amphocin, Fungizone

IOM: 100-02, 15, 50

⊛ **J0287** Injection, amphotericin B lipid complex, **10 mg** Ⓑ Ⓑ   K2 K

NDC: Abelcet

IOM: 100-02, 15, 50

⊛ **J0288** Injection, amphotericin B cholesteryl sulfate complex, **10 mg** Ⓑ Ⓑ   N1 N

IOM: 100-02, 15, 50

⊛ **J0289** Injection, amphotericin B liposome, **10 mg** Ⓑ Ⓑ Qp Qh   K2 K

NDC: AmBisome

IOM: 100-02, 15, 50

⊛ **J0290** Injection, ampicillin sodium, **500 mg** Ⓑ Ⓑ   N1 N

Other: Omnipen-N, Polycillin-N, Totacillin-N

IOM: 100-02, 15, 50

⊛ **J0295** Injection, ampicillin sodium/sulbactam sodium, **per 1.5 gm** Ⓑ Ⓑ   N1 N

NDC: Unasyn

Other: Omnipen-N, Polycillin-N, Totacillin-N

IOM: 100-02, 15, 50

⊛ **J0300** Injection, amobarbital, **up to 125 mg** Ⓑ Ⓑ Qp Qh   K2 K

Other: Amytal

IOM: 100-02, 15, 50

⊛ **J0330** Injection, succinylcholine chloride, **up to 20 mg** Ⓑ Ⓑ   N1 N

Other: Anectine, Quelicin

IOM: 100-02, 15, 50

＊ **J0348** Injection, anidulafungin, **1 mg** Ⓑ Ⓑ Qp Qh   N1 N

NDC: Eraxis

⊛ **J0350** Injection, anistreplase, **per 30 units** Ⓑ Ⓑ Qp Qh   E

Other: Eminase

IOM: 100-02, 15, 50

⊛ **J0360** Injection, hydralazine hydrochloride, **up to 20 mg** Ⓑ Ⓑ Qp Qh   N1 N

Other: Apresoline

IOM: 100-02, 15, 50

＊ **J0364** Injection, apomorphine hydrochloride, **1 mg** Ⓑ Ⓑ Qp Qh   E

⊛ **J0365** Injection, aprotinin, **10,000 KIU** Ⓑ Ⓑ   K

NDC: Trasylol

IOM: 100-02, 15, 50

⊛ **J0380** Injection, metaraminol bitartrate, **per 10 mg** Ⓑ Ⓑ   N1 N

Other: Aramine

IOM: 100-02, 15, 50

⊛ **J0390** Injection, chloroquine hydrochloride, **up to 250 mg** Ⓑ Ⓑ   N1 N

Benefit only for diagnosed malaria or amebiasis

Other: Aralen

IOM: 100-02, 15, 50

↻ ⊛ **J0395** Injection, arbutamine HCL, **1 mg** Ⓑ Ⓑ   E

IOM: 100-02, 15, 50

＊ **J0400** Injection, aripiprazole, intramuscular, **0.25 mg** Ⓑ Ⓑ   N1 N

Other: Abilify

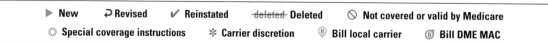

▶ New   ↻ Revised   ✔ Reinstated   ~~deleted~~ Deleted   ⊘ Not covered or valid by Medicare
⊛ Special coverage instructions   ＊ Carrier discretion   Ⓑ Bill local carrier   Ⓑ Bill DME MAC

J0270 – J0400   DRUGS OTHER THAN CHEMOTHERAPY

❋ **J0401** Injection, aripiprazole, extended
release, **1 mg** ⒷⒷ   K2 K

NDC: Abilify

⊛ **J0456** Injection, azithromycin,
500 mg ⒷⒷ Qp Qh   N1 N

NDC: Zithromax

IOM: 100-02, 15, 50

⊛ **J0461** Injection, atropine sulfate,
0.01 mg ⒷⒷ   N1 N

IOM: 100-02, 15, 50

⊛ **J0470** Injection, dimercaprol, per
100 mg ⒷⒷ   N1 N

NDC: BAL In Oil

IOM: 100-02, 15, 50

⊛ **J0475** Injection, baclofen,
10 mg ⒷⒷ Qp Qh   K2 K

NDC: Gablofen, Lioresal

IOM: 100-02, 15, 50

⊛ **J0476** Injection, baclofen **50 mcg** for
intrathecal trial ⒷⒷ   K2 K

NDC: Gablofen, Lioresal

IOM: 100-02, 15, 50

⊛ **J0480** Injection, basiliximab,
20 mg ⒷⒷ   K2 K

NDC: Simulect

IOM: 100-02, 15, 50

❋ **J0485** Injection, belatacept,
1 mg ⒷⒷ Qp Qh   K2 K

NDC: Nulojix

❋ **J0490** Injection, belimumab,
10 mg ⒷⒷ Qp Qh   K2 K

NDC: Benlysta

Coding Clinic: 2012, Q1, P9

⊛ **J0500** Injection, dicyclomine HCL, **up to
20 mg** ⒷⒷ   N1 N

NDC: Bentyl

*Other: Antispas, Dibent, Dicyclocot,
Dilomine, Di-Spaz, Neoquess, Or-Tyl,
Spasmoject*

IOM: 100-02, 15, 50

⊛ **J0515** Injection, benztropine mesylate, **per
1 mg** ⒷⒷ   N1 N

NDC: Cogentin

IOM: 100-02, 15, 50

⊛ **J0520** Injection, bethanechol chloride,
myotonachol or urecholine, **up to
5 mg** ⒷⒷ   N1 N

IOM: 100-02, 15, 50

❋ **J0558** Injection, penicillin G benzathine and
penicillin G procaine,
100,000 units ⒷⒷ   N1 N

NDC: Bicillin C-R

Coding Clinic: 2011, Q1, P8

⊛ **J0561** Injection, penicillin G benzathine,
100,000 units ⒷⒷ   N1 N

NDC: Bicillin L-A

IOM: 100-02, 15, 50

Coding Clinic: 2013: Q2, P3; 2011, Q1, P8

▶ ⊛ **J0571** Buprenorphine, oral, 1 mg   E

▶ ⊛ **J0572** Buprenorphine/naloxone, oral, less
than or equal to 3 mg   E

▶ ⊛ **J0573** Buprenorphine/naloxone, oral, greater
than 3 mg, but less than or equal to
6 mg   E

▶ ⊛ **J0574** Buprenorphine/naloxone, oral, greater
than 6 mg, but less than or equal to
10 mg   E

▶ ⊛ **J0575** Buprenorphine/naloxone, oral, greater
than 10 mg   E

❋ **J0583** Injection, bivalirudin,
1 mg ⒷⒷ   K2 K

NDC: Angiomax

❋ **J0585** Injection, onabotulinumtoxinA,
1 unit ⒷⒷ   K2 K

NDC: Botox, Botox Cosmetic

Other: Oculinum

IOM: 100-02, 15, 50

❋ **J0586** Injection, abobotulinumtoxinA,
5 units ⒷⒷ   K2 K

NDC: Dysport

❋ **J0587** Injection, rimabotulinumtoxinB,
100 units ⒷⒷ   K2 K

NDC: Myobloc

IOM: 100-02, 15, 50

❋ **J0588** Injection, incobotulinumtoxin A,
1 unit ⒷⒷ   K2 K

NDC: Xeomin

Coding Clinic: 2012, Q1, P9

⊛ **J0592** Injection, buprenorphine
hydrochloride, **0.1 mg** ⒷⒷ   N1 N

IOM: 100-02, 15, 50

❋ **J0594** Injection, busulfan, **1 mg** ⒷⒷ   K2 K

❋ **J0595** Injection, butorphanol tartrate,
1 mg ⒷⒷ   N1 N

NDC: Stadol

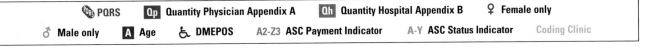

ⓟ PQRS	Qp Quantity Physician Appendix A	Qh Quantity Hospital Appendix B	♀ Female only
♂ Male only	Ⓐ Age	♿ DMEPOS	A2-Z3 ASC Payment Indicator	A-Y ASC Status Indicator	Coding Clinic

* **J0597** Injection, C-1 esterase inhibitor (human), Berinet, **10 units** Ⓑ Ⓑ **Qp Qh** K2 K

  Coding Clinic: 2011, Q1, P7

* **J0598** Injection, C1 esterase inhibitor (human), cinryze, **10 units** Ⓑ Ⓑ K2 K

⊘ **J0600** Injection, edetate calcium disodium, **up to 1000 mg** Ⓑ Ⓑ K2 K

  Other: Calcium Disodium Versenate

  IOM: 100-02, 15, 50

⊘ **J0610** Injection, calcium gluconate, **per 10 ml** Ⓑ Ⓑ N1 N

  Other: Kaleinate

  IOM: 100-02, 15, 50

⊘ **J0620** Injection, calcium glycerophosphate and calcium lactate, **per 10 ml** Ⓑ Ⓑ N1 N

  Other: Calphosan

  MCM 2049

  IOM: 100-02, 15, 50

⊘ **J0630** Injection, calcitonin (salmon), **up to 400 units** Ⓑ Ⓑ K2 K

  NDC: Miacalcin

  Other: Calcimar, Calcitonin-salmon

  IOM: 100-02, 15, 50

⊘ **J0636** Injection, calcitriol, **0.1 mcg** Ⓑ Ⓑ N1 N

  Non-dialysis use

  NDC: Calcijex

  Other: Calcitriol in almond oil

  IOM: 100-02, 15, 50

* **J0637** Injection, caspofungin acetate, **5 mg** Ⓑ Ⓑ K2 K

  NDC: Cancidas

* **J0638** Injection, canakinumab, **1 mg** Ⓑ Ⓑ **Qp Qh** K2 K

  NDC: Ilaris

⊘ **J0640** Injection, leucovorin calcium, **per 50 mg** Ⓑ Ⓑ N1 N

  NDC: Calcium Folinate (Hungarian import)

  Other: Wellcovorin

  IOM: 100-02, 15, 50

  Coding Clinic: 2009, Q1, P10

⊘ **J0641** Injection, levoleucovorin calcium, **0.5 mg** Ⓑ Ⓑ K2 K

  Part of treatment regimen for osteosarcoma

⊘ **J0670** Injection, mepivacaine HCL, **per 10 ml** Ⓑ Ⓑ N1 N

  NDC: Polocaine, Polocaine-MPF

  Other: Carbocaine, Isocaine HCl

  IOM: 100-02, 15, 50

⊘ **J0690** Injection, cefezolin sodium, **500 mg** Ⓑ Ⓑ N1 N

  Other: Ancef, Kefzol

  IOM: 100-02, 15, 50

* **J0692** Injection, cefepime HCL, **500 mg** Ⓑ Ⓑ N1 N

  NDC: Maxipime

⊘ **J0694** Injection, cefoxitin sodium, **1 gm** Ⓑ Ⓑ N1 N

  NDC: Mefoxin

  IOM: 100-02, 15, 50,

  Cross Reference Q0090

⊘ **J0696** Injection, ceftriaxone sodium, **per 250 mg** Ⓑ Ⓑ N1 N

  NDC: Rocephin

  IOM: 100-02, 15, 50

⊘ **J0697** Injection, sterile cefuroxime sodium, **per 750 mg** Ⓑ Ⓑ **Qp Qh** N1 N

  NDC: Zinacef

  Other: Kefurox

  IOM: 100-02, 15, 50

⊘ **J0698** Injection, cefotaxime sodium, **per g** Ⓑ Ⓑ N1 N

  NDC: Claforan

  IOM: 100-02, 15, 50

⊘ **J0702** Injection, betamethasone acetate **3 mg** and betamethasone sodium phosphate **3 mg** Ⓑ Ⓑ N1 N

  NDC: Celestone Soluspan

  Other: Betameth

  IOM: 100-02, 15, 50

* **J0706** Injection, caffeine citrate, **5 mg** Ⓑ Ⓑ N1 N

  Other: Cafcit, Cipro IV, Ciprofloxacin

⊘ **J0710** Injection, cephapirin sodium, **up to 1 gm** Ⓑ Ⓑ N

  Other: Cefadyl

  IOM: 100-02, 15, 50

* **J0712** Injection, ceftaroline fosamil, **10 mg** Ⓑ Ⓑ **Qp Qh** N1 E

  NDC: Teflaro

  Coding Clinic: 2012, Q1, P9

▶ **New**   ↻ **Revised**   ✔ **Reinstated**   ~~deleted~~ **Deleted**   ⊘ **Not covered or valid by Medicare**
⊘ **Special coverage instructions**   * **Carrier discretion**   Ⓑ **Bill local carrier**   Ⓑ **Bill DME MAC**

⚙ **J0713** Injection, ceftazidime, **per 500 mg** Ⓑ Ⓑ   N1 N

NDC: Fortaz, Tazicef

IOM: 100-02, 15, 50

⚙ **J0715** Injection, ceftizoxime sodium, **per 500 mg** Ⓑ Ⓑ   N1 N

Other: Cefizox

IOM: 100-02, 15, 50

✳ **J0716** Injection, centruroides immune F(ab)2, up to 120 milligrams Ⓑ Ⓑ   K2 K

✳ **J0717** Injection, certolizumab pegol, **1 mg** (code may be used for Medicare when drug administered under the direct supervision of a physician, not for use when drug is self administered) Ⓑ Ⓑ **Qp** **Qh**   K2 K

⚙ **J0720** Injection, chloramphenicol sodium succinate, **up to 1 gm** Ⓑ Ⓑ   N1 N

IOM: 100-02, 15, 50

↻⚙ **J0725** Injection, chorionic gonadotropin, **per 1,000 USP units** Ⓑ Ⓑ   K2 K

NDC: Novarel

Other: A.P.L., Chorex-5, Chorex-10, Chorignon, Choron-10, Corgonject-5, Follutein, Glukor, Gonic, Pregnyl, Profasi HP

IOM: 100-02, 15, 50

⚙ **J0735** Injection, clonidine hydrochloride (HCL), **1 mg** Ⓑ Ⓑ   N1 N

NDC: Duraclon

IOM: 100-02, 15, 50

⚙ **J0740** Injection, cidofovir, **375 mg** Ⓑ Ⓑ   K2 K

NDC: Vistide

IOM: 100-02, 15, 50

⚙ **J0743** Injection, cilastatin sodium; imipenem, **per 250 mg** Ⓑ Ⓑ   N1 N

NDC: Primaxin

IOM: 100-02, 15, 50

✳ **J0744** Injection, ciprofloxacin for intravenous infusion, **200 mg** Ⓑ Ⓑ   N1 N

Other: Cipro IV

⚙ **J0745** Injection, codeine phosphate, **per 30 mg** Ⓑ Ⓑ **Qp** **Qh**   N1 N

IOM: 100-02, 15, 50

⚙ **J0760** Injection, colchicine, **per 1 mg** Ⓑ Ⓑ **Qp** **Qh**   N1 N

IOM: 100-02, 15, 50

⚙ **J0770** Injection, colistimethate sodium, **up to 150 mg** Ⓑ Ⓑ **Qp** **Qh**   N1 N

NDC: Coly-Mycin M Parenteral

IOM: 100-02, 15, 50

✳ **J0775** Injection, collagenase, clostridium histolyticum, **0.01 mg** Ⓑ Ⓑ   K2 K

NDC: Xiaflex

Coding Clinic: 2011, Q1, P7

⚙ **J0780** Injection, prochlorperazine, **up to 10 mg** Ⓑ Ⓑ **Qp** **Qh**   N1 N

Other: Compa-Z, Compazine, Cotranzine, Ultrazine-10

IOM: 100-02, 15, 50

⚙ **J0795** Injection, corticorelin ovine triflutate, **1 microgram** Ⓑ Ⓑ   K2 K

NDC: Acthrel

IOM: 100-02, 15, 50

⚙ **J0800** Injection, corticotropin, **up to 40 units** Ⓑ Ⓑ **Qp** **Qh**   K2 K

NDC: Acthar H.P.

Other: Acthar, ACTH

IOM: 100-02, 15, 50

✳ **J0833** Injection, cosyntropin, not otherwise specified, **0.25 mg** Ⓑ Ⓑ **Qp** **Qh**   K2 K

✳ **J0834** Injection, cosyntropin (Cortrosyn), **0.25 mg** Ⓑ Ⓑ   N1 N

✳ **J0840** Injection, crotalidae polyvalent immune fab (ovine), **up to 1 gram** Ⓑ Ⓑ   K2 K

NDC: Crofab Powder for Solution

Coding Clinic: 2012, Q1, P9

⚙ **J0850** Injection, cytomegalovirus immune globulin intravenous (human), **per vial** Ⓑ Ⓑ   K2 K

Prophylaxis to prevent cytomegalovirus disease associated with transplantation of kidney, lung, liver, pancreas, and heart.

NDC: CytoGam

IOM: 100-02, 15, 50

✳ **J0878** Injection, daptomycin, **1 mg** Ⓑ Ⓑ   K2 K

NDC: Cubicin

⚙ **J0881** Injection, darbepoetin alfa, **1 microgram (non-ESRD use)** Ⓑ Ⓑ   K2 K

NDC: Aranesp

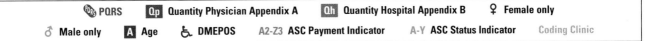

ⓅPQRS PQRS	**Qp** Quantity Physician Appendix A	**Qh** Quantity Hospital Appendix B	♀ Female only
♂ **Male only**	**A** Age	♿ **DMEPOS**	A2-Z3 **ASC Payment Indicator** A-Y **ASC Status Indicator** Coding Clinic

⊘ **J0882** Injection, darbepoetin alfa, **1 microgram (for ESRD on dialysis)** Ⓑ Ⓑ   K

NDC: Aranesp

IOM: 100-02, 6, 10; 100-04, 4, 240

⊘ **J0885** Injection, epoetin alfa, (for non-ESRD use), **1000 units** Ⓑ Ⓑ   K2   K

NDC: Epogen, Procrit

IOM: 100-02, 15, 50

Coding Clinic: 2006, Q2, P5

⊘ **J0886** Injection, epoetin alfa, **1000 units (for ESRD on dialysis)** Ⓑ Ⓑ   N

NDC: Epogen, Procrit

IOM: 100-02, 6, 10; 100-04, 4, 240

Coding Clinic: 2006, Q2, P5

▶ ⊘ **J0887** Injection, epoetin beta, 1 microgram, (for ESRD on dialysis)   N

▶ ⊘ **J0888** Injectin, epoetin beta, 1 microgram, (for non ESRD use)   N1   N

✳ **J0890** Injection, peginesatide, 0.1 mg (for ESRD on dialysis) Ⓑ Ⓑ **Qp** **Qh**   E

NDC: Omontys

✳ **J0894** Injection, decitabine, **1 mg** Ⓑ Ⓑ   K2   K

Indicated for treatment of myelodysplastic syndromes (MDS)

⊘ **J0895** Injection, deferoxamine mesylate, **500 mg** Ⓑ Ⓑ   N1   N

NDC: Desferal

Other: Desferal mesylate

IOM: 100-02, 15, 50,

Cross Reference Q0087

✳ **J0897** Injection, denosumab, **1 mg** Ⓑ Ⓑ **Qp** **Qh**   K2   K

NDC: Prolia, Xgeva

Coding Clinic: 2012, Q1, P9

~~J0900~~ ~~Injection, testosterone enanthate and estradiol valerate, up to 1 cc~~ ✖

⊘ **J0945** Injection, brompheniramine maleate, **per 10 mg** Ⓑ Ⓑ **Qp** **Qh**   N1   N

Other: Codimal-A, Cophene-B, Dehist, Histaject, Nasahist B, ND Stat, Oraminic II, Sinusol-B

IOM: 100-02, 15, 50

⊘ **J1000** Injection, depo-estradiol cypionate, **up to 5 mg** Ⓑ Ⓑ   N1   N

Other: DepGynogen, Depogen, Dura-Estrin, Estra-D, Estro-Cyp, Estroject LA, Estronol-LA

IOM: 100-02, 15, 50

⊘ **J1020** Injection, methylprednisolone acetate, **20 mg** Ⓑ Ⓑ   N1   N

NDC: Depo-Medrol, Methylpred

Other: DepMedalone, Depoject, Depopred, D-Med 80, Duralone, Medralone, M-Prednisol, Rep-Pred

IOM: 100-02, 15, 50

Coding Clinic: 2005, Q3, P10

⊘ **J1030** Injection, methylprednisolone acetate, **40 mg** Ⓑ Ⓑ   N1   N

NDC: Depo-Medrol

Other: DepMedalone, Depoject, Depopred, D-Med 80, Duralone, Medralone, M-Prednisol, Rep-Pred

IOM: 100-02, 15, 50

Coding Clinic: 2005, Q3, P10

⊘ **J1040** Injection, methylprednisolone acetate, **80 mg** Ⓑ Ⓑ   N1   N

NDC: Depo-Medrol

Other: DepMedalone, Depoject, Depopred, D-Med 80, Duralone, Medralone, M-Prednisol, Rep-Pred

IOM: 100-02, 15, 50

✳ **J1050** Injection, medroxyprogesterone acetate, **1 mg** Ⓑ Ⓑ **Qp** **Qh**   N1   N

Other: Depo-Provera Contraceptive

~~J1060~~ ~~Injection, testosterone cypionate and estradiol cypionate, up to 1 ml~~ ✖

~~J1070~~ ~~Injection, testosterone cypionate, up to 100 mg~~ ✖

▶ ⊘ **J1071** Injection, testosterone cypionate, **1 mg**   N1   N

~~J1080~~ ~~Injection, testosterone cypionate, 1 cc, 200 mg~~ ✖

⊘ **J1094** Injection, dexamethasone acetate, **1 mg** Ⓑ Ⓑ   N1   N

Other: Dalalone LA, Decadron LA, Decaject LA, Dexacen-LA-8, Dexamethasone Micronized, Dexasone L.A., Dexone-LA

IOM: 100-02, 15, 50

▶ **New**   ↻ **Revised**   ✔ **Reinstated**   ~~deleted~~ **Deleted**   ⊘ **Not covered or valid by Medicare**

⊘ **Special coverage instructions**   ✳ **Carrier discretion**   Ⓑ **Bill local carrier**   Ⓑ **Bill DME MAC**

⊛ **J1100** Injection, dexamethasone sodium
phosphate, **1 mg** Ⓑ Ⓑ   N1 N

*Other: Dalalone, Decadron Phosphate,
Decaject, Dexacen-4, Dexone, Hexadrol
Phosphate, Solurex*

IOM: 100-02, 15, 50

⊛ **J1110** Injection, dihydroergotamine mesylate,
per 1 mg Ⓑ Ⓑ   N1 N

NDC: D.H.E. 45

IOM: 100-02, 15, 50

⊛ **J1120** Injection, acetazolamide sodium, **up to
500 mg** Ⓑ Ⓑ   N1 N

Other: Diamox

IOM: 100-02, 15, 50

⊛ **J1160** Injection, digoxin, **up to
0.5 mg** Ⓑ Ⓑ   N1 N

NDC: Lanoxin

IOM: 100-02, 15, 50

⊛ **J1162** Injection, digoxin immune Fab (ovine),
per vial Ⓑ Ⓑ **Qp Qh**   K2 K

NDC: Digibind, DigiFab

IOM: 100-02, 15, 50

⊛ **J1165** Injection, phenytoin sodium, **per
50 mg** Ⓑ Ⓑ   N1 N

Other: Dilantin

IOM: 100-02, 15, 50

⊛ **J1170** Injection, hydromorphone, **up to
4 mg** Ⓑ Ⓑ   N1 N

Other: Dilaudid

IOM: 100-02, 15, 50

⊛ **J1180** Injection, dyphylline, **up to
500 mg** Ⓑ Ⓑ   E

Other: Dilor, Lufyllin

IOM: 100-02, 15, 50

⊛ **J1190** Injection, dexrazoxane hydrochloride,
per 250 mg Ⓑ Ⓑ   K2 K

NDC: Totect, Zinecard

IOM: 100-02, 15, 50

⊛ **J1200** Injection, diphenhydramine HCL, **up
to 50 mg** Ⓑ Ⓑ   N1 N

NDC: Benadryl

Other: Bena-D, Truxadryl

IOM: 100-02, 15, 50

⊛ **J1205** Injection, chlorothiazide sodium, **per
500 mg** Ⓑ Ⓑ   K2 K

NDC: Diuril

IOM: 100-02, 15, 50

⊛ **J1212** Injection, DMSO, dimethyl sulfoxide,
50%, **50 ml** Ⓑ Ⓑ   N1 N

NDC: Rimso-50

IOM: 100-02, 15, 50; 100-03, 4, 230.12

⊛ **J1230** Injection, methadone HCL, **up to
10 mg** Ⓑ Ⓑ   N1 N

MCM 2049

IOM: 100-02, 15, 50

⊛ **J1240** Injection, dimenhydrinate, **up to
50 mg** Ⓑ Ⓑ   N1 N

*Other: Dinate, Dommanate, Dramamine,
Dramanate, Dramilin, Dramocen,
Dramoject, Dymenate, Hydrate,
Marmine, Wehamine*

IOM: 100-02, 15, 50

⊛ **J1245** Injection, dipyridamole, **per
10 mg** Ⓑ Ⓑ   N1 N

Other: Persantine

IOM: 100-04, 15, 50; 100-04, 12, 30.6

⊛ **J1250** Injection, dobutamine HCL, **per
250 mg** Ⓑ Ⓑ   N1 N

Other: Dobutrex

IOM: 100-02, 15, 50

⊛ **J1260** Injection, dolasetron mesylate,
10 mg Ⓑ Ⓑ   N1 N

NDC: Anzemet

IOM: 100-02, 15, 50

✳ **J1265** Injection, dopamine HCL,
40 mg Ⓑ Ⓑ   N1 N

✳ **J1267** Injection, doripenem,
10 mg Ⓑ Ⓑ   N1 N

NDC: Doribax

✳ **J1270** Injection, doxercalciferol,
1 mcg Ⓑ Ⓑ   N1 N

NDC: Hectorol

✳ **J1290** Injection, ecallantide,
1 mg Ⓑ Ⓑ   K2 K

NDC: Kalbitor

Coding Clinic: 2011, Q1, P7

✳ **J1300** Injection, eculizumab,
10 mg Ⓑ Ⓑ   K2 K

NDC: Soliris

🄟🄦🄡🅂 **PQRS**   **Qp** Quantity Physician Appendix A   **Qh** Quantity Hospital Appendix B   ♀ **Female only**
♂ **Male only**   **A** Age   ♿ **DMEPOS**   A2-Z3 **ASC Payment Indicator**   A-Y **ASC Status Indicator**   *Coding Clinic*

⊛ **J1320**   Injection, amitriptyline HCL, **up to 20 mg** Ⓑ Ⓑ   N1 N

Other: Elavil, Enovil

IOM: 100-02, 15, 50

▶ ✳ **J1322**   Injection, elosulfase alfa, **1 mg**   K2 G

✳ **J1324**   Injection, enfuvirtide, **1 mg** Ⓑ Ⓑ   K2 K

Other: Fuzeon

⊛ **J1325**   Injection, epoprostenol, **0.5 mg** Ⓑ Ⓑ   N1 N

NDC: Flolan, Veletri

IOM: 100-02, 15, 50

⊛ **J1327**   Injection, eptifibatide, **5 mg** Ⓑ Ⓑ   K2 K

Other: Integrilin

IOM: 100-02, 15, 50

⊛ **J1330**   Injection, ergonovine maleate, **up to 0.2 mg** Ⓑ Ⓑ   N1 N

Benefit limited to obstetrical diagnosis

IOM: 100-02, 15, 50

✳ **J1335**   Injection, ertapenem sodium, **500 mg** Ⓑ Ⓑ   N1 N

NDC: Invanz

↻⊛ **J1364**   Injection, erythromycin lactobionate, **per 500 mg** Ⓑ Ⓑ   K2 N

IOM: 100-02, 15, 50

⊛ **J1380**   Injection, estradiol valerate, **up to 10 mg** Ⓑ Ⓑ   N1 N

NDC: Delestrogen

Other: Dioval, Duragen, Estra-L, Gynogen L.A., L.A.E. 20, Valergen

IOM: 100-02, 15, 50

Coding Clinic: 2011, Q1, P8

⊛ **J1410**   Injection, estrogen conjugated, **per 25 mg** Ⓑ Ⓑ   K2 K

NDC: Premarin

IOM: 100-02, 15, 50

⊛ **J1430**   Injection, ethanolamine oleate, **100 mg** Ⓑ Ⓑ   K2 K

Other: Ethamolin

IOM: 100-02, 15, 50

↻⊛ **J1435**   Injection, estrone, **per 1 mg** Ⓑ Ⓑ   E

Other: Estragyn, Estronol, Kestrone 5, Theelin Aqueous

IOM: 100-02, 15, 50

⊛ **J1436**   Injection, etidronate disodium, **per 300 mg** Ⓑ Ⓑ   N1 N

Other: Didronel

IOM: 100-02, 15, 50

⊛ **J1438**   Injection, etanercept, **25 mg** (Code may be used for Medicare when drug administered under the direct supervision of a physician, not for use when drug is self-administered.) Ⓑ Ⓑ   K2 K

NDC: Enbrel

IOM: 100-02, 15, 50

▶ ✳ **J1439**   Injection, ferric carboxymaltose, **1 mg**   K2 G

⊛ **J1442**   Injection, filgrastim (G-CSF), **1 microgram** Ⓑ Ⓑ **Qp Qh**   K2 K

NDC: Neupogen

⊛ **J1446**   Injection, TBO-filgrastim, **5 micrograms** Ⓑ Ⓑ **Qp Qh**   K2 G

NDC: Granix

⊛ **J1450**   Injection, fluconazole, **200 mg** Ⓑ Ⓑ   N1 N

NDC: Diflucan

IOM: 100-02, 15, 50

⊛ **J1451**   Injection, fomepizole, **15 mg** Ⓑ Ⓑ   K2 K

IOM: 100-02, 15, 50

⊛ **J1452**   Injection, fomivirsen sodium, intraocular, **1.65 mg** Ⓑ Ⓑ   N1 N

IOM: 100-02, 15, 50

✳ **J1453**   Injection, fosaprepitant, **1 mg** Ⓑ Ⓑ   K2 K

Prevents chemotherapy-induced nausea and vomiting

NDC: Emend

↻⊛ **J1455**   Injection, foscarnet sodium, **per 1000 mg** Ⓑ Ⓑ   N1 N

Other: Foscavir

IOM: 100-02, 15, 50

✳ **J1457**   Injection, gallium nitrate, **1 mg** Ⓑ Ⓑ **Qp Qh**   N1 N

NDC: Ganite

✳ **J1458**   Injection, galsulfase, **1 mg** Ⓑ Ⓑ   K2 K

NDC: Naglazyme

✳ **J1459**   Injection, immune globulin (Privigen), intravenous, non-lyophilized (e.g., liquid), **500 mg** Ⓑ Ⓑ   K2 K

▶ **New**   ↻ **Revised**   ✔ **Reinstated**   ~~deleted~~ **Deleted**   ⊘ **Not covered or valid by Medicare**

⊛ **Special coverage instructions**   ✳ **Carrier discretion**   Ⓑ **Bill local carrier**   Ⓑ **Bill DME MAC**

J1460 Injection, gamma globulin, intramuscular, **1 cc** Ⓑ Ⓑ **Qp** **Qh** N1 N

NDC: GamaSTAN

Other: Gammar

IOM: 100-02, 15, 50

Coding Clinic: 2011, Q1, P8

J1556 Injection, immune globulin (Bivigam), **500 mg** Ⓑ Ⓑ K2 G

J1557 Injection, immune globulin, (gammaplex), intravenous, non-lyophilized (e.g., liquid), **500 mg** Ⓑ Ⓑ K2 K

Coding Clinic: 2012, Q1, P9

J1559 Injection, immune globulin, (hizentra), **100 mg** Ⓑ Ⓑ K2 K

Coding Clinic: 2011, Q1, P6

J1560 Injection, gamma globulin, intramuscular, **over 10 cc** Ⓑ Ⓑ N1 N

NDC: GamaSTAN

Other: Gammar

IOM: 100-02, 15, 50

J1561 Injection, immune globulin, (Gamunex-C/Gammaked), non-lyophilized (e.g. liquid), **500 mg** Ⓑ Ⓑ K2 K

NDC: Gamunex

IOM: 100-02, 15, 50

Coding Clinic: 2012, Q1, P9

J1562 Injection, immune globulin (Vivaglobin), **100 mg** Ⓑ Ⓑ E

J1566 Injection, immune globulin, intravenous, lyophilized (e.g., powder), not otherwise specified, **500 mg** Ⓑ Ⓑ K2 K

NDC: Carimune, Gammagard S/D

Other: Polygam

IOM: 100-02, 15, 50

J1568 Injection, immune globulin, (Octagam), intravenous, non-lyophilized (e.g., liquid), **500 mg** Ⓑ Ⓑ **Qp** **Qh** K2 K

J1569 Injection, immune globulin, (Gammagard Liquid), non-lyophilized, (e.g. liquid), **500 mg** Ⓑ Ⓑ **Qp** **Qh** K2 K

IOM: 100-02, 15, 50

J1570 Injection, ganciclovir sodium, **500 mg** Ⓑ Ⓑ N1 N

NDC: Cytovene

IOM: 100-02, 15, 50

J1571 Injection, hepatitis B immune globulin (HepaGam B), intramuscular, **0.5 ml** Ⓑ Ⓑ K2 K

IOM: 100-02, 15, 50

Coding Clinic: 2008, Q3, P7-8

J1572 Injection, immune globulin, (flebogamma/flebogamma DIF) intravenous, non-lyophilized (e.g. liquid), **500 mg** Ⓑ Ⓑ **Qp** **Qh** K2 K

IOM: 100-02, 15, 50

J1573 Injection, hepatitis B immune globulin (HepaGam B), intravenous, **0.5 ml** Ⓑ Ⓑ K2 K

Coding Clinic: 2008, Q3, P8

J1580 Injection, Garamycin, gentamicin, **up to 80 mg** Ⓑ Ⓑ N1 N

NDC: Gentamicin Sulfate

Other: Jenamicin

IOM: 100-02, 15, 50

J1590 Injection, gatifloxacin, **10 mg** Ⓑ Ⓑ N1 N

Other: Tequin

J1595 Injection, glatiramer acetate, **20 mg** Ⓑ Ⓑ K2 K

Other: Copaxone

IOM: 100-02, 15, 50

J1599 Injection, immune globulin, intravenous, non-lyophilized (e.g., liquid), not otherwise specified, **500 mg** Ⓑ Ⓑ N1 N

Coding Clinic: 2011, P1, Q6

J1600 Injection, gold sodium thiomalate, **up to 50 mg** Ⓑ Ⓑ K2 K

NDC: Myochrysine

IOM: 100-02, 15, 50

J1602 Injection, golimumab, **1 mg,** for intravenous use Ⓑ Ⓑ K2 G

NDC: Simponi Aria

J1610 Injection, glucagon hydrochloride, **per 1 mg** Ⓑ Ⓑ K2 K

NDC: GlucaGen, Glucagon Emergency

IOM: 100-02, 15, 50

J1620 Injection, gonadorelin hydrochloride, **per 100 mcg** Ⓑ Ⓑ E

Other: Factrel

IOM: 100-02, 15, 50

J1626 Injection, granisetron hydrochloride, **100 mcg** Ⓑ Ⓑ N1 N

Other: Kytril

IOM: 100-02, 15, 50

PQRS PQRS **Qp** Quantity Physician Appendix A **Qh** Quantity Hospital Appendix B ♀ Female only ♂ Male only **A** Age ♿ DMEPOS A2-Z3 ASC Payment Indicator A-Y ASC Status Indicator Coding Clinic

⚙ **J1630** Injection, haloperidol, **up to 5 mg** Ⓑ Ⓑ   N1 N

NDC: Haldol, Haloperidol Lactate

IOM: 100-02, 15, 50

⚙ **J1631** Injection, haloperidol decanoate, **per 50 mg** Ⓑ Ⓑ   N1 N

IOM: 100-02, 15, 50

⚙ **J1640** Injection, hemin, **1 mg** Ⓑ Ⓑ   K2 K

NDC: Panhematin

IOM: 100-02, 15, 50

⚙ **J1642** Injection, heparin sodium, (heparin lock flush), **per 10 units** Ⓑ Ⓑ   N1 N

NDC: Heparin (Porcine) Lock Flush, Heparin Sodium Flush

Other: Hep-Lock U/P

IOM: 100-02, 15, 50

⚙ **J1644** Injection, heparin sodium, **per 1000 units** Ⓑ Ⓑ   N1 N

NDC: Heparin (Porcine), Heparin Sodium (Porcine)

Other: Liquaemin Sodium

IOM: 100-02, 15, 50

⚙ **J1645** Injection, dalteparin sodium, **per 2500 IU** Ⓑ Ⓑ   N1 N

NDC: Fragmin

IOM: 100-02, 15, 50

✳ **J1650** Injection, enoxaparin sodium, **10 mg** Ⓑ Ⓑ   N1 N

NDC: Lovenox

⚙ **J1652** Injection, fondaparinux sodium, **0.5 mg** Ⓑ Ⓑ   N1 N

NDC: Arixtra

IOM: 100-02, 15, 50

✳ **J1655** Injection, tinzaparin sodium, **1000 IU** Ⓑ Ⓑ   E

Other: Innohep

⚙ **J1670** Injection, tetanus immune globulin, human, **up to 250 units** Ⓑ Ⓑ   K2 K

Indicated for transient protection against tetanus post-exposure to tetanus (V03.7).

NDC: Hypertet S/D

Other: Hyper-tet

IOM: 100-02, 15, 50

⚙ **J1675** Injection, histrelin acetate, **10 micrograms** Ⓑ Ⓑ   B

IOM: 100-02, 15, 50

⚙ **J1700** Injection, hydrocortisone acetate, **up to 25 mg** Ⓑ Ⓑ   N1 N

Other: Hydrocortone Acetate

IOM: 100-02, 15, 50

⚙ **J1710** Injection, hydrocortisone sodium phosphate, **up to 50 mg** Ⓑ Ⓑ   N1 N

Other: A-hydroCort, Hydrocortone phosphate, Solu-Cortef

IOM: 100-02, 15, 50

⚙ **J1720** Injection, hydrocortisone sodium succinate, **up to 100 mg** Ⓑ Ⓑ   N1 N

NDC: Solu-Cortef

Other: A-Hydrocort

IOM: 100-02, 15, 50

✳ **J1725** Injection, hydroxyprogesterone caproate, **1 mg** Ⓑ Ⓑ **Qp Qh**   K2 K

Coding Clinic: 2012, Q1, P9

⚙ **J1730** Injection, diazoxide, **up to 300 mg** Ⓑ Ⓑ   E

Other: Hyperstat

IOM: 100-02, 15, 50

✳ **J1740** Injection, ibandronate sodium, **1 mg** Ⓑ Ⓑ   K2 K

NDC: Boniva

✳ **J1741** Injection, ibuprofen, **100 mg** Ⓑ Ⓑ   N1 N

⚙ **J1742** Injection, ibutilide fumarate, **1 mg** Ⓑ Ⓑ   K2 K

NDC: Corvert

IOM: 100-02, 15, 50

✳ **J1743** Injection, idursulfase, **1 mg** Ⓑ Ⓑ   K2 K

NDC: Elaprase

✳ **J1744** Injection, icatibant, **1 mg** Ⓑ Ⓑ **Qp Qh**   K2 K

⚙ **J1745** Injection, infliximab, **10 mg** Ⓑ Ⓑ   K2 K

Report total number of 10 mg increments administered

NDC: Remicade

IOM: 100-02, 15, 50

⚙ **J1750** Injection, iron dextran, **50 mg** Ⓑ Ⓑ   K2 K

IOM: 100-02, 15, 50

NDC: Dexferrum, Infed

✳ **J1756** Injection, iron sucrose, **1 mg** Ⓑ Ⓑ   N1 N

NDC: Venofer

▶ **New**	↻ **Revised**	✔ **Reinstated**	~~deleted~~ **Deleted**	⊘ **Not covered or valid by Medicare**
⚙ **Special coverage instructions**		✳ **Carrier discretion**	Ⓑ **Bill local carrier**	Ⓑ **Bill DME MAC**

○ **J1786** Injection, imiglucerase,
10 units Ⓑ Ⓑ   K2 K

NDC: Cerezyme

IOM: 100-02, 15, 50

Coding Clinic: 2011, Q1, P8

○ **J1790** Injection, droperidol, **up to**
5 mg Ⓑ Ⓑ   N1 N

NDC: Inapsine

IOM: 100-02, 15, 50

○ **J1800** Injection, propranolol HCL, **up to**
1 mg Ⓑ Ⓑ   N1 N

Other: Inderal

IOM: 100-02, 15, 50

○ **J1810** Injection, droperidol and fentanyl citrate, **up to 2 ml ampule** Ⓟ Ⓑ   E

Other: Innovar

IOM: 100-02, 15, 50

○ **J1815** Injection, insulin, **per**
5 units Ⓑ Ⓑ   N1 N

NDC: Humalog, Humulin, Lantus, Novolin, Novolog

IOM: 100-02, 15, 50; 100-03, 4, 280.14

✳ **J1817** Insulin for administration through
DME (i.e., insulin pump) **per**
50 units Ⓑ Ⓑ   N1 N

NDC: Humalog, Humulin, Novolin, Novolog

Other: Apidra Solostar, Insulin Lispro

⊘ **J1826** Injection, interferon beta-1a,
30 mcg Ⓑ Ⓑ   E

Coding Clinic: 2011, Q2, P9; Q1, P8

○ **J1830** Injection interferon beta-1b, **0.25 mg**
(Code may be used for Medicare
when drug administered under the
direct supervision of a physician,
not for use when drug is self
administered) Ⓑ Ⓑ   K2 K

Other: Betaseron

IOM: 100-02, 15, 50

✳ **J1835** Injection, itraconazole,
50 mg Ⓑ Ⓑ   E

Other: Sporanox

○ **J1840** Injection, kanamycin sulfate, **up to**
500 mg Ⓑ Ⓑ   N1 N

Other: Kantrex, Klebcil

IOM: 100-02, 15, 50

○ **J1850** Injection, kanamycin sulfate, **up to**
75 mg Ⓑ Ⓑ   N1 N

Other: Kantrex, Klebcil

IOM: 100-02, 15, 50

Coding Clinic: 2013: Q2, P3

○ **J1885** Injection, ketorolac tromethamine, **per**
15 mg Ⓑ Ⓑ   N1 N

Other: Toradol

IOM: 100-02, 15, 50

○ **J1890** Injection, cephalothin sodium, **up to**
1 gram Ⓑ Ⓑ   N1 N

IOM: 100-02, 15, 50

↺✳ **J1930** Injection, lanreotide,
1 mg Ⓑ Ⓑ   K2 K

Treats acromegaly and symptoms
caused by neuroendocrine tumors

NDC: Somatuline Depot

✳ **J1931** Injection, laronidase,
0.1 mg Ⓑ Ⓑ   K2 K

NDC: Aldurazyme

○ **J1940** Injection, furosemide, **up to**
20 mg Ⓑ Ⓑ   N1 N

Other: Lasix

MCM 2049

IOM: 100-02, 15, 50

○ **J1945** Injection, lepirudin,
50 mg Ⓟ Ⓑ   K2 K

IOM: 100-02, 15, 50

○ **J1950** Injection, leuprolide acetate (for depot
suspension), **per 3.75 mg** Ⓑ Ⓑ K2 K

NDC: Lupron Depot, Lupron Depot-Ped

IOM: 100-02, 15, 50

✳ **J1953** Injection, levetiracetam,
10 mg Ⓑ Ⓑ   N1 N

○ **J1955** Injection, levocarnitine, **per 1**
gm Ⓑ Ⓑ   B

NDC: Carnitor

Other: L-Carnitine

IOM: 100-02, 15, 50

○ **J1956** Injection, levofloxacin,
250 mg Ⓑ Ⓑ   N1 N

NDC: Levaquin

IOM: 100-02, 15, 50

○ **J1960** Injection, levorphanol tartrate, **up to**
2 mg Ⓑ Ⓑ   N1 N

Other: Levo-Dromoran

MCM 2049

IOM: 100-02, 15, 50

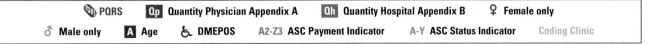

○ **J1980** Injection, hyoscyamine sulfate, **up to 0.25 mg** Ⓑ Ⓑ   N1 N

NDC: Levsin

IOM: 100-02, 15, 50

○ **J1990** Injection, chlordiazepoxide HCL, **up to 100 mg** Ⓑ Ⓑ   N1 N

Other: Librium

IOM: 100-02, 15, 50

○ **J2001** Injection, lidocaine HCL for intravenous infusion, **10 mg** Ⓑ Ⓑ   N1 N

NDC: Lidocaine in D5W

Other: Anestacaine, Caine-1, Dilocaine, L-Caine, Lidoject, Nervocaine, Nulicaine, Xylocaine

IOM: 100-02, 15, 50

○ **J2010** Injection, lincomycin HCL, **up to 300 mg** Ⓑ Ⓑ   N1 N

NDC: Lincocin

IOM: 100-02, 15, 50

✱ **J2020** Injection, linezolid, **200 mg** Ⓑ Ⓑ   K2 K

NDC: Zyvox

○ **J2060** Injection, lorazepam, **2 mg** Ⓟ Ⓑ   N1 N

NDC: Ativan

IOM: 100-02, 15, 50

○ **J2150** Injection, mannitol, **25% in 50 ml** Ⓑ Ⓑ   N1 N

MCM 2049

IOM: 100-02, 15, 50

✱ **J2170** Injection, mecasermin, **1 mg** Ⓟ Ⓑ Ⓑ   N1 N

Other: Increlex

○ **J2175** Injection, meperidine hydrochloride, **per 100 mg** Ⓑ Ⓑ   N1 N

NDC: Demerol

IOM: 100-02, 15, 50

○ **J2180** Injection, meperidine and promethazine HCL, **up to 50 mg** Ⓑ Ⓑ   N1 N

Other: Mepergan

IOM: 100-02, 15, 50

✱ **J2185** Injection, meropenem, **100 mg** Ⓑ Ⓑ   N1 N

NDC: Merrem

○ **J2210** Injection, methylergonovine maleate, **up to 0.2 mg** Ⓑ Ⓑ   N1 N

Benefit limited to obstetrical diagnoses for prevention and control of post-partum hemorrhage

NDC: Methergine

IOM: 100-02, 15, 50

↻✱ **J2212** Injection, methylnaltrexone, **0.1 mg** Ⓑ Ⓑ **Qp** **Qh**   N1 N

✱ **J2248** Injection, micafungin sodium, **1 mg** Ⓑ Ⓑ   K2 K

Other: Mycamine

○ **J2250** Injection, midazolam hydrochloride, **per 1 mg** Ⓑ Ⓑ   N1 N

Other: Versed

IOM: 100-02, 15, 50

○ **J2260** Injection, milrinone lactate, **5 mg** Ⓑ Ⓑ   N1 N

Other: Primacor

IOM: 100-02, 15, 50

✱ **J2265** Injection, minocycline hydrochloride, **1 mg** Ⓑ Ⓑ **Qp** **Qh**   N1 N

○ **J2270** Injection, morphine sulfate, **up to 10 mg** Ⓑ Ⓑ   N1 N

Other: Astromorph PF, Duramorph

IOM: 100-02, 15, 50

Coding Clinic: 2013, Q2, P4

~~J2271~~ ~~Injection, morphine sulfate, 100 mg~~   ✖

▶ ○ **J2274** Injection, morphine sulfate, preservative-free for epidural or intrathecal use, **10 mg**   N1 N

IOM: 100-03, 4, 280.1; 100-02, 15, 50

~~J2275~~ ~~Injection, morphine sulfate (preservative-free sterile solution), per 10 mg~~   ✖

○ **J2278** Injection, ziconotide, **1 microgram** Ⓑ Ⓟ   K2 K

NDC: Prialt

✱ **J2280** Injection, moxifloxacin, **100 mg** Ⓟ Ⓑ   N1 N

NDC: Avelox

○ **J2300** Injection, nalbuphine hydrochloride, **per 10 mg** Ⓟ Ⓑ   N1 N

Other: Nubain

IOM: 100-02, 15, 50

▶ **New**   ↻ **Revised**   ✔ **Reinstated**   ~~deleted~~ **Deleted**   ⊘ **Not covered or valid by Medicare**

○ **Special coverage instructions**   ✱ **Carrier discretion**   Ⓑ **Bill local carrier**   Ⓑ **Bill DME MAC**

✿ **J2310** Injection, naloxone hydrochloride, **per 1 mg** Ⓑ Ⓑ   N1 N

Other: Narcan

IOM: 100-02, 15, 50

✳ **J2315** Injection, naltrexone, depot form, **1 mg** Ⓑ Ⓑ   K2 K

NDC: Vivitrol

↻✿ **J2320** Injection, nandrolone decanoate, **up to 50 mg** Ⓑ Ⓑ   K2 K

Other: Anabolin LA 100, Androlone, Deca-Durabolin, Decolone, Hybolin Decanoate, Nandrobolic LA, Neo-Durabolic

IOM: 100-02, 15, 50

Coding Clinic: 2011, Q1, P8

✳ **J2323** Injection, natalizumab, **1 mg** Ⓑ Ⓑ   K2 K

NDC: Tysabri

✿ **J2325** Injection, nesiritide, **0.1 mg** Ⓑ Ⓑ   K2 K

Other: Natrecor

IOM: 100-02, 15, 50

✳ **J2353** Injection, octreotide, depot form for intramuscular injection, **1 mg** Ⓑ Ⓑ   K2 K

NDC: Sandostatin LAR Depot

✳ **J2354** Injection, octreotide, non-depot form for subcutaneous or intravenous injection, **25 mcg** Ⓑ Ⓑ   N1 N

Other: Sandostatin LAR Depot

✿ **J2355** Injection, oprelvekin, **5 mg** Ⓑ Ⓑ   K2 K

NDC: Neumega

IOM: 100-02, 15, 50

✳ **J2357** Injection, omalizumab, **5 mg** Ⓑ Ⓑ   K2 K

NDC: Xolair

✳ **J2358** Injection, olanzapine, long-acting, **1 mg** Ⓑ Ⓑ   K2 K

NDC: Zyprexa, Relprevv

Coding Clinic: 2011, Q1, P6

✿ **J2360** Injection, orphenadrine citrate, **up to 60 mg** Ⓑ Ⓑ   N1 N

Other: Antiflex, Banflex, Flexoject, Flexon, K-Flex, Mio-Rel, Neocyten, Norflex, O-Flex, Orfro, Orphenate

IOM: 100-02, 15, 50

✿ **J2370** Injection, phenylephrine HCL, **up to 1 ml** Ⓑ Ⓑ   N1 N

Other: Neo-Synephrine

IOM: 100-02, 15, 50

✿ **J2400** Injection, chloroprocaine hydrochloride, **per 30 ml** Ⓑ Ⓑ   N1 N

NDC: Nesacaine, Nesacaine-MPF

IOM: 100-02, 15, 50

✿ **J2405** Injection, ondansetron hydrochloride, **per 1 mg** Ⓑ Ⓑ   N1 N

NDC: Zofran

IOM: 100-02, 15, 50

✿ **J2410** Injection, oxymorphone HCL, **up to 1 mg** Ⓑ Ⓑ   N1 N

NDC: Opana

Other: Numorphan

IOM: 100-02, 15, 50

✳ **J2425** Injection, palifermin, **50 micrograms** Ⓑ Ⓑ   K2 K

NDC: Kepivance

✳ **J2426** Injection, paliperidone palmitate extended release, **1 mg** Ⓑ Ⓑ   K2 K

NDC: Invega Sustenna

Coding Clinic: 2011, Q1, P7

✿ **J2430** Injection, pamidronate disodium, **per 30 mg** Ⓑ Ⓑ   N1 N

Other: Aredia

IOM: 100-02, 15, 50

✿ **J2440** Injection, papaverine HCL, **up to 60 mg** Ⓑ Ⓑ   N1 N

IOM: 100-02, 15, 50

✿ **J2460** Injection, oxytetracycline HCL, **up to 50 mg** Ⓑ Ⓑ   E

Other: Terramycin IM

IOM: 100-02, 15, 50

✳ **J2469** Injection, palonosetron HCL, **25 mcg** Ⓑ Ⓑ   K2 K

Example: 0.25 mgm dose = 10 units. Example of use is acute, delayed, nausea and vomiting due to chemotherapy

NDC: Aloxi

✿ **J2501** Injection, paricalcitol, **1 mcg** Ⓑ Ⓑ   N1 N

NDC: Zemplar

IOM: 100-02, 15, 50

✳ **J2503** Injection, pegaptanib sodium, **0.3 mg** Ⓑ Ⓑ   K2 K

NDC: Macugen

⚙ **J2504** Injection, pegademase bovine,
25 IU Ⓑ Ⓑ   K2 K

NDC: Adagen

IOM: 100-02, 15, 50

✳ **J2505** Injection, pegfilgrastim,
6 mg Ⓑ Ⓑ   K2 K

Report 1 unit per 6 mg.

NDC: Neulasta

✳ **J2507** Injection, pegloticase,
1 mg Ⓑ Ⓑ **Qp** **Qh**   K2 K

NDC: Krystexxa

Coding Clinic: 2012, Q1, P9

⚙ **J2510** Injection, penicillin G
procaine, aqueous, **up to
600,000 units** Ⓑ Ⓑ   N1 N

*Other: Crysticillin, Duracillin AS,
Pfizerpen AS, Wycillin*

IOM: 100-02, 15, 50

⚙ **J2513** Injection, pentastarch, 10% solution,
100 ml Ⓑ Ⓑ   E

IOM: 100-02, 15, 50

⚙ **J2515** Injection, pentobarbital sodium, **per
50 mg** Ⓑ Ⓑ   K2 K

NDC: Nembutal

IOM: 100-02, 15, 50

⚙ **J2540** Injection, penicillin G potassium, **up to
600,000 units** Ⓑ Ⓑ   N1 N

NDC: Pfizerpen-G

IOM: 100-02, 15, 50

⚙ **J2543** Injection, piperacillin sodium/
tazobactam sodium, **1 gram/
0.125 grams
(1.125 grams)** Ⓑ Ⓑ   N1 N

NDC: Zosyn

IOM: 100-02, 15, 50

⚙ **J2545** Pentamidine isethionate, inhalation
solution, FDA-approved final product,
non-compounded, administered
through DME, unit dose form, **per
300 mg** Ⓑ Ⓑ   B

NDC: Nebupent

⚙ **J2550** Injection, promethazine HCL, **up to
50 mg** Ⓑ Ⓑ   N1 N

Administration of phenergan
suppository considered part of E/M
encounter

NDC: Phenergan

*Other: Anergan, Phenazine, Prorex,
Prothazine*

IOM: 100-02, 15, 50

⚙ **J2560** Injection, phenobarbital sodium, **up to
120 mg** Ⓑ Ⓑ   N1 N

IOM: 100-02, 15, 50

✳ **J2562** Injection, plerixafor, **1 mg** Ⓑ Ⓑ   K2 K

FDA approved for non-Hodgkin
lymphoma and multiple myeloma in
2008.

NDC: Mozobil

⚙ **J2590** Injection, oxytocin, **up to
10 units** Ⓑ Ⓑ   N1 N

Other: Pitocin, Syntocinon

IOM: 100-02, 15, 50

⚙ **J2597** Injection, desmopressin acetate, **per
1 mcg** Ⓑ Ⓑ   K2 K

NDC: DDAVP

IOM: 100-02, 15, 50

⚙ **J2650** Injection, prednisolone acetate, **up to
1 ml** Ⓑ Ⓑ   N1 N

*Other: Cotolone, Key-Pred, Predalone,
Predcor, Predicort*

IOM: 100-02, 15, 50

⚙ **J2670** Injection, tolazoline HCL, **up to
25 mg** Ⓑ Ⓑ   K

Other: Priscoline Hydrochloride

IOM: 100-02, 15, 50

⚙ **J2675** Injection, progesterone, **per
50 mg** Ⓑ Ⓑ   N1 N

Other: Gesterol 50, Progestaject

IOM: 100-02, 15, 50

⚙ **J2680** Injection, fluphenazine decanoate, **up
to 25 mg** Ⓑ Ⓑ   N1 N

Other: Prolixin Decanoate

MCM 2049

IOM: 100-02, 15, 50

⚙ **J2690** Injection, procainamide HCL, **up to
1 gm** Ⓑ Ⓑ ♀   N1 N

Benefit limited to obstetrical diagnoses

Other: Pronestyl, Prostaphlin

IOM: 100-02, 15, 50

⚙ **J2700** Injection, oxacillin sodium, **up to
250 mg** Ⓑ Ⓑ   N1 N

NDC: Bactocill

IOM: 100-02, 15, 50

▶✳ **J2704** Injection, propofol, **10 mg**   N1 N

⚙ **J2710** Injection, neostigmine methylsulfate,
up to 0.5 mg Ⓑ Ⓑ   N1 N

Other: Prostigmin

IOM: 100-02, 15, 50

▶ New   ↺ Revised   ✔ Reinstated   deleted Deleted   ⊘ Not covered or valid by Medicare
⚙ Special coverage instructions   ✳ Carrier discretion   Ⓑ Bill local carrier   Ⓑ Bill DME MAC

⊛ **J2720** Injection, protamine sulfate, **per 10 mg** ⓑ Ⓑ   N1 N

IOM: 100-02, 15, 50

✳ **J2724** Injection, protein C concentrate, intravenous, human, **10 IU** ⓑ Ⓑ   K2 K

NDC: Ceprotin

↩ ⊛ **J2725** Injection, protirelin, **per 250 mcg** ⓑ Ⓑ   E

Other: Relefact TRH, Thypinone

IOM: 100-02, 15, 50

⊛ **J2730** Injection, pralidoxime chloride, **up to 1 gm** ⓑ Ⓑ   K2 K

NDC: Protopam Chloride

IOM: 100-02, 15, 50

⊛ **J2760** Injection, phentolamine mesylate, **up to 5 mg** ⓑ Ⓑ   K2 K

Other: Regitine

IOM: 100-02, 15, 50

⊛ **J2765** Injection, metoclopramide HCL, **up to 10 mg** ⓑ Ⓑ   N1 N

Other: Reglan

IOM: 100-02, 15, 50

⊛ **J2770** Injection, quinupristin/dalfopristin, **500 mg (150/350)** ⓑ Ⓑ   K2 K

NDC: Synercid

IOM: 100-02, 15, 50

✳ **J2778** Injection, ranibizumab, **0.1 mg** ⓑ Ⓑ   K2 K

May be reported for exudative senile macular degeneration (wet AMD) with 67028 (RT or LT)

Other: Lucentis

⊛ **J2780** Injection, ranitidine hydrochloride, **25 mg** ⓑ Ⓑ   N1 N

NDC: Zantac

IOM: 100-02, 15, 50

✳ **J2783** Injection, rasburicase, **0.5 mg** ⓑ Ⓑ   K2 K

NDC: Elitek

✳ **J2785** Injection, regadenoson, **0.1 mg** ⓑ Ⓑ   N1 N

One billing unit equal to 0.1 mg of regadenoson

⊛ **J2788** Injection, Rho D immune globulin, human, minidose, **50 mcg (250 IU)** ⓑ Ⓑ   N1 N

NDC: MicRhoGAM

Other: HypRho-D, RhoGam

IOM: 100-02, 15, 50

⊛ **J2790** Injection, Rho D immune globulin, human, full dose, **300 mcg (1500 IU)** ⓑ Ⓑ   N1 N

Administered to pregnant female to prevent hemolistic disease of newborn. Report 90384 to private payer

NDC: Hyperrho S/D, RhoGAM

Other: Gamulin Rh, HypRho-D, Rhesonativ

IOM: 100-02, 15, 50

⊛ **J2791** Injection, Rho(D) immune globulin (human), (Rhophylac), intramuscular or intravenous, **100 IU** ⓑ Ⓑ   K2 K

Agent must be billed per 100 IU in both physician office and hospital outpatient settings

Other: HypRho-D

IOM: 100-02, 15, 50

⊛ **J2792** Injection, Rho D immune globulin intravenous, human, solvent detergent, **100 IU** ⓑ Ⓑ   K2 K

NDC: WinRHo-SDF

Other: Gamulin RH, Hyperrho S/D

IOM: 100-02, 15, 50

⊛ **J2793** Injection, rilonacept, **1 mg** ⓑ Ⓑ   K2 K

IOM: 100-02, 15, 50

✳ **J2794** Injection, risperidone, long acting, **0.5 mg** ⓑ Ⓑ   K2 K

NDC: Risperdal Costa

✳ **J2795** Injection, ropivacaine hydrochloride, **1 mg** ⓑ Ⓑ   N1 N

NDC: Naropin

✳ **J2796** Injection, romiplostim, **10 micrograms** ⓑ Ⓑ   K2 K

Stimulates bone marrow megakarocytes to produce platelets (i.e., ITP).

NDC: Nplate

⊛ **J2800** Injection, methocarbamol, **up to 10 ml** ⓑ Ⓑ   N1 N

NDC: Robaxin

IOM: 100-02, 15, 50

✳ **J2805** Injection, sincalide, **5 micrograms** ⓑ Ⓑ   N1 N

ⓅQRS PQRS	Qp Quantity Physician Appendix A	Qh Quantity Hospital Appendix B	♀ Female only
♂ Male only Ⓐ Age ♿ DMEPOS A2-Z3 ASC Payment Indicator A-Y ASC Status Indicator Coding Clinic			

⊛ **J2810**   Injection, theophylline, **per 40 mg** Ⓑ Ⓑ   N1   N

IOM: 100-02, 15, 50

⊛ **J2820**   Injection, sargramostim (GM-CSF), **50 mcg** Ⓑ Ⓑ   K2   K

NDC: Leukine

Other: Prokine

IOM: 100-02, 15, 50

⊛ **J2850**   Injection, secretin, synthetic, human, **1 microgram** Ⓑ Ⓑ   K2   K

NDC: Chirhostim

IOM: 100-02, 15, 50

⊛ **J2910**   Injection, aurothioglucose, **up to 50 mg** Ⓑ Ⓑ   N1   N

Other: Solganal

IOM: 100-02, 15, 50

⊛ **J2916**   Injection, sodium ferric gluconate complex in sucrose injection, **12.5 mg** Ⓑ Ⓑ   N1   N

NDC: Ferrlecit, Nulecit

IOM: 100-02, 15, 50

⊛ **J2920**   Injection, methylprednisolone sodium succinate, **up to 40 mg** Ⓑ Ⓑ   N1   N

NDC: Solu-Medrol

Other: A-MethaPred

IOM: 100-02, 15, 50

⊛ **J2930**   Injection, methylprednisolone sodium succinate, **up to 125 mg** Ⓑ Ⓑ   N1   N

NDC: Solu-Medrol

Other: A-MethaPred

IOM: 100-02, 15, 50

⊛ **J2940**   Injection, somatrem, **1 mg** Ⓑ Ⓑ   K2   E

IOM: 100-02, 15, 50,

Medicare Statute 1861s2b

↻ ⊛ **J2941**   Injection, somatropin, **1 mg** Ⓑ Ⓑ   K2   K

Other: Genotropin, Humatrope, Nutropin, Omnitrope, Saizen, Serostim, Trev-Tropin, Zorbtive

IOM: 100-02, 15, 50,

Medicare Statute 1861s2b

⊛ **J2950**   Injection, promazine HCL, **up to 25 mg** Ⓑ Ⓑ   N1   N

Other: Prozine-50, Sparine

IOM: 100-02, 15, 50

⊛ **J2993**   Injection, reteplase, **18.1 mg** Ⓑ Ⓑ   K2   K

NDC: Retavase

IOM: 100-02, 15, 50

⊛ **J2995**   Injection, streptokinase, **per 250,000 IU** Ⓑ Ⓑ Qp Qh   N1   N

Bill 1 unit for each 250,000 IU

Other: Kabikinase, Streptase

IOM: 100-02, 15, 50

⊛ **J2997**   Injection, alteplase recombinant, **1 mg** Ⓑ Ⓑ   K2   K

Thrombolytic agent, treatment of occluded catheters. Bill units of 1 mg administered

NDC: Activase, Cathflo Activase

IOM: 100-02, 15, 50

Coding Clinic: 2014, Q1, P4

⊛ **J3000**   Injection, streptomycin, **up to 1 gm** Ⓑ Ⓑ   N1   N

IOM: 100-02, 15, 50

⊛ **J3010**   Injection, fentanyl citrate, **0.1 mg** Ⓑ Ⓑ Qp Qh   N1   N

NDC: Sublimaze

IOM: 100-02, 15, 50

⊛ **J3030**   Injection, sumatriptan succinate, **6 mg** (Code may be used for Medicare when drug administered under the direct supervision of a physician, not for use when drug is self administered) Ⓑ Ⓑ   N1   N

Other: Imitrex

IOM: 100-02, 15, 150

✳ **J3060**   Injection, taliglucerace alfa, **10 units** Ⓑ Ⓑ Qp Qh   K2   G

NDC: Elelyso

↻ ⊛ **J3070**   Injection, pentazocine, **30 mg** Ⓑ Ⓑ   K2   K

Other: Talwin

IOM: 100-02, 15, 50

▶ **New**   ↻ **Revised**   ✔ **Reinstated**   ~~deleted~~ **Deleted**   ⊘ **Not covered or valid by Medicare**
⊛ **Special coverage instructions**   ✳ **Carrier discretion**   Ⓑ **Bill local carrier**   Ⓑ **Bill DME MAC**

✳ **J3095** Injection, televancin, **10 mg** ⓑ ⓑ   K2 K

Prescribed for the treatment of adults with complicated skin and skin structure infections (cSSSI) of the following Gram-positive microorganisms: Staphylococcus aureus; *Streptococcus pyogenes, Streptococcus agalactiae, Streptococcus anginosus* group. Separately payable under the ASC payment system.

NDC: Vibativ

Coding Clinic: 2011, Q1, P7

✳ **J3101** Injection, tenecteplase, **1 mg** ⓑ ⓑ   K2 K

NDC: TNKase

☼ **J3105** Injection, terbutaline sulfate, **up to 1 mg** ⓑ ⓑ   N1 N

Other: Brethine

IOM: 100-02, 15, 50

☼ **J3110** Injection, teriparatide, **10 mcg** ⓑ ⓑ ⓑ   B

Other: Forteo

~~J3120~~ ~~Injection, testosterone enanthate, up to 100 mg~~   ✖

▶ ☼ **J3121** Injection, testosterone enanthate, **1 mg**   N1 N

~~J3130~~ ~~Injection, testosterone enanthate, up to 200 mg~~   ✖

~~J3140~~ ~~Injection, testosterone suspension, up to 50 mg~~   ✖

▶ ☼ **J3145** Injection, testosterone undecanoate, **1 mg**   K2 G

~~J3150~~ ~~Injection, testosterone propionate, up to 100 mg~~   ✖

☼ **J3230** Injection, chlorpromazine HCL, **up to 50 mg** ⓑ ⓑ   N1 N

Other: Ormazine, Thorazine

IOM: 100-02, 15, 50

☼ **J3240** Injection, thyrotropin alfa, **0.9 mg provided in 1.1 mg vial** ⓑ ⓑ   K2 K

NDC: Thyrogen

IOM: 100-02, 15, 50

✳ **J3243** Injection, tigecycline, **1 mg** ⓑ ⓑ   K2 K

✳ **J3246** Injection, tirofiban HCL, **0.25 mg** ⓑ ⓑ   K2 K

Other: Aggrastat

☼ **J3250** Injection, trimethobenzamide HCL, **up to 200 mg** ⓑ ⓑ   N1 N

NDC: Ticon, Tigan

Other: Arrestin, Tiject 20

IOM: 100-02, 15, 50

☼ **J3260** Injection, tobramycin sulfate, **up to 80 mg** ⓑ ⓑ   N1 N

Other: Nebcin

IOM: 100-02, 15, 50

✳ **J3262** Injection, tocilizumab, **1 mg** ⓑ ⓑ   K2 K

Indicated for the treatment of adult patients with moderately to severely active rheumatoid arthritis (RA) who have had an inadequate response to one or more tumor necrosis factor (TNF) antagonist therapies.

NDC: Actemra

Coding Clinic: 2011, Q1, P7

☼ **J3265** Injection, torsemide, **10 mg/ml** ⓑ ⓑ   N1 N

Other: Demadex

IOM: 100-02, 15, 50

☼ **J3280** Injection, thiethylperazine maleate, **up to 10 mg** ⓑ ⓑ   N1 N

Other: Norzine, Torecan

IOM: 100-02, 15, 50

✳ **J3285** Injection, treprostinil, **1 mg** ⓑ ⓑ **Qp** **Qh**   K2 K

NDC: Remodulin

☼ **J3300** Injection, triamcinolone acetonide, preservative free, **1 mg** ⓑ ⓑ   K2 K

Other: Triam-A, Triesence, Tri-Kort, Trilog

☼ **J3301** Injection, triamcinolone acetonide, **not otherwise specified, 10 mg** ⓑ ⓑ   N1 N

NDC: Kenalog

Other: Cenacort A-40, Kenaject-40, Triam A, Triesence, Tri-Kort, Trilog

IOM: 100-02, 15, 50

Coding Clinic: 2013, Q2, P4

🅟 PQRS	**Qp** Quantity Physician Appendix A	**Qh** Quantity Hospital Appendix B	♀ Female only
♂ **Male only**	**A** **Age**	♿ **DMEPOS**	**A2-Z3 ASC Payment Indicator**	**A-Y ASC Status Indicator**	Coding Clinic

⊗ **J3302** Injection, triamcinolone diacetate, **per 5 mg** Ⓑ Ⓑ   N1   N

Other: Amcort, Aristocort Forte, Cenacort Forte, Clinacort, Triamcot, Trilone

IOM: 100-02, 15, 50

⊗ **J3303** Injection, triamcinolone hexacetonide, **per 5 mg** Ⓑ Ⓑ   N1   N

NDC: Aristospan

IOM: 100-02, 15, 50

⊗ **J3305** Injection, trimetrexate glucuronate, **per 25 mg** Ⓑ Ⓑ   E

Other: NeuTrexin

IOM: 100-02, 15, 50

⊗ **J3310** Injection, perphenazine, **up to 5 mg** Ⓑ Ⓑ   N1   N

Other: Trilafon

IOM: 100-02, 15, 50

⊗ **J3315** Injection, triptorelin pamoate, **3.75 mg** Ⓑ Ⓑ   K2   K

NDC: Trelstar

IOM: 100-02, 15, 50

⊗ **J3320** Injection, spectinomycin dihydrochloride, **up to 2 gm** Ⓑ Ⓑ   N

Other: Trobicin

IOM: 100-02, 15, 50

⊗ **J3350** Injection, urea, **up to 40 gm** Ⓑ Ⓑ   K2   K

Other: Ureaphil

IOM: 100-02, 15, 50

⊗ **J3355** Injection, urofollitropin, **75 IU** Ⓑ Ⓑ   K2   K

Other: Bravelle, Metrodin

IOM: 100-02, 15, 50

✳ **J3357** Injection, ustekinumab, **1 mg** Ⓑ Ⓑ   K2   K

Other: Stelara

Coding Clinic: 2011, Q1, P7

⊗ **J3360** Injection, diazepam, **up to 5 mg** Ⓑ Ⓑ   N1   N

Other: Valium, Zetran

IOM: 100-02, 15, 50

Coding Clinic: 2007, Q2, P6-7

⊗ **J3364** Injection, urokinase, **5000 IU vial** Ⓑ Ⓑ   N1   N

NDC: Abbokinase

IOM: 100-02, 15, 50

↻ ⊗ **J3365** Injection, IV, urokinase, **250,000 IU vial** Ⓑ Ⓑ   E

Other: Abbokinase

IOM: 100-02, 15, 50,

Cross Reference Q0089

⊗ **J3370** Injection, vancomycin HCL, **500 mg** Ⓑ Ⓑ   N1   N

NDC: Vancocin

Other: Vancoled

IOM: 100-02, 15, 50; 100-03, 4, 280.14

↻✳ **J3385** Injection, velaglucerase alfa, **100 units** Ⓑ Ⓑ   K2   K

Enzyme replacement therapy in Gaucher Disease that results from a specific enzyme deficiency in the body, caused by a genetic mutation received from both parents. Type 1 is the most prevalent Ashkenazi Jewish genetic disease, occurring in one in every 1,000.

NDC: VPRIV

Coding Clinic: 2011, Q1, P7

⊗ **J3396** Injection, verteporfin, **0.1 mg** Ⓑ Ⓑ   K2   K

NDC: Visudyne

IOM: 100-03, 1, 80.2; 100-03, 1, 80.3

⊗ **J3400** Injection, triflupromazine HCL, **up to 20 mg** Ⓑ Ⓑ   E

Other: Vesprin

IOM: 100-02, 15, 50

⊗ **J3410** Injection, hydroxyzine HCL, **up to 25 mg** Ⓑ Ⓑ   N1   N

Other: Hyzine-50, Vistacot, Vistaject 25

IOM: 100-02, 15, 50

✳ **J3411** Injection, thiamine HCL, **100 mg** Ⓑ Ⓑ   N1   N

✳ **J3415** Injection, pyridoxine HCL, **100 mg** Ⓑ Ⓑ   N1   N

Other: Rodex

▶ **New**   ↻ **Revised**   ✔ **Reinstated**   ~~deleted~~ **Deleted**   ⊘ **Not covered or valid by Medicare**

⊗ **Special coverage instructions**   ✳ **Carrier discretion**   Ⓑ **Bill local carrier**   Ⓑ **Bill DME MAC**

⚙ **J3420** Injection, vitamin B-12 cyanocobalamin, **up to 1000 mcg** Ⓑ Ⓖ   N1   N

Medicare carriers may have local coverage decisions regarding vitamin B_{12} injections that provide reimbursement only for patients with certain types of anemia and other conditions

Other: Cobolin-M, Hydroxocobalamin, Neuroforte-R, Redisol, Rubramin PC, Sytobex, Vita #12

IOM: 100-02, 15, 50; 100-03, 2, 150.6

⚙ **J3430** Injection, phytonadione (vitamin K), **per 1 mg** Ⓑ Ⓖ   N1   N

NDC: Vitamin K1

Other: AquaMephyton, Konakion, Menadione, Synkavite

IOM: 100-02, 15, 50

⚙ **J3465** Injection, voriconazole, **10 mg** Ⓑ Ⓖ Ⓠp Ⓠh   K2   K

NDC: VFEND

IOM: 100-02, 15, 50

⚙ **J3470** Injection, hyaluronidase, **up to 150 units** Ⓑ Ⓖ   N1   N

Other: Wydase

IOM: 100-02, 15, 50

⚙ **J3471** Injection, hyaluronidase, ovine, preservative free, **per 1 USP unit (up to 999 USP units)** Ⓑ Ⓖ   N1   N

⚙ **J3472** Injection, hyaluronidase, ovine, preservative free, **per 1000 USP units** Ⓑ Ⓖ   N1   N

⚙ **J3473** Injection, hyaluronidase, recombinant, **1 USP unit** Ⓑ Ⓖ   N1   N

IOM: 100-02, 15, 50

⚙ **J3475** Injection, magnesium sulfate, **per 500 mg** Ⓑ Ⓖ   N1   N

IOM: 100-02, 15, 50

⚙ **J3480** Injection, potassium chloride, **per 2 meq** Ⓑ Ⓖ   N1   N

IOM: 100-02, 15, 50

⚙ **J3485** Injection, zidovudine, **10 mg** Ⓑ Ⓖ   K2   K

NDC: Retrovir

IOM: 100-02, 15, 50

✳ **J3486** Injection, ziprasidone mesylate, **10 mg** Ⓑ Ⓖ   N1   N

NDC: Geodon

✳ **J3489** Injection, zoledronic acid, **1 mg** Ⓑ Ⓖ Ⓠp Ⓠh   K2   K

NDC: Reclast, Zometra

⚙ **J3490** Unclassified drugs Ⓑ Ⓖ   N1   N

Bill on paper. Bill one unit. Identify drug and total dosage in "Remarks" field.

Other: Acthib, Aminocaproic Acid, Baciim, Bacitracin, Benzocaine, Betamethasone Acetate, Brevital Sodium, Bumetanide, Bupivacaine, Cefotetan, Cimetidine, Ciprofloxacin, Cleocin Phosphate, Clindamycin, Cortisone Acetate, Definity, Diprivan, Engerix-B, Ethanolamine, Famotidine, Ganirelix, Gonal-F, Hyaluronic Acid, Marcaine, Metronidazole, Nafcillin, Naltrexone, Ovidrel, Pegasys, Peg-Intron, Penicillin G Sodium, Propofol, Protonix, Recombivax, Rifadin, Rifampin, Sensorcaine-MPF, Smz-TMP, Sodium Hyaluronate, Sufentanil Citrate, Timentin, Treanda, Twinrix, Valcyte, Veritas Collagen Matrix

IOM: 100-02, 15, 50

Coding Clinic: 2014, Q2, P6; 2013, Q2, P3-4

⊘ **J3520** Edetate disodium, **per 150 mg** Ⓑ Ⓖ   E

Other: Chealamide, Disotate, Endrate ethylenediamine-tetra-acetic

IOM: 100-03, 1, 20.21; 100-03, 1, 20.22

⚙ **J3530** Nasal vaccine inhalation Ⓑ Ⓖ   N1   N

IOM: 100-02, 15, 50

⊘ **J3535** Drug administered through a metered dose inhaler Ⓑ Ⓖ   E

Other: Ipratropium bromide

IOM: 100-02, 15, 50

⊘ **J3570** Laetrile, amygdalin, vitamin B-17 Ⓑ Ⓖ   E

IOM: 100-03, 1, 30.7

✳ **J3590** Unclassified biologics Ⓑ   N1   N

Bill on paper. Bill one unit. Identify drug and total dosage in "Remarks" field.

Other: Bayhep B, Hyperhep-B, NABI-HB

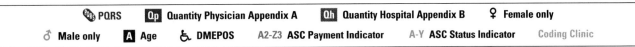

🅟 PQRS	Ⓠp Quantity Physician Appendix A	Ⓠh Quantity Hospital Appendix B	♀ Female only
♂ Male only	Ⓐ Age	🦽 DMEPOS	A2-Z3 ASC Payment Indicator	A-Y ASC Status Indicator	Coding Clinic

Miscellaneous Drugs and Solutions

⊛ **J7030** Infusion, normal saline solution, **1000 cc** Ⓑ Ⓓ   N1 N

Bill local carrier (Ⓑ) if incident to a physician's service or used in an implanted infusion pump. If other, bill DME MAC (Ⓓ).

NDC: Sodium Chloride

IOM: 100-02, 15, 50

⊛ **J7040** Infusion, normal saline solution, sterile **(500 ml = 1 unit)** Ⓑ Ⓓ   N1 N

Bill local carrier (Ⓑ) if incident to a physician's service or used in an implanted infusion pump. If other, bill DME MAC (Ⓓ).

NDC: Sodium Chloride

IOM: 100-02, 15, 50

⊛ **J7042** 5% dextrose/normal saline **(500 ml = 1 unit)** Ⓑ Ⓓ   N1 N

Bill local carrier (Ⓑ) if incident to a physician's service or used in an implanted infusion pump. If other, bill DME MAC (Ⓓ).

NDC: Dextrose-Nacl

IOM: 100-02, 15, 50

⊛ **J7050** Infusion, normal saline solution, **250 cc** Ⓑ Ⓓ   N1 N

Bill local carrier (Ⓑ) if incident to a physician's service or used in an implanted infusion pump. If other, bill DME MAC (Ⓓ).

NDC: Sodium Chloride

IOM: 100-02, 15, 50

⊛ **J7060** 5% dextrose/water **(500 ml = 1 unit)** Ⓑ Ⓓ   N1 N

Bill local carrier (Ⓑ) if incident to a physician's service or used in an implanted infusion pump. If other, bill DME MAC (Ⓓ).

IOM: 100-02, 15, 50

⊛ **J7070** Infusion, D 5 W, **1000 cc** Ⓑ Ⓓ   N1 N

Bill local carrier (Ⓑ) if incident to a physician's service or used in an implanted infusion pump. If other, bill DME MAC (Ⓓ).

NDC: Dextrose

IOM: 100-02, 15, 50

⊛ **J7100** Infusion, dextran 40, **500 ml** Ⓑ Ⓓ   N1 N

Bill local carrier (Ⓑ) if incident to a physician's service or used in an implanted infusion pump. If other, bill DME MAC (Ⓓ).

Other: Gentran, LMD, Rheomacrodex

IOM: 100-02, 15, 50

⊛ **J7110** Infusion, dextran 75, **500 ml** Ⓑ Ⓓ   N1 N

Bill local carrier (Ⓑ) if incident to a physician's service or used in an implanted infusion pump. If other, bill DME MAC (Ⓓ).

Other: Gentran

IOM: 100-02, 15, 50

⊛ **J7120** Ringer's lactate infusion, **up to 1000 cc** Ⓑ Ⓓ   N1 N

Bill local carrier (Ⓑ) 20if incident to a physician's service or used in an implanted infusion pump. If other, bill DME MAC (Ⓓ).

Replacement fluid or electrolytes.

NDC: Lactated Ringers

IOM: 100-02, 15, 50

⊛ **J7131** Hypertonic saline solution, **1 ml**   N1 N

IOM: 100-02, 15, 50

Coding Clinic: 2012, Q1, P9

⮂ ✳ **J7178** Injection, human fibrinogen concentrate, 1 mg Ⓑ   K2 K

⮂ ✳ **J7180** Injection, factor XIII (antihemophilic factor, human), 1 i.u.   N1 N

Coding Clinic: 2012, Q1, P8

▶ ✳ **J7181** Injection, factor XIII a-subunit, (recombinant), **per iu**   K2 G

▶ ✳ **J7182** Injection, factor VIII, (antihemophilic factor, recombinant), (novoeight), **per iu**   E

⊛ **J7183** Injection, von Willebrand factor complex (human), wilate, **1 i.u. vwf:rco**   K2 K

IOM: 100-02, 15, 50

Coding Clinic: 2012, Q1, P9

✳ **J7185** Injection, Factor VIII (antihemophilic factor, recombinant) (Xyntha), **per IU**   K2 K

Reported in place of temporary code Q2023.

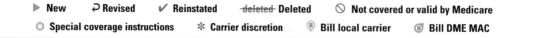

▶ **New**   ⮂ **Revised**   ✔ **Reinstated**   ~~deleted~~ **Deleted**   ⊘ **Not covered or valid by Medicare**
⊛ **Special coverage instructions**   ✳ **Carrier discretion**   Ⓑ **Bill local carrier**   Ⓓ **Bill DME MAC**

⊛ **J7186** Injection, anti-hemophilic factor VIII/von Willebrand factor complex (human), **per factor VIII IU** ⓑ K2 K

NDC: Alphanate

IOM: 100-02, 15, 50

⊛ **J7187** Injection, von Willebrand factor complex (HUMATE-P), **per IU VWF:RCO** ⓑ K2 K

NDC: Humate-P Low Dilutent

Other: Wilate

IOM: 100-02, 15, 50

⊛ **J7189** Factor VIIa (anti-hemophilic factor, recombinant), **per 1 microgram** ⓑ K2 K

NDC: NovoSeven

IOM: 100-02, 15, 50

⊛ **J7190** Factor VIII anti-hemophilic factor, human, **per IU** ⓑ K2 K

NDC: Alphanate/von Willebrand factor complex, Hemofil M, Koate DVI, Monoclate-P

Other: Koate-HP, Kogenate, Recombinate

IOM: 100-02, 15, 50

⊛ **J7191** Factor VIII, anti-hemophilic factor (porcine), **per IU** ⓑ K2 K

Other: Hyate C, Koate-HP, Kogenate, Monoclate-P, Recombinate

IOM: 100-02, 15, 50

✳ **J7192** Factor VIII (anti-hemophilic factor, recombinant) **per IU, not otherwise specified** ⓑ K2 K

NDC: Advate, Helixate FS, Kogenate FS, Recombinate

Other: Koate-HP, Refacto

IOM: 100-02, 15, 50

⊛ **J7193** Factor IX (anti-hemophilic factor, purified, non-recombinant) **per IU** ⓑ K2 K

NDC: AlphaNine SD, Mononine, Profiline, Proplex T

IOM: 100-02, 15, 50

⊛ **J7194** Factor IX, complex, **per IU** ⓑ K2 K

NDC: Profilnine SD

Other: Bebulin VH, Konyne-80, Profilnine Heat-treated, Proplex SX-T, Proplex T

IOM: 100-02, 15, 50

↻ ⊛ **J7195** Injection, Factor IX (anti-hemophilic factor, recombinant) **per IU**, not otherwise specified ⓑ K2 K

NDC: Benefix

Other: Konyne 80, Profiline, Proplex T

IOM: 100-02, 15, 50

✳ **J7196** Injection, antithrombin recombinant, **50 i.u.** Qp Qh K2 K

Other: ATryn

Coding Clinic: 2011, Q1, P6

⊛ **J7197** Anti-thrombin III (human), **per IU** ⓑ K2 K

NDC: Thrombate III

IOM: 100-02, 15, 50

⊛ **J7198** Anti-inhibitor, **per IU** ⓑ K2 K

Diagnosis examples: 286.0 Congenital Factor VIII disorder; 286.1 Congenital Factor IX disorder; 286.4 VonWillebrand's disease

Other: Autoplex T, Feiba VH Immuno, Hemophilia clotting factors

IOM: 100-02, 15, 50; 100-03, 2, 110.3

⊛ **J7199** Hemophilia clotting factor, not otherwise classified ⓑ B

Other: Autoplex T

IOM: 100-02, 15, 50; 100-03, 2, 110.3

▶ ⊛ **J7200** Injection, factor IX, (antihemophilic factor, recombinant), rixubis, **per iu** K2 G

IOM: 100-02, 15, 50

▶ ⊛ **J7201** Injection, factor IX, fc fusion protein (recombinant), **per iu** K2 G

IOM: 100-02, 15, 50

⊘ **J7300** Intrauterine copper contraceptive ⓑ E

Report IVD insertion with 58300. Bill usual and customary charge.

Other: Paragard T 380 A

Medicare Statute 1862a1

↻ ⊘ **J7301** Levonorgestrel-releasing intrauterine contraceptive system, **13.5 mg** ⓑ Qp Qh E

Medicare Statute 1862(a)(1)

↻ ⊘ **J7302** Levonorgestrel-releasing intrauterine contraceptive system, **52 mg** ⓑ ♀ E

Other: Mirena

Medicare Statute 1862a1

⊘ **J7303** Contraceptive supply, hormone containing vaginal ring, each ⓑ ♀ E

Medicare Statute 1862.1

⊘ **J7304** Contraceptive supply, hormone containing patch, each Ⓑ ♀   E

Only billed by Family Planning Clinics

Medicare Statute 1862.1

⊘ **J7306** Levonorgestrel (contraceptive) implant system, including implants and supplies Ⓑ   E

⊘ **J7307** Etonogestrel (contraceptive) implant system, including implant and supplies Ⓑ   E

⚹ **J7308** Aminolevulinic acid HCL for topical administration, 20%, single unit dosage form **(354 mg)** Ⓑ   K2 K

NDC: Levulan Kerastick

☼ **J7309** Methyl aminolevulinate (MAL) for topical administration, 16.8%, **1 gram** Ⓑ Ⓑ   K2 K

NDC: Metvixia

Coding Clinic: 2011, Q1, P6

☼ **J7310** Ganciclovir, **4.5 mg,** long-acting implant Ⓑ **Qp** **Qh**   K2 K

NDC: Vitrasert

IOM: 100-02, 15, 50

⚹ **J7311** Fluocinolone acetonide, intravitreal implant Ⓑ   K2 K

Treatment of chronic noninfectious posterior segment uveitis

Other: Retisert

⚹ **J7312** Injection, dexamethasone, intravitreal implant, **0.1 mg** Ⓑ Ⓑ   K2 K

To bill for Ozurdex services submit the following codes: J7312 and 67028 with the modifier -22 (for the increased work difficulty and increased risk). Indicated for the treatment of macular edema occurring after branch retinal vein occlusion (BRVO) or central retinal vein occlusion (CRVO) and non-infectious uveitis affecting the posterior segment of the eye.

NDC: Ozurdex

Coding Clinic: 2011, Q1, P7

⚹ **J7315** Mitomycin, ophthalmic, 0.2 mg Ⓑ   K2 G

Coding Clinic: 2014, Q2, P6

⚹ **J7316** Injection, ocriplasmin, 0.125 mg Ⓑ Ⓑ **Qp** **Qh**   K2 G

NDC: Jetrea

⚹ **J7321** Hyaluronan or derivative, Hyalgan or Supartz, for intra-articular injection, **per dose** Ⓑ   K2 K

Therapeutic goal is to restore visco-elasticity of synovial hyaluronan, thereby decreasing pain, improving mobility and restoring natural protective functions of hyaluronan in joint

⚹ **J7323** Hyaluronan or derivative, Euflexxa, for intra-articular injection, **per dose** Ⓑ   K2 K

⚹ **J7324** Hyaluronan or derivative, Orthovisc, for intra-articular injection, **per dose** Ⓑ   K2 K

⚹ **J7325** Hyaluronan or derivative, Synvisc or Synvisc-One, for intra-articular injection, **1 mg** Ⓑ Ⓑ   K2 K

⚹ **J7326** Hyaluronan or derivative, Gel-One, for intra-articular injection, **per dose** Ⓑ Ⓑ **Qp** **Qh**   K2 K

Coding Clinic: 2012, Q1, P8

▶ ⚹ **J7327** Hyaluronan or derivative, monovisc, for intra-articular injection, per dose **Qp** **Qh**   K2 K

⚹ **J7330** Autologous cultured chondrocytes, **implant** Ⓑ   B

Other: Carticel

Coding Clinic: 2010, Q4, P3

~~J7335~~   ~~Capsaicin 8% patch, per 10 square centimeters~~   ✖

▶ ⚹ **J7336** Capsaicin 8% patch, **per square centimeter**   K2 K

Immunosuppressive Drugs (Includes Non-injectibles)

J7500-J7599: Bill local carrier (Ⓑ) if incident to a physician's service or used in an implanted infusion pump. If other, bill DME MAC (Ⓑ).

☼ **J7500** Azathioprine, oral, **50 mg** Ⓑ Ⓑ   N1 N

NDC: Azasan

Other: Imuran

IOM: 100-02, 15, 50

☼ **J7501** Azathioprine, parenteral, **100 mg** Ⓑ Ⓑ   K2 K

Other: Imuran

IOM: 100-02, 15, 50

☼ **J7502** Cyclosporine, oral, **100 mg** Ⓑ Ⓑ   N1 N

NDC: Gengraf, Neoral, Sandimmune

IOM: 100-02, 15, 50

▶ **New**   ⟳ **Revised**   ✔ **Reinstated**   ~~deleted~~ **Deleted**   ⊘ **Not covered or valid by Medicare**
☼ **Special coverage instructions**   ⚹ **Carrier discretion**   Ⓑ **Bill local carrier**   Ⓑ **Bill DME MAC**

⚙ **J7504** Lymphocyte immune globulin, antithymocyte globulin, equine, parenteral, **250 mg** ⒷⒷ   **K2** **K**

NDC: Atgam

IOM: 100-02, 15, 50; 100-03, 2, 110.3

↻⚙ **J7505** Muromonab-CD3, parenteral, **5 mg** ⒷⒷ   **N1** **N**

Other: Monoclonal antibodies (parenteral)

IOM: 100-02, 15, 50

⚙ **J7506** Prednisone, oral, **per 5 mg** ⒷⒷ   **N1** **N**

Unit billing example, fifty 10 mg prednisone tablets dispensed, report J7506, 100 units (1 unit of J7506 = 5 mg)

Other: Prednicot, Sterapred DS

IOM: 100-02, 15, 50

⚙ **J7507** Tacrolimus, immediate release, oral, **1 mg** ⒷⒷ   **N1** **N**

NDC: Prograf

IOM: 100-02, 15, 50

⚙ **J7508** Tacrolimus, extended release, oral, **0.1 mg** ⒷⒷ   **K2** **G**

NDC: Astagraf XL

IOM: 100-02, 15, 50

⚙ **J7509** Methylprednisolone oral, **per 4 mg** ⒷⒷ   **N1** **N**

Other: Medrol, Methylpred DP

IOM: 100-02, 15, 50

⚙ **J7510** Prednisolone oral, **per 5 mg** ⒷⒷ   **N1** **N**

NDC: Flo-Pred

Other: Cotolone, Delta-Cortef, Orapred, Pediapred, Prelone

IOM: 100-02, 15, 50

✳ **J7511** Lymphocyte immune globulin, antithymocyte globulin, rabbit, parenteral, **25 mg** ⒷⒷ   **K2** **K**

NDC: Thymoglobulin

⚙ **J7513** Daclizumab, parenteral, **25 mg** ⒷⒷ   **K**

Other: Zenapax

IOM: 100-02, 15, 50

✳ **J7515** Cyclosporine, oral, **25 mg** ⒷⒷ   **N1** **N**

NDC: Gengraf, Neoral, Sandimmune

✳ **J7516** Cyclosporin, parenteral, **250 mg** ⒷⒷ   **N1** **N**

NDC: Sandimmune

✳ **J7517** Mycophenolate mofetil, oral, **250 mg** ⒷⒷ   **N1** **N**

NDC: CellCept

⚙ **J7518** Mycophenolic acid, oral, **180 mg** ⒷⒷ   **N1** **N**

NDC: Myfortic

IOM: 100-04, 4, 240; 100-4, 17, 80.3.1

⚙ **J7520** Sirolimus, oral, **1 mg** ⒷⒷ   **N1** **N**

NDC: Rapamune

IOM: 100-02, 15, 50

⚙ **J7525** Tacrolimus, parenteral, **5 mg** ⒷⒷ   **K2** **K**

NDC: Prograf

IOM: 100-02, 15, 50

⚙ **J7527** Everolimus, oral, 0.25 mg ⒷⒷ   **N1** **N**

NDC: Zortress

IOM 100-02, 15, 50

⚙ **J7599** Immunosuppressive drug, not otherwise classified ⒷⒷ   **N1** **N**

Bill on paper. Bill one unit. Identify drug and total dosage in "Remarks" field.

IOM: 100-02, 15, 50

Inhalation Solutions

✳ **J7604** Acetylcysteine, inhalation solution, compounded product, administered through DME, unit dose form, **per gram** Ⓑ **Qp** **Qh**   **M**

If "incident to" a physician's service, do not bill.

Other: Mucomyst (unit dose form), Mucosol

✳ **J7605** Arformoterol, inhalation solution, FDA approved final product, non-compounded, administered through DME, unit dose form, **15 micrograms** Ⓑ   **M**

Maintenance treatment of bronchoconstriction in patients with chronic obstructive pulmonary disease (COPD) Ⓑ

If "incident to" a physician's service, do not bill.

Other: Brovana

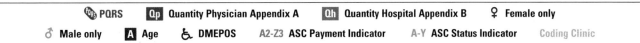

* **J7606** Formoterol fumarate, inhalation solution, FDA approved final product, non-compounded, administered through DME, unit dose form, **20 micrograms** Ⓑ   M

If "incident to" a physician's service, do not bill.

NDC: Perforomist

* **J7607** Levalbuterol, inhalation solution, compounded product, administered through DME, concentrated form, **0.5 mg** Ⓑ Qp Qh   M

If "incident to" a physician's service, do not bill.

☺ **J7608** Acetylcysteine, inhalation solution, FDA-approved final product, non-compounded, administered through DME, unit dose form, **per gram** Ⓑ   M

Other: Mucomyst, Mucosol

If "incident to" a physician's service, do not bill.

* **J7609** Albuterol, inhalation solution, compounded product, administered through DME, unit dose, **1 mg** Ⓑ Qp Qh   M

If "incident to" a physician's service, do not bill.

Patient's home, medications—such as albuterol when administered through a nebulizer—are considered DME and are payable under Part B.

Other: Proventil, Xopenex, Ventolin

* **J7610** Albuterol, inhalation solution, compounded product, administered through DME, concentrated form, **1 mg** Ⓑ Qp Qh   M

If "incident to" a physician's service, do not bill.

Other: Proventil, Xopenex, Ventolin

☺ **J7611** Albuterol, inhalation solution, FDA-approved final product, non-compounded, administered through DME, concentrated form, **1 mg** Ⓑ   M

If "incident to" a physician's service, do not bill.

Report once for each milligram administered. For example, 2 mg of concentrated albuterol (usually diluted with saline), reported with J7611×2

Other: Proventil, Xopenex

☺ **J7612** Levalbuterol, inhalation solution, FDA-approved final product, non-compounded, administered through DME, concentrated form, **0.5 mg** Ⓑ   M

If "incident to" a physician's service, do not bill.

NDC: Xopenex

☺ **J7613** Albuterol, inhalation solution, FDA-approved final product, non-compounded, administered through DME, unit dose, **1 mg** Ⓑ   M

If "incident to" a physician's service, do not bill.

NDC: Accuneb, Proventil, Ventolin

☺ **J7614** Levalbuterol, inhalation solution, FDA-approved final product, non-compounded, administered through DME, unit dose, **0.5 mg** Ⓑ   M

If "incident to" a physician's service, do not bill.

NDC: Xopenex

* **J7615** Levalbuterol, inhalation solution, compounded product, administered through DME, unit dose, **0.5 mg** Ⓑ Qp Qh   M

If "incident to" a physician's service, do not bill.

☺ **J7620** Albuterol, **up to 2.5 mg** and ipratropium bromide, **up to 0.5 mg**, FDA-approved final product, non-compounded, administered through DME Ⓑ   M

If "incident to" a physician's service, do not bill.

NDC: DuoNeb

* **J7622** Beclomethasone, inhalation solution, compounded product, administered through DME, unit dose form, **per milligram** Ⓑ Qp Qh   M

If "incident to" a physician's service, do not bill.

* **J7624** Betamethasone, inhalation solution, compounded product, administered through DME, unit dose form, **per mg** Ⓑ Qp Qh   M

If "incident to" a physician's service, do not bill.

Other: Celestone Soluspan

▶ **New**   ↻ **Revised**   ✔ **Reinstated**   ~~deleted~~ **Deleted**   ⊘ **Not covered or valid by Medicare**
☺ **Special coverage instructions**   * **Carrier discretion**   Ⓑ **Bill local carrier**   Ⓑ **Bill DME MAC**

✳ **J7626** Budesonide inhalation solution, FDA-approved final product, non-compounded, administered through DME, unit dose form, **up to 0.5 mg** Ⓑ   M

If "incident to" a physician's service, do not bill.

NDC: Pulmicort

✳ **J7627** Budesonide, inhalation solution, compounded product, administered through DME, unit dose form, **up to 0.5 mg** Ⓑ 𝐐𝐩 𝐐𝐡   M

If "incident to" a physician's service, do not bill.

Other: Pulmicort Respulses

◎ **J7628** Bitolterol mesylate, inhalation solution, compounded product, administered through DME, concentrated form, **per milligram** Ⓑ 𝐐𝐩 𝐐𝐡   M

If "incident to" a physician's service, do not bill.

Other: Tornalate

◎ **J7629** Bitolterol mesylate, inhalation solution, compounded product, administered through DME, unit dose form, **per milligram** Ⓑ 𝐐𝐩 𝐐𝐡   M

If "incident to" a physician's service, do not bill.

Other: Tornalate

◎ **J7631** Cromolyn sodium, inhalation solution, FDA-approved final product, non-compounded, administered through DME, unit dose form, **per 10 milligrams** Ⓑ   M

If "incident to" a physician's service, do not bill.

Other: Intal

✳ **J7632** Cromolyn sodium, inhalation solution, compounded product, administered through DME, unit dose form, **per 10 milligrams** Ⓑ 𝐐𝐩 𝐐𝐡   M

If "incident to" a physician's service, do not bill.

Other: Intal

✳ **J7633** Budesonide, inhalation solution, FDA-approved final product, non-compounded, administered through DME, concentrated form, **per 0.25 milligram** Ⓑ   M

If "incident to" a physician's service, do not bill.

Other: Pulmicort Respules

✳ **J7634** Budesonide, inhalation solution, compounded product, administered through DME, concentrated form, **per 0.25 milligram** Ⓑ 𝐐𝐩 𝐐𝐡   M

If "incident to" a physician's service, do not bill.

◎ **J7635** Atropine, inhalation solution, compounded product, administered through DME, concentrated form, **per milligram** Ⓑ 𝐐𝐩 𝐐𝐡   M

If "incident to" a physician's service, do not bill.

◎ **J7636** Atropine, inhalation solution, compounded product, administered through DME, unit dose form, **per milligram** Ⓑ 𝐐𝐩 𝐐𝐡   M

If "incident to" a physician's service, do not bill.

◎ **J7637** Dexamethasone, inhalation solution, compounded product, administered through DME, concentrated form, **per milligram** Ⓑ 𝐐𝐩 𝐐𝐡   M

If "incident to" a physician's service, do not bill.

◎ **J7638** Dexamethasone, inhalation solution, compounded product, administered through DME, unit dose form, **per milligram** Ⓑ 𝐐𝐩 𝐐𝐡   M

If "incident to" a physician's service, do not bill.

◎ **J7639** Dornase alfa, inhalation solution, FDA-approved final product, non-compounded, administered through DME, unit dose form, **per milligram** Ⓑ   M

If "incident to" a physician's service, do not bill.

NDC: Pulmozyme

✳ **J7640** Formoterol, inhalation solution, compounded product, administered through DME, unit dose form, **12 micrograms** Ⓑ 𝐐𝐩 𝐐𝐡   E

If "incident to" a physician's service, do not bill.

✳ **J7641** Flunisolide, inhalation solution, compounded product, administered through DME, unit dose, **per milligram** Ⓑ 𝐐𝐩 𝐐𝐡   M

If "incident to" a physician's service, do not bill.

℗ᵩ PQRS	𝐐𝐩 Quantity Physician Appendix A	𝐐𝐡 Quantity Hospital Appendix B	♀ Female only
♂ Male only	🅰 Age	♿ DMEPOS	A2-Z3 ASC Payment Indicator A-Y ASC Status Indicator Coding Clinic

⚙ **J7642** Glycopyrrolate, inhalation solution, compounded product, administered through DME, concentrated form, **per milligram** Ⓑ Qp Qh M

If "incident to" a physician's service, do not bill.

⚙ **J7643** Glycopyrrolate, inhalation solution, compounded product, administered through DME, unit dose form, **per milligram** Ⓑ Qp Qh M

If "incident to" a physician's service, do not bill.

Other: Robinul

⚙ **J7644** Ipratropium bromide, inhalation solution, FDA-approved final product, non-compounded, administered through DME, unit dose form, **per milligram** Ⓑ M

If "incident to" a physician's service, do not bill.

Other: Atrovent

✳ **J7645** Ipratropium bromide, inhalation solution, compounded product, administered through DME, unit dose form, **per milligram** Ⓑ Qp Qh M

If "incident to" a physician's service, do not bill.

Other: Atrovent

✳ **J7647** Isoetharine HCL, inhalation solution, compounded product, administered through DME, concentrated form, **per milligram** Ⓑ Qp Qh M

If "incident to" a physician's service, do not bill.

Other: Bronkosol

⚙ **J7648** Isoetharine HCL, inhalation solution, FDA-approved final product, non-compounded, administered through DME, concentrated form, **per milligram** Ⓑ M

If "incident to" a physician's service, do not bill.

Other: Bronkosol

⚙ **J7649** Isoetharine HCL, inhalation solution, FDA-approved final product, non-compounded, administered through DME, unit dose form, **per milligram** Ⓑ M

If "incident to" a physician's service, do not bill.

Other: Bronkosol

✳ **J7650** Isoetharine HCL, inhalation solution, compounded product, administered through DME, unit dose form, **per milligram** Ⓑ Qp Qh M

If "incident to" a physician's service, do not bill.

Other: Bronkosol

✳ **J7657** Isoproterenol HCL, inhalation solution, compounded product, administered through DME, concentrated form, **per milligram** Ⓑ Qp Qh M

If "incident to" a physician's service, do not bill.

Other: Isuprel

⚙ **J7658** Isoproterenol HCL inhalation solution, FDA-approved final product, non-compounded, administered through DME, concentrated form, **per milligram** Ⓑ M

If "incident to" a physician's service, do not bill.

Other: Isuprel

⚙ **J7659** Isoproterenol HCL, inhalation solution, FDA-approved final product, non-compounded, administered through DME, unit dose form, **per milligram** Ⓑ M

If "incident to" a physician's service, do not bill.

Other: Isuprel

✳ **J7660** Isoproterenol HCL, inhalation solution, compounded product, administered through DME, unit dose form, **per milligram** Ⓑ Qp Qh M

If "incident to" a physician's service, do not bill.

Other: Isuprel

✳ **J7665** Mannitol, administered through an inhaler, **5 mg** Ⓑ Qp Qh N1 N

If "incident to" a physician's service, do not bill.

NDC: Aridol

✳ **J7667** Metaproterenol sulfate, inhalation solution, compounded product, concentrated form, **per 10 milligrams** Ⓑ Qp Qh M

If "incident to" a physician's service, do not bill.

Other: Alupent, Metaprel

▶ New   ⟳ Revised   ✔ Reinstated   ~~deleted~~ Deleted   ⊘ Not covered or valid by Medicare
⚙ Special coverage instructions   ✳ Carrier discretion   Ⓑ Bill local carrier   Ⓓ Bill DME MAC

◌ **J7668** Metaproterenol sulfate, inhalation solution, FDA-approved final product, non-compounded, administered through DME, concentrated form, **per 10 milligrams** ⑱ M

If "incident to" a physician's service, do not bill.

Other: Alupent, Metaprel

◌ **J7669** Metaproterenol sulfate, inhalation solution, FDA-approved final product, non-compounded, administered through DME, unit dose form, **per 10 milligrams** ⑱ M

If "incident to" a physician's service, do not bill.

Other: Alupent, Metaprel

✳ **J7670** Metaproterenol sulfate, inhalation solution, compounded product, administered through DME, unit dose form, **per 10 milligrams** ⑱ **Qp Qh** M

If "incident to" a physician's service, do not bill.

Other: Alupent, Metaprel

✳ **J7674** Methacholine chloride administered as inhalation solution through a nebulizer, **per 1 mg** ⑱ N1 N

If "incident to" a physician's service, do not bill.

NDC: Provocholine

✳ **J7676** Pentamidine isethionate, inhalation solution, compounded product, administered through DME, unit dose form, **per 300 mg** ⑱ **Qp Qh** M

If "incident to" a physician's service, do not bill.

Other: NebuPent, Pentam

◌ **J7680** Terbutaline sulfate, inhalation solution, compounded product, administered through DME, concentrated form, **per milligram** ⑱ **Qp Qh** M

If "incident to" a physician's service, do not bill.

Other: Brethine

◌ **J7681** Terbutaline sulfate, inhalation solution, compounded product, administered through DME, unit dose form, **per milligram** ⑱ **Qp Qh** M

If "incident to" a physician's service, do not bill.

Other: Brethine

◌ **J7682** Tobramycin, inhalation solution, FDA-approved final product, non-compounded unit dose form, administered through DME, **per 300 milligrams** ⑱ M

If "incident to" a physician's service, do not bill.

NDC: Bethkis, Tobi

Other: Nebcin

◌ **J7683** Triamcinolone, inhalation solution, compounded product, administered through DME, concentrated form, **per milligram** ⑱ **Qp Qh** M

If "incident to" a physician's service, do not bill.

◌ **J7684** Triamcinolone, inhalation solution, compounded product, administered through DME, unit dose form, **per milligram** ⑱ **Qp Qh** M

If "incident to" a physician's service, do not bill.

Other: Triamcinolone acetonide

✳ **J7685** Tobramycin, inhalation solution, compounded product, administered through DME, unit dose form, **per 300 milligrams** ⑱ **Qp Qh** M

If "incident to" a physician's service, do not bill.

✳ **J7686** Treprostinil, inhalation solution, FDA-approved final product, non-compounded, administered through DME, unit dose form, **1.74 mg** ⑱ M

If "incident to" a physician's service, do not bill.

NDC: Tyvaso

◌ **J7699** NOC drugs, inhalation solution administered through DME ⑱ M

If "incident to" a physician's service, do not bill.

Other: Gentamicin Sulfate, Sodium chloride

◌ **J7799** NOC drugs, other than inhalation drugs, administered through DME ⑱ N1 N

If "incident to" a physician's service, do not bill.

Bill on paper. Bill one unit and identify drug and total dosage in the "Remark" field.

Other: Epinephrine, Mannitol, Osmitrol, Phenylephrine, Resectisol, Sodium chloride

IOM: 100-02, 15, 110.3

PQRS | **Qp** Quantity Physician Appendix A | **Qh** Quantity Hospital Appendix B | ♀ **Female only** | ♂ **Male only** | **A** Age | 🦽 **DMEPOS** | A2-Z3 **ASC Payment Indicator** | A-Y **ASC Status Indicator** | Coding Clinic

DRUGS OTHER THAN CHEMOTHERAPY J7668 — J7799

279

Other

⊛ **J8498** Antiemetic drug, rectal/suppository, not otherwise specified ⓑ   B

Other: Compazine, Compro, Phenadoz, Phenergan, Prochlorperazine, Promethazine, Promethegan, Thorazine

Medicare Statute 1861(s)2t

⊘ **J8499** Prescription drug, oral, non chemotherapeutic, NOS ⓑ   E

If "incident to" a physician's service, do not bill.

Other: Acyclovir, Zovirax

IOM: 100-02, 15, 50

Coding Clinic: 2013, Q2, P4

⊛ **J8501** Aprepitant, oral, **5 mg** ⓑ   K2 K

NDC: Emend

⊛ **J8510** Busulfan; oral, **2 mg** ⓑ   N1 N

NDC: Myleran

IOM 100-02, 15, 50; 100-04, 4, 240; 100-04, 17, 80.1.1

⊘ **J8515** Cabergoline, oral, **0.25 mg** ⓑ   E

IOM: 100-02, 15, 50; 100-04, 4, 240

⊛ **J8520** Capecitabine, oral, **150 mg** ⓑ   K2 K

NDC: Xeloda

IOM: 100-02, 15, 50; 100-04, 4, 240; 100-04, 17, 80.1.1

⊛ **J8521** Capecitabine, oral, **500 mg** ⓑ   K2 K

NDC: Xeloda

IOM: 100-02, 15, 50; 100-04, 4, 240; 100-04, 17, 80.1.1

⊛ **J8530** Cyclophosphamide; oral, **25 mg** ⓑ   N1 N

Other: Cytoxan

IOM: 100-02, 15, 50; 100-04, 4, 240; 100-04, 17, 80.1.1

⊛ **J8540** Dexamethasone, oral, **0.25** ⓑ   N1 N

Other: Decadron, Dexone, Dexpak

Medicare Statute 1861(s)2t

⊛ **J8560** Etoposide; oral, **50 mg** ⓑ   K2 K

NDC: VePesid

IOM: 100-02, 15, 50; 100-04, 4, 230.1; 100-04, 4, 240; 100-04, 17, 80.1.1

✳ **J8562** Fludarabine phosphate, oral, **10 mg** ⓑ   E

Other: Oforta

Coding Clinic: 2011, Q1, P9

↻⊛ **J8565** Gefitinib, oral, **250 mg** ⓑ   E

Other: Iressa

⊛ **J8597** Antiemetic drug, oral, not otherwise specified ⓑ   N1 N

Medicare Statute 1861(s)2t

⊛ **J8600** Melphalan; oral, **2 mg** ⓑ   N1 N

NDC: Alkeran

IOM: 100-02, 15, 50; 100-04, 4, 240; 100-04, 17, 80.1.1

⊛ **J8610** Methotrexate; oral, **2.5 mg** ⓑ   N1 N

NDC: Rheumatrex, Trexall

IOM: 100-02, 15, 50; 100-04, 4, 240; 100-04, 17, 80.1.1

✳ **J8650** Nabilone, oral, **1 mg** ⓑ   K2 K

⊛ **J8700** Temozolomide, oral, **5 mg** ⓑ   K2 K

NDC: Temodar

IOM: 100-02, 15, 50; 100-04, 4, 240

✳ **J8705** Topotecan, oral, **0.25 mg** ⓑ   K2 K

Treatment for ovarian and lung cancers, etc. Report J9350 (Topotecan, 4 mg) for intravenous version

⊛ **J8999** Prescription drug, oral, chemotherapeutic, NOS ⓑ   B

Other: Arimidex, Aromasin, Droxia, Flutamide, Hydrea, Hydroxyurea, Leukeran, Malulane, Megace, Megestrol Acetate, Mercaptopurine, Nolvadex, Purinethol, Tamoxifen Citrate

IOM: 100-02, 15, 50; 100-04, 4, 250; 100-04, 17, 80.1.1; 100-04, 17, 80.1.2

CHEMOTHERAPY DRUGS (J9000-J9999)

NOTE: These codes cover the cost of the chemotherapy drug only, not to include the administration

J9000-J9999: Bill local carrier (ⓑ) if incident to a physician's service or used in an implanted infusion pump. If other, bill DME MAC (ⓑ).

⊛ **J9000** Injection, doxorubicin hydrochloride, **10 mg** ⓑ ⓑ   N1 N

NDC: Adriamycin

Other: Rubex

IOM: 100-02, 15, 50

Coding Clinic: 2007, Q4, P5

↻⊘ **J9010** Injection, alemtuzumab, **10 mg** ⓑ ⓑ   E

⊛ **J9015** Injection, aldesleukin, **per single use vial** ⓑ ⓑ   K2 K

NDC: Proleukin

IOM: 100-02, 15, 50

▶ **New**   ↻ **Revised**   ✔ **Reinstated**   ~~deleted~~ **Deleted**   ⊘ **Not covered or valid by Medicare**

⊛ **Special coverage instructions**   ✳ **Carrier discretion**   ⓑ **Bill local carrier**   ⓑ **Bill DME MAC**

✴ **J9017** Injection, arsenic trioxide,
1 mg Ⓑ Ⓑ   K2   K

NDC: Trisenox

✪ **J9019** Injection, asparaginase (Erwinaze),
1,000 iu Ⓑ Ⓑ **Qp** **Qh**   K2   K

IOM 100-02, 15, 50

✪ **J9020** Injection, asparaginase, not otherwise
specified **10,000 units** Ⓑ Ⓑ   K2   K

NDC: Elspar

IOM: 100-02, 15, 50

✴ **J9025** Injection, azacitidine, **1 mg** Ⓑ Ⓑ   K2   K

NDC: Vidaza

✴ **J9027** Injection, clofarabine, **1 mg** Ⓑ Ⓑ   K2   K

NDC: Clolar

✪ **J9031** BCG (intravesical), **per
instillation** Ⓑ Ⓑ   K2   K

NDC: TheraCys, Tice BCG

IOM: 100-02, 15, 50

✴ **J9033** Injection, bendamustine HCL,
1 mg Ⓑ Ⓑ   K2   K

Treatment for form of non-Hodgkin's
lymphoma; standard administration
time is as an intravenous infusion over
30 minutes

NDC: Treanda

✴ **J9035** Injection, bevacizumab,
10 mg Ⓟ Ⓑ   K2   K

For malignant neoplasm of breast,
considered J9207.

NDC: Avastin

Coding Clinic: 2013, Q3, P9, Q2, P8

✪ **J9040** Injection, bleomycin sulfate,
15 units Ⓑ Ⓑ   N1   N

Other: Blenoxane

IOM: 100-02, 15, 50

✴ **J9041** Injection, bortezomib,
0.1 mg Ⓑ Ⓑ   K2   K

NDC: Velcade

✴ **J9042** Injection, brentuximab vedotin,
1 mg Ⓟ Ⓑ **Qp** **Qh**   K2   K

NDC: Adcetris

✴ **J9043** Injection, cabazitaxel, **1 mg** Ⓑ Ⓑ   K2   K

NDC: Jertana

Coding Clinic: 2012, Q1, P9

✪ **J9045** Injection, carboplatin,
50 mg Ⓑ Ⓑ   N1   N

Other: Paraplatin

IOM: 100-02, 15, 50

✴ **J9047** Injection, carfilzomib,
1 mg Ⓑ Ⓑ **Qp** **Qh**   K2   G

NDC: Kyprolis

✪ **J9050** Injection, carmustine,
100 mg Ⓑ Ⓑ   K2   K

NDC: BiCNU

IOM: 100-02, 15, 50

✴ **J9055** Injection, cetuximab,
10 mg Ⓑ Ⓑ   K2   K

NDC: Erbitux

✪ **J9060** Injection, cisplatin, powder or solution,
10 mg Ⓑ Ⓑ   N1   N

Other: Plantinol AQ

IOM: 100-02, 15, 50

Coding Clinic: 2013, Q2, P6; 2011, Q1, P8

✪ **J9065** Injection, cladribine, **per
1 mg** Ⓑ Ⓑ   K2   K

NDC: Leustatin

IOM: 100-02, 15, 50

✪ **J9070** Cyclophosphamide,
100 mg Ⓑ Ⓑ   K2   K

Other: Cytoxan, Neosar

IOM: 100-02, 15, 50

Coding Clinic: 2011, Q1, P8-9

✴ **J9098** Injection, cytarabine liposome,
10 mg Ⓑ Ⓑ   K2   K

NDC: DepoCyt

⊘ **J9100** Injection, cytarabine,
100 mg Ⓑ Ⓑ   N1   N

Other: Cytosar-U

IOM: 100-02, 15, 50

Coding Clinic: 2011, Q1, P9

✪ **J9120** Injection, dactinomycin,
0.5 mg Ⓑ Ⓑ   K2   K

NDC: Cosmegen

IOM: 100-02, 15, 50

✪ **J9130** Dacarbazine, **100 mg** Ⓑ Ⓑ   N1   N

Other: DTIC-Dome

IOM: 100-02, 15, 50

Coding Clinic: 2011, Q1, P9

✪ **J9150** Injection, daunorubicin,
10 mg Ⓑ Ⓑ   K2   K

NDC: Cerubidine

IOM: 100-02, 15, 50

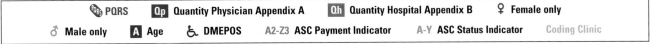

⊛ **J9151** Injection, daunorubicin
citrate, liposomal formulation,
10 mg ⑧ ⑧   K2 K

Other: Daunoxome

IOM: 100-02, 15, 50

✳ **J9155** Injection, degarelix, **1 mg** ⑧ ⑧   K2 K

Report 1 unit for every 1 mg.

NDC: Firmagon

↻✳ **J9160** Injection, denileukin diftitox,
300 micrograms ⑧ ⑧   E

⊛ **J9165** Injection, diethylstilbestrol
diphosphate, **250 mg** ⑧ ⑧   E

Other: Stilphostrol

IOM: 100-02, 15, 50

⊛ **J9171** Injection, docetaxel,
1 mg ⑧ ⑧   K2 K

Report 1 unit for every 1 mg.

NDC: Docefrez, Taxotere

IOM: 100-02, 15, 50

Coding Clinic: 2012, Q1, P9

⊛ **J9175** Injection, Elliott's B solution,
1 ml ⑧ ⑧   N1 N

Other: Elliott's B

IOM: 100-02, 15, 50

✳ **J9178** Injection, epirubicin HCL,
2 mg ⑧ ⑧   N1 N

NDC: Ellence

✳ **J9179** Injection, eribulin mesylate,
0.1 mg ⑧ ⑧ **Qp** **Qh**   K2 K

NDC: Halaven

⊛ **J9181** Injection, etoposide, **10 mg** ⑧ ⑧   N1 N

NDC: Etopophos, Toposar, VePesid

⊛ **J9185** Injection, fludarabine phosphate,
50 mg ⑧ ⑧   K2 K

NDC: Fludara

IOM: 100-02, 15, 50

⊛ **J9190** Injection, fluorouracil,
500 mg ⑧ ⑧   N1 N

NDC: Adrucil

IOM: 100-02, 15, 50

⊛ **J9200** Injection, floxuridine,
500 mg ⑧ ⑧   K2 K

Other: FUDR

IOM: 100-02, 15, 50

⊛ **J9201** Injection, gemcitabine hydrochloride,
200 mg ⑧ ⑧   N1 N

NDC: Gemzar

IOM: 100-02, 15, 50

⊛ **J9202** Goserelin acetate implant, **per
3.6 mg** ⑧ ⑧   K2 K

NDC: Zoladex

IOM: 100-02, 15, 50

⊛ **J9206** Injection, irinotecan,
20 mg ⑧ ⑧   N1 N

NDC: Camptosar

IOM: 100-02, 15, 50

✳ **J9207** Injection, ixabepilone,
1 mg ⑧ ⑧   K2 K

⊛ **J9208** Injection, ifosfamide, **1
gm** ⑧ ⑧   K2 K

NDC: Ifex

IOM: 100-02, 15, 50

⊛ **J9209** Injection, mesna, **200 mg** ⑧ ⑧   N1 N

NDC: Mesnex

IOM: 100-02, 15, 50

⊛ **J9211** Injection, idarubicin hydrochloride,
5 mg ⑧ ⑧   K2 K

NDC: Idamycin PFS

IOM: 100-02, 15, 50

⊛ **J9212** Injection, interferon alfacon-1,
recombinant, **1 mcg** ⑧ ⑧   E

Other: Infergen

IOM: 100-02, 15, 50

⊛ **J9213** Injection, interferon, alfa-2a,
recombinant, **3 million
units** ⑧ ⑧   K2 K

IOM: 100-02, 15, 50

⊛ **J9214** Injection, interferon, alfa-2b,
recombinant, **1 million
units** ⑧ ⑧   K2 K

NDC: Intron-A

IOM: 100-02, 15, 50

↻⊛ **J9215** Injection, interferon, alfa-n3
(human leukocyte derived), **250,000
IU** ⑧ ⑧   N1 N

Other: Alferon N

IOM: 100-02, 15, 50

⊛ **J9216** Injection, interferon, gamma-1B,
3 million units ⑧ ⑧   K2 K

Other: Actimmune

IOM: 100-02, 15, 50

⊛ **J9217** Leuprolide acetate (for depot
suspension), **7.5 mg** ⑧ ⑧   K2 K

NDC: Eligard, Lupron Depot

IOM: 100-02, 15, 50

▶ **New**   ↻ **Revised**   ✔ **Reinstated**   ~~deleted~~ **Deleted**   ⊘ **Not covered or valid by Medicare**

⊛ **Special coverage instructions**   ✳ **Carrier discretion**   ⑧ **Bill local carrier**   ⑧ **Bill DME MAC**

↻ ✲ **J9218** Leuprolide acetate, **per 1 mg** ⒷⒷ N1 N

Other: Lupron

IOM: 100-02, 15, 50

↻ ✲ **J9219** Leuprolide acetate implant, **65 mg** ⒷⒷ E

Other: Viadur

IOM: 100-02, 15, 50

✲ **J9225** Histrelin implant (Vantas), **50 mg** ⒷⒷ K2 K

IOM: 100-02, 15, 50

✲ **J9226** Histrelin implant (Supprelin LA), **50 mg** ⒷⒷ K2 K

Other: Vantas

IOM: 100-02, 15, 50

✳ **J9228** Injection, ipilimumab, **1 mg** ⒷⒸ Qp Qh K2 K

NDC: Yervoy

Coding Clinic: 2012, Q1, P9

✲ **J9230** Injection, mechlorethamine hydrochloride, (nitrogen mustard), **10 mg** ⒷⒷ K2 K

NDC: Mustargen

IOM: 100-02, 15, 50

✲ **J9245** Injection, melphalan hydrochloride, **50 mg** ⒷⒷ K2 K

NDC: Alkeran

IOM: 100-02, 15, 50

✲ **J9250** Methotrexate sodium, **5 mg** ⒷⒷ N1 N

Other: Folex

IOM: 100-02, 15, 50

✲ **J9260** Methotrexate sodium, **50 mg** ⒷⒷ N1 N

Other: Folex

IOM: 100-02, 15, 50

✳ **J9261** Injection, nelarabine, **50 mg** ⒸⒷ K2 K

NDC: Arranon

✳ **J9262** Injection, omacetaxine mepesuccinate, **0.01 mg** ⒷⒸ Qp Qh K2 G

✳ **J9263** Injection, oxaliplatin, **0.5 mg** ⒸⒷ K2 K

Eloxatin, platinum-based anticancer drug that destroys cancer cells

NDC: Eloxatin

Coding Clinic: 2009, Q1, P10

✳ **J9264** Injection, paclitaxel protein-bound particles, **1 mg** ⒷⒷ K2 K

NDC: Abraxane

~~J9265   Injection, paclitaxel, 30 mg~~ ✖

✲ **J9266** Injection, pegaspargase, **per single dose vial** ⒷⒸ K2 K

NDC: Oncaspar

IOM: 100-02, 15, 50

▶ ✲ **J9267** Injection, paclitaxel, **1 mg** N1 N

✲ **J9268** Injection, pentostatin, **10 mg** ⒸⒷ K2 K

NDC: Nipent

IOM: 100-02, 15, 50

✲ **J9270** Injection, plicamycin, **2.5 mg** ⒷⒷ N1 N

Other: Mithracin

IOM: 100-02, 15, 50

✲ **J9280** Injection, mitomycin, **5 mg** ⒸⒷ K2 K

NDC: Mutamycin

IOM: 100-02, 15, 50

Coding Clinic: 2014, Q2, P6; 2011, Q1, P9

✲ **J9293** Injection, mitoxantrone hydrochloride, **per 5 mg** ⒷⒸ K2 K

Other: Novantrone

IOM: 100-02, 15, 50

↻ ✳ **J9300** Injection, gemtuzumab ozogamicin, **5 mg** ⒸⒷ E

Other: Mylotarg

▶ ✳ **J9301** Injection, obinutuzumab, **10 mg** K2 G

✳ **J9302** Injection, ofatumumab, **10 mg** ⒸⒷ K2 K

NDC: Arzerra

Coding Clinic: 2011, Q1, P7

✳ **J9303** Injection, panitumumab, **10 mg** ⒸⒷ K2 K

Other: Vectibix

✳ **J9305** Injection, pemetrexed, **10 mg** ⒷⒷ K2 K

NDC: Alimta

✳ **J9306** Injection, pertuzumab, **1 mg** ⒷⒸ Qp Qh K2 K

NDC: Perjeta

✳ **J9307** Injection, pralatrexate, **1 mg** ⒷⒸ K2 K

NDC: Folotyn

Coding Clinic: 2011, Q1, P7

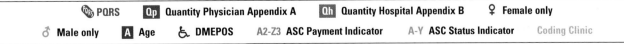

| ⒫ᵠᴿˢ PQRS | Qp Quantity Physician Appendix A | Qh Quantity Hospital Appendix B | ♀ Female only |
| ♂ Male only | Ⓐ Age | ♿ DMEPOS | A2-Z3 ASC Payment Indicator | A-Y ASC Status Indicator | Coding Clinic |

CHEMOTHERAPY DRUGS   J9218 — J9307

283

⚙ **J9310** Injection, rituximab,
100 mg ⒷⒷ   K2 K

NDC: RituXan

IOM: 100-02, 15, 50

Coding Clinic: 2013, Q3, P9

✳ **J9315** Injection, romidepsin,
1 mg ⒷⒷ   K2 K

NDC: Istodax

Coding Clinic: 2011, Q1, P7

⚙ **J9320** Injection, streptozocin,
1 gram ⒷⒷ   K2 K

NDC: Zanosar

IOM: 100-02, 15, 50

✳ **J9328** Injection, temozolomide,
1 mg ⒷⒷ   K2 K

Intravenous formulation, not for oral administration

NDC: Temodar

✳ **J9330** Injection, temsirolimus,
1 mg ⒷⒷ   K2 K

Treatment for advanced renal cell carcinoma; standard administration is intravenous infusion greater than 30-60 minutes

Other: Torisel

⚙ **J9340** Injection, thiotepa,
15 mg ⒷⒷ   K2 K

Other: Thiethylenethiophosphoramide/T

IOM: 100-02, 15, 50

✳ **J9351** Injection, topotecan,
0.1 mg ⒷⒷ   K2 K

NDC: Hycamtin

Coding Clinic: 2011, Q1, P9

✳ **J9354** Injection, ado-trastuzumab emtansine,
1 mg ⒷⒷ Qp Qh   K2 G

NDC: Kadcyla

✳ **J9355** Injection, trastuzumab,
10 mg ⒷⒷ Qp Qh   K2 K

NDC: Herceptin

⚙ **J9357** Injection, valrubicin, intravesical,
200 mg ⒷⒷ   K2 K

NDC: Valstar

IOM: 100-02, 15, 50

⚙ **J9360** Injection, vinblastine sulfate,
1 mg ⒷⒷ   N1 N

Other: Alkaban-AQ, Velban, Velsar

IOM: 100-02, 15, 50

⚙ **J9370** Vincristine sulfate, **1 mg** ⒷⒷ   N1 N

Other: Oncovin, Vincasar PFS

IOM: 100-02, 15, 50

Coding Clinic: 2011, Q1, P9

✳ **J9371** Injection, vincristine sulfate liposome,
1 mg ⒷⒷ   K2 G

↻⚙ **J9390** Injection, vinorelbine tartrate,
10 mg ⒷⒷ   N1 N

NDC: Navelbine

IOM: 100-02, 15, 50

✳ **J9395** Injection, fulvestrant,
25 mg ⒷⒷ   K2 K

NDC: Faslodex

✳ **J9400** Injection, ziv-aflibercept,
1 mg ⒷⒷ Qp Qh   K2 G

NDC: Zaltrap

⚙ **J9600** Injection, porfimer sodium,
75 mg ⒷⒷ   K2 K

Other: Photofrin

IOM: 100-02, 15, 50

⚙ **J9999** Not otherwise classified, antineoplastic drugs ⒷⒷ   N1 N

Bill on paper, bill one unit, and identify drug and total dosage in "Remarks" field. Include invoice of cost or NDC number in "Remarks" field.

Other: Allopurinol Sodium, Ifosfamide/ Mesna

IOM: 100-02, 15, 50; 100-03, 2, 110.2

Coding Clinic: 2013, Q2, P3

▶ **New**   ↻ **Revised**   ✔ **Reinstated**   ~~deleted~~ **Deleted**   ⊘ **Not covered or valid by Medicare**

⚙ **Special coverage instructions**   ✳ **Carrier discretion**   Ⓑ **Bill local carrier**   Ⓑ **Bill DME MAC**

TEMPORARY CODES ASSIGNED TO DME REGIONAL CARRIERS (K0000-K9999)

Wheelchairs and Accessories

NOTE: This section contains national codes assigned by CMS on a temporary basis and for the exclusive use of the durable medical equipment regional carriers (DMERC).

⁂ **K0001** Standard wheelchair ⑧ Qp Qh ♿   Y

Capped rental

DMEPOS Modifier(s): RR

⁂ **K0002** Standard hemi (low seat) wheelchair ⑧ Qp Qh ♿   Y

Capped rental

DMEPOS Modifier(s): RR

⁂ **K0003** Lightweight wheelchair ⑧ Qp Qh ♿   Y

Capped rental

DMEPOS Modifier(s): RR

⁂ **K0004** High strength, lightweight wheelchair ⑧ Qp Qh ♿   Y

Capped rental

DMEPOS Modifier(s): RR

⁂ **K0005** Ultralightweight wheelchair ⑧ Qp Qh ♿   Y

Capped rental. Inexpensive and routinely purchased DME

DMEPOS Modifier(s): NU, RR, UE

⁂ **K0006** Heavy duty wheelchair ⑧ Qp Qh ♿   Y

Capped rental

DMEPOS Modifier(s): RR

⁂ **K0007** Extra heavy duty wheelchair ⑧ Qp Qh ♿   Y

Capped rental

DMEPOS Modifier(s): RR

⊙ **K0008** Custom manual wheelchair/ base Qh   Y

⁂ **K0009** Other manual wheelchair/ base Qp Qh ♿   Y

Not Otherwise Classified.

DMEPOS Modifier(s): RR

⁂ **K0010** Standard - weight frame motorized/ power wheelchair ♿   Y

Capped rental. Codes K0010-K0014 are not for manual wheelchairs with add-on power packs. Use the appropriate code for the manual wheelchair base provided (K0001-K0009) and code K0460

DMEPOS Modifier(s): RR

⁂ **K0011** Standard - weight frame motorized/power wheelchair with programmable control parameters for speed adjustment, tremor dampening, acceleration control and braking ♿   Y

Capped rental. A patient who requires a power wheelchair usually is totally nonambulatory and has severe weakness of the upper extremities due to a neurologic or muscular disease/ condition

DMEPOS Modifier(s): KF, RR

⁂ **K0012** Lightweight portable motorized/power wheelchair ♿   Y

Capped rental

DMEPOS Modifier(s): RR

⊙ **K0013** Custom motorized/power wheelchair base Qh   Y

⁂ **K0014** Other motorized/power wheelchair base   Y

Capped rental

⁂ **K0015** Detachable, non-adjustable height armrest, each Qp Qh ♿   Y

Inexpensive and routinely purchased DME

DMEPOS Modifier(s): KE, NU, RR, UE

⁂ **K0017** Detachable, adjustable height armrest, base, each Qp Qh ♿   Y

Inexpensive and routinely purchased DME

DMEPOS Modifier(s): KE, NU, RR, UE

⁂ **K0018** Detachable, adjustable height armrest, upper portion, each Qp Qh ♿   Y

Inexpensive and routinely purchased DME

DMEPOS Modifier(s): KE, NU, RR, UE

⁂ **K0019** Arm pad, each Qp Qh ♿   Y

Inexpensive and routinely purchased DME

DMEPOS Modifier(s): KE, NU, RR, UE

⁂ **K0020** Fixed, adjustable height armrest, pair Qp Qh ♿   Y

Inexpensive and routinely purchased DME

DMEPOS Modifier(s): KE, NU, RR, UE

⁂ **K0037** High mount flip-up footrest, each Qp Qh ♿   Y

Inexpensive and routinely purchased DME

DMEPOS Modifier(s): KE, NU, RR, UE

℘ PQRS	Qp Quantity Physician Appendix A	Qh Quantity Hospital Appendix B	♀ Female only
♂ Male only	A Age	♿ DMEPOS	A2-Z3 ASC Payment Indicator A-Y ASC Status Indicator Coding Clinic

✳ **K0038** Leg strap, each **Qp** **Qh** &♿ Y

Inexpensive and routinely purchased DME

DMEPOS Modifier(s): KE, NU, RR, UE

✳ **K0039** Leg strap, H style, each **Qp** **Qh** &♿ Y

Inexpensive and routinely purchased DME

DMEPOS Modifier(s): KE, NU, RR, UE

✳ **K0040** Adjustable angle footplate, each **Qp** **Qh** &♿ Y

Inexpensive and routinely purchased DME

DMEPOS Modifier(s): KE, NU, RR, UE

✳ **K0041** Large size footplate, each **Qp** **Qh** &♿ Y

Inexpensive and routinely purchased DME

DMEPOS Modifier(s): KE, NU, RR, UE

✳ **K0042** Standard size footplate, each **Qp** **Qh** &♿ Y

Inexpensive and routinely purchased DME

DMEPOS Modifier(s): KE, NU, RR, UE

✳ **K0043** Footrest, lower extension tube, each **Qp** **Qh** &♿ Y

Inexpensive and routinely purchased DME

DMEPOS Modifier(s): KE, NU, RR, UE

✳ **K0044** Footrest, upper hanger bracket, each **Qp** **Qh** &♿ Y

Inexpensive and routinely purchased DME

DMEPOS Modifier(s): KE, NU, RR, UE

✳ **K0045** Footrest, complete assembly **Qp** **Qh** &♿ Y

Inexpensive and routinely purchased DME

DMEPOS Modifier(s): KE, NU, RR, UE

✳ **K0046** Elevating legrest, lower extension tube, each **Qp** **Qh** &♿ Y

Inexpensive and routinely purchased DME

DMEPOS Modifier(s): KE, NU, RR, UE

✳ **K0047** Elevating legrest, upper hanger bracket, each **Qp** **Qh** &♿ Y

Inexpensive and routinely purchased DME

DMEPOS Modifier(s): KE, NU, RR, UE

✳ **K0050** Ratchet assembly **Qp** **Qh** &♿ Y

Inexpensive and routinely purchased DME

DMEPOS Modifier(s): KE, NU, RR, UE

✳ **K0051** Cam release assembly, footrest or legrests, each **Qp** **Qh** &♿ Y

Inexpensive and routinely purchased DME

DMEPOS Modifier(s): KE, NU, RR, UE

✳ **K0052** Swing-away, detachable footrests, each **Qp** **Qh** &♿ Y

Inexpensive and routinely purchased DME

DMEPOS Modifier(s): KE, NU, RR, UE

✳ **K0053** Elevating footrests, articulating (telescoping), each **Qp** **Qh** &♿ Y

Inexpensive and routinely purchased DME

DMEPOS Modifier(s): KE, NU, RR, UE

✳ **K0056** Seat height less than 17″ or equal to or greater than 21″ for a high strength, lightweight, or ultralightweight wheelchair **Qp** **Qh** &♿ Y

Inexpensive and routinely purchased DME

DMEPOS Modifier(s): NU, RR, UE

✳ **K0065** Spoke protectors, each **Qp** **Qh** &♿ Y

Inexpensive and routinely purchased DME

DMEPOS Modifier(s): NU, RR, UE

✳ **K0069** Rear wheel assembly, complete, with solid tire, spokes or molded, each **Qp** **Qh** &♿ Y

Inexpensive and routinely purchased DME

DMEPOS Modifier(s): NU, RR, UE

✳ **K0070** Rear wheel assembly, complete, with pneumatic tire, spokes or molded, each **Qp** **Qh** &♿ Y

Inexpensive and routinely purchased DME

DMEPOS Modifier(s): NU, RR, UE

✳ **K0071** Front caster assembly, complete, with pneumatic tire, each **Qp** **Qh** &♿ Y

Caster assembly includes a caster fork (E2396), wheel rim, and tire. Inexpensive and routinely purchased DME

DMEPOS Modifier(s): NU, RR, UE

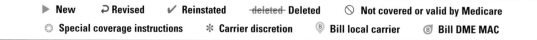

▶ **New**   ↻ **Revised**   ✔ **Reinstated**   ~~deleted~~ **Deleted**   ⊘ **Not covered or valid by Medicare**
Ⓢ **Special coverage instructions**   ✳ **Carrier discretion**   Ⓑ **Bill local carrier**   Ⓑ **Bill DME MAC**

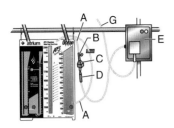

Figure 20 Infusion pump.

✳ **K0072** Front caster assembly, complete, with semi-pneumatic tire, each Qp Qh ♿   Y

Inexpensive and routinely purchased DME

DMEPOS Modifier(s): NU, RR, UE

✳ **K0073** Caster pin lock, each Qp Qh ♿   Y

Inexpensive and routinely purchased DME

DMEPOS Modifier(s): NU, RR, UE

✳ **K0077** Front caster assembly, complete, with solid tire, each Qp Qh ♿   Y

DMEPOS Modifier(s): NU, RR, UE

✳ **K0098** Drive belt for power wheelchair ♿   Y

Inexpensive and routinely purchased DME

DMEPOS Modifier(s): KE, NU, RR, UE

✳ **K0105** IV hanger, each Qp Qh ♿   Y

Inexpensive and routinely purchased DME

DMEPOS Modifier(s): NU, RR, UE

✳ **K0108** Wheelchair component or accessory, not otherwise specified   Y

⊛ **K0195** Elevating leg rests, pair (for use with capped rental wheelchair base) ⑧ Qp Qh ♿   Y

Medically necessary replacement items are covered if rollabout chair or transport chair covered

IOM: 100-03, 4, 280.1

DMEPOS Modifier(s): KE, RR

⊛ **K0455** Infusion pump used for uninterrupted parenteral administration of medication (e.g., epoprostenol or treprostinol) ⑧ Qp Qh ♿   Y

An EIP may also be referred to as an external insulin pump, ambulatory pump, or mini-infuser. CMN/DIF required. Frequent and substantial service DME

IOM: 100-03, 1, 50.3

DMEPOS Modifier(s): RR

⊛ **K0462** Temporary replacement for patient owned equipment being repaired, any type ⑧ Qp Qh   Y

Only report for maintenance and service for an item for which initial claim was paid. The term power mobility device (PMD) includes power operated vehicles (POVs) and power wheelchairs (PWCs). Not Otherwise Classified.

IOM: 100-04, 20, 40.1

⊛ **K0552** Supplies for external drug infusion pump, syringe type cartridge, sterile, each ⑧ Qh ♿   Y

Supplies.

IOM: 100-03, 1, 50.3

✳ **K0601** Replacement battery for external infusion pump owned by patient, silver oxide, 1.5 volt, each ⑧ Qh ♿   Y

Inexpensive and routinely purchased DME

DMEPOS Modifier(s): NU

✳ **K0602** Replacement battery for external infusion pump owned by patient, silver oxide, 3 volt, each ⑧ Qp Qh ♿   Y

Inexpensive and routinely purchased DME

DMEPOS Modifier(s): NU

✳ **K0603** Replacement battery for external infusion pump owned by patient, alkaline, 1.5 volt, each ⑧ Qh ♿   Y

Inexpensive and routinely purchased DME

DMEPOS Modifier(s): NU

✳ **K0604** Replacement battery for external infusion pump owned by patient, lithium, 3.6 volt, each ⑧ Qh ♿   Y

Inexpensive and routinely purchased DME

DMEPOS Modifier(s): NU

✳ **K0605** Replacement battery for external infusion pump owned by patient, lithium, 4.5 volt, each ⑧ Qp Qh ♿   Y

Inexpensive and routinely purchased DME

DMEPOS Modifier(s): NU

✳ **K0606** Automatic external defibrillator, with integrated electrocardiogram analysis, garment type ⑧ Qp Qh ♿   Y

Capped rental

DMEPOS Modifier(s): KE, RR

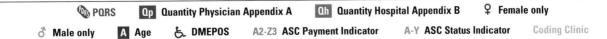

ⓅQRS PQRS	Qp **Quantity Physician Appendix A**	Qh **Quantity Hospital Appendix B**	♀ **Female only**
♂ **Male only**	A **Age**	♿ **DMEPOS**	A2-Z3 **ASC Payment Indicator** A-Y **ASC Status Indicator** Coding Clinic

↻ ✳ **K0607** Replacement battery for automated external defibrillator, garment type only, each Ⓑ Qp Qh ♿   Y

Inexpensive and routinely purchased DME

DMEPOS Modifier(s): RR, KF

✳ **K0608** Replacement garment for use with automated external defibrillator, each Ⓑ Qp Qh ♿   Y

Inexpensive and routinely purchased DME

DMEPOS Modifier(s): KF, NU, RR, UE

✳ **K0609** Replacement electrodes for use with automated external defibrillator, garment type only, each Ⓑ Qp Qh ♿   Y

Supplies.

DMEPOS Modifier(s): KF

✳ **K0669** Wheelchair accessory, wheelchair seat or back cushion, does not meet specific code criteria or no written coding verification from DME PDAC Ⓓ   Y

Inexpensive and routinely purchased DME

✳ **K0672** Addition to lower extremity orthosis, removable soft interface, all components, replacement only, each Ⓑ Qp ♿   A

Prosthetics/Orthotics

↻ ✳ **K0730** Controlled dose inhalation drug delivery system Ⓑ Qp Qh ♿   Y

Inexpensive and routinely purchased DME

DMEPOS Modifier(s): RR

✳ **K0733** Power wheelchair accessory, 12 to 24 amp hour sealed lead acid battery, each (e.g., gel cell, absorbed glassmat) Ⓑ Qp Qh ♿   Y

Inexpensive and routinely purchased DME

DMEPOS Modifier(s): KF, NU, RR, UE

✳ **K0738** Portable gaseous oxygen system, rental; home compressor used to fill portable oxygen cylinders; includes portable containers, regulator, flowmeter, humidifier, cannula or mask, and tubing Ⓑ Qp Qh ♿   Y

Oxygen and oxygen equipment

DMEPOS Modifier(s): RR

✳ **K0739** Repair or nonroutine service for durable medical equipment other than oxygen equipment requiring the skill of a technician, labor component, per 15 minutes Ⓑ   Y

Local carrier (Ⓑ) if used with implanted DME.

⊘ **K0740** Repair or nonroutine service for oxygen equipment requiring the skill of a technician, labor component, per 15 minutes Ⓑ   E

✳ **K0743** Suction pump, home model, portable, for use on wounds Ⓑ Qp Qh   Y

✳ **K0744** Absorptive wound dressing for use with suction pump, home model, portable, pad size 16 square inches or less Ⓑ Qp   A

✳ **K0745** Absorptive wound dressing for use with suction pump, home model, portable, pad size more than 16 square inches but less than or equal to 48 square inches Ⓑ Qp   A

✳ **K0746** Absorptive wound dressing for use with suction pump, home model, portable, pad size greater than 48 square inches Ⓑ Qp   A

✳ **K0800** Power operated vehicle, group 1 standard, patient weight capacity up to and including 300 pounds Ⓑ Qp Qh ♿   Y

Power mobility device (PMD) includes power operated vehicles (POVs) and power wheelchairs (PWCs). Inexpensive and routinely purchased DME

DMEPOS Modifier(s): NU, RR, UE

✳ **K0801** Power operated vehicle, group 1 heavy duty, patient weight capacity 301 to 450 pounds Ⓑ Qp Qh ♿   Y

Inexpensive and routinely purchased DME

DMEPOS Modifier(s): NU, RR, UE

✳ **K0802** Power operated vehicle, group 1 very heavy duty, patient weight capacity 451 to 600 pounds Ⓑ Qp Qh ♿   Y

Inexpensive and routinely purchased DME

DMEPOS Modifier(s): NU, RR, UE

✳ **K0806** Power operated vehicle, group 2 standard, patient weight capacity up to and including 300 pounds Ⓑ Qp Qh ♿   Y

Inexpensive and routinely purchased DME

DMEPOS Modifier(s): NU, RR, UE

▶ **New**   ↻ **Revised**   ✔ **Reinstated**   ~~deleted~~ **Deleted**   ⊘ **Not covered or valid by Medicare**
⊘ **Special coverage instructions**   ✳ **Carrier discretion**   Ⓑ **Bill local carrier**   Ⓑ **Bill DME MAC**

＊ **K0807** Power operated vehicle, group 2 heavy duty, patient weight capacity 301 to 450 pounds ⑧ **Qp** **Qh** ᕻ   Y

Inexpensive and routinely purchased DME

DMEPOS Modifier(s): NU, RR, UE

＊ **K0808** Power operated vehicle, group 2 very heavy duty, patient weight capacity 451 to 600 pounds ⑧ **Qp** **Qh** ᕻ   Y

Inexpensive and routinely purchased DME

DMEPOS Modifier(s): NU, RR, UE

＊ **K0812** Power operated vehicle, not otherwise classified ⑧ **Qp** **Qh**   Y

Not Otherwise Classified.

＊ **K0813** Power wheelchair, group 1 standard, portable, sling/solid seat and back, patient weight capacity up to and including 300 pounds ⑧ **Qp** **Qh** ᕻ   Y

Capped rental

DMEPOS Modifier(s): RR

＊ **K0814** Power wheelchair, group 1 standard, portable, captains chair, patient weight capacity up to and including 300 pounds ⑧ **Qp** **Qh** ᕻ   Y

Capped rental

DMEPOS Modifier(s): RR

＊ **K0815** Power wheelchair, group 1 standard, sling/solid seat and back, patient weight capacity up to and including 300 pounds ⑧ **Qp** **Qh** ᕻ   Y

Capped rental

DMEPOS Modifier(s): RR

＊ **K0816** Power wheelchair, group 1 standard, captains chair, patient weight capacity up to and including 300 pounds ⑧ **Qp** **Qh** ᕻ   Y

Capped rental

DMEPOS Modifier(s): RR

＊ **K0820** Power wheelchair, group 2 standard, portable, sling/solid seat/back, patient weight capacity up to and including 300 pounds ⑧ **Qp** **Qh** ᕻ   Y

Capped rental

DMEPOS Modifier(s): RR

＊ **K0821** Power wheelchair, group 2 standard, portable, captains chair, patient weight capacity up to and including 300 pounds ⑧ **Qp** **Qh** ᕻ   Y

Capped rental

DMEPOS Modifier(s): RR

＊ **K0822** Power wheelchair, group 2 standard, sling/solid seat/back, patient weight capacity up to and including 300 pounds ⑧ **Qp** **Qh** ᕻ   Y

Capped rental

DMEPOS Modifier(s): RR

＊ **K0823** Power wheelchair, group 2 standard, captains chair, patient weight capacity up to and including 300 pounds ⑧ **Qp** **Qh** ᕻ   Y

Capped rental

DMEPOS Modifier(s): RR

＊ **K0824** Power wheelchair, group 2 heavy duty, sling/solid seat/back, patient weight capacity 301 to 450 pounds ⑧ **Qp** **Qh** ᕻ   Y

Capped rental

DMEPOS Modifier(s): RR

＊ **K0825** Power wheelchair, group 2 heavy duty, captains chair, patient weight capacity 301 to 450 pounds ⑧ **Qp** **Qh** ᕻ   Y

Capped rental

DMEPOS Modifier(s): RR

＊ **K0826** Power wheelchair, group 2 very heavy duty, sling/solid seat/back, patient weight capacity 451 to 600 pounds ⑧ **Qp** **Qh** ᕻ   Y

Capped rental

DMEPOS Modifier(s): RR

＊ **K0827** Power wheelchair, group 2 very heavy duty, captains chair, patient weight capacity 451 to 600 pounds ⑧ **Qp** **Qh** ᕻ   Y

Capped rental

DMEPOS Modifier(s): RR

＊ **K0828** Power wheelchair, group 2 extra heavy duty, sling/solid seat/back, patient weight capacity 601 pounds or more ⑧ **Qp** **Qh** ᕻ   Y

Capped rental

DMEPOS Modifier(s): RR

＊ **K0829** Power wheelchair, group 2 extra heavy duty, captains chair, patient weight 601 pounds or more ⑧ **Qp** **Qh** ᕻ   Y

Capped rental

DMEPOS Modifier(s): RR

＊ **K0830** Power wheelchair, group 2 standard, seat elevator, sling/solid seat/back, patient weight capacity up to and including 300 pounds ⑧ **Qp** **Qh**   Y

Capped rental

DMEPOS Modifier(s): NU, RR, UE

PQRS PQRS   **Qp** Quantity Physician Appendix A   **Qh** Quantity Hospital Appendix B   ♀ Female only

♂ Male only   **A** Age   ᕻ DMEPOS   A2-Z3 ASC Payment Indicator   A-Y ASC Status Indicator   Coding Clinic

* **K0831** Power wheelchair, group 2 standard, seat elevator, captains chair, patient weight capacity up to and including 300 pounds Ⓑ **Qp** **Qh**   Y

  DMEPOS Modifier(s): NU, RR, UE

* **K0835** Power wheelchair, group 2 standard, single power option, sling/solid seat/back, patient weight capacity up to and including 300 pounds Ⓑ **Qp** **Qh** ♿   Y

  Capped rental

  DMEPOS Modifier(s): RR

* **K0836** Power wheelchair, group 2 standard, single power option, captains chair, patient weight capacity up to and including 300 pounds Ⓑ **Qp** **Qh** ♿   Y

  Capped rental

  DMEPOS Modifier(s): RR

* **K0837** Power wheelchair, group 2 heavy duty, single power option, sling/solid seat/back, patient weight capacity 301 to 450 pounds Ⓑ **Qp** **Qh** ♿   Y

  Capped rental

  DMEPOS Modifier(s): RR

* **K0838** Power wheelchair, group 2 heavy duty, single power option, captains chair, patient weight capacity 301 to 450 pounds Ⓑ **Qp** **Qh** ♿   Y

  Capped rental

  DMEPOS Modifier(s): RR

* **K0839** Power wheelchair, group 2 very heavy duty, single power option sling/solid seat/back, patient weight capacity 451 to 600 pounds Ⓑ **Qp** **Qh** ♿   Y

  Capped rental

  DMEPOS Modifier(s): RR

* **K0840** Power wheelchair, group 2 extra heavy duty, single power option, sling/solid seat/back, patient weight capacity 601 pounds or more Ⓑ **Qp** **Qh** ♿   Y

  Capped rental

  DMEPOS Modifier(s): RR

* **K0841** Power wheelchair, group 2 standard, multiple power option, sling/solid seat/back, patient weight capacity up to and including 300 pounds Ⓑ **Qp** **Qh** ♿   Y

  Capped rental

  DMEPOS Modifier(s): RR

* **K0842** Power wheelchair, group 2 standard, multiple power option, captains chair, patient weight capacity up to and including 300 pounds Ⓑ **Qp** **Qh** ♿   Y

  Capped rental

  DMEPOS Modifier(s): RR

* **K0843** Power wheelchair, group 2 heavy duty, multiple power option, sling/solid seat/back, patient weight capacity 301 to 450 pounds Ⓑ **Qp** **Qh** ♿   Y

  Capped rental

  DMEPOS Modifier(s): RR

* **K0848** Power wheelchair, group 3 standard, sling/solid seat/back, patient weight capacity up to and including 300 pounds Ⓑ **Qp** **Qh** ♿   Y

  Capped rental

  DMEPOS Modifier(s): RR

* **K0849** Power wheelchair, group 3 standard, captains chair, patient weight capacity up to and including 300 pounds Ⓑ **Qp** **Qh** ♿   Y

  Capped rental

  DMEPOS Modifier(s): RR

* **K0850** Power wheelchair, group 3 heavy duty, sling/solid seat/back, patient weight capacity 301 to 450 pounds Ⓑ **Qp** **Qh** ♿   Y

  Capped rental

  DMEPOS Modifier(s): RR

* **K0851** Power wheelchair, group 3 heavy duty, captains chair, patient weight capacity 301 to 450 pounds Ⓑ **Qp** **Qh** ♿   Y

  Capped rental

  DMEPOS Modifier(s): RR

* **K0852** Power wheelchair, group 3 very heavy duty, sling/solid seat/back, patient weight capacity 451 to 600 pounds Ⓑ **Qp** **Qh** ♿   Y

  Capped rental

  DMEPOS Modifier(s): RR

* **K0853** Power wheelchair, group 3 very heavy duty, captains chair, patient weight capacity 451 to 600 pounds Ⓑ **Qp** **Qh** ♿   Y

  Capped rental

  DMEPOS Modifier(s): RR

▶ New   ↻ Revised   ✔ Reinstated   ~~deleted~~ Deleted   ⊘ Not covered or valid by Medicare

⊛ Special coverage instructions   * Carrier discretion   Ⓑ Bill local carrier   Ⓑ Bill DME MAC

* **K0854** Power wheelchair, group 3 extra heavy duty, sling/solid seat/back, patient weight capacity 601 pounds or more Ⓑ Qp Qh ♿   Y

Capped rental

DMEPOS Modifier(s): RR

* **K0855** Power wheelchair, group 3 extra heavy duty, captains chair, patient weight capacity 601 pounds or more Ⓑ Qp Qh ♿   Y

Capped rental

DMEPOS Modifier(s): RR

* **K0856** Power wheelchair, group 3 standard, single power option, sling/solid seat/back, patient weight capacity up to and including 300 pounds Ⓑ Qp Qh ♿   Y

Capped rental

DMEPOS Modifier(s): RR

* **K0857** Power wheelchair, group 3 standard, single power option, captains chair, patient weight capacity up to and including 300 pounds Ⓑ Qp Qh ♿   Y

Capped rental

DMEPOS Modifier(s): RR

* **K0858** Power wheelchair, group 3 heavy duty, single power option, sling/solid seat/back, patient weight 301 to 450 pounds Ⓑ Qp Qh ♿   Y

Capped rental

DMEPOS Modifier(s): RR

* **K0859** Power wheelchair, group 3 heavy duty, single power option, captains chair, patient weight capacity 301 to 450 pounds Ⓑ Qp Qh ♿   Y

Capped rental

DMEPOS Modifier(s): RR

* **K0860** Power wheelchair, group 3 very heavy duty, single power option, sling/solid seat/back, patient weight capacity 451 to 600 pounds Ⓑ Qp Qh ♿   Y

Capped rental

DMEPOS Modifier(s): RR

* **K0861** Power wheelchair, group 3 standard, multiple power option, sling/solid seat/back, patient weight capacity up to and including 300 pounds Ⓑ Qp Qh ♿   Y

Capped rental

DMEPOS Modifier(s): KF, RR

* **K0862** Power wheelchair, group 3 heavy duty, multiple power option, sling/solid seat/back, patient weight capacity 301 to 450 pounds Ⓑ Qp Qh ♿   Y

Capped rental

DMEPOS Modifier(s): RR

* **K0863** Power wheelchair, group 3 very heavy duty, multiple power option, sling/solid seat/back, patient weight capacity 451 to 600 pounds Ⓑ Qp Qh ♿   Y

Capped rental

DMEPOS Modifier(s): RR

* **K0864** Power wheelchair, group 3 extra heavy duty, multiple power option, sling/solid seat/back, patient weight capacity 601 pounds or more Ⓑ Qp Qh ♿   Y

Capped rental

DMEPOS Modifier(s): RR

* **K0868** Power wheelchair, group 4 standard, sling/solid seat/back, patient weight capacity up to and including 300 pounds Ⓑ Qp Qh   Y

Capped rental

* **K0869** Power wheelchair, group 4 standard, captains chair, patient weight capacity up to and including 300 pounds Ⓑ Qp Qh   Y

Capped rental

* **K0870** Power wheelchair, group 4 heavy duty, sling/solid seat/back, patient weight capacity 301 to 450 pounds Ⓑ Qp Qh   Y

Capped rental

* **K0871** Power wheelchair, group 4 very heavy duty, sling/solid seat/back, patient weight capacity 451 to 600 pounds Ⓑ Qp Qh   Y

Capped rental

* **K0877** Power wheelchair, group 4 standard, single power option, sling/solid seat/back, patient weight capacity up to and including 300 pounds Ⓑ Qp Qh   Y

Capped rental

* **K0878** Power wheelchair, group 4 standard, single power option, captains chair, patient weight capacity up to and including 300 pounds Ⓑ Qp Qh   Y

Capped rental

* **K0879** Power wheelchair, group 4 heavy duty, single power option, sling/solid seat/back, patient weight capacity 301 to 450 pounds Ⓑ Qp Qh   Y

Capped rental

* **K0880** Power wheelchair, group 4 very heavy duty, single power option, sling/solid seat/back, patient weight 451 to 600 pounds ⑧ **Qp** **Qh**   Y

  Capped rental

* **K0884** Power wheelchair, group 4 standard, multiple power option, sling/solid seat/back, patient weight capacity up to and including 300 pounds ⑧ **Qp** **Qh**   Y

  Capped rental

* **K0885** Power wheelchair, group 4 standard, multiple power option, captains chair, patient weight capacity up to and including 300 pounds ⑧ **Qp** **Qh**   Y

  Capped rental

* **K0886** Power wheelchair, group 4 heavy duty, multiple power option, sling/solid seat/back, patient weight capacity 301 to 450 pounds ⑧ **Qp** **Qh**   Y

  Capped rental

* **K0890** Power wheelchair, group 5 pediatric, single power option, sling/solid seat/back, patient weight capacity up to and including 125 pounds ⑧ **Qp** **Qh** **A**   Y

  Capped rental

* **K0891** Power wheelchair, group 5 pediatric, multiple power option, sling/solid seat/back, patient weight capacity up to and including 125 pounds ⑧ **Qp** **Qh** **A**   Y

  Capped rental

* **K0898** Power wheelchair, not otherwise classified ⑧ **Qp** **Qh**   Y

* **K0899** Power mobility device, not coded by DME PDAC or does not meet criteria ⑧   Y

○ **K0900** Customized durable medical equipment, other than wheelchair ⑧ **Qp** **Qh**   Y

▶ * **K0901** Knee orthosis (KO), single upright, thigh and calf, with adjustable flexion and extension joint (unicentric or polycentric), medial-lateral and rotation control, with or without varus/valgus adjustment, prefabricated, off-the-shelf ♿   A

▶ * **K0902** Knee orthosis (KO), double upright, thigh and calf, with adjustable flexion and extension joint (unicentric or polycentric), medial-lateral and rotation control, with or without varus/valgus adjustment, prefabricated, off-the-shelf ♿   A

▶ **New**   ↻ **Revised**   ✔ **Reinstated**   ~~deleted~~ **Deleted**   ⊘ **Not covered or valid by Medicare**
○ **Special coverage instructions**   * **Carrier discretion**   ⑧ **Bill local carrier**   ⑧ **Bill DME MAC**

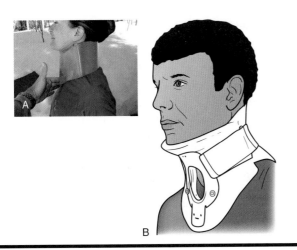

Figure 21 A. Flexible cervical collar. **B.** Adjustable cervical collar.

ORTHOTICS (L0100-L4999)

DMEPOS fee schedule:

www.cms.gov/DMEPOSFeeSched/LSDMEPOSFEE/list.asp#TopOfPage

Orthotic Devices: Spinal

Cervical

✳ **L0112** Cranial cervical orthosis, congenital torticollis type, with or without soft interface material, adjustable range of motion joint, custom fabricated Ⓑ Qp Qh ᜶   A

✳ **L0113** Cranial cervical orthosis, torticollis type, with or without joint, with or without soft interface material, prefabricated, includes fitting and adjustment Ⓑ Qp Qh ᜶   A

✳ **L0120** Cervical, flexible, non-adjustable, prefabricated, off-the-shelf (foam collar)t Ⓑ Qp Qh ᜶   A

Cervical orthoses, including soft and rigid devices may be used as nonoperative management for cervical trauma

✳ **L0130** Cervical, flexible, thermoplastic collar, molded to patient Ⓑ Qp Qh ᜶   A

✳ **L0140** Cervical, semi-rigid, adjustable (plastic collar) Ⓑ Qp Qh ᜶   A

✳ **L0150** Cervical, semi-rigid, adjustable molded chin cup (plastic collar with mandibular/occipital piece) Ⓑ Qp Qh ᜶   A

✳ **L0160** Cervical, semi-rigid, wire frame occipital/mandibular support, prefabricated, off-the-shelf Ⓑ Qp Qh ᜶   A

✳ **L0170** Cervical, collar, molded to patient model Ⓑ Qp Qh ᜶   A

✳ **L0172** Cervical, collar, semi-rigid thermoplastic foam, two-piece, prefabricated, off-the-shelf Ⓑ Qp Qh ᜶   A

✳ **L0174** Cervical, collar, semi-rigid, thermoplastic foam, two piece with thoracic extension, prefabricated, off-the-shelf Ⓑ Qp Qh ᜶   A

Multiple Post Collar

✳ **L0180** Cervical, multiple post collar, occipital/mandibular supports, adjustable Ⓑ Qp Qh ᜶   A

✳ **L0190** Cervical, multiple post collar, occipital/mandibular supports, adjustable cervical bars (SOMI, Guilford, Taylor types) Ⓑ Qp Qh ᜶   A

✳ **L0200** Cervical, multiple post collar, occipital/mandibular supports, adjustable cervical bars, and thoracic extension Ⓑ Qp Qh ᜶   A

Thoracic

✳ **L0220** Thoracic, rib belt, custom fabricated Ⓑ Qp Qh ᜶   A

Thoracic-Lumbar-Sacral

Anterior-Posterior-Lateral Rotary-Control

✳ **L0450** TLSO, flexible, provides trunk support, upper thoracic region, produces intracavitary pressure to reduce load on the intervertebral disks with rigid stays or panel(s), includes shoulder straps and closures, prefabricated, off-the-shelf Ⓑ Qp Qh ᜶   A

Used to immobilize specified area of spine, and is generally worn under clothing

✳ **L0452** TLSO, flexible, provides trunk support, upper thoracic region, produces intracavitary pressure to reduce load on the intervertebral disks with rigid stays or panel(s), includes shoulder straps and closures, custom fabricated Ⓑ Qp Qh ᜶   A

⁽ᴾᴼᴿˢ⁾ PQRS	Qp **Quantity Physician Appendix A**	Qh **Quantity Hospital Appendix B**	♀ **Female only**
♂ **Male only**	A **Age**	᜶ **DMEPOS**	A2-Z3 **ASC Payment Indicator**	A-Y **ASC Status Indicator**	Coding Clinic

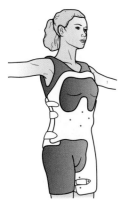

Figure 22 Thoracic-Lumbar-Sacral orthosis (TLSO).

✳ **L0454** TLSO flexible, provides trunk support, extends from sacrococcygeal junction to above T-9 vertebra, restricts gross trunk motion in the sagittal plane, produces intracavitary pressure to reduce load on the intervertebral disks with rigid stays or panel(s), includes shoulder straps and closures, prefabricated item that has been trimmed, bent, molded, assembled, or otherwise customized to fit a specific patient by an individual with expertise ⑧ **Qp** **Qh** ⟱   A

Used to immobilize specified areas of spine; and is generally designed to be worn under clothing; not specifically designed for patients in wheelchairs

✳ **L0455** TLSO, flexible, provides trunk support, extends from sacrococcygeal junction to above T-9 vertebra, restricts gross trunk motion in the sagittal plane, produces intracavitary pressure to reduce load on the intervertebral disks with rigid stays or panel(s), includes shoulder straps and closures, prefabricated, off-the-shelf ⑧ **Qp** **Qh**   A

✳ **L0456** TLSO, flexible, provides trunk support, thoracic region, rigid posterior panel and soft anterior apron, extends from the sacrococcygeal junction and terminates just inferior to the scapular spine, restricts gross trunk motion in the sagittal plane, produces intracavitary pressure to reduce load on the intervertebral disks, includes straps and closures, prefabricated item that has been trimmed, bent, molded, assembled, or otherwise customized to fit a specific patient by an individual with expertise ⑧ **Qp** **Qh** ⟱   A

✳ **L0457** TLSO, flexible, provides trunk support, thoracic region, rigid posterior panel and soft anterior apron, extends from the sacrococcygeal junction and terminates just inferior to the scapular spine, restricts gross trunk motion in the sagittal plane, produces intracavitary pressure to reduce load on the intervertebral disks, includes straps and closures, prefabricated, off-the-shelf ⑧ **Qp** **Qh**   A

✳ **L0458** TLSO, triplanar control, modular segmented spinal system, two rigid plastic shells, posterior extends from the sacrococcygeal junction and terminates just inferior to the scapular spine, anterior extends from the symphysis pubis to the xiphoid, soft liner, restricts gross trunk motion in the sagittal, coronal, and transverse planes, lateral strength is provided by overlapping plastic and stabilizing closures, includes straps and closures, prefabricated, includes fitting and adjustment ⑧ **Qp** **Qh** ⟱   A

To meet Medicare's definition of body jacket, orthosis has to have rigid plastic shell that circles trunk with overlapping edges and stabilizing closures, and entire circumference of shell must be made of same rigid material

✳ **L0460** TLSO, triplanar control, modular segmented spinal system, two rigid plastic shells, posterior extends from the sacrococcygeal junction and terminates just inferior to the scapular spine, anterior extends from the symphysis pubis to the sternal notch, soft liner, restricts gross trunk motion in the sagittal, coronal, and transverse planes, lateral strength is provided by overlapping plastic and stabilizing closures, includes straps and closures, prefabricated item that has been trimmed, bent, molded, assembled, or otherwise customized to fit a specific patient by an individual with expertise ⑧ **Qp** **Qh** ⟱   A

▶ **New**   ↻ **Revised**   ✔ **Reinstated**   ~~deleted~~ **Deleted**   ⊘ **Not covered or valid by Medicare**
⟳ **Special coverage instructions**   ✳ **Carrier discretion**   ⑧ **Bill local carrier**   ⑧ **Bill DME MAC**

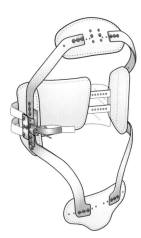

Figure 23 Thoracic-Lumbar-Sacral orthosis (TLSO) Jewett flexion control.

✳ **L0462** TLSO, triplanar control, modular segmented spinal system, three rigid plastic shells, posterior extends from the sacrococcygeal junction and terminates just inferior to the scapular spine, anterior extends from the symphysis pubis to the sternal notch, soft liner, restricts gross trunk motion in the sagittal, coronal, and transverse planes, lateral strength is provided by overlapping plastic and stabilizing closures, includes straps and closures, prefabricated, includes fitting and adjustment Ⓑ Qp Qh   A

✳ **L0464** TLSO, triplanar control, modular segmented spinal system, four rigid plastic shells, posterior extends from sacrococcygeal junction and terminates just inferior to scapular spine, anterior extends from symphysis pubis to the sternal notch, soft liner, restricts gross trunk motion in sagittal, coronal, and transverse planes, lateral strength is provided by overlapping plastic and stabilizing closures, includes straps and closures, prefabricated, includes fitting and adjustment Ⓑ Qp Qh   A

✳ **L0466** TLSO, sagittal control, rigid posterior frame and flexible soft anterior apron with straps, closures and padding, restricts gross trunk motion in sagittal plane, produces intracavitary pressure to reduce load on intervertebral disks, prefabricated item that has been trimmed, bent, molded, assembled, or otherwise customized to fit a specific patient by an individual with expertise Ⓑ Qp Qh   A

✳ **L0467** TLSO, sagittal control, rigid posterior frame and flexible soft anterior apron with straps, closures and padding, restricts gross trunk motion in sagittal plane, produces intracavitary pressure to reduce load on intervertebral disks, prefabricated, off-the-shelf Ⓑ Qp Qh   A

✳ **L0468** TLSO, sagittal-coronal control, rigid posterior frame and flexible soft anterior apron with straps, closures and padding, extends from sacrococcygeal junction over scapulae, lateral strength provided by pelvic, thoracic, and lateral frame pieces, restricts gross trunk motion in sagittal, and coronal planes, produces intracavitary pressure to reduce load on intervertebral disks, prefabricated item that has been trimmed, bent, molded, assembled, or otherwise customized to fit a specific patient by an individual with expertise Ⓑ Qp Qh   A

✳ **L0469** TLSO, sagittal-coronal control, rigid posterior frame and flexible soft anterior apron with straps, closures and padding, extends from sacrococcygeal junction over scapulae, lateral strength provided by pelvic, thoracic, and lateral frame pieces, restricts gross trunk motion in sagittal and coronal planes, produces intracavitary pressure to reduce load on intervertebral disks, prefabricated, off-the-shelf Ⓑ Qp Qh   A

✳ **L0470** TLSO, triplanar control, rigid posterior frame and flexible soft anterior apron with straps, closures and padding, extends from sacrococcygeal junction to scapula, lateral strength provided by pelvic, thoracic, and lateral frame pieces, rotational strength provided by subclavicular extensions, restricts gross trunk motion in sagittal, coronal, and transverse planes, provides intracavitary pressure to reduce load on the intervertebral disks, includes fitting and shaping the frame, prefabricated, includes fitting and adjustment Ⓑ Qp Qh   A

✳ **L0472** TLSO, triplanar control, hyperextension, rigid anterior and lateral frame extends from symphysis pubis to sternal notch with two anterior components (one pubic and one sternal), posterior and lateral pads with straps and closures, limits spinal flexion, restricts gross trunk motion in sagittal, coronal, and transverse planes, includes fitting and shaping the frame, prefabricated, includes fitting and adjustment Ⓑ Qp Qh   A

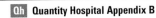

✳ **L0480** TLSO, triplanar control, one piece rigid plastic shell without interface liner, with multiple straps and closures, posterior extends from sacrococcygeal junction and terminates just inferior to scapular spine, anterior extends from symphysis pubis to sternal notch, anterior or posterior opening, restricts gross trunk motion in sagittal, coronal, and transverse planes, includes a carved plaster or CAD-CAM model, custom fabricated Ⓑ Qp Qh ♿　　　A

✳ **L0482** TLSO, triplanar control, one piece rigid plastic shell with interface liner, multiple straps and closures, posterior extends from sacrococcygeal junction and terminates just inferior to scapular spine, anterior extends from symphysis pubis to sternal notch, anterior or posterior opening, restricts gross trunk motion in sagittal, coronal, and transverse planes, includes a carved plaster or CAD-CAM model, custom fabricated Ⓑ Qp Qh ♿　　　A

✳ **L0484** TLSO, triplanar control, two piece rigid plastic shell without interface liner, with multiple straps and closures, posterior extends from sacrococcygeal junction and terminates just inferior to scapular spine, anterior extends from symphysis pubis to sternal notch, lateral strength is enhanced by overlapping plastic, restricts gross trunk motion in the sagittal, coronal, and transverse planes, includes a carved plaster or CAD-CAM model, custom fabricated Ⓑ Qp Qh ♿　　　A

✳ **L0486** TLSO, triplanar control, two piece rigid plastic shell with interface liner, multiple straps and closures, posterior extends from sacrococcygeal junction and terminates just inferior to scapular spine, anterior extends from symphysis pubis to sternal notch, lateral strength is enhanced by overlapping plastic, restricts gross trunk motion in the sagittal, coronal, and transverse planes, includes a carved plaster or CAD-CAM model, custom fabricated Ⓑ Qp Qh ♿　　　A

✳ **L0488** TLSO, triplanar control, one piece rigid plastic shell with interface liner, multiple straps and closures, posterior extends from sacrococcygeal junction and terminates just inferior to scapular spine, anterior extends from symphysis pubis to sternal notch, anterior or posterior opening, restricts gross trunk motion in sagittal, coronal, and transverse planes, prefabricated, includes fitting and adjustment Ⓑ Qp Qh ♿　　　A

✳ **L0490** TLSO, sagittal-coronal control, one piece rigid plastic shell, with overlapping reinforced anterior, with multiple straps and closures, posterior extends from sacrococcygeal junction and terminates at or before the T-9 vertebra, anterior extends from symphysis pubis to xiphoid, anterior opening, restricts gross trunk motion in sagittal and coronal planes, prefabricated, includes fitting and adjustment Ⓑ Qp Qh ♿　　　A

✳ **L0491** TLSO, sagittal-coronal control, modular segmented spinal system, two rigid plastic shells, posterior extends from the sacrococcygeal junction and terminates just inferior to the scapular spine, anterior extends from the symphysis pubis to the xiphoid, soft liner, restricts gross trunk motion in the sagittal and coronal planes, lateral strength is provided by overlapping plastic and stabilizing closures, includes straps and closures, prefabricated, includes fitting and adjustment Ⓑ Qp Qh ♿　　　A

✳ **L0492** TLSO, sagittal-coronal control, modular segmented spinal system, three rigid plastic shells, posterior extends from the sacrococcygeal junction and terminates just inferior to the scapular spine, anterior extends from the symphysis pubis to the xiphoid, soft liner, restricts gross trunk motion in the sagittal and coronal planes, lateral strength is provided by overlapping plastic and stabilizing closures, includes straps and closures, prefabricated, includes fitting and adjustment Ⓑ Qp Qh ♿　　　A

Sacroilliac, Lumbar, Sacral Orthosis

✳ **L0621** Sacroiliac orthosis, flexible, provides pelvic-sacral support, reduces motion about the sacroiliac joint, includes straps, closures, may include pendulous abdomen design, prefabricated, off-the-shelf Ⓑ Qp Qh ♿　　　A

✳ **L0622** Sacroiliac orthosis, flexible, provides pelvic-sacral support, reduces motion about the sacroiliac joint, includes straps, closures, may include pendulous abdomen design, custom fabricated Ⓑ Qp Qh ♿　　　A

Type of custom-fabricated device for which impression of specific body part is made (e.g., by means of plaster cast, or CAD-CAM [computer-aided design] technology); impression then used to make specific patient model

---

▶ **New**　　↻ **Revised**　　✔ **Reinstated**　　~~deleted~~ **Deleted**　　⊘ **Not covered or valid by Medicare**
⊙ **Special coverage instructions**　　✳ **Carrier discretion**　　Ⓛ **Bill local carrier**　　Ⓑ **Bill DME MAC**

* **L0623** Sacroiliac orthosis, provides pelvic-sacral support, with rigid or semi-rigid panels over the sacrum and abdomen, reduces motion about the sacroiliac joint, includes straps, closures, may include pendulous abdomen design, prefabricated, off-the-shelf Ⓑ 𝐐𝐩 𝐐𝐡 🦽   A

* **L0624** Sacroiliac orthosis, provides pelvic-sacral support, with rigid or semi-rigid panels placed over the sacrum and abdomen, reduces motion about the sacroiliac joint, includes straps, closures, may include pendulous abdomen design, custom fabricated Ⓑ 𝐐𝐩 𝐐𝐡 🦽   A

Custom fitted

* **L0625** Lumbar orthosis, flexible, provides lumbar support, posterior extends from L-1 to below L-5 vertebra, produces intracavitary pressure to reduce load on the intervertebral discs, includes straps, closures, may include pendulous abdomen design, shoulder straps, stays, prefabricated, off-the-shelf Ⓑ 𝐐𝐩 𝐐𝐡 🦽   A

* **L0626** Lumbar orthosis, sagittal control, with rigid posterior panel(s), posterior extends from L-1 to below L-5 vertebra, produces intracavitary pressure to reduce load on the intervertebral discs, includes straps, closures, may include padding, stays, shoulder straps, pendulous abdomen design, prefabricated item that has been trimmed, bent, molded, assembled, or otherwise customized to fit a specific patient by an individual with expertise Ⓑ 𝐐𝐩 𝐐𝐡 🦽   A

* **L0627** Lumbar orthosis, sagittal control, with rigid anterior and posterior panels, posterior extends from L-1 to below L-5 vertebra, produces intracavitary pressure to reduce load on the intervertebral discs, includes straps, closures, may include padding, shoulder straps, pendulous abdomen design, prefabricated item that has been trimmed, bent, molded, assembled, or otherwise customized to fit a specific patient by an individual with expertise Ⓑ 𝐐𝐩 𝐐𝐡 🦽   A

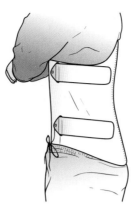

Figure 24 Lumbar-sacral orthosis.

* **L0628** Lumbar-sacral orthosis, flexible, provides lumbo-sacral support, posterior extends from sacrococcygeal junction to T-9 vertebra, produces intracavitary pressure to reduce load on the intervertebral discs, includes straps, closures, may include stays, shoulder straps, pendulous abdomen design, prefabricated, off-the-shelf Ⓑ 𝐐𝐩 𝐐𝐡 🦽   A

* **L0629** Lumbar-sacral orthosis, flexible, provides lumbo-sacral support, posterior extends from sacrococcygeal junction to T-9 vertebra, produces intracavitary pressure to reduce load on the intervertebral discs, includes straps, closures, may include stays, shoulder straps, pendulous abdomen design, custom fabricated Ⓑ 𝐐𝐩 𝐐𝐡 🦽   A

Custom fitted

* **L0630** Lumbar-sacral orthosis, sagittal control, with rigid posterior panel(s), posterior extends from sacrococcygeal junction to T-9 vertebra, produces intracavitary pressure to reduce load on the intervertebral discs, includes straps, closures, may include padding, stays, shoulder straps, pendulous abdomen design, prefabricated item that has been trimmed, bent, molded, assembled, or otherwise customized to fit a specific patient by an individual with expertise Ⓑ 𝐐𝐩 𝐐𝐡 🦽   A

* **L0631** Lumbar-sacral orthosis, sagittal control, with rigid anterior and posterior panels, posterior extends from sacrococcygeal junction to T-9 vertebra, produces intracavitary pressure to reduce load on the intervertebral discs, includes straps, closures, may include padding, shoulder straps, pendulous abdomen design, prefabricated item that has been trimmed, bent, molded, assembled, or otherwise customized to fit a specific patient by an individual with expertise Ⓑ 𝐐𝐩 𝐐𝐡 🦽   A

| 🄿 PQRS | 𝐐𝐩 Quantity Physician Appendix A | 𝐐𝐡 Quantity Hospital Appendix B | ♀ Female only |
| ♂ Male only | A Age | 🦽 DMEPOS | A2-Z3 ASC Payment Indicator | A-Y ASC Status Indicator | Coding Clinic |

ORTHOTICS L0623 – L0631

297

* **L0632** Lumbar-sacral orthosis, sagittal control, with rigid anterior and posterior panels, posterior extends from sacrococcygeal junction to T-9 vertebra, produces intracavitary pressure to reduce load on the intervertebral discs, includes straps, closures, may include padding, shoulder straps, pendulous abdomen design, custom fabricated Ⓑ Qp Qh ♿   A

Custom fitted

* **L0633** Lumbar-sacral orthosis, sagittal-coronal control, with rigid posterior frame/panel(s), posterior extends from sacrococcygeal junction to T-9 vertebra, lateral strength provided by rigid lateral frame/panels, produces intracavitary pressure to reduce load on intervertebral discs, includes straps, closures, may include padding, stays, shoulder straps, pendulous abdomen design, prefabricated item that has been trimmed, bent, molded, assembled, or otherwise customized to fit a specific patient by an individual with expertise Ⓑ Qp Qh ♿   A

* **L0634** Lumbar-sacral orthosis, sagittal-coronal control, with rigid posterior frame/panel(s), posterior extends from sacrococcygeal junction to T-9 vertebra, lateral strength provided by rigid lateral frame/panel(s), produces intracavitary pressure to reduce load on intervertebral discs, includes straps, closures, may include padding, stays, shoulder straps, pendulous abdomen design, custom fabricated Ⓑ Qp Qh ♿   A

Custom fitted

* **L0635** Lumbar-sacral orthosis, sagittal-coronal control, lumbar flexion, rigid posterior frame/panel(s), lateral articulating design to flex the lumbar spine, posterior extends from sacrococcygeal junction to T-9 vertebra, lateral strength provided by rigid lateral frame/panel(s), produces intracavitary pressure to reduce load on intervertebral discs, includes straps, closures, may include padding, anterior panel, pendulous abdomen design, prefabricated, includes fitting and adjustment Ⓑ Qp Qh ♿   A

* **L0636** Lumbar sacral orthosis, sagittal-coronal control, lumbar flexion, rigid posterior frame/panels, lateral articulating design to flex the lumbar spine, posterior extends from sacrococcygeal junction to T-9 vertebra, lateral strength provided by rigid lateral frame/panels, produces intracavitary pressure to reduce load on intervertebral discs, includes straps, closures, may include padding, anterior panel, pendulous abdomen design, custom fabricated Ⓑ Qp Qh ♿   A

Custom fitted

* **L0637** Lumbar-sacral orthosis, sagittal-coronal control, with rigid anterior and posterior frame/panels, posterior extends from sacrococcygeal junction to T-9 vertebra, lateral strength provided by rigid lateral frame/panels, produces intracavitary pressure to reduce load on intervertebral discs, includes straps, closures, may include padding, shoulder straps, pendulous abdomen design, prefabricated item that has been trimmed, bent, molded, assembled, or otherwise customized to fit a specific patient by an individual with expertise Ⓑ Qp Qh ♿   A

* **L0638** Lumbar-sacral orthosis, sagittal-coronal control, with rigid anterior and posterior frame/panels, posterior extends from sacrococcygeal junction to T-9 vertebra, lateral strength provided by rigid lateral frame/panels, produces intracavitary pressure to reduce load on intervertebral discs, includes straps, closures, may include padding, shoulder straps, pendulous abdomen design, custom fabricated Ⓑ Qp Qh ♿   A

* **L0639** Lumbar-sacral orthosis, sagittal-coronal control, rigid shell(s)/panel(s), posterior extends from sacrococcygeal junction to T-9 vertebra, anterior extends from symphysis pubis to xyphoid, produces intracavitary pressure to reduce load on the intervertebral discs, overall strength is provided by overlapping rigid material and stabilizing closures, includes straps, closures, may include soft interface, pendulous abdomen design, prefabricated item that has been trimmed, bent, molded, assembled, or otherwise customized to fit a specific patient by an individual with expertise Ⓑ Qp Qh ♿   A

Characterized by rigid plastic shell that encircles trunk with overlapping edges and stabilizing closures and provides high degree of immobility

---

▶ **New**   ↻ **Revised**   ✔ **Reinstated**   deleted **Deleted**   ⊘ **Not covered or valid by Medicare**

✪ **Special coverage instructions**   ✳ **Carrier discretion**   Ⓢ **Bill local carrier**   Ⓑ **Bill DME MAC**

* **L0640** Lumbar-sacral orthosis, sagittal-coronal control, rigid shell(s)/panel(s), posterior extends from sacrococcygeal junction to T-9 vertebra, anterior extends from symphysis pubis to xyphoid, produces intracavitary pressure to reduce load on the intervertebral discs, overall strength is provided by overlapping rigid material and stabilizing closures, includes straps, closures, may include soft interface, pendulous abdomen design, custom fabricated Ⓑ **Qp** **Qh** ♿ A

Custom fitted

* **L0641** Lumbar orthosis, sagittal control, with rigid posterior panel(s), posterior extends from L-1 to below L-5 vertebra, produces intracavitary pressure to reduce load on the intervertebral discs, includes straps, closures, may include padding, stays, shoulder straps, pendulous abdomen design, prefabricated, off-the-shelf **Qp** **Qh** A

* **L0642** Lumbar orthosis, sagittal control, with rigid anterior and posterior panels, posterior extends from L-1 to below L-5 vertebra, produces intracavitary pressure to reduce load on the intervertebral discs, includes straps, closures, may include padding, shoulder straps, pendulous abdomen design, prefabricated, off-the-shelf **Qp** **Qh** A

* **L0643** Lumbar-sacral orthosis, sagittal control, with rigid posterior panel(s), posterior extends from sacrococcygeal junction to T-9 vertebra, produces intracavitary pressure to reduce load on the intervertebral discs, includes straps, closures, may include padding, stays, shoulder straps, pendulous abdomen design, prefabricated, off-the-shelf **Qp** **Qh** A

* **L0648** Lumbar-sacral orthosis, sagittal control, with rigid anterior and posterior panels, posterior extends from sacrococcygeal junction to T-9 vertebra, produces intracavitary pressure to reduce load on the intervertebral discs, includes straps, closures, may include padding, shoulder straps, pendulous abdomen design, prefabricated, off-the-shelf **Qp** **Qh** A

* **L0649** Lumbar-sacral orthosis, sagittal-coronal control, with rigid posterior frame/panel(s), posterior extends from sacrococcygeal junction to T-9 vertebra, lateral strength provided by rigid lateral frame/panels, produces intracavitary pressure to reduce load on intervertebral discs, includes straps, closures, may include padding, stays, shoulder straps, pendulous abdomen design, prefabricated, off-the-shelf **Qp** **Qh** A

* **L0650** Lumbar-sacral orthosis, sagittal-coronal control, with rigid anterior and posterior frame/panel(s), posterior extends from sacrococcygeal junction to T-9 vertebra, lateral strength provided by rigid lateral frame/panel(s), produces intracavitary pressure to reduce load on intervertebral discs, includes straps, closures, may include padding, shoulder straps, pendulous abdomen design, prefabricated, off-the-shelf **Qp** **Qh** A

* **L0651** Lumbar-sacral orthosis, sagittal-coronal control, rigid shell(s)/panel(s), posterior extends from sacrococcygeal junction to T-9 vertebra, anterior extends from symphysis pubis to xyphoid, produces intracavitary pressure to reduce load on the intervertebral discs, overall strength is provided by overlapping rigid material and stabilizing closures, includes straps, closures, may include soft interface, pendulous abdomen design, prefabricated, off-the-shelf **Qp** **Qh** A

Cervical-Thoracic-Lumbar-Sacral

Anterior-Posterior-Lateral Control

* **L0700** Cervical-thoracic-lumbar-sacral-orthoses (CTLSO), anterior-posterior-lateral control, molded to patient model, (Minerva type) Ⓑ **Qp** **Qh** ♿ A

* **L0710** CTLSO, anterior-posterior-lateral-control, molded to patient model, with interface material, (Minerva type) Ⓑ **Qp** **Qh** ♿ A

HALO Procedure

* **L0810** HALO procedure, cervical halo incorporated into jacket vest Ⓑ **Qp** **Qh** ♿ A

* **L0820** HALO procedure, cervical halo incorporated into plaster body jacket Ⓑ **Qp** **Qh** ♿ A

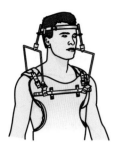

Figure 25 Halo device.

* **L0830** HALO procedure, cervical halo incorporated into Milwaukee type orthosis ⑧ **Qp** **Qh** ⚕️   A

* **L0859** Addition to HALO procedure, magnetic resonance image compatible systems, rings and pins, any material ⑧ **Qp** **Qh** ⚕️   A

* **L0861** Addition to HALO procedure, replacement liner/interface material ⑧ **Qp** **Qh** ⚕️   A

Additions to Spinal Orthoses

TLSO - Thoraci-lumbar-sacral orthoses

Spinal orthoses may be prefabricated, prefitted, or custom fabricated. Conservative treatment for back pain may include the use of spinal orthoses.

* **L0970** TLSO, corset front ⑧ **Qp** **Qh** ⚕️   A
* **L0972** LSO, corset front ⑧ **Qp** **Qh** ⚕️   A
* **L0974** TLSO, full corset ⑧ **Qp** **Qh** ⚕️   A
* **L0976** LSO, full corset ⑧ **Qp** **Qh** ⚕️   A
* **L0978** Axillary crutch extension ⑧ **Qp** **Qh** ⚕️ A
* **L0980** Peroneal straps, prefabricated, off-the-shelf, pair ⑧ **Qp** **Qh** ⚕️   A
* **L0982** Stocking supporter grips, prefabricated, off-the-shelf, set of four (4) ⑧ **Qp** **Qh** ⚕️   A

Convenience item

* **L0984** Protective body sock, prefabricated, off-the-shelf, each ⑧ **Qp** **Qh** ⚕️   A

Convenience item

Garment made of cloth or similar material that is worn under spinal orthosis and is not primarily medical in nature

* **L0999** Addition to spinal orthosis, not otherwise specified ⑧   A

Orthotic Devices: Scoliosis Procedures (L1000-L1520)

NOTE: Orthotic care of scoliosis differs from other orthotic care in that the treatment is more dynamic in nature and uses ongoing continual modification of the orthosis to the patient's changing condition. This coding structure uses the proper names, or eponyms, of the procedures because they have historic and universal acceptance in the profession. It should be recognized that variations to the basic procedures described by the founders/developers are accepted in various medical and orthotic practices throughout the country. All procedures include a model of patient when indicated.

Scoliosis: Cervical-Thoracic-Lumbar-Sacral (CTLSO) (Milwaukee)

* **L1000** Cervical-thoracic-lumbar-sacral orthosis (CTLSO) (Milwaukee), inclusive of furnishing initial orthosis, including model ⑧ **Qp** **Qh** ⚕️   A

* **L1001** Cervical thoracic lumbar sacral orthosis, immobilizer, infant size, prefabricated, includes fitting and adjustment ⑧ **Qp** **Qh** ⚕️   A

* **L1005** Tension based scoliosis orthosis and accessory pads, includes fitting and adjustment ⑧ **Qp** **Qh** ⚕️   A

* **L1010** Addition to cervical-thoracic-lumbar-sacral orthosis (CTLSO) or scoliosis orthosis, axilla sling ⑧ **Qp** **Qh** ⚕️   A

Correction Pads

* **L1020** Addition to CTLSO or scoliosis orthosis, kyphosis pad ⑧ **Qp** **Qh** ⚕️   A

* **L1025** Addition to CTLSO or scoliosis orthosis, kyphosis pad, floating ⑧ **Qp** **Qh** ⚕️   A

* **L1030** Addition to CTLSO or scoliosis orthosis, lumbar bolster pad ⑧ **Qp** **Qh** ⚕️   A

* **L1040** Addition to CTLSO or scoliosis orthosis, lumbar or lumbar rib pad ⑧ **Qp** **Qh** ⚕️   A

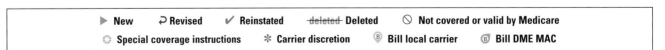

▶ New   ↻ Revised   ✔ Reinstated   ~~deleted~~ Deleted   ⊘ Not covered or valid by Medicare
⊙ Special coverage instructions   ✱ Carrier discretion   ⑧ Bill local carrier   ⑦ Bill DME MAC

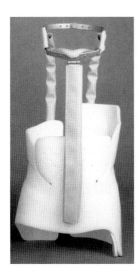

Figure 26 Milwaukee CTLSO.

* **L1050** Addition to CTLSO or scoliosis orthosis, sternal pad Ⓑ Qp Qh ♿ A

* **L1060** Addition to CTLSO or scoliosis orthosis, thoracic pad Ⓑ Qp Qh ♿ A

* **L1070** Addition to CTLSO or scoliosis orthosis, trapezius sling Ⓑ Qp Qh ♿ A

* **L1080** Addition to CTLSO or scoliosis orthosis, outrigger Ⓑ Qp Qh ♿ A

* **L1085** Addition to CTLSO or scoliosis orthosis, outrigger, bilateral with vertical extensions Ⓑ Qp Qh ♿ A

* **L1090** Addition to CTLSO or scoliosis orthosis, lumbar sling Ⓑ Qp Qh ♿ A

* **L1100** Addition to CTLSO or scoliosis orthosis, ring flange, plastic or leather Ⓑ Qh ♿ A

* **L1110** Addition to CTLSO or scoliosis orthosis, ring flange, plastic or leather, molded to patient model Ⓑ Qp Qh ♿ A

* **L1120** Addition to CTLSO, scoliosis orthosis, cover for upright, each Ⓑ Qp Qh ♿ A

Scoliosis: Thoracic-Lumbar-Sacral (Low Profile)

* **L1200** Thoracic-lumbar-sacral-orthosis (TLSO), inclusive of furnishing initial orthosis only Ⓑ Qp Qh ♿ A

* **L1210** Addition to TLSO, (low profile), lateral thoracic extension Ⓑ Qp Qh ♿ A

* **L1220** Addition to TLSO, (low profile), anterior thoracic extension Ⓑ Qp Qh ♿ A

* **L1230** Addition to TLSO, (low profile), Milwaukee type superstructure Ⓑ Qp Qh ♿ A

* **L1240** Addition to TLSO, (low profile), lumbar derotation pad Ⓑ Qp Qh ♿ A

* **L1250** Addition to TLSO, (low profile), anterior ASIS pad Ⓑ Qp Qh ♿ A

* **L1260** Addition to TLSO, (low profile), anterior thoracic derotation pad Ⓑ Qp Qh ♿ A

* **L1270** Addition to TLSO, (low profile), abdominal pad Ⓑ Qp Qh ♿ A

* **L1280** Addition to TLSO, (low profile), rib gusset (elastic), each Ⓑ Qp Qh ♿ A

* **L1290** Addition to TLSO, (low profile), lateral trochanteric pad Ⓑ Qp Qh ♿ A

Other Scoliosis Procedures

* **L1300** Other scoliosis procedure, body jacket molded to patient model Ⓑ Qp Qh ♿ A

* **L1310** Other scoliosis procedure, postoperative body jacket Ⓑ Qp Qh ♿ A

* **L1499** Spinal orthosis, not otherwise specified Ⓑ Qp Qh A

Orthotic Devices: Lower Limb

NOTE: the procedures in L1600-L2999 are considered as base or basic procedures and may be modified by listing procedure from the Additions Sections and adding them to the base procedure.

Hip: Flexible

* **L1600** Hip orthosis, abduction control of hip joints, flexible, frejka type with cover, prefabricated item that has been trimmed, bent, molded, assembled, or otherwise customized to fit a specific patient by an individual with expertise Ⓑ Qp Qh ♿ A

* **L1610** Hip orthosis, abduction control of hip joints, flexible, (frejka cover only), prefabricated item that has been trimmed, bent, molded, assembled, or otherwise customized to fit a specific patient by an individual with expertise Ⓑ Qp Qh ♿ A

* **L1620** Hip orthosis, abduction control of hip joints, flexible, (Pavlik harness), prefabricated item that has been trimmed, bent, molded, assembled, or otherwise customized to fit a specific patient by an individual with expertise Ⓑ Qp Qh ♿ A

* **L1630** Hip orthosis, abduction control of hip joints, semi-flexible (Von Rosen type), custom-fabricated Ⓑ Qp Qh ♿ A

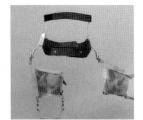

Figure 27 Thoracic-hip-knee-ankle orthosis (THKAO).

＊ **L1640** Hip orthosis, abduction control of hip joints, static, pelvic band or spreader bar, thigh cuffs, custom-fabricated Ⓑ Qp Qh 🦽 A

＊ **L1650** Hip orthosis, abduction control of hip joints, static, adjustable, (Ilfled type), prefabricated, includes fitting and adjustment Ⓑ Qp Qh 🦽 A

＊ **L1652** Hip orthosis, bilateral thigh cuffs with adjustable abductor spreader bar, adult size, prefabricated, includes fitting and adjustment, any type Ⓑ Qp Qh A 🦽 A

＊ **L1660** Hip orthosis, abduction control of hip joints, static, plastic, prefabricated, includes fitting and adjustment Ⓑ Qp Qh 🦽 A

＊ **L1680** Hip orthosis, abduction control of hip joints, dynamic, pelvic control, adjustable hip motion control, thigh cuffs (Rancho hip action type), custom fabrication Ⓑ Qp Qh 🦽 A

＊ **L1685** Hip orthosis, abduction control of hip joint, postoperative hip abduction type, custom fabricated Ⓑ Qp Qh 🦽 A

＊ **L1686** Hip orthosis, abduction control of hip joint, postoperative hip abduction type, prefabricated, includes fitting and adjustment Ⓑ Qp Qh 🦽 A

＊ **L1690** Combination, bilateral, lumbo-sacral, hip, femur orthosis providing adduction and internal rotation control, prefabricated, includes fitting and adjustment Ⓑ Qp Qh 🦽 A

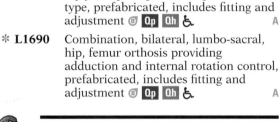

Figure 28 Hip orthosis.

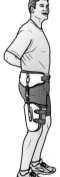

Legg Perthes

＊ **L1700** Legg-Perthes orthosis, (Toronto type), custom-fabricated Ⓑ Qp Qh 🦽 A

＊ **L1710** Legg-Perthes orthosis, (Newington type), custom-fabricated Ⓑ Qp Qh 🦽 A

＊ **L1720** Legg-Perthes orthosis, trilateral, (Tachdjian type), custom-fabricated Ⓑ Qp Qh 🦽 A

＊ **L1730** Legg-Perthes orthosis, (Scottish Rite type), custom-fabricated Ⓑ Qp Qh 🦽 A

＊ **L1755** Legg-Perthes orthosis, (Patten bottom type), custom-fabricated Ⓑ Qp Qh 🦽 A

Knee (KO)

＊ **L1810** Knee orthosis, elastic with joints, prefabricated item that has been trimmed, bent, molded, assembled, or otherwise customized to fit a specific patient by an individual with expertise Ⓑ Qp Qh 🦽 A

＊ **L1812** Knee orthosis, elastic with joints, prefabricated, off-the-shelf Ⓑ Qp Qh A

＊ **L1820** Knee orthosis, elastic with condylar pads and joints, with or without patellar control, prefabricated, includes fitting and adjustment Ⓑ Qp Qh 🦽 A

＊ **L1830** Knee orthosis, immobilizer, canvas longitudinal, prefabricated, off-the-shelf Ⓑ Qp Qh 🦽 A

＊ **L1831** Knee orthosis, locking knee joint(s), positional orthosis, prefabricated, includes fitting and adjustment Ⓑ Qp Qh 🦽 A

＊ **L1832** Knee orthosis, adjustable knee joints (unicentric or polycentric), positional orthosis, rigid support, prefabricated item that has been trimmed, bent, molded, assembled, or otherwise customized to fit a specific patient by an individual with expertise Ⓑ Qp Qh 🦽 A

▶ **New** ↻ **Revised** ✔ **Reinstated** ~~deleted~~ **Deleted** ⊘ **Not covered or valid by Medicare** ⊙ **Special coverage instructions** ＊ **Carrier discretion** Ⓛ **Bill local carrier** Ⓑ **Bill DME MAC**

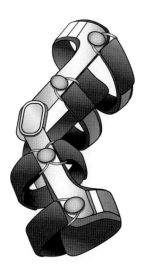

Figure 29 Knee Orthosis.

✳ **L1833** Knee orthosis, adjustable knee joints (unicentric or polycentric), positional orthosis, rigid support, prefabricated, off-the-shelf ⓑ Qp Qh   A

✳ **L1834** Knee orthosis, without knee joint, rigid, custom-fabricated ⓑ Qp Qh �   A

✳ **L1836** Knee orthosis, rigid, without joint(s), includes soft interface material, prefabricated, off-the-shelf ⓑ Qp Qh ⅟   A

✳ **L1840** Knee orthosis, derotation, medial-lateral, anterior cruciate ligament, custom fabricated ⓑ Qp Qh ⅟   A

✳ **L1843** Knee orthosis, single upright, thigh and calf, with adjustable flexion and extension joint (unicentric or polycentric), medial-lateral and rotation control, with or without varus/valgus adjustment, prefabricated item that has been trimmed, bent, molded, assembled, or otherwise customized to fit a specific patient by an individual with expertise ⓑ Qp Qh ⅟   A

✳ **L1844** Knee orthosis, single upright, thigh and calf, with adjustable flexion and extension joint (unicentric or polycentric), medial-lateral and rotation control, with or without varus/ valgus adjustment, custom fabricated ⓑ Qp Qh ⅟   A

✳ **L1845** Knee orthosis, double upright, thigh and calf, with adjustable flexion and extension joint (unicentric or polycentric), medial-lateral and rotation control, with or without varus/valgus adjustment, prefabricated item that has been trimmed, bent, molded, assembled, or otherwise customized to fit a specific patient by an individual with expertise ⓑ Qp Qh ⅟   A

✳ **L1846** Knee orthrosis, double upright, thigh and calf, with adjustable flexion and extension joint (unicentric or polycentric), medial-lateral and rotation control, with or without varus/ valgus adjustment, custom fabricated ⓑ Qp Qh ⅟   A

✳ **L1847** Knee orthosis, double upright with adjustable joint, with inflatable air support chamber(s), prefabricated item that has been trimmed, bent, molded, assembled, or otherwise customized to fit a specific patient by an individual with expertise ⓑ Qp Qh ⅟   A

✳ **L1848** Knee orthosis, double upright with adjustable joint, with inflatable air support chamber(s), prefabricated, off-the-shelf Qp Qh   A

✳ **L1850** Knee orthosis, Swedish type, prefabricated, off-the-shelf ⓑ Qp Qh ⅟   A

✳ **L1860** Knee orthosis, modification of supracondylar prosthetic socket, custom fabricated (SK) ⓑ Qp Qh ⅟   A

Ankle-Foot (AFO)

✳ **L1900** Ankle foot orthosis (AFO), spring wire, dorsiflexion assist calf band, custom-fabricated ⓑ Qp Qh ⅟   A

✳ **L1902** Ankle foot orthosis, ankle gauntlet, prefabricated, off-the-shelf ⓑ Qp Qh ⅟   A

✳ **L1904** Ankle orthosis, ankle gauntlet, custom-fabricated ⓑ Qp Qh ⅟   A

✳ **L1906** Ankle foot orthosis, multiligamentus ankle support, prefabricated, off-the-shelf ⓑ Qp Qh ⅟   A

✳ **L1907** Ankle orthosis, supramalleolar with straps, with or without interface/pads, custom fabricated ⓑ Qp Qh ⅟   A

✳ **L1910** Ankle foot orthosis, posterior, single bar, clasp attachment to shoe counter, prefabricated, includes fitting and adjustment ⓑ Qp Qh ⅟   A

✳ **L1920** Ankle foot orthosis, single upright with static or adjustable stop (Phelps or Perlstein type), custom-fabricated ⓑ Qp Qh ⅟   A

✳ **L1930** Ankle-foot orthosis, plastic or other material, prefabricated, includes fitting and adjustment ⓑ Qp Qh ⅟   A

✳ **L1932** AFO, rigid anterior tibial section, total carbon fiber or equal material, prefabricated, includes fitting and adjustment ⓑ Qp Qh ⅟   A

PQRS PQRS	Qp Quantity Physician Appendix A	Qh Quantity Hospital Appendix B	♀ Female only
♂ Male only	A Age	⅟ DMEPOS	A2-Z3 ASC Payment Indicator	A-Y ASC Status Indicator	Coding Clinic

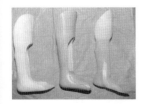

Figure 30 Ankle foot orthosis (AFO).

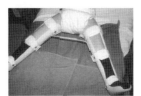

Figure 31 Knee ankle foot orthosis (KAFO).

* **L1940** Ankle foot orthosis, plastic or other material, custom-fabricated ⑧ Qp Qh 🔥   A

* **L1945** Ankle foot orthosis, plastic, rigid anterior tibial section (floor reaction), custom-fabricated ⑧ Qp Qh 🔥   A

* **L1950** Ankle foot orthosis, spiral, (Institute of Rehabilitation Medicine type), plastic, custom-fabricated ⑧ Qp Qh 🔥   A

* **L1951** Ankle foot orthosis, spiral, (Institute of Rehabilitative Medicine type), plastic or other material, prefabricated, includes fitting and adjustment ⑧ Qp Qh 🔥   A

* **L1960** Ankle foot orthosis, posterior solid ankle, plastic, custom-fabricated ⑧ Qp Qh 🔥   A

* **L1970** Ankle foot orthosis, plastic, with ankle joint, custom-fabricated ⑧ Qp Qh 🔥   A

* **L1971** Ankle foot orthosis, plastic or other material with ankle joint, prefabricated, includes fitting and adjustment ⑧ Qp Qh 🔥   A

* **L1980** Ankle foot orthosis, single upright free plantar dorsiflexion, solid stirrup, calf band/cuff (single bar 'BK' orthosis), custom-fabricated ⑧ Qp Qh 🔥   A

* **L1990** Ankle foot orthosis, double upright free plantar dorsiflexion, solid stirrup, calf band/cuff (double bar 'BK' orthosis), custom-fabricated ⑧ Qp Qh 🔥   A

Hip-Knee-Ankle-Foot (or Any Combination)

NOTE: L2000, L2020, and L2036 are base procedures to be used with any knee joint. L2010 and L2030 are to be used only with no knee joint.

* **L2000** Knee ankle foot orthosis, single upright, free knee, free ankle, solid stirrup, thigh and calf bands/cuffs (single bar 'AK' orthosis), custom-fabricated ⑧ Qp Qh 🔥   A

* **L2005** Knee ankle foot orthosis, any material, single or double upright, stance control, automatic lock and swing phase release, any type activation; includes ankle joint, any type, custom fabricated ⑧ Qp Qh 🔥   A

* **L2010** Knee ankle foot orthosis, single upright, free ankle, solid stirrup, thigh and calf bands/cuffs (single bar 'AK' orthosis), without knee joint, custom-fabricated ⑧ Qp Qh 🔥   A

* **L2020** Knee ankle foot orthosis, double upright, free knee, free ankle, solid stirrup, thigh and calf bands/cuffs (double bar 'AK' orthosis), custom-fabricated ⑧ Qp Qh 🔥   A

* **L2030** Knee ankle foot orthosis, double upright, free ankle, solid stirrup, thigh and calf bands/cuffs (double bar 'AK' orthosis), without knee joint, custom fabricated ⑧ Qp Qh 🔥   A

* **L2034** Knee ankle foot orthosis, full plastic, single upright, with or without free motion knee, medial lateral rotation control, with or without free motion ankle, custom fabricated ⑧ Qp Qh 🔥   A

* **L2035** Knee ankle foot orthosis, full plastic, static (pediatric size), without free motion ankle, prefabricated, includes fitting and adjustment ⑧ Qp Qh A 🔥   A

* **L2036** Knee ankle foot orthosis, full plastic, double upright, with or without free motion knee, with or without free motion ankle, custom fabricated ⑧ Qp Qh 🔥   A

* **L2037** Knee ankle foot orthosis, full plastic, single upright, with or without free motion knee, with or without free motion ankle, custom fabricated ⑧ Qp Qh 🔥   A

* **L2038** Knee ankle foot orthosis, full plastic, with or without free motion knee, multi-axis ankle, custom fabricated ⑧ Qp Qh 🔥   A

Torsion Control

* **L2040** Hip knee ankle foot orthosis, torsion control, bilateral rotation straps, pelvic band/belt, custom fabricated ⑧ Qp Qh 🔥   A

* **L2050** Hip knee ankle foot orthosis, torsion control, bilateral torsion cables, hip joint, pelvic band/belt, custom-fabricated ⑧ Qp Qh 🔥   A

▶ New   ↻ Revised   ✔ Reinstated   ~~deleted~~ Deleted   ⃠ Not covered or valid by Medicare

○ Special coverage instructions   * Carrier discretion   ⑧ Bill local carrier   ⑥ Bill DME MAC

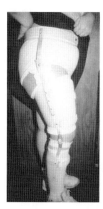

Figure 32 Hip-knee-ankle-foot orthosis (HKAFO).

* **L2060**   Hip knee ankle foot orthosis, torsion control, bilateral torsion cables, ball bearing hip joint, pelvic band/belt, custom-fabricated Ⓑ Qp Qh &   A

* **L2070**   Hip knee ankle foot orthosis, torsion control, unilateral rotation straps, pelvic band/belt, custom-fabricated Ⓑ Qp Qh &   A

* **L2080**   Hip knee ankle foot orthosis, torsion control, unilateral torsion cable, hip joint, pelvic band/belt, custom-fabricated Ⓑ Qp Qh &   A

* **L2090**   Hip knee ankle foot orthosis, torsion control, unilateral torsion cable, ball bearing hip joint, pelvic band/belt, custom-fabricated Ⓑ Qp Qh &   A

Fracture Orthoses

* **L2106**   Ankle foot orthosis, fracture orthosis, tibial fracture cast orthosis, thermoplastic type casting material, custom-fabricated Ⓑ Qp Qh &   A

* **L2108**   Ankle foot orthosis, fracture orthosis, tibial fracture cast orthosis, custom-fabricated Ⓑ Qp Qh &   A

* **L2112**   Ankle foot orthosis, fracture orthosis, tibial fracture orthosis, soft, prefabricated, includes fitting and adjustment Ⓑ Qp Qh &   A

* **L2114**   Ankle foot orthosis, fracture orthosis, tibial fracture orthosis, semi-rigid, prefabricated, includes fitting and adjustment Ⓑ Qp Qh &   A

* **L2116**   Ankle foot orthosis, fracture orthosis, tibial fracture orthosis, rigid, prefabricated, includes fitting and adjustment Ⓑ Qp Qh &   A

* **L2126**   Knee ankle foot orthosis, fracture orthosis, femoral fracture cast orthosis, thermoplastic type casting material, custom-fabricated Ⓑ Qp Qh &   A

* **L2128**   Knee ankle foot orthosis, fracture orthosis, femoral fracture cast orthosis, custom-fabricated Ⓑ Qp Qh &   A

* **L2132**   KAFO, femoral fracture cast orthosis, soft, prefabricated, includes fitting and adjustment Ⓑ Qp Qh &   A

* **L2134**   KAFO, femoral fracture cast orthosis, semi-rigid, prefabricated, includes fitting and adjustment Ⓑ Qp Qh &   A

* **L2136**   KAFO, fracture orthosis, femoral fracture cast orthosis, rigid, prefabricated, includes fitting and adjustment Ⓑ Qp Qh &   A

Additions to Fracture Orthosis

* **L2180**   Addition to lower extremity fracture orthosis, plastic shoe insert with ankle joints Ⓑ Qp Qh &   A

* **L2182**   Addition to lower extremity fracture orthosis, drop lock knee joint Ⓑ Qp Qh &   A

* **L2184**   Addition to lower extremity fracture orthosis, limited motion knee joint Ⓑ Qp Qh &   A

* **L2186**   Addition to lower extremity fracture orthosis, adjustable motion knee joint, Lerman type Ⓑ Qp Qh &   A

* **L2188**   Addition to lower extremity fracture orthosis, quadrilateral brim Ⓑ Qp Qh &   A

* **L2190**   Addition to lower extremity fracture orthosis, waist belt Ⓑ Qp Qh &   A

* **L2192**   Addition to lower extremity fracture orthosis, hip joint, pelvic band, thigh flange, and pelvic belt Ⓑ Qp Qh &   A

Additions to Lower Extremity Orthosis

Shoe-Ankle-Shin-Knee

* **L2200**   Addition to lower extremity, limited ankle motion, each joint Ⓑ Qp Qh &   A

* **L2210**   Addition to lower extremity, dorsiflexion assist (plantar flexion resist), each joint Ⓑ Qp Qh &   A

* **L2220**   Addition to lower extremity, dorsiflexion and plantar flexion assist/resist, each joint Ⓑ Qp Qh &   A

* **L2230**   Addition to lower extremity, split flat caliper stirrups and plate attachment Ⓑ Qp Qh &   A

ᴾ◯ᴿˢ **PQRS**   Qp **Quantity Physician Appendix A**   Qh **Quantity Hospital Appendix B**   ♀ **Female only**

♂ **Male only**   A **Age**   & **DMEPOS**   A2-Z3 **ASC Payment Indicator**   A-Y **ASC Status Indicator**   Coding Clinic

* **L2232** Addition to lower extremity orthosis, rocker bottom for total contact ankle foot orthosis, for custom fabricated orthosis only ⑧ Qp Qh ♿   A

* **L2240** Addition to lower extremity, round caliper and plate attachment ⑧ Qp Qh ♿   A

* **L2250** Addition to lower extremity, foot plate, molded to patient model, stirrup attachment ⑧ Qp Qh ♿   A

* **L2260** Addition to lower extremity, reinforced solid stirrup (Scott-Craig type) ⑧ Qp Qh ♿   A

* **L2265** Addition to lower extremity, long tongue stirrup ⑧ Qp Qh ♿   A

* **L2270** Addition to lower extremity, varus/ valgus correction ('T') strap, padded/lined or malleolus pad ⑧ Qp Qh ♿   A

* **L2275** Addition to lower extremity, varus/ valgus correction, plastic modification, padded/lined ⑧ Qp Qh ♿   A

* **L2280** Addition to lower extremity, molded inner boot ⑧ Qp Qh ♿   A

* **L2300** Addition to lower extremity, abduction bar (bilateral hip involvement), jointed, adjustable ⑧ Qp Qh ♿   A

* **L2310** Addition to lower extremity, abduction bar-straight ⑧ Qp Qh ♿   A

* **L2320** Addition to lower extremity, non-molded lacer, for custom fabricated orthosis only ⑧ Qp Qh ♿   A

* **L2330** Addition to lower extremity, lacer molded to patient model, for custom fabricated orthosis only ⑧ Qp Qh ♿   A

      Used whether closure is lacer or Velcro

* **L2335** Addition to lower extremity, anterior swing band ⑧ Qp Qh ♿   A

* **L2340** Addition to lower extremity, pre-tibial shell, molded to patient model ⑧ Qp Qh ♿   A

* **L2350** Addition to lower extremity, prosthetic type, (BK) socket, molded to patient model, (used for 'PTB' and 'AFO' orthoses) ⑧ Qp Qh ♿   A

* **L2360** Addition to lower extremity, extended steel shank ⑧ Qp Qh ♿   A

* **L2370** Addition to lower extremity, Patten bottom ⑧ Qp Qh ♿   A

* **L2375** Addition to lower extremity, torsion control, ankle joint and half solid stirrup ⑧ Qp Qh ♿   A

* **L2380** Addition to lower extremity, torsion control, straight knee joint, each joint ⑧ Qp Qh ♿   A

* **L2385** Addition to lower extremity, straight knee joint, heavy duty, each joint ⑧ Qp ♿   A

* **L2387** Addition to lower extremity, polycentric knee joint, for custom fabricated knee ankle foot orthosis, each joint ⑧ Qp ♿   A

* **L2390** Addition to lower extremity, offset knee joint, each joint ⑧ Qp ♿   A

* **L2395** Addition to lower extremity, offset knee joint, heavy duty, each joint ⑧ Qp ♿   A

* **L2397** Addition to lower extremity orthosis, suspension sleeve ⑧ Qp ♿   A

Additions to Straight Knee or Offset Knee Joints

* **L2405** Addition to knee joint, drop lock, each ⑧ Qp ♿   A

* **L2415** Addition to knee lock with integrated release mechanism (bail, cable, or equal), any material, each joint ⑧ Qp ♿   A

* **L2425** Addition to knee joint, disc or dial lock for adjustable knee flexion, each joint ⑧ Qp ♿   A

* **L2430** Addition to knee joint, ratchet lock for active and progressive knee extension, each joint ⑧ Qp ♿   A

* **L2492** Addition to knee joint, lift loop for drop lock ring ⑧ Qp ♿   A

Additions to Thigh/Weight Bearing

Gluteal/Ischial Weight Bearing

* **L2500** Addition to lower extremity, thigh/ weight bearing, gluteal/ischial weight bearing, ring ⑧ Qp Qh ♿   A

* **L2510** Addition to lower extremity, thigh/ weight bearing, quadri-lateral brim, molded to patient model ⑧ Qp Qh ♿   A

* **L2520** Addition to lower extremity, thigh/ weight bearing, quadri-lateral brim, custom fitted ⑧ Qp Qh ♿   A

* **L2525** Addition to lower extremity, thigh/ weight bearing, ischial containment/ narrow M-L brim molded to patient model ⑧ Qp Qh ♿   A

* **L2526** Addition to lower extremity, thigh/ weight bearing, ischial containment/ narrow M-L brim, custom fitted ⑧ Qp Qh ♿   A

▶ New   ⟳ Revised   ✔ Reinstated   ~~deleted~~ Deleted   ⊘ Not covered or valid by Medicare

⊛ Special coverage instructions   ✳ Carrier discretion   ⑧ Bill local carrier   ⑧ Bill DME MAC

※ **L2530** Addition to lower extremity, thigh-weight bearing, lacer, non-molded ⑧ Qp Qh ⛷   A

※ **L2540** Addition to lower extremity, thigh/weight bearing, lacer, molded to patient model ⑧ Qp Qh ⛷   A

※ **L2550** Addition to lower extremity, thigh/weight bearing, high roll cuff ⑧ Qp Qh ⛷   A

Additions to Pelvic and Thoracic Control

※ **L2570** Addition to lower extremity, pelvic control, hip joint, Clevis type two position joint, each ⑧ Qp Qh ⛷   A

※ **L2580** Addition to lower extremity, pelvic control, pelvic sling ⑧ Qp Qh ⛷   A

※ **L2600** Addition to lower extremity, pelvic control, hip joint, Clevis type, or thrust bearing, free, each ⑧ Qp Qh ⛷   A

※ **L2610** Addition to lower extremity, pelvic control, hip joint, Clevis or thrust bearing, lock, each ⑧ Qp Qh ⛷   A

※ **L2620** Addition to lower extremity, pelvic control, hip joint, heavy duty, each ⑧ Qp Qh ⛷   A

※ **L2622** Addition to lower extremity, pelvic control, hip joint, adjustable flexion, each ⑧ Qp Qh ⛷   A

※ **L2624** Addition to lower extremity, pelvic control, hip joint, adjustable flexion, extension, abduction control, each ⑧ Qp Qh ⛷   A

※ **L2627** Addition to lower extremity, pelvic control, plastic, molded to patient model, reciprocating hip joint and cables ⑧ Qp Qh ⛷   A

※ **L2628** Addition to lower extremity, pelvic control, metal frame, reciprocating hip joint and cables ⑧ Qp Qh ⛷   A

※ **L2630** Addition to lower extremity, pelvic control, band and belt, unilateral ⑧ Qp Qh ⛷   A

※ **L2640** Addition to lower extremity, pelvic control, band and belt, bilateral ⑧ Qp Qh ⛷   A

※ **L2650** Addition to lower extremity, pelvic and thoracic control, gluteal pad, each ⑧ Qp Qh ⛷   A

※ **L2660** Addition to lower extremity, thoracic control, thoracic band ⑧ Qp Qh ⛷   A

※ **L2670** Addition to lower extremity, thoracic control, paraspinal uprights ⑧ Qp Qh ⛷   A

※ **L2680** Addition to lower extremity, thoracic control, lateral support uprights ⑧ Qp Qh ⛷   A

General Additions

※ **L2750** Addition to lower extremity orthosis, plating chrome or nickel, per bar ⑧ Qp ⛷   A

※ **L2755** Addition to lower extremity orthosis, high strength, lightweight material, all hybrid lamination/prepreg composite, per segment, for custom fabricated orthosis only ⑧ Qp ⛷   A

※ **L2760** Addition to lower extremity orthosis, extension, per extension, per bar (for lineal adjustment for growth) ⑧ Qp ⛷   A

※ **L2768** Orthotic side bar disconnect device, per bar ⑧ Qp ⛷   A

※ **L2780** Addition to lower extremity orthosis, non-corrosive finish, per bar ⑧ Qp ⛷   A

※ **L2785** Addition to lower extremity orthosis, drop lock retainer, each ⑧ Qp ⛷   A

※ **L2795** Addition to lower extremity orthosis, knee control, full kneecap ⑧ Qp Qh ⛷   A

※ **L2800** Addition to lower extremity orthosis, knee control, knee cap, medial or lateral pull, for use with custom fabricated orthosis only ⑧ Qp Qh ⛷   A

※ **L2810** Addition to lower extremity orthosis, knee control, condylar pad ⑧ Qp ⛷   A

※ **L2820** Addition to lower extremity orthosis, soft interface for molded plastic, below knee section ⑧ Qp Qh ⛷   A

Only report if soft interface provided, either leather or other material

※ **L2830** Addition to lower extremity orthosis, soft interface for molded plastic, above knee section ⑧ Qp Qh ⛷   A

※ **L2840** Addition to lower extremity orthosis, tibial length sock, fracture or equal, each ⑧ ⛷   A

※ **L2850** Addition to lower extremity orthosis, femoral length sock, fracture or equal, each ⑧ ⛷   A

⊘ **L2861** Addition to lower extremity joint, knee or ankle, concentric adjustable torsion style mechanism for custom fabricated orthotics only, each ⑧   E

※ **L2999** Lower extremity orthoses, not otherwise specified ⑧   A

| PQRS PQRS | Qp Quantity Physician Appendix A | Qh Quantity Hospital Appendix B | ♀ Female only |
| ♂ Male only | A Age | ⛷ DMEPOS | A2-Z3 ASC Payment Indicator | A-Y ASC Status Indicator | Coding Clinic |

ORTHOTICS   L2530 – L2999

307

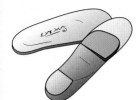

Figure 33 Foot inserts.

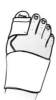

Figure 35 Hallux valgus splint.

Foot (Orthopedic Shoes)

Insert, Removable, Molded to Patient Model

⊛ **L3000** Foot, insert, removable, molded to patient model, 'UCB' type, Berkeley shell, each Ⓑ Qp Qh ⅖   A

If both feet casted and supplied with an orthosis, bill L3000-LT and L3000-RT

IOM: 100-02, 15, 290

⊛ **L3001** Foot, insert, removable, molded to patient model, Spenco, each Ⓑ Qp Qh ⅖   A

IOM: 100-02, 15, 290

⊛ **L3002** Foot, insert, removable, molded to patient model, Plastazote or equal, each Ⓑ Qp Qh ⅖   A

IOM: 100-02, 15, 290

⊛ **L3003** Foot, insert, removable, molded to patient model, silicone gel, each Ⓑ Qp Qh ⅖   A

IOM: 100-02, 15, 290

⊛ **L3010** Foot, insert, removable, molded to patient model, longitudinal arch support, each Ⓑ Qp Qh ⅖   A

IOM: 100-02, 15, 290

⊛ **L3020** Foot, insert, removable, molded to patient model, longitudinal/metatarsal support, each Ⓑ Qp Qh ⅖   A

IOM: 100-02, 15, 290

⊛ **L3030** Foot, insert, removable, formed to patient foot, each Ⓑ Qp Qh ⅖   A

IOM: 100-02, 15, 290

✳ **L3031** Foot, insert/plate, removable, addition to lower extremity orthosis, high strength, lightweight material, all hybrid lamination/prepreg composite, each Ⓑ Qp Qh ⅖   A

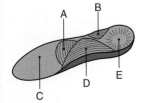

Figure 34 Arch support.

Arch Support, Removable, Premolded

⊛ **L3040** Foot, arch support, removable, premolded, longitudinal, each Ⓑ Qp Qh ⅖   A

IOM: 100-02, 15, 290

⊛ **L3050** Foot, arch support, removable, premolded, metatarsal, each Ⓑ Qp Qh ⅖   A

IOM: 100-02, 15, 290

⊛ **L3060** Foot, arch support, removable, premolded, longitudinal/metatarsal, each Ⓑ Qp Qh ⅖   A

IOM: 100-02, 15, 290

Arch Support, Non-removable, Attached to Shoe

⊛ **L3070** Foot, arch support, non-removable attached to shoe, longitudinal, each Ⓑ Qp Qh ⅖   A

IOM: 100-02, 15, 290

⊛ **L3080** Foot, arch support, non-removable attached to shoe, metatarsal, each Ⓑ Qp Qh ⅖   A

IOM: 100-02, 15, 290

⊛ **L3090** Foot, arch support, non-removable attached to shoe, longitudinal/metatarsal, each Ⓑ Qp Qh ⅖   A

IOM: 100-02, 15, 290

⊛ **L3100** Hallus-valgus night dynamic splint, prefabricated, off-the-shelf Ⓑ Qp Qh ⅖   A

IOM: 100-02, 15, 290

Abduction and Rotation Bars

⊛ **L3140** Foot, abduction rotation bar, including shoes Ⓑ Qp Qh ⅖   A

IOM: 100-02, 15, 290

⊛ **L3150** Foot, abduction rotation bar, without shoes Ⓑ Qp Qh ⅖   A

IOM: 100-02, 15, 290

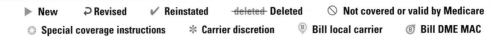

▶ **New**   ⟲ **Revised**   ✔ **Reinstated**   ~~deleted~~ **Deleted**   ⊘ **Not covered or valid by Medicare**
⊛ **Special coverage instructions**   ✳ **Carrier discretion**   Ⓑ **Bill local carrier**   Ⓑ **Bill DME MAC**

* **L3160** Foot, adjustable shoe-styled positioning device ⑧ **Qp** **Qh**   A

⊘ **L3170** Foot, plastic, silicone or equal, heel stabilizer, prefabricated, off-the-shelf, each ⑧ **Qp** **Qh** ⑉   A

IOM: 100-02, 15, 290

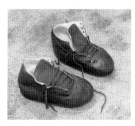

Figure 36   Molded custom shoe.

Orthopedic Footwear

⊛ **L3201** Orthopedic shoe, oxford with supinator or pronator, infant ⑧ **A**   A

IOM: 100-02, 15, 290

⊛ **L3202** Orthopedic shoe, oxford with supinator or pronator, child ⑧ **A**   A

IOM: 100-02, 15, 290

⊛ **L3203** Orthopedic shoe, oxford with supinator or pronator, junior ⑧ **A**   A

IOM: 100-02, 15, 290

⊛ **L3204** Orthopedic shoe, hightop with supinator or pronator, infant ⑧ **A**   A

IOM: 100-02, 15, 290

⊛ **L3206** Orthopedic shoe, hightop with supinator or pronator, child ⑧ **A**   A

IOM: 100-02, 15, 290

⊛ **L3207** Orthopedic shoe, hightop with supinator or pronator, junior ⑧ **A**   A

IOM: 100-02, 15, 290

⊛ **L3208** Surgical boot, infant, each ⑧ **A**   A

IOM: 100-02, 15, 100

⊛ **L3209** Surgical boot, each, child ⑧ **A**   A

IOM: 100-02, 15, 100

⊛ **L3211** Surgical boot, each, junior ⑧ **A**   A

IOM: 100-02, 15, 100

⊛ **L3212** Benesch boot, pair, infant ⑧ **A**   A

IOM: 100-02, 15, 100

⊛ **L3213** Benesch boot, pair, child ⑧ **A**   A

IOM: 100-02, 15, 100

⊛ **L3214** Benesch boot, pair, junior ⑧ **A**   A

IOM: 100-02, 15, 100

⊘ **L3215** Orthopedic footwear, ladies shoe, oxford, each ⑧ **Qp** **Qh** ♀   E

Medicare Statute 1862a8

⊘ **L3216** Orthopedic footwear, ladies shoe, depth inlay, each ⑧ **Qp** **Qh** ♀   E

Medicare Statute 1862a8

⊘ **L3217** Orthopedic footwear, ladies shoe, hightop, depth inlay, each ⑧ **Qp** **Qh** ♀   E

Medicare Statute 1862a8

⊘ **L3219** Orthopedic footwear, mens shoe, oxford, each ⑧ **Qp** **Qh** ♂   E

Medicare Statute 1862a8

⊘ **L3221** Orthopedic footwear, mens shoe, depth inlay, each ⑧ **Qp** **Qh** ♂   E

Medicare Statute 1862a8

⊘ **L3222** Orthopedic footwear, mens shoe, hightop, depth inlay, each ⑧ **Qp** **Qh** ♂   E

Medicare Statute 1862a8

⊛ **L3224** Orthopedic footwear, ladies shoe, oxford, used as an integral part of a brace (orthosis) ⑧ **Qp** **Qh** ♀ ⑉   A

IOM: 100-02, 15, 290

⊛ **L3225** Orthopedic footwear, mens shoe, oxford, used as an integral part of a brace (orthosis) ⑧ **Qp** **Qh** ♀ ⑉   A

IOM: 100-02, 15, 290

⊛ **L3230** Orthopedic footwear, custom shoe, depth inlay, each ⑧ **Qp** **Qh**   A

IOM: 100-02, 15, 290

⊛ **L3250** Orthopedic footwear, custom molded shoe, removable inner mold, prosthetic shoe, each ⑧ **Qp** **Qh**   A

IOM: 100-02, 15, 290

⊛ **L3251** Foot, shoe molded to patient model, silicone shoe, each ⑧ **Qp** **Qh**   A

IOM: 100-02, 15, 290

⊛ **L3252** Foot, shoe molded to patient model, Plastazote (or similar), custom fabricated, each ⑧ **Qp** **Qh**   A

IOM: 100-02, 15, 290

⊛ **L3253** Foot, molded shoe Plastazote (or similar), custom fitted, each ⑧ **Qp** **Qh**   A

IOM: 100-02, 15, 290

⊛ **L3254** Non-standard size or width ⑧   A

IOM: 100-02, 15, 290

⊛ **L3255** Non-standard size or length ⑧   A

IOM: 100-02, 15, 290

PQRS   **Qp** Quantity Physician Appendix A   **Qh** Quantity Hospital Appendix B   ♀ Female only
♂ **Male only**   **A** Age   ⑉ DMEPOS   A2-Z3 ASC Payment Indicator   A-Y ASC Status Indicator   Coding Clinic

⊙ **L3257** Orthopedic footwear, additional charge for split size ⑧   A

IOM: 100-02, 15, 290

⊙ **L3260** Surgical boot/shoe, each ⑧   E

IOM: 100-02, 15, 100

✳ **L3265** Plastazote sandal, each ⑧   A

Shoe Modifications

Lifts

⊙ **L3300** Lift, elevation, heel, tapered to metatarsals, per inch ⑧ Qp   A

IOM: 100-02, 15, 290

⊙ **L3310** Lift, elevation, heel and sole, Neoprene, per inch ⑧ Qp   A

IOM: 100-02, 15, 290

⊙ **L3320** Lift, elevation, heel and sole, cork, per inch ⑧   A

IOM: 100-02, 15, 290

⊙ **L3330** Lift, elevation, metal extension (skate) ⑧ Qp Qh   A

IOM: 100-02, 15, 290

⊙ **L3332** Lift, elevation, inside shoe, tapered, up to one-half inch ⑧ Qp Qh   A

IOM: 100-02, 15, 290

⊙ **L3334** Lift, elevation, heel, per inch ⑧ Qp   A

IOM: 100-02, 15, 290

Wedges

⊙ **L3340** Heel wedge, SACH ⑧ Qp Qh   A

IOM: 100-02, 15, 290

⊙ **L3350** Heel wedge ⑧ Qp Qh   A

IOM: 100-02, 15, 290

⊙ **L3360** Sole wedge, outside sole ⑧ Qp Qh   A

IOM: 100-02, 15, 290

⊙ **L3370** Sole wedge, between sole ⑧ Qp Qh   A

IOM: 100-02, 15, 290

⊙ **L3380** Clubfoot wedge ⑧ Qp Qh   A

IOM: 100-02, 15, 290

⊙ **L3390** Outflare wedge ⑧ Qp Qh   A

IOM: 100-02, 15, 290

⊙ **L3400** Metatarsal bar wedge, rocker ⑧ Qp Qh   A

IOM: 100-02, 15, 290

⊙ **L3410** Metatarsal bar wedge, between sole ⑧ Qp Qh   A

IOM: 100-02, 15, 290

⊙ **L3420** Full sole and heel wedge, between sole ⑧ Qp Qh   A

IOM: 100-02, 15, 290

Heels

⊙ **L3430** Heel, counter, plastic reinforced ⑧ Qp Qh   A

IOM: 100-02, 15, 290

⊙ **L3440** Heel, counter, leather reinforced ⑧ Qp Qh   A

IOM: 100-02, 15, 290

⊙ **L3450** Heel, SACH cushion type ⑧ Qp Qh   A

IOM: 100-02, 15, 290

⊙ **L3455** Heel, new leather, standard ⑧ Qp Qh   A

IOM: 100-02, 15, 290

⊙ **L3460** Heel, new rubber, standard ⑧ Qp Qh   A

IOM: 100-02, 15, 290

⊙ **L3465** Heel, Thomas with wedge ⑧ Qp Qh   A

IOM: 100-02, 15, 290

⊙ **L3470** Heel, Thomas extended to ball ⑧ Qp Qh   A

IOM: 100-02, 15, 290

⊙ **L3480** Heel, pad and depression for spur ⑧ Qp Qh   A

IOM: 100-02, 15, 290

⊙ **L3485** Heel, pad, removable for spur ⑧ Qp Qh   A

IOM: 100-02, 15, 290

Additions to Orthopedic Shoes

⊙ **L3500** Orthopedic shoe addition, insole, leather ⑧ Qp Qh   A

IOM: 100-02, 15, 290

⊙ **L3510** Orthopedic shoe addition, insole, rubber ⑧ Qp Qh   A

IOM: 100-02, 15, 290

⊙ **L3520** Orthopedic shoe addition, insole, felt covered with leather ⑧ Qp Qh   A

IOM: 100-02, 15, 290

⊙ **L3530** Orthopedic shoe addition, sole, half ⑧ Qp Qh   A

IOM: 100-02, 15, 290

▶ **New**   ↻ **Revised**   ✔ **Reinstated**   ~~deleted~~ **Deleted**   ⊘ **Not covered or valid by Medicare**

⊙ **Special coverage instructions**   ✳ **Carrier discretion**   ⑧ **Bill local carrier**   ⑧ **Bill DME MAC**

⊛ **L3540** Orthopedic shoe addition, sole, full Ⓑ Qp Qh &   A

IOM: 100-02, 15, 290

⊛ **L3550** Orthopedic shoe addition, toe tap standard Ⓑ Qp Qh &   A

IOM: 100-02, 15, 290

⊛ **L3560** Orthopedic shoe addition, toe tap, horseshoe Ⓑ Qp Qh &   A

IOM: 100-02, 15, 290

⊛ **L3570** Orthopedic shoe addition, special extension to instep (leather with eyelets) Ⓑ Qp Qh &   A

IOM: 100-02, 15, 290

⊛ **L3580** Orthopedic shoe addition, convert instep to Velcro closure Ⓑ Qp Qh &   A

IOM: 100-02, 15, 290

⊛ **L3590** Orthopedic shoe addition, convert firm shoe counter to soft counter Ⓑ Qp Qh &   A

IOM: 100-02, 15, 290

⊛ **L3595** Orthopedic shoe addition, March bar Ⓑ Qp Qh &   A

IOM: 100-02, 15, 290

Transfer or Replacement

⊛ **L3600** Transfer of an orthosis from one shoe to another, caliper plate, existing Ⓑ Qp Qh &   A

IOM: 100-02, 15, 290

⊛ **L3610** Transfer of an orthosis from one shoe to another, caliper plate, new Ⓑ Qp Qh &   A

IOM: 100-02, 15, 290

⊛ **L3620** Transfer of an orthosis from one shoe to another, solid stirrup, existing Ⓑ Qp Qh &   A

IOM: 100-02, 15, 290

⊛ **L3630** Transfer of an orthosis from one shoe to another, solid stirrup, new Ⓑ Qp Qh &   A

IOM: 100-02, 15, 290

⊛ **L3640** Transfer of an orthosis from one shoe to another, Dennis Browne splint (Riveton), both shoes Ⓑ Qp Qh &   A

IOM: 100-02, 15, 290

⊛ **L3649** Orthopedic shoe, modification, addition or transfer, not otherwise specified Ⓑ   A

IOM: 100-02, 15, 290

Orthotic Devices: Upper Limb

NOTE: The procedures in this section are considered as base or basic procedures and may be modified by listing procedures from the Additions section and adding them to the base procedure.

Shoulder

✳ **L3650** Shoulder orthosis, figure of eight design abduction restrainer, prefabricated, off-the-shelf Ⓑ Qp Qh &   A

✳ **L3660** Shoulder orthosis, figure of eight design abduction restrainer, canvas and webbing, prefabricated, off-the-shelf Ⓑ Qp Qh &   A

✳ **L3670** Shoulder orthosis, acromio/clavicular (canvas and webbing type), prefabricated, off-the-shelf Ⓑ Qp Qh &   A

✳ **L3671** Shoulder orthosis, shoulder joint design, without joints, may include soft interface, straps, custom fabricated, includes fitting and adjustment Ⓑ Qp Qh &   A

✳ **L3674** Shoulder orthosis, abduction positioning (airplane design), thoracic component and support bar, with or without nontorsion joint/turnbuckle, may include soft interface, straps, custom fabricated, includes fitting and adjustment Ⓑ Qp Qh   A

✳ **L3675** Shoulder orthosis, vest type abduction restrainer, canvas webbing type or equal, prefabricated, off-the-shelf Ⓑ Qp Qh &   A

⊛ **L3677** Shoulder orthosis, shoulder joint design, without joints, may include soft interface, straps, prefabricated item that has been trimmed, bent, molded, assembled, or otherwise customized to fit a specific patient by an individual with expertise Ⓑ Qp Qh   A

✳ **L3678** Shoulder orthosis, shoulder joint design, without joints, may include soft interface, straps, prefabricated, off-the-shelf Ⓑ Qp Qh   A

Elbow

✳ **L3702** Elbow orthosis, without joints, may include soft interface, straps, custom fabricated, includes fitting and adjustment Ⓑ Qp Qh &   A

✳ **L3710** Elbow orthosis, elastic with metal joints, prefabricated, off-the-shelf Ⓑ Qp Qh &   A

| ⊛ PQRS | Qp Quantity Physician Appendix A | Qh Quantity Hospital Appendix B | ♀ Female only |
| ♂ Male only | A Age | & DMEPOS | A2-Z3 ASC Payment Indicator | A-Y ASC Status Indicator | Coding Clinic |

ORTHOTICS L3540 – L3710

311

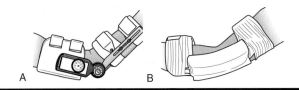

Figure 37 Elbow orthoses.

✳ **L3720** Elbow orthosis, double upright with forearm/arm cuffs, free motion, custom-fabricated Ⓑ Qp Qh &   A

✳ **L3730** Elbow orthosis, double upright with forearm/arm cuffs, extension/flexion assist, custom-fabricated Ⓑ Qp Qh &   A

✳ **L3740** Elbow orthosis, double upright with forearm/arm cuffs, adjustable position lock with active control, custom-fabricated Ⓑ Qp Qh &   A

✳ **L3760** Elbow orthosis, with adjustable position locking joint(s), prefabricated, includes fitting and adjustments, any type Ⓑ Qp Qh &   A

✳ **L3762** Elbow orthosis, rigid, without joints, includes soft interface material, prefabricated, off-the-shelf Ⓑ Qp Qh &   A

✳ **L3763** Elbow wrist hand orthosis, rigid, without joints, may include soft interface, straps, custom fabricated, includes fitting and adjustment Ⓑ Qp Qh &   A

✳ **L3764** Elbow wrist hand orthosis, includes one or more nontorsion joints, elastic bands, turnbuckles, may include soft interface, straps, custom fabricated, includes fitting and adjustment Ⓑ Qp Qh &   A

✳ **L3765** Elbow wrist hand finger orthosis, rigid, without joints, may include soft interface, straps, custom fabricated, includes fitting and adjustment Ⓑ Qp Qh &   A

✳ **L3766** Elbow wrist hand finger orthosis, includes one or more nontorsion joints, elastic bands, turnbuckles, may include soft interface, straps, custom fabricated, includes fitting and adjustment Ⓑ Qp Qh &   A

Wrist-Hand-Finger Orthosis (WHFO)

✳ **L3806** Wrist hand finger orthosis, includes one or more nontorsion joint(s), turnbuckles, elastic bands/springs, may include soft interface material, straps, custom fabricated, includes fitting and adjustment Ⓑ Qp Qh &   A

✳ **L3807** Wrist hand finger orthosis, without joint(s), prefabricated item that has been trimmed, bent, molded, assembled, or otherwise customized to fit a specific patient by an individual with expertise Ⓑ Qp Qh &   A

✳ **L3808** Wrist hand finger orthosis, rigid without joints, may include soft interface material; straps, custom fabricated, includes fitting and adjustment Ⓑ Qp Qh &   A

✳ **L3809** Wrist hand finger orthosis, without joint(s), prefabricated, off-the-shelf, any type Ⓑ Qp Qh   A

Additions and Extensions

⊘ **L3891** Addition to upper extremity joint, wrist or elbow, concentric adjustable torsion style mechanism for custom fabricated orthotics only, each Ⓑ   E

✳ **L3900** Wrist hand finger orthosis, dynamic flexor hinge, reciprocal wrist extension/flexion, finger flexion/extension, wrist or finger driven, custom-fabricated Ⓑ Qp Qh &   A

✳ **L3901** Wrist hand finger orthosis, dynamic flexor hinge, reciprocal wrist extension/flexion, finger flexion/extension, cable driven, custom-fabricated Ⓑ Qp Qh &   A

External Power

✳ **L3904** Wrist hand finger orthosis, external powered, electric, custom-fabricated Ⓑ Qp Qh &   A

✳ **L3905** Wrist hand orthosis, includes one or more nontorsion joints, elastic bands, turnbuckles, may include soft interface, straps, custom fabricated, includes fitting and adjustment Ⓑ Qp Qh &   A

Other Wrist-Hand-Finger Orthoses: Custom Fitted

✳ **L3906** Wrist hand orthosis, without joints, may include soft interface, straps, custom fabricated, includes fitting and adjustment Ⓑ Qp Qh &   A

✳ **L3908** Wrist hand orthosis, wrist extension control cock-up, non-molded, prefabricated, off-the-shelf Ⓑ Qp Qh &   A

✳ **L3912** Hand finger orthosis (HFO), flexion glove with elastic finger control, prefabricated, off-the-shelf Ⓑ Qp Qh &   A

▶ New   ⟳ Revised   ✔ Reinstated   ~~deleted~~ Deleted   ⊘ Not covered or valid by Medicare

⊙ Special coverage instructions   ✳ Carrier discretion   Ⓑ Bill local carrier   Ⓑ Bill DME MAC

✳ **L3913** Hand finger orthosis, without joints, may include soft interface, straps, custom fabricated, includes fitting and adjustment Ⓑ Ⓠp Ⓠh 🦽   A

✳ **L3915** Wrist hand orthosis, includes one or more nontorsion joint(s), elastic bands, turnbuckles, may include soft interface, straps, prefabricated item that has been trimmed, bent, molded, assembled, or otherwise customized to fit a specific patient by an individual with expertise Ⓑ Ⓠp Ⓠh 🦽   A

✳ **L3916** Wrist hand orthosis, includes one or more nontorsion joint(s), elastic bands, turnbuckles, may include soft interface, straps, prefabricated, off-the-shelf Ⓑ Ⓠp Ⓠh   A

✳ **L3917** Hand orthosis, metacarpal fracture orthosis, prefabricated item that has been trimmed, bent, molded, assembled, or otherwise customized to fit a specific patient by an individual with expertise Ⓑ Ⓠp Ⓠh 🦽   A

✳ **L3918** Hand orthosis, metacarpal fracture orthosis, prefabricated, off-the-shelf Ⓑ Ⓠp Ⓠh   A

✳ **L3919** Hand orthosis, without joints, may include soft interface, straps, custom fabricated, includes fitting and adjustment Ⓑ Ⓠp Ⓠh 🦽   A

✳ **L3921** Hand finger orthosis, includes one or more nontorsion joints, elastic bands, turnbuckles, may include soft interface, straps, custom fabricated, includes fitting and adjustment Ⓑ Ⓠp Ⓠh 🦽   A

✳ **L3923** Hand finger orthosis, without joints, may include soft interface, straps, prefabricated item that has been trimmed, bent, molded, assembled, or otherwise customized to fit a specific patient by an individual with expertise Ⓑ Ⓠp Ⓠh 🦽   A

✳ **L3924** Hand finger orthosis, without joints, may include soft interface, straps, prefabricated, off-the-shelf Ⓑ Ⓠp Ⓠh   A

✳ **L3925** Finger orthosis, proximal interphalangeal (PIP)/distal interphalangeal (DIP), non torsion joint/spring, extension/flexion, may include soft interface material, prefabricated, off-the-shelf Ⓑ Ⓠp Ⓠh 🦽   A

✳ **L3927** Finger orthosis, proximal interphalangeal (PIP)/distal interphalangeal (DIP), without joint/spring, extension/flexion (e.g. static or ring type), may include soft interface material, prefabricated, off-the-shelf Ⓑ Ⓠp Ⓠh 🦽   A

✳ **L3929** Hand finger orthosis, includes one or more nontorsion joint(s), turnbuckles, elastic bands/springs, may include soft interface material, straps, prefabricated item that has been trimmed, bent, molded, assembled, or otherwise customized to fit a specific patient by an individual with expertise Ⓑ Ⓠp Ⓠh 🦽   A

✳ **L3930** Hand finger orthosis, includes one or more nontorsion joint(s), turnbuckles, elastic bands/springs, may include soft interface material, straps, prefabricated, off-the-shelf Ⓑ Ⓠp Ⓠh   A

✳ **L3931** Wrist hand finger orthosis, includes one or more nontorsion joint(s), turnbuckles, elastic bands/springs, may include soft interface material, straps, prefabricated, includes fitting and adjustment Ⓑ Ⓠp Ⓠh 🦽   A

✳ **L3933** Finger orthosis, without joints, may include soft interface, custom fabricated, includes fitting and adjustment Ⓑ Ⓠp Ⓠh 🦽   A

✳ **L3935** Finger orthosis, nontorsion joint, may include soft interface, custom fabricated, includes fitting and adjustment Ⓑ Ⓠp Ⓠh 🦽   A

✳ **L3956** Addition of joint to upper extremity orthosis, any material, per joint Ⓑ Ⓠp 🦽   A

Shoulder-Elbow-Wrist-Hand Orthosis (SEWHO)

Abduction Positioning: Custom Fitted

✳ **L3960** Shoulder elbow wrist hand orthosis, abduction positioning, airplane design, prefabricated, includes fitting and adjustment Ⓑ Ⓠp Ⓠh 🦽   A

✳ **L3961** Shoulder elbow wrist hand orthosis, shoulder cap design, without joints, may include soft interface, straps, custom fabricated, includes fitting and adjustment Ⓑ Ⓠp Ⓠh 🦽   A

✳ **L3962** Shoulder elbow wrist hand orthosis, abduction positioning, Erbs palsy design, prefabricated, includes fitting and adjustment Ⓑ Ⓠp Ⓠh 🦽   A

| ⓅQRS PQRS | Ⓠp Quantity Physician Appendix A | Ⓠh Quantity Hospital Appendix B | ♀ Female only |
| ♂ Male only | Ⓐ Age | 🦽 DMEPOS | A2-Z3 ASC Payment Indicator | A-Y ASC Status Indicator | Coding Clinic |

313

ORTHOTICS   L3913 — L3962

✳ **L3967** Shoulder elbow wrist hand orthosis, abduction positioning (airplane design), thoracic component and support bar, without joints, may include soft interface, straps, custom fabricated, includes fitting and adjustment Ⓑ Qp Qh ♿   A

Additions to Mobile Arm Supports and SEWHO

✳ **L3971** Shoulder elbow wrist hand orthosis, shoulder cap design, includes one or more nontorsion joints, elastic bands, turnbuckles, may include soft interface, straps, custom fabricated, includes fitting and adjustment Ⓑ Qp Qh ♿   A

✳ **L3973** Shoulder elbow wrist hand orthosis, abduction positioning (airplane design), thoracic component and support bar, includes one or more nontorsion joints, elastic bands, turnbuckles, may include soft interface, straps, custom fabricated, includes fitting and adjustment Ⓑ Qp Qh ♿   A

✳ **L3975** Shoulder elbow wrist hand finger orthosis, shoulder cap design, without joints, may include soft interface, straps, custom fabricated, includes fitting and adjustment Ⓑ Qp Qh ♿   A

✳ **L3976** Shoulder elbow wrist hand finger orthosis, abduction positioning (airplane design), thoracic component and support bar, without joints, may include soft interface, straps, custom fabricated, includes fitting and adjustment Ⓑ Qp Qh ♿   A

✳ **L3977** Shoulder elbow wrist hand finger orthosis, shoulder cap design, includes one or more nontorsion joints, elastic bands, turnbuckles, may include soft interface, straps, custom fabricated, includes fitting and adjustment Ⓑ Qp Qh ♿   A

✳ **L3978** Shoulder elbow wrist hand finger orthosis, abduction positioning (airplane design), thoracic component and support bar, includes one or more nontorsion joints, elastic bands, turnbuckles, may include soft interface, straps, custom fabricated, includes fitting and adjustment Ⓑ Qp Qh ♿   A

Fracture Orthoses

↻✳ **L3980** Upper extremity fracture orthosis, humeral, prefabricated, includes fitting and adjustment Ⓑ Qp Qh ♿   A

▶✳ **L3981** Upper extremity fracture orthosis, humeral, prefabricated, includes shoulder cap design, with or without joints, forearm section, may include soft interface, straps, includes fitting and adjustments   A

✳ **L3982** Upper extremity fracture orthosis, radius/ulnar, prefabricated, includes fitting and adjustment Ⓑ Qp Qh ♿   A

✳ **L3984** Upper extremity fracture orthosis, wrist, prefabricated, includes fitting and adjustment Ⓑ Qp Qh ♿   A

✳ **L3995** Addition to upper extremity orthosis, sock, fracture or equal, each Ⓑ ♿   A

✳ **L3999** Upper limb orthosis, not otherwise specified Ⓑ   A

Specific Repair

✳ **L4000** Replace girdle for spinal orthosis (CTLSO or SO) Ⓑ Qp Qh ♿   A

✳ **L4002** Replacement strap, any orthosis, includes all components, any length, any type Ⓑ Qp ♿   A

✳ **L4010** Replace trilateral socket brim Ⓑ Qp Qh ♿   A

✳ **L4020** Replace quadrilateral socket brim, molded to patient model Ⓑ Qp Qh ♿   A

✳ **L4030** Replace quadrilateral socket brim, custom fitted Ⓑ Qp Qh ♿   A

✳ **L4040** Replace molded thigh lacer, for custom fabricated orthosis only Ⓑ Qp Qh ♿   A

✳ **L4045** Replace non-molded thigh lacer, for custom fabricated orthosis only Ⓑ Qp Qh ♿   A

✳ **L4050** Replace molded calf lacer, for custom fabricated orthosis only Ⓑ Qp Qh ♿   A

✳ **L4055** Replace non-molded calf lacer, for custom fabricated orthosis only Ⓑ Qp Qh ♿   A

✳ **L4060** Replace high roll cuff Ⓑ Qp Qh ♿   A

✳ **L4070** Replace proximal and distal upright for KAFO Ⓑ Qp Qh ♿   A

✳ **L4080** Replace metal bands KAFO, proximal thigh Ⓑ Qp Qh ♿   A

✳ **L4090** Replace metal bands KAFO-AFO, calf or distal thigh Ⓑ Qp ♿   A

▶ **New**   ↻ **Revised**   ✔ **Reinstated**   ~~deleted~~ **Deleted**   ⊘ **Not covered or valid by Medicare**

⊛ **Special coverage instructions**   ✳ **Carrier discretion**   Ⓑ **Bill local carrier**   Ⓑ **Bill DME MAC**

✳ **L4100** Replace leather cuff KAFO, proximal thigh Ⓑ Qp Qh ♿ A

✳ **L4110** Replace leather cuff KAFO-AFO, calf or distal thigh Ⓑ Qp ♿ A

✳ **L4130** Replace pretibial shell Ⓑ Qp Qh ♿ A

Repairs

⊗ **L4205** Repair of orthotic device, labor component, per 15 minutes Ⓑ Qp A

IOM: 100-02, 15, 110.2

⊗ **L4210** Repair of orthotic device, repair or replace minor parts Ⓑ Qp A

IOM: 100-02, 15, 110.2; 100-02, 15, 120

Ancillary Orthotic Services

✳ **L4350** Ankle control orthosis, stirrup style, rigid, includes any type interface (e.g., pneumatic, gel), prefabricated, off-the-shelf Ⓑ Qp Qh ♿ A

✳ **L4360** Walking boot, pneumatic and/or vacuum, with or without joints, with or without interface material, prefabricated item that has been trimmed, bent, molded, assembled, or otherwise customized to fit a specific patient by an individual with expertise Ⓑ Qp Qh ♿ A

Noncovered when walking boots used primarily to relieve pressure, especially on sole of foot, or are used for patients with foot ulcers

✳ **L4361** Walking boot, pneumatic and/or vacuum, with or without joints, with or without interface material, prefabricated, off-the-shelf Ⓑ Qp Qh A

✳ **L4370** Pneumatic full leg splint, prefabricated, off-the-shelf Ⓑ Qp Qh ♿ A

✳ **L4386** Walking boot, non-pneumatic, with or without joints, with or without interface material, prefabricated item that has been trimmed, bent, molded, assembled, or otherwise customized to fit a specific patient by an individual with expertise Ⓑ Qp Qh ♿ A

✳ **L4387** Walking boot, non-pneumatic, with or without joints, with or without interface material, prefabricated, off-the-shelf Ⓑ Qp Qh A

✳ **L4392** Replacement, soft interface material, static AFO Ⓑ Qp Qh ♿ A

✳ **L4394** Replace soft interface material, foot drop splint Ⓑ Qp Qh ♿ A

✳ **L4396** Static or dynamic ankle foot orthosis, including soft interface material, adjustable for fit, for positioning, may be used for minimal ambulation, prefabricated item that has been trimmed, bent, molded, assembled, or otherwise customized to fit a specific patient by an individual with expertise Ⓑ Qp Qh ♿ A

✳ **L4397** Static or dynamic ankle foot orthosis, including soft interface material, adjustable for fit, for positioning, may be used for minimal ambulation, prefabricated, off-the-shelf Ⓑ Qp Qh A

✳ **L4398** Foot drop splint, recumbent positioning device, prefabricated, off-the-shelf Ⓑ Qp Qh ♿ A

✳ **L4631** Ankle foot orthosis, walking boot type, varus/valgus correction, rocker bottom, anterior tibial shell, soft interface, custom arch support, plastic or other material, includes straps and closures, custom fabricated Ⓑ Qp Qh ♿ A

PROSTHETICS (L5000-L9999)

Lower Limb (L5000-L5999)

NOTE: The procedures in this section are considered as base or basic procedures and may be modified by listing items/procedures or special materials from the Additions section and adding them to the base procedure.

Partial Foot

⊗ **L5000** Partial foot, shoe insert with longitudinal arch, toe filler Ⓑ Qp Qh ♿ A

IOM: 100-02, 15, 290

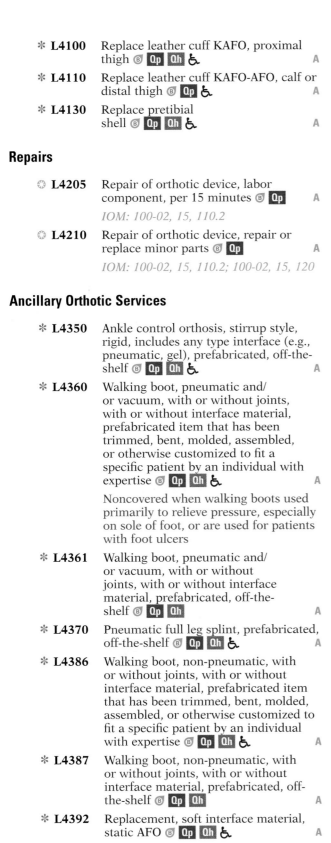

Figure 38 Partial foot.

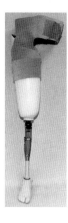

Figure 39 Above knee.

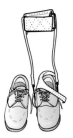

Figure 40 Ankle Symes.

⊛ **L5010** Partial foot, molded socket, ankle height, with toe filler ⑧ **Qp** **Qh** ⅗ A

IOM: 100-02, 15, 290

⊛ **L5020** Partial foot, molded socket, tibial tubercle height, with toe filler ⑧ **Qp** **Qh** ⅗ A

IOM: 100-02, 15, 290

Ankle

* **L5050** Ankle, Symes, molded socket, SACH foot ⑧ **Qp** **Qh** ⅗ A

* **L5060** Ankle, Symes, metal frame, molded leather socket, articulated ankle/foot ⑧ **Qp** **Qh** ⅗ A

Below Knee

* **L5100** Below knee, molded socket, shin, SACH foot ⑧ **Qp** **Qh** ⅗ A

* **L5105** Below knee, plastic socket, joints and thigh lacer, SACH foot ⑧ **Qp** **Qh** ⅗ A

Knee Disarticulation

* **L5150** Knee disarticulation (or through knee), molded socket, external knee joints, shin, SACH foot ⑧ **Qp** **Qh** ⅗ A

* **L5160** Knee disarticulation (or through knee), molded socket, bent knee configuration, external knee joints, shin, SACH foot ⑧ **Qp** **Qh** ⅗ A

Above Knee

* **L5200** Above knee, molded socket, single axis constant friction knee, shin, SACH foot ⑧ **Qp** **Qh** ⅗ A

* **L5210** Above knee, short prosthesis, no knee joint ('stubbies'), with foot blocks, no ankle joints, each ⑧ **Qp** **Qh** ⅗ A

* **L5220** Above knee, short prosthesis, no knee joint ('stubbies'), with articulated ankle/foot, dynamically aligned, each ⑧ **Qp** **Qh** ⅗ A

* **L5230** Above knee, for proximal femoral focal deficiency, constant friction knee, shin, SACH foot ⑧ **Qp** **Qh** ⅗ A

Hip Disarticulation

* **L5250** Hip disarticulation, Canadian type; molded socket, hip joint, single axis constant friction knee, shin, SACH foot ⑧ **Qp** **Qh** ⅗ A

* **L5270** Hip disarticulation, tilt table type; molded socket, locking hip joint, single axis constant friction knee, shin, SACH foot ⑧ **Qp** **Qh** ⅗ A

Hemipelvectomy

* **L5280** Hemipelvectomy, Canadian type; molded socket, hip joint, single axis constant friction knee, shin, SACH foot ⑧ **Qp** **Qh** ⅗ A

Endoskeleton: Below Knee

* **L5301** Below knee, molded socket, shin, SACH foot, endoskeletal system ⑧ **Qp** **Qh** ⅗ A

* **L5312** Knee disarticulation (or through knee), molded socket, single axis knee, pylon, sach foot, endoskeletal system ⑧ **Qp** **Qh** ⅗ A

Endoskeletal: Above Knee

* **L5321** Above knee, molded socket, open end, SACH foot, endoskeletal system, single axis knee ⑧ **Qp** **Qh** ⅗ A

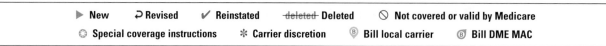

▶ **New**   ↻ **Revised**   ✔ **Reinstated**   ~~deleted~~ **Deleted**   ⊘ **Not covered or valid by Medicare**
⊛ **Special coverage instructions**   ✳ **Carrier discretion**   Ⓛ **Bill local carrier**   ⑧ **Bill DME MAC**

Endoskeletal: Hip Disarticulation

✳ **L5331**   Hip disarticulation, Canadian type, molded socket, endoskeletal system, hip joint, single axis knee, SACH foot ⒷⓆⓅⓆⓗ ♿   A

Endoskeletal: Hemipelvectomy

✳ **L5341**   Hemipelvectomy, Canadian type, molded socket, endoskeletal system, hip joint, single axis knee, SACH foot ⒷⓆⓅⓆⓗ ♿   A

Immediate Postsurgical or Early Fitting Procedures

✳ **L5400**   Immediate post surgical or early fitting, application of initial rigid dressing, including fitting, alignment, suspension, and one cast change, below knee ⒷⓆⓅⓆⓗ ♿   A

✳ **L5410**   Immediate post surgical or early fitting, application of initial rigid dressing, including fitting, alignment and suspension, below knee, each additional cast change and realignment ⒷⓆⓅⓆⓗ ♿   A

✳ **L5420**   Immediate post surgical or early fitting, application of initial rigid dressing, including fitting, alignment and suspension and one cast change 'AK' or knee disarticulation ⒷⓆⓅⓆⓗ ♿   A

✳ **L5430**   Immediate postsurgical or early fitting, application of initial rigid dressing, including fitting, alignment, and suspension, 'AK' or knee disarticulation, each additional cast change and realignment ⒷⓆⓅⓆⓗ ♿   A

✳ **L5450**   Immediate post surgical or early fitting, application of non-weight bearing rigid dressing, below knee ⒷⓆⓅⓆⓗ ♿   A

✳ **L5460**   Immediate post surgical or early fitting, application of non-weight bearing rigid dressing, above knee ⒷⓆⓅⓆⓗ ♿   A

Initial Prosthesis

✳ **L5500**   Initial, below knee 'PTB' type socket, non-alignable system, pylon, no cover, SACH foot, plaster socket, direct formed ⒷⓆⓅⓆⓗ ♿   A

✳ **L5505**   Initial, above knee–knee disarticulation, ischial level socket, non-alignable system, pylon, no cover, SACH foot, plaster socket, direct formed ⒷⓆⓅⓆⓗ ♿   A

Preparatory Prosthesis

✳ **L5510**   Preparatory, below knee 'PTB' type socket, non-alignable system, pylon, no cover, SACH foot, plaster socket, molded to model ⒷⓆⓅⓆⓗ ♿   A

✳ **L5520**   Preparatory, below knee 'PTB' type socket, non-alignable system, pylon, no cover, SACH foot, thermoplastic or equal, direct formed ⒷⓆⓅⓆⓗ ♿   A

✳ **L5530**   Preparatory, below knee 'PTB' type socket, non-alignable system, pylon, no cover, SACH foot, thermoplastic or equal, molded to model ⒷⓆⓅⓆⓗ ♿   A

✳ **L5535**   Preparatory, below knee 'PTB' type socket, non-alignable system, no cover, SACH foot, prefabricated, adjustable open end socket ⒷⓆⓅⓆⓗ ♿   A

✳ **L5540**   Preparatory, below knee 'PTB' type socket, non-alignable system, pylon, no cover, SACH foot, laminated socket, molded to model ⒷⓆⓅⓆⓗ ♿   A

✳ **L5560**   Preparatory, above knee - knee disarticulation, ischial level socket, non-alignable system, pylon, no cover, SACH foot, plaster socket, molded to model ⒷⓆⓅⓆⓗ ♿   A

✳ **L5570**   Preparatory, above knee - knee disarticulation, ischial level socket, non-alignable system, pylon, no cover, SACH foot, thermoplastic or equal, direct formed ⒷⓆⓅⓆⓗ ♿   A

✳ **L5580**   Preparatory, above knee - knee disarticulation, ischial level socket, non-alignable system, pylon, no cover, SACH foot, thermoplastic or equal, molded to model ⒷⓆⓅⓆⓗ ♿   A

✳ **L5585**   Preparatory, above knee - knee disarticulation, ischial level socket, non-alignable system, pylon, no cover, SACH foot, prefabricated adjustable open end socket ⒷⓆⓅⓆⓗ ♿   A

✳ **L5590**   Preparatory, above knee - knee disarticulation, ischial level socket, non-alignable system, pylon, no cover, SACH foot, laminated socket, molded to model ⒷⓆⓅⓆⓗ ♿   A

✳ **L5595**   Preparatory, hip disarticulation-hemipelvectomy, pylon, no cover, SACH foot, thermoplastic or equal, molded to patient model ⒷⓆⓅⓆⓗ ♿   A

✳ **L5600**   Preparatory, hip disarticulation-hemipelvectomy, pylon, no cover, SACH foot, laminated socket, molded to patient model ⒷⓆⓅⓆⓗ ♿   A

Additions to Lower Extremity

* **L5610** Addition to lower extremity, endoskeletal system, above knee, hydracadence system ⑧ Qp Qh ♿ A

* **L5611** Addition to lower extremity, endoskeletal system, above knee- knee disarticulation, 4 bar linkage, with friction swing phase control ⑧ Qp Qh ♿ A

* **L5613** Addition to lower extremity, endoskeletal system, above knee-knee disarticulation, 4 bar linkage, with hydraulic swing phase control ⑧ Qp Qh ♿ A

* **L5614** Addition to lower extremity, exoskeletal system, above knee-knee disarticulation, 4 bar linkage, with pneumatic swing phase control ⑧ Qp Qh ♿ A

* **L5616** Addition to lower extremity, endoskeletal system, above knee, universal multiplex system, friction swing phase control ⑧ Qp Qh ♿ A

* **L5617** Addition to lower extremity, quick change self-aligning unit, above knee or below knee, each ⑧ Qp Qh ♿ A

Additions to Test Sockets

* **L5618** Addition to lower extremity, test socket, Symes ⑧ Qp ♿ A

* **L5620** Addition to lower extremity, test socket, below knee ⑧ Qp ♿ A

* **L5622** Addition to lower extremity, test socket, knee disarticulation ⑧ Qp ♿ A

* **L5624** Addition to lower extremity, test socket, above knee ⑧ Qp ♿ A

* **L5626** Addition to lower extremity, test socket, hip disarticulation ⑧ Qp ♿ A

* **L5628** Addition to lower extremity, test socket, hemipelvectomy ⑧ Qp Qh ♿ A

* **L5629** Addition to lower extremity, below knee, acrylic socket ⑧ Qp Qh ♿ A

Additions to Socket Variations

* **L5630** Addition to lower extremity, Symes type, expandable wall socket ⑧ Qp Qh ♿ A

* **L5631** Addition to lower extremity, above knee or knee disarticulation, acrylic socket ⑧ Qp Qh ♿ A

* **L5632** Addition to lower extremity, Symes type, 'PTB' brim design socket ⑧ Qp Qh ♿ A

* **L5634** Addition to lower extremity, Symes type, posterior opening (Canadian) socket ⑧ Qp Qh ♿ A

* **L5636** Addition to lower extremity, Symes type, medial opening socket ⑧ Qp Qh ♿ A

* **L5637** Addition to lower extremity, below knee, total contact ⑧ Qp Qh ♿ A

* **L5638** Addition to lower extremity, below knee, leather socket ⑧ Qp Qh ♿ A

* **L5639** Addition to lower extremity, below knee, wood socket ⑧ Qp Qh ♿ A

* **L5640** Addition to lower extremity, knee disarticulation, leather socket ⑧ Qp Qh ♿ A

* **L5642** Addition to lower extremity, above knee, leather socket ⑧ Qp Qh ♿ A

* **L5643** Addition to lower extremity, hip disarticulation, flexible inner socket, external frame ⑧ Qp Qh ♿ A

* **L5644** Addition to lower extremity, above knee, wood socket ⑧ Qp Qh ♿ A

* **L5645** Addition to lower extremity, below knee, flexible inner socket, external frame ⑧ Qp Qh ♿ A

* **L5646** Addition to lower extremity, below knee, air, fluid, gel or equal, cushion socket ⑧ Qp Qh ♿ A

* **L5647** Addition to lower extremity, below knee, suction socket ⑧ Qp Qh ♿ A

* **L5648** Addition to lower extremity, above knee, air, fluid, gel or equal, cushion socket ⑧ Qp Qh ♿ A

* **L5649** Addition to lower extremity, ischial containment/narrow M-L socket ⑧ Qp Qh ♿ A

* **L5650** Additions to lower extremity, total contact, above knee or knee disarticulation socket ⑧ Qp Qh ♿ A

* **L5651** Addition to lower extremity, above knee, flexible inner socket, external frame ⑧ Qp Qh ♿ A

* **L5652** Addition to lower extremity, suction suspension, above knee or knee disarticulation socket ⑧ Qp Qh ♿ A

* **L5653** Addition to lower extremity, knee disarticulation, expandable wall socket ⑧ Qp Qh ♿ A

Additions to Socket Insert and Suspension

* **L5654** Addition to lower extremity, socket insert, Symes, (Kemblo, Pelite, Aliplast, Plastazote or equal) ⑧ Qp Qh ♿ A

▶ New ↻ Revised ✔ Reinstated ~~deleted~~ Deleted ⊘ Not covered or valid by Medicare
✪ Special coverage instructions * Carrier discretion Ⓑ Bill local carrier ⑧ Bill DME MAC

* **L5655** Addition to lower extremity, socket insert, below knee (Kemblo, Pelite, Aliplast, Plastazote or equal) Ⓑ Ⓠp Ⓠh ♿ A

* **L5656** Addition to lower extremity, socket insert, knee disarticulation (Kemblo, Pelite, Aliplast, Plastazote or equal) Ⓑ Ⓠp Ⓠh ♿ A

* **L5658** Addition to lower extremity, socket insert, above knee (Kemblo, Pelite, Aliplast, Plastazote or equal) Ⓑ Ⓠp Ⓠh ♿ A

* **L5661** Addition to lower extremity, socket insert, multi-durometer Symes Ⓑ Ⓠp Ⓠh ♿ A

* **L5665** Addition to lower extremity, socket insert, multi-durometer, below knee Ⓑ Ⓠp Ⓠh ♿ A

* **L5666** Addition to lower extremity, below knee, cuff suspension Ⓑ Ⓠp Ⓠh ♿ A

* **L5668** Addition to lower extremity, below knee, molded distal cushion Ⓑ Ⓠp Ⓠh ♿ A

* **L5670** Addition to lower extremity, below knee, molded supracondylar suspension ('PTS' or similar) Ⓑ Ⓠp Ⓠh ♿ A

* **L5671** Addition to lower extremity, below knee/above knee suspension locking mechanism (shuttle, lanyard or equal), excludes socket insert Ⓑ Ⓠp Ⓠh ♿ A

* **L5672** Addition to lower extremity, below knee, removable medial brim suspension Ⓑ Ⓠp Ⓠh ♿ A

* **L5673** Addition to lower extremity, below knee/above knee, custom fabricated from existing mold or prefabricated, socket insert, silicone gel, elastomeric or equal, for use with locking mechanism Ⓑ Ⓠp ♿ A

* **L5676** Additions to lower extremity, below knee, knee joints, single axis, pair Ⓑ Ⓠp Ⓠh ♿ A

* **L5677** Additions to lower extremity, below knee, knee joints, polycentric, pair Ⓑ Ⓠp Ⓠh ♿ A

* **L5678** Additions to lower extremity, below knee, joint covers, pair Ⓑ Ⓠp Ⓠh ♿ A

* **L5679** Addition to lower extremity, below knee/above knee, custom fabricated from existing mold or prefabricated, socket insert, silicone gel, elastomeric or equal, not for use with locking mechanism Ⓑ Ⓠp ♿ A

* **L5680** Addition to lower extremity, below knee, thigh lacer, non-molded Ⓑ Ⓠp Ⓠh ♿ A

* **L5681** Addition to lower extremity, below knee/above knee, custom fabricated socket insert for congenital or atypical traumatic amputee, silicone gel, elastomeric or equal, for use with or without locking mechanism, initial only (for other than initial, use code L5673 or L5679) Ⓑ Ⓠp Ⓠh ♿ A

* **L5682** Addition to lower extremity, below knee, thigh lacer, gluteal/ischial, molded Ⓑ Ⓠp Ⓠh ♿ A

* **L5683** Addition to lower extremity, below knee/above knee, custom fabricated socket insert for other than congenital or atypical traumatic amputee, silicone gel, elastomeric, or equal, for use with or without locking mechanism, initial only (for other than initial, use code L5673 or L5679) Ⓑ Ⓠp Ⓠh ♿ A

* **L5684** Addition to lower extremity, below knee, fork strap Ⓑ Ⓠp Ⓠh ♿ A

* **L5685** Addition to lower extremity prosthesis, below knee, suspension/sealing sleeve, with or without valve, any material, each Ⓑ Ⓠp ♿ A

* **L5686** Addition to lower extremity, below knee, back check (extension control) Ⓑ Ⓠp Ⓠh ♿ A

* **L5688** Addition to lower extremity, below knee, waist belt, webbing Ⓑ Ⓠp Ⓠh ♿ A

* **L5690** Addition to lower extremity, below knee, waist belt, padded and lined Ⓑ Ⓠp Ⓠh ♿ A

* **L5692** Addition to lower extremity, above knee, pelvic control belt, light Ⓑ Ⓠp Ⓠh ♿ A

* **L5694** Addition to lower extremity, above knee, pelvic control belt, padded and lined Ⓑ Ⓠp Ⓠh ♿ A

* **L5695** Addition to lower extremity, above knee, pelvic control, sleeve suspension, neoprene or equal, each Ⓑ Ⓠp Ⓠh ♿ A

* **L5696** Addition to lower extremity, above knee or knee disarticulation, pelvic joint Ⓑ Ⓠp Ⓠh ♿ A

* **L5697** Addition to lower extremity, above knee or knee disarticulation, pelvic band Ⓑ Ⓠp Ⓠh ♿ A

* **L5698** Addition to lower extremity, above knee or knee disarticulation, Silesian bandage Ⓑ Ⓠp Ⓠh ♿ A

* **L5699** All lower extremity prostheses, shoulder harness Ⓑ Ⓠp Ⓠh ♿ A

Additions/Replacements to Feet-Ankle Units

* **L5700** Replacement, socket, below knee, molded to patient model ⑧ **Qp** **Qh** ♿   A

* **L5701** Replacement, socket, above knee/knee disarticulation, including attachment plate, molded to patient model ⑧ **Qp** **Qh** ♿   A

* **L5702** Replacement, socket, hip disarticulation, including hip joint, molded to patient model ⑧ **Qp** **Qh** ♿   A

* **L5703** Ankle, Symes, molded to patient model, socket without solid ankle cushion heel (SACH) foot, replacement only ⑧ **Qp** **Qh** ♿   A

* **L5704** Custom shaped protective cover, below knee ⑧ **Qp** **Qh** ♿   A

* **L5705** Custom shaped protective cover, above knee ⑧ **Qp** **Qh** ♿   A

* **L5706** Custom shaped protective cover, knee disarticulation ⑧ **Qp** **Qh** ♿   A

* **L5707** Custom shaped protective cover, hip disarticulation ⑧ **Qp** **Qh** ♿   A

Additions to Exoskeletal–Knee-Shin System

* **L5710** Addition, exoskeletal knee-shin system, single axis, manual lock ⑧ **Qp** **Qh** ♿ A

* **L5711** Additions exoskeletal knee-shin system, single axis, manual lock, ultra-light material ⑧ **Qp** **Qh** ♿   A

* **L5712** Addition, exoskeletal knee-shin system, single axis, friction swing and stance phase control (safety knee) ⑧ **Qp** **Qh** ♿   A

* **L5714** Addition, exoskeletal knee-shin system, single axis, variable friction swing phase control ⑧ **Qp** **Qh** ♿   A

* **L5716** Addition, exoskeletal knee-shin system, polycentric, mechanical stance phase lock ⑧ **Qp** **Qh** ♿   A

* **L5718** Addition, exoskeletal knee-shin system, polycentric, friction swing and stance phase control ⑧ **Qp** **Qh** ♿   A

* **L5722** Addition, exoskeletal knee-shin system, single axis, pneumatic swing, friction stance phase control ⑧ **Qp** **Qh** ♿   A

* **L5724** Addition, exoskeletal knee-shin system, single axis, fluid swing phase control ⑧ **Qp** **Qh** ♿   A

* **L5726** Addition, exoskeletal knee-shin system, single axis, external joints, fluid swing phase control ⑧ **Qp** **Qh** ♿   A

* **L5728** Addition, exoskeletal knee-shin system, single axis, fluid swing and stance phase control ⑧ **Qp** **Qh** ♿   A

* **L5780** Addition, exoskeletal knee-shin system, single axis, pneumatic/hydra pneumatic swing phase control ⑧ **Qp** **Qh** ♿   A

* **L5781** Addition to lower limb prosthesis, vacuum pump, residual limb volume management and moisture evacuation system ⑧ **Qp** **Qh** ♿   A

* **L5782** Addition to lower limb prosthesis, vacuum pump, residual limb volume management and moisture evacuation system, heavy duty ⑧ **Qp** **Qh** ♿   A

Component Modification

* **L5785** Addition, exoskeletal system, below knee, ultra-light material (titanium, carbon fiber, or equal) ⑧ **Qp** **Qh** ♿   A

* **L5790** Addition, exoskeletal system, above knee, ultra-light material (titanium, carbon fiber, or equal) ⑧ **Qp** **Qh** ♿   A

* **L5795** Addition, exoskeletal system, hip disarticulation, ultra-light material (titanium, carbon fiber, or equal) ⑧ **Qp** **Qh** ♿   A

Endoskeletal

* **L5810** Addition, endoskeletal knee-shin system, single axis, manual lock ⑧ **Qp** **Qh** ♿   A

* **L5811** Addition, endoskeletal knee-shin system, single axis, manual lock, ultralight material ⑧ **Qp** **Qh** ♿   A

* **L5812** Addition, endoskeletal knee-shin system, single axis, friction swing and stance phase control (safety knee) ⑧ **Qp** **Qh** ♿   A

* **L5814** Addition, endoskeletal knee-shin system, polycentric, hydraulic swing phase control, mechanical stance phase lock ⑧ **Qp** **Qh** ♿   A

* **L5816** Addition, endoskeletal knee-shin system, polycentric, mechanical stance phase lock ⑧ **Qp** **Qh** ♿   A

* **L5818** Addition, endoskeletal knee-shin system, polycentric, friction swing, and stance phase control ⑧ **Qp** **Qh** ♿   A

* **L5822** Addition, endoskeletal knee-shin system, single axis, pneumatic swing, friction stance phase control ⑧ **Qp** **Qh** ♿   A

► New	⤺ Revised	✔ Reinstated	̶d̶e̶l̶e̶t̶e̶d̶ Deleted	⊘ Not covered or valid by Medicare
♲ Special coverage instructions		✳ Carrier discretion	⑧ Bill local carrier	⑧ Bill DME MAC

✳ **L5824** Addition, endoskeletal knee-shin system, single axis, fluid swing phase control Ⓑ Qp Qh ♿ A

✳ **L5826** Addition, endoskeletal knee-shin system, single axis, hydraulic swing phase control, with miniature high activity frame Ⓑ Qp Qh ♿ A

✳ **L5828** Addition, endoskeletal knee-shin system, single axis, fluid swing and stance phase control Ⓑ Qp Qh ♿ A

✳ **L5830** Addition, endoskeletal knee-shin system, single axis, pneumatic/swing phase control Ⓑ Qp Qh ♿ A

✳ **L5840** Addition, endoskeletal knee/ shin system, 4-bar linkage or multiaxial, pneumatic swing phase control Ⓑ Qp Qh ♿ A

✳ **L5845** Addition, endoskeletal, knee-shin system, stance flexion feature, adjustable Ⓑ Qp Qh ♿ A

✳ **L5848** Addition to endoskeletal, knee-shin system, fluid stance extension, dampening feature, with or without adjustability Ⓑ Qp Qh ♿ A

✳ **L5850** Addition, endoskeletal system, above knee or hip disarticulation, knee extension assist Ⓑ Qp Qh ♿ A

✳ **L5855** Addition, endoskeletal system, hip disarticulation, mechanical hip extension assist Ⓑ Qp Qh ♿ A

✳ **L5856** Addition to lower extremity prosthesis, endoskeletal knee-shin system, microprocessor control feature, swing and stance phase; includes electronic sensor(s), any type Ⓑ Qp Qh ♿ A

✳ **L5857** Addition to lower extremity prosthesis, endoskeletal knee-shin system, microprocessor control feature, swing phase only; includes electronic sensor(s), any type Ⓑ Qp Qh ♿ A

✳ **L5858** Addition to lower extremity prosthesis, endoskeletal knee shin system, microprocessor control feature, stance phase only, includes electronic sensor(s), any type Ⓑ Qp Qh ♿ A

✳ **L5859** Addition to lower extremity prosthesis, endoskeletal knee-shin system, powered and programmable flexion/extension assist control, includes any type motor(s) Ⓑ Qp Qh ♿ A

✳ **L5910** Addition, endoskeletal system, below knee, alignable system Ⓑ Qp Qh ♿ A

✳ **L5920** Addition, endoskeletal system, above knee or hip disarticulation, alignable system Ⓑ Qp Qh ♿ A

✳ **L5925** Addition, endoskeletal system, above knee, knee disarticulation or hip disarticulation, manual lock Ⓑ Qp Qh ♿ A

✳ **L5930** Addition, endoskeletal system, high activity knee control frame Ⓑ Qp Qh ♿ A

✳ **L5940** Addition, endoskeletal system, below knee, ultra-light material (titanium, carbon fiber or equal) Ⓑ Qp Qh ♿ A

✳ **L5950** Addition, endoskeletal system, above knee, ultra-light material (titanium, carbon fiber or equal) Ⓑ Qp Qh ♿ A

✳ **L5960** Addition, endoskeletal system, hip disarticulation, ultra-light material (titanium, carbon fiber, or equal) Ⓑ Qp Qh ♿ A

✳ **L5961** Addition, endoskeletal system, polycentric hip joint, pneumatic or hydraulic control, rotation control, with or without flexion, and/or extension control Ⓑ Qp Qh ♿ A

✳ **L5962** Addition, endoskeletal system, below knee, flexible protective outer surface covering system Ⓑ Qp Qh ♿ A

✳ **L5964** Addition, endoskeletal system, above knee, flexible protective outer surface covering system Ⓑ Qp Qh ♿ A

✳ **L5966** Addition, endoskeletal system, hip disarticulation, flexible protective outer surface covering system Ⓑ Qp Qh ♿ A

✳ **L5968** Addition to lower limb prosthesis, multiaxial ankle with swing phase active dorsiflexion feature Ⓑ Qp Qh ♿ A

✳ **L5969** Addition, endoskeletal ankle-foot or ankle system, power assist, includes any type motor(s) Ⓑ Qp Qh A

✳ **L5970** All lower extremity prostheses, foot, external keel, SACH foot Ⓑ Qp Qh ♿ A

✳ **L5971** All lower extremity prosthesis, solid ankle cushion keel (SACH) foot, replacement only Ⓑ Qp Qh ♿ A

✳ **L5972** All lower extremity prostheses (foot, flexible keel) Ⓑ Qp Qh ♿ A

✳ **L5973** Endoskeletal ankle foot system, microprocessor controlled feature, dorsiflexion and/or plantar flexion control, includes power source Ⓑ Qh ♿ A

✳ **L5974** All lower extremity prostheses, foot, single axis ankle/foot Ⓑ Qp Qh ♿ A

✳ **L5975** All lower extremity prostheses, combination single axis ankle and flexible keel foot Ⓑ Qp Qh ♿ A

🅟 PQRS	Qp Quantity Physician Appendix A	Qh Quantity Hospital Appendix B	♀ Female only
♂ Male only	A Age	♿ DMEPOS	A2-Z3 ASC Payment Indicator A-Y ASC Status Indicator Coding Clinic

* **L5976** All lower extremity prostheses, energy storing foot (Seattle Carbon Copy II or equal) ⑧ Qp Qh ♿   A

* **L5978** All lower extremity prostheses, foot, multiaxial ankle/foot ⑧ Qp Qh ♿   A

* **L5979** All lower extremity prostheses, multiaxial ankle, dynamic response foot, one piece system ⑧ Qp Qh ♿   A

* **L5980** All lower extremity prostheses, flex foot system ⑧ Qp Qh ♿   A

* **L5981** All lower extremity prostheses, flexwalk system or equal ⑧ Qp Qh ♿   A

* **L5982** All exoskeletal lower extremity prostheses, axial rotation unit ⑧ Qp Qh ♿   A

* **L5984** All endoskeletal lower extremity prostheses, axial rotation unit, with or without adjustability ⑧ Qp Qh ♿   A

* **L5985** All endoskeletal lower extremity prostheses, dynamic prosthetic pylon ⑧ Qp Qh ♿   A

* **L5986** All lower extremity prostheses, multiaxial rotation unit ('MCP' or equal) ⑧ Qp Qh ♿   A

* **L5987** All lower extremity prostheses, shank foot system with vertical loading pylon ⑧ Qp Qh ♿   A

* **L5988** Addition to lower limb prosthesis, vertical shock reducing pylon feature ⑧ Qp Qh ♿   A

* **L5990** Addition to lower extremity prosthesis, user adjustable heel height ⑧ Qp Qh ♿   A

* **L5999** Lower extremity prosthesis, not otherwise specified ⑧   A

Upper Limb

NOTE: The procedures in L6000-L6599 are considered as base or basic procedures and may be modified by listing procedures from the additions sections. The base procedures include only standard friction wrist and control cable system unless otherwise specified.

Partial Hand

* **L6000** Partial hand, thumb remaining ⑧ Qp Qh ♿   A

* **L6010** Partial hand, little and/or ring finger remaining ⑧ Qp Qh ♿   A

* **L6020** Partial hand, no finger remaining ⑧ Qp Qh ♿   A

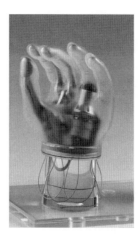

Figure 41 Partial hand.

~~L6025 Transcarpal/metacarpal or partial hand disarticulation prosthesis, external power, self-suspended, inner socket with removable forearm section, electrodes and cables, two batteries, charger, myoelectric control of terminal device~~ ✖

▶ * **L6026** Transcarpal/metacarpal or partial hand disarticulation prosthesis, external power, self-suspended, inner socket with removable forearm section, electrodes and cables, two batteries, charger, myoelectric control of terminal device, excludes terminal device(s)   A

Wrist Disarticulation

* **L6050** Wrist disarticulation, molded socket, flexible elbow hinges, triceps pad ⑧ Qp Qh ♿   A

* **L6055** Wrist disarticulation, molded socket with expandable interface, flexible elbow hinges, triceps pad ⑧ Qp Qh ♿ A

Below Elbow

* **L6100** Below elbow, molded socket, flexible elbow hinge, triceps pad ⑧ Qp Qh ♿   A

* **L6110** Below elbow, molded socket, (Muenster or Northwestern suspension types) ⑧ Qp Qh ♿   A

* **L6120** Below elbow, molded double wall split socket, step-up hinges, half cuff ⑧ Qp Qh ♿   A

* **L6130** Below elbow, molded double wall split socket, stump activated locking hinge, half cuff ⑧ Qp Qh ♿   A

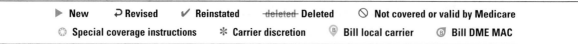

▶ New   ⟲ Revised   ✔ Reinstated   ~~deleted~~ Deleted   ⊘ Not covered or valid by Medicare
☼ Special coverage instructions   * Carrier discretion   Ⓛ Bill local carrier   ⑧ Bill DME MAC

Elbow Disarticulation

✳ **L6200** Elbow disarticulation, molded socket, outside locking hinge, forearm Ⓑ **Qp** **Qh** ♿   A

✳ **L6205** Elbow disarticulation, molded socket with expandable interface, outside locking hinges, forearm Ⓑ **Qp** **Qh** ♿   A

Above Elbow

✳ **L6250** Above elbow, molded double wall socket, internal locking elbow, forearm Ⓑ **Qp** **Qh** ♿   A

Shoulder Disarticulation

✳ **L6300** Shoulder disarticulation, molded socket, shoulder bulkhead, humeral section, internal locking elbow, forearm Ⓑ **Qp** **Qh** ♿   A

✳ **L6310** Shoulder disarticulation, passive restoration (complete prosthesis) Ⓑ **Qp** **Qh** ♿   A

✳ **L6320** Shoulder disarticulation, passive restoration (shoulder cap only) Ⓑ **Qp** **Qh** ♿   A

Interscapular Thoracic

✳ **L6350** Interscapular thoracic, molded socket, shoulder bulkhead, humeral section, internal locking elbow, forearm Ⓑ **Qp** **Qh** ♿   A

✳ **L6360** Interscapular thoracic, passive restoration (complete prosthesis) Ⓑ **Qp** **Qh** ♿   A

✳ **L6370** Interscapular thoracic, passive restoration (shoulder cap only) Ⓑ **Qp** **Qh** ♿   A

Immediate and Early Postsurgical Procedures

✳ **L6380** Immediate post surgical or early fitting, application of initial rigid dressing, including fitting alignment and suspension of components, and one cast change, wrist disarticulation or below elbow Ⓑ **Qp** **Qh** ♿   A

✳ **L6382** Immediate post surgical or early fitting, application of initial rigid dressing including fitting alignment and suspension of components, and one cast change, elbow disarticulation or above elbow Ⓑ **Qp** **Qh** ♿   A

✳ **L6384** Immediate post surgical or early fitting, application of initial rigid dressing including fitting alignment and suspension of components, and one cast change, shoulder disarticulation or interscapular thoracic Ⓑ **Qp** **Qh** ♿   A

✳ **L6386** Immediate post surgical or early fitting, each additional cast change and realignment Ⓑ **Qp** **Qh** ♿   A

✳ **L6388** Immediate post surgical or early fitting, application of rigid dressing only Ⓑ **Qp** **Qh** ♿   A

Endoskeletal: Below Elbow

✳ **L6400** Below elbow, molded socket, endoskeletal system, including soft prosthetic tissue shaping Ⓑ **Qp** **Qh** ♿ A

Endoskeletal: Elbow Disarticulation

✳ **L6450** Elbow disarticulation, molded socket, endoskeletal system, including soft prosthetic tissue shaping Ⓑ **Qp** **Qh** ♿ A

Endoskeletal: Above Elbow

✳ **L6500** Above elbow, molded socket, endoskeletal system, including soft prosthetic tissue shaping Ⓑ **Qp** **Qh** ♿ A

Endoskeletal: Shoulder Disarticulation

✳ **L6550** Shoulder disarticulation, molded socket, endoskeletal system, including soft prosthetic tissue shaping Ⓑ **Qp** **Qh** ♿   A

Endoskeletal: Interscapular Thoracic

✳ **L6570** Interscapular thoracic, molded socket, endoskeletal system, including soft prosthetic tissue shaping Ⓑ **Qp** **Qh** ♿ A

✳ **L6580** Preparatory, wrist disarticulation or below elbow, single wall plastic socket, friction wrist, flexible elbow hinges, figure of eight harness, humeral cuff, Bowden cable control, USMC or equal pylon, no cover, molded to patient model Ⓑ **Qp** **Qh** ♿   A

✳ **L6582** Preparatory, wrist disarticulation or below elbow, single wall socket, friction wrist, flexible elbow hinges, figure of eight harness, humeral cuff, Bowden cable control, USMC or equal pylon, no cover, direct formed Ⓑ **Qp** **Qh** ♿   A

🅟 PQRS	**Qp** Quantity Physician Appendix A	**Qh** Quantity Hospital Appendix B	♀ Female only
♂ Male only	**A** Age	♿ DMEPOS	A2-Z3 ASC Payment Indicator A-Y ASC Status Indicator Coding Clinic

✳ **L6584** Preparatory, elbow disarticulation or above elbow, single wall plastic socket, friction wrist, locking elbow, figure of eight harness, fair lead cable control, USMC or equal pylon, no cover, molded to patient model Ⓑ Qp Qh ♿   A

✳ **L6586** Preparatory, elbow disarticulation or above elbow, single wall socket, friction wrist, locking elbow, figure of eight harness, fair lead cable control, USMC or equal pylon, no cover, direct formed Ⓑ Qp Qh ♿   A

✳ **L6588** Preparatory, shoulder disarticulation or interscapular thoracic, single wall plastic socket, shoulder joint, locking elbow, friction wrist, chest strap, fair lead cable control, USMC or equal pylon, no cover, molded to patient model Ⓑ Qp Qh ♿   A

✳ **L6590** Preparatory, shoulder disarticulation or interscapular thoracic, single wall socket, shoulder joint, locking elbow, friction wrist, chest strap, fair lead cable control, USMC or equal pylon, no cover, direct formed Ⓑ Qp Qh ♿   A

Additions to Upper Limb

NOTE: The following procedures/modifications/components may be added to other base procedures. The items in this section should reflect the additional complexity of each modification procedure, in addition to base procedure, at the time of the original order.

✳ **L6600** Upper extremity additions, polycentric hinge, pair Ⓑ Qp Qh ♿   A

✳ **L6605** Upper extremity additions, single pivot hinge, pair Ⓑ Qp Qh ♿   A

✳ **L6610** Upper extremity additions, flexible metal hinge, pair Ⓑ Qp Qh ♿   A

✳ **L6611** Addition to upper extremity prosthesis, external powered, additional switch, any type Ⓑ Qp Qh ♿   A

✳ **L6615** Upper extremity addition, disconnect locking wrist unit Ⓑ Qp Qh ♿   A

✳ **L6616** Upper extremity addition, additional disconnect insert for locking wrist unit, each Ⓑ Qp Qh ♿   A

✳ **L6620** Upper extremity addition, flexion/extension wrist unit, with or without friction Ⓑ Qp Qh ♿   A

✳ **L6621** Upper extremity prosthesis addition, flexion/extension wrist with or without friction, for use with external powered terminal device Ⓑ Qp Qh ♿   A

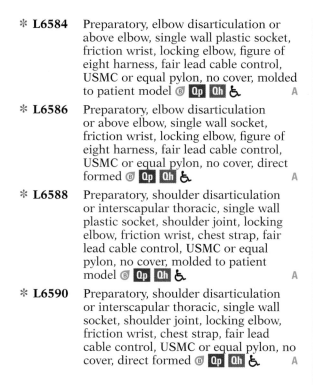
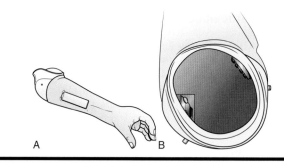

Figure 42 Upper extremity addition.

✳ **L6623** Upper extremity addition, spring assisted rotational wrist unit with latch release Ⓑ Qp Qh ♿   A

✳ **L6624** Upper extremity addition, flexion/extension and rotation wrist unit Ⓑ Qp Qh ♿   A

✳ **L6625** Upper extremity addition, rotation wrist unit with cable lock Ⓑ Qp Qh ♿   A

✳ **L6628** Upper extremity addition, quick disconnect hook adapter, Otto Bock or equal Ⓑ Qp Qh ♿   A

✳ **L6629** Upper extremity addition, quick disconnect lamination collar with coupling piece, Otto Bock or equal Ⓑ Qp Qh ♿   A

✳ **L6630** Upper extremity addition, stainless steel, any wrist Ⓑ Qp Qh ♿   A

✳ **L6632** Upper extremity addition, latex suspension sleeve, each Ⓑ Qp ♿   A

✳ **L6635** Upper extremity addition, lift assist for elbow Ⓑ Qp Qh ♿   A

✳ **L6637** Upper extremity addition, nudge control elbow lock Ⓑ Qp Qh ♿   A

✳ **L6638** Upper extremity addition to prosthesis, electric locking feature, only for use with manually powered elbow Ⓑ Qp Qh ♿   A

✳ **L6640** Upper extremity additions, shoulder abduction joint, pair Ⓑ Qp Qh ♿   A

✳ **L6641** Upper extremity addition, excursion amplifier, pulley type Ⓑ Qp Qh ♿   A

✳ **L6642** Upper extremity addition, excursion amplifier, lever type Ⓑ Qp Qh ♿   A

✳ **L6645** Upper extremity addition, shoulder flexion-abduction joint, each Ⓑ Qp Qh ♿   A

✳ **L6646** Upper extremity addition, shoulder joint, multipositional locking, flexion, adjustable abduction friction control, for use with body powered or external powered system Ⓑ Qp Qh ♿   A

▶ **New**   ⟲ **Revised**   ✔ **Reinstated**   ~~deleted~~ **Deleted**   ⊘ **Not covered or valid by Medicare**
   ⊛ **Special coverage instructions**   ✳ **Carrier discretion**   Ⓛ **Bill local carrier**   Ⓑ **Bill DME MAC**

* **L6647** Upper extremity addition, shoulder lock mechanism, body powered actuator Ⓑ Qp Qh &   A

* **L6648** Upper extremity addition, shoulder lock mechanism, external powered actuator Ⓑ Qp Qh &   A

* **L6650** Upper extremity addition, shoulder universal joint, each Ⓑ Qp Qh &   A

* **L6655** Upper extremity addition, standard control cable, extra Ⓑ Qp &   A

* **L6660** Upper extremity addition, heavy duty control cable Ⓑ Qp &   A

* **L6665** Upper extremity addition, Teflon, or equal, cable lining Ⓑ Qp &   A

* **L6670** Upper extremity addition, hook to hand, cable adapter Ⓑ Qp Qh &   A

* **L6672** Upper extremity addition, harness, chest or shoulder, saddle type Ⓑ Qp Qh &   A

* **L6675** Upper extremity addition, harness, (e.g. figure of eight type), single cable design Ⓑ Qp Qh &   A

* **L6676** Upper extremity addition, harness, (e.g. figure of eight type), dual cable design Ⓑ Qp Qh &   A

* **L6677** Upper extremity addition, harness, triple control, simultaneous operation of terminal device and elbow Ⓑ Qp Qh &   A

* **L6680** Upper extremity addition, test socket, wrist disarticulation or below elbow Ⓑ Qp &   A

* **L6682** Upper extremity addition, test socket, elbow disarticulation or above elbow Ⓑ Qp &   A

* **L6684** Upper extremity addition, test socket, shoulder disarticulation or interscapular thoracic Ⓑ Qp &   A

* **L6686** Upper extremity addition, suction socket Ⓑ Qp Qh &   A

* **L6687** Upper extremity addition, frame type socket, below elbow or wrist disarticulation Ⓑ Qp Qh &   A

* **L6688** Upper extremity addition, frame type socket, above elbow or elbow disarticulation Ⓑ Qp Qh &   A

* **L6689** Upper extremity addition, frame type socket, shoulder disarticulation Ⓑ Qp Qh &   A

* **L6690** Upper extremity addition, frame type socket, interscapular-thoracic Ⓑ Qp Qh &   A

* **L6691** Upper extremity addition, removable insert, each Ⓑ Qp &   A

* **L6692** Upper extremity addition, silicone gel insert or equal, each Ⓑ Qp &   A

* **L6693** Upper extremity addition, locking elbow, forearm counterbalance Ⓑ Qp Qh &   A

* **L6694** Addition to upper extremity prosthesis, below elbow/above elbow, custom fabricated from existing mold or prefabricated, socket insert, silicone gel, elastomeric or equal, for use with locking mechanism Ⓑ Qp Qh &   A

* **L6695** Addition to upper extremity prosthesis, below elbow/above elbow, custom fabricated from existing mold or prefabricated, socket insert, silicone gel, elastomeric or equal, not for use with locking mechanism Ⓑ Qp Qh &   A

* **L6696** Addition to upper extremity prosthesis, below elbow/above elbow, custom fabricated socket insert for congenital or atypical traumatic amputee, silicone gel, elastomeric or equal, for use with or without locking mechanism, initial only (for other than initial, use code L6694 or L6695) Ⓑ Qp Qh &   A

* **L6697** Addition to upper extremity prosthesis, below elbow/above elbow, custom fabricated socket insert for other than congenital or atypical traumatic amputee, silicone gel, elastomeric or equal, for use with or without locking mechanism, initial only (for other than initial, use code L6694 or L6695) Ⓑ Qp Qh &   A

* **L6698** Addition to upper extremity prosthesis, below elbow/above elbow, lock mechanism, excludes socket insert Ⓑ Qp Qh &   A

Terminal Devices

Hooks

* **L6703** Terminal device, passive hand/mitt, any material, any size Ⓑ Qp Qh &   A

* **L6704** Terminal device, sport/recreational/ work attachment, any material, any size Ⓑ Qp Qh &   A

* **L6706** Terminal device, hook, mechanical, voluntary opening, any material, any size, lined or unlined Ⓑ Qp Qh &   A

* **L6707** Terminal device, hook, mechanical, voluntary closing, any material, any size, lined or unlined Ⓑ Qp Qh &   A

* **L6708** Terminal device, hand, mechanical, voluntary opening, any material, any size Ⓑ Qp Qh &   A

| ℗ℚℝ℞ PQRS | Qp Quantity Physician Appendix A | Qh Quantity Hospital Appendix B | ♀ Female only |
| ♂ Male only | A Age | & DMEPOS | A2-Z3 ASC Payment Indicator | A-Y ASC Status Indicator | Coding Clinic |

PROSTHETICS L6647 – L6708

325

❋ **L6709** Terminal device, hand, mechanical, voluntary closing, any material, any size ⑧ Qp Qh 🚹　　　A

❋ **L6711** Terminal device, hook, mechanical, voluntary opening, any material, any size, lined or unlined, pediatric ⑧ Qp Qh A 🚹　　　A

❋ **L6712** Terminal device, hook, mechanical, voluntary closing, any material, any size, lined or unlined, pediatric ⑧ Qp Qh A 🚹　　　A

❋ **L6713** Terminal device, hand, mechanical, voluntary opening, any material, any size, pediatric ⑧ Qp Qh A 🚹　　　A

❋ **L6714** Terminal device, hand, mechanical, voluntary closing, any material, any size, pediatric ⑧ Qp Qh A 🚹　　　A

❋ **L6715** Terminal device, multiple articulating digit, includes motor(s), initial issue or replacement ⑧ Qp Qh 🚹　　　A

❋ **L6721** Terminal device, hook or hand, heavy duty, mechanical, voluntary opening, any material, any size, lined or unlined ⑧ Qp Qh 🚹　　　A

❋ **L6722** Terminal device, hook or hand, heavy duty, mechanical, voluntary closing, any material, any size, lined or unlined ⑧ Qp Qh 🚹　　　A

✪ **L6805** Addition to terminal device, modifier wrist unit ⑧ Qp Qh 🚹　　　A

　　　IOM: 100-02, 15, 120; 100-04, 3, 10.4

✪ **L6810** Addition to terminal device, precision pinch device ⑧ Qp Qh 🚹　　　A

　　　IOM: 100-02, 15, 120; 100-04, 3, 10.4

Hands

❋ **L6880** Electric hand, switch or myoelectric controlled, independently articulating digits, any grasp pattern or combination of grasp patterns, includes motor(s) ⑧ Qp Qh 🚹　　　A

❋ **L6881** Automatic grasp feature, addition to upper limb electric prosthetic terminal device ⑧ Qp Qh 🚹　　　A

✪ **L6882** Microprocessor control feature, addition to upper limb prosthetic terminal device ⑧ Qp Qh 🚹　　　A

　　　IOM: 100-02, 15, 120; 100-04, 3, 10.4

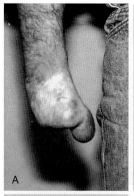
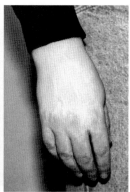
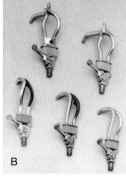

Figure 43 Terminal devices, **(A)** hand and **(B)** hook.

Replacement Sockets

❋ **L6883** Replacement socket, below elbow/wrist disarticulation, molded to patient model, for use with or without external power ⑧ Qp Qh 🚹　　　A

❋ **L6884** Replacement socket, above elbow/elbow disarticulation, molded to patient model, for use with or without external power ⑧ Qp Qh 🚹　　　A

❋ **L6885** Replacement socket, shoulder disarticulation/interscapular thoracic, molded to patient model, for use with or without external power ⑧ Qp Qh 🚹　　　A

Gloves for Above Hands

❋ **L6890** Addition to upper extremity prosthesis, glove for terminal device, any material, prefabricated, includes fitting and adjustment ⑧ Qp Qh 🚹　　　A

❋ **L6895** Addition to upper extremity prosthesis, glove for terminal device, any material, custom fabricated ⑧ Qp Qh 🚹　　　A

▶ **New**　　↻ **Revised**　　✔ **Reinstated**　　deleted **Deleted**　　⊘ **Not covered or valid by Medicare**

✪ **Special coverage instructions**　　❋ **Carrier discretion**　　⑧ **Bill local carrier**　　⑧ **Bill DME MAC**

Hand Restoration

* **L6900** Hand restoration (casts, shading and measurements included), partial hand, with glove, thumb or one finger remaining Ⓑ Qp Qh ♿   A

* **L6905** Hand restoration (casts, shading and measurements included), partial hand, with glove, multiple fingers remaining Ⓑ Qp Qh ♿   A

* **L6910** Hand restoration (casts, shading and measurements included), partial hand, with glove, no fingers remaining Ⓑ Qp Qh ♿   A

* **L6915** Hand restoration (shading, and measurements included), replacement glove for above Ⓑ Qp Qh ♿   A

External Power

Base Devices

* **L6920** Wrist disarticulation, external power, self-suspended inner socket, removable forearm shell, Otto Bock or equal switch, cables, two batteries and one charger, switch control of terminal device Ⓑ Qp Qh ♿   A

* **L6925** Wrist disarticulation, external power, self-suspended inner socket, removable forearm shell, Otto Bock or equal electrodes, cables, two batteries and one charger, myoelectronic control of terminal device Ⓑ Qp Qh ♿   A

* **L6930** Below elbow, external power, self-suspended inner socket, removable forearm shell, Otto Bock or equal switch, cables, two batteries and one charger, switch control of terminal device Ⓑ Qp Qh ♿   A

* **L6935** Below elbow, external power, self-suspended inner socket, removable forearm shell, Otto Bock or equal electrodes, cables, two batteries and one charger, myoelectronic control of terminal device Ⓑ Qp Qh ♿   A

* **L6940** Elbow disarticulation, external power, molded inner socket, removable humeral shell, outside locking hinges, forearm, Otto Bock or equal switch, cables, two batteries and one charger, switch control of terminal device Ⓑ Qp Qh ♿   A

* **L6945** Elbow disarticulation, external power, molded inner socket, removable humeral shell, outside locking hinges, forearm, Otto Bock or equal electrodes, cables, two batteries and one charger, myoelectronic control of terminal device Ⓑ Qp Qh ♿   A

* **L6950** Above elbow, external power, molded inner socket, removable humeral shell, internal locking elbow, forearm, Otto Bock or equal switch, cables, two batteries and one charger, switch control of terminal device Ⓑ Qp Qh ♿   A

* **L6955** Above elbow, external power, molded inner socket, removable humeral shell, internal locking elbow, forearm, Otto Bock or equal electrodes, cables, two batteries and one charger, myoelectronic control of terminal device Ⓑ Qp Qh ♿   A

* **L6960** Shoulder disarticulation, external power, molded inner socket, removable shoulder shell, shoulder bulkhead, humeral section, mechanical elbow, forearm, Otto Bock or equal switch, cables, two batteries and one charger, switch control of terminal device Ⓑ Qp Qh ♿   A

* **L6965** Shoulder disarticulation, external power, molded inner socket, removable shoulder shell, shoulder bulkhead, humeral section, mechanical elbow, forearm, Otto Bock or equal electrodes, cables, two batteries and one charger, myoelectronic control of terminal device Ⓑ Qp Qh ♿   A

* **L6970** Interscapular-thoracic, external power, molded inner socket, removable shoulder shell, shoulder bulkhead, humeral section, mechanical elbow, forearm, Otto Bock or equal switch, cables, two batteries and one charger, switch control of terminal device Ⓑ Qp Qh ♿   A

* **L6975** Interscapular-thoracic, external power, molded inner socket, removable shoulder shell, shoulder bulkhead, humeral section, mechanical elbow, forearm, Otto Bock or equal electrodes, cables, two batteries and one charger, myoelectronic control of terminal device Ⓑ Qp Qh ♿   A

Terminal Devices

* **L7007** Electric hand, switch or myoelectric controlled, adult Ⓑ Qp Qh A ♿   A

* **L7008** Electric hand, switch or myoelectric controlled, pediatric Ⓑ Qp Qh A ♿   A

ⓅQRS PQRS	Qp Quantity Physician Appendix A	Qh Quantity Hospital Appendix B	♀ Female only
♂ Male only A Age ♿ DMEPOS	A2-Z3 ASC Payment Indicator	A-Y ASC Status Indicator	Coding Clinic

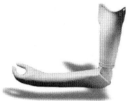

Figure 44 Electronic elbow.

※ **L7009** Electric hook, switch or myoelectric controlled, adult ⑧ Qp Qh A ⅙   A

※ **L7040** Prehensile actuator, switch controlled ⑧ Qp Qh &   A

※ **L7045** Electric hook, switch or myoelectric controlled, pediatric ⑧ Qp Qh A &   A

Elbow

※ **L7170** Electronic elbow, Hosmer or equal, switch controlled ⑧ Qp Qh &   A

※ **L7180** Electronic elbow, microprocessor sequential control of elbow and terminal device ⑧ Qp Qh &   A

※ **L7181** Electronic elbow, microprocessor simultaneous control of elbow and terminal device ⑧ Qp Qh &   A

※ **L7185** Electronic elbow, adolescent, Variety Village or equal, switch controlled ⑧ Qp Qh &   A

※ **L7186** Electronic elbow, child, Variety Village or equal, switch controlled ⑧ Qp Qh A &   A

※ **L7190** Electronic elbow, adolescent, Variety Village or equal, myoelectronically controlled ⑧ Qp Qh &   A

※ **L7191** Electronic elbow, child, Variety Village or equal, myoelectronically controlled ⑧ Qp Qh A &   A

Wrist

▶ ※ **L7259** Electronic wrist rotator, any type   A

~~L7260~~ ~~Electronic wrist rotator, Otto Bock or equal~~ ✖

~~L7261~~ ~~Electronic wrist rotator, for Utah arm~~ ✖

Battery Components

※ **L7360** Six volt battery, each ⑧ Qp &   A

※ **L7362** Battery charger, six volt, each ⑧ Qp Qh &   A

※ **L7364** Twelve volt battery, each ⑧ Qp &   A

※ **L7366** Battery charger, twelve volt, each ⑧ Qp Qh &   A

↻※ **L7367** Lithium ion battery, rechargeable, replacement ⑧ Qp &   A

※ **L7368** Lithium ion battery charger, replacement only ⑧ Qp Qh &   A

Other/Repair

※ **L7400** Addition to upper extremity prosthesis, below elbow/wrist disarticulation, ultralight material (titanium, carbon fiber or equal) ⑧ Qp Qh &   A

※ **L7401** Addition to upper extremity prosthesis, above elbow disarticulation, ultralight material (titanium, carbon fiber or equal) ⑧ Qp Qh &   A

※ **L7402** Addition to upper extremity prosthesis, shoulder disarticulation/interscapular thoracic, ultralight material (titanium, carbon fiber or equal) ⑧ Qp Qh &   A

※ **L7403** Addition to upper extremity prosthesis, below elbow/wrist disarticulation, acrylic material ⑧ Qp Qh &   A

※ **L7404** Addition to upper extremity prosthesis, above elbow disarticulation, acrylic material ⑧ Qp Qh &   A

※ **L7405** Addition to upper extremity prosthesis, shoulder disarticulation/interscapular thoracic, acrylic material ⑧ Qp Qh & A

※ **L7499** Upper extremity prosthesis, not otherwise specified ⑧   A

◎ **L7510** Repair of prosthetic device, repair or replace minor parts ⑧   A

Bill local carrier (⑧) if repair of implanted prosthetic device.

IOM: 100-02, 15, 110.2; 100-02, 15, 120; 100-04, 32, 100

※ **L7520** Repair prosthetic device, labor component, per 15 minutes ⑧   A

Bill local carrier (⑧) if repair of implanted prosthetic device.

⊘ **L7600** Prosthetic donning sleeve, any material, each ⑧   E

Medicare Statute 1862(1)(a)

General

※ **L7900** Male vacuum erection system ⑧ Qp Qh ♂ &   A

※ **L7902** Tension ring, for vacuum erection device, any type, replacement only, each ⑧ Qp Qh &   A

▶ New	↻ Revised	✔ Reinstated	~~deleted~~ Deleted	⊘ Not covered or valid by Medicare
◎ Special coverage instructions		※ Carrier discretion	⑧ Bill local carrier	⑧ Bill DME MAC

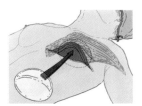

Figure 45 Implant breast prosthesis.

Breast Prostheses

⊛ **L8000** Breast prosthesis, mastectomy bra, without integrated breast prosthesis form, any size, any type Ⓑ Qp ♀   A
IOM: 100-02, 15, 120

⊛ **L8001** Breast prosthesis, mastectomy bra, with integrated breast prosthesis form, unilateral, any size, any type Ⓑ Qp ♀   A
IOM: 100-02, 15, 120

⊛ **L8002** Breast prosthesis, mastectomy bra, with integrated breast prosthesis form, bilateral, any size, any type Ⓑ Qp ♀   A
IOM: 100-02, 15, 120

⊛ **L8010** Breast prosthesis, mastectomy sleeve Ⓑ ♀   A
IOM: 100-02, 15, 120

⊛ **L8015** External breast prosthesis garment, with mastectomy form, post mastectomy Ⓑ Qp ♀   A
IOM: 100-02, 15, 120

⊛ **L8020** Breast prosthesis, mastectomy form Ⓑ Qp ♀   A
IOM: 100-02, 15, 120

✳ **L8030** Breast prosthesis, silicone or equal, without integral adhesive Ⓑ Qp Qh ♀   A
IOM: 100-02, 15, 120

⊛ **L8031** Breast prosthesis, silicone or equal, with integral adhesive Ⓑ Qp Qh   A
IOM: 100-02, 15, 120

✳ **L8032** Nipple prosthesis, reusable, any type, each Ⓑ Qp Qh   A

⊛ **L8035** Custom breast prosthesis, post mastectomy, molded to patient model Ⓑ Qp Qh ♀   A
IOM: 100-02, 15, 120

✳ **L8039** Breast prosthesis, not otherwise specified Ⓑ Qp Qh ♀   A

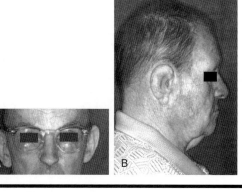

Figure 46 **A.** Nasal prosthesis. **B.** Auricular prosthesis.

Nasal, Orbital, Auricular Prosthesis

✳ **L8040** Nasal prosthesis, provided by a non-physician Ⓑ Qp Qh   A
DMEPOS Modifier(s): KM, KN

✳ **L8041** Midfacial prosthesis, provided by a non-physician Ⓑ Qp Qh   A
DMEPOS Modifier(s): KM, KN

✳ **L8042** Orbital prosthesis, provided by a non-physician Ⓑ Qp Qh   A
DMEPOS Modifier(s): KM, KN

✳ **L8043** Upper facial prosthesis, provided by a non-physician Ⓑ Qp Qh   A
DMEPOS Modifier(s): KM, KN

✳ **L8044** Hemi-facial prosthesis, provided by a non-physician Ⓑ Qp Qh   A
DMEPOS Modifier(s): KM, KN

✳ **L8045** Auricular prosthesis, provided by a non-physician Ⓑ Qp Qh   A
DMEPOS Modifier(s): KM, KN

✳ **L8046** Partial facial prosthesis, provided by a non-physician Ⓑ Qp Qh   A
DMEPOS Modifier(s): KM, KN

✳ **L8047** Nasal septal prosthesis, provided by a non-physician Ⓑ Qp Qh   A
DMEPOS Modifier(s): KM, KN

✳ **L8048** Unspecified maxillofacial prosthesis, by report, provided by a non-physician Ⓑ Qp Qh   A

✳ **L8049** Repair or modification of maxillofacial prosthesis, labor component, 15 minute increments, provided by a non-physician Ⓑ Qp   A

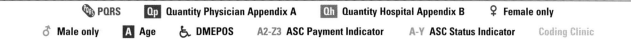
PQRS   Qp Quantity Physician Appendix A   Qh Quantity Hospital Appendix B   ♀ Female only   ♂ Male only   A Age   & DMEPOS   A2-Z3 ASC Payment Indicator   A-Y ASC Status Indicator   Coding Clinic

Trusses

⊛ **L8300** Truss, single with standard
pad ⑧ **Qp** **Qh** &♿;   A
IOM: 100-02, 15, 120; 100-03, 4, 280.11;
100-03, 4, 280.12; 100-04, 4, 240

⊛ **L8310** Truss, double with standard
pads ⑧ **Qp** **Qh** ♿   A
IOM: 100-02, 15, 120; 100-03, 4, 280.11;
100-03, 4, 280.12; 100-04, 4, 240

⊛ **L8320** Truss, addition to standard pad, water
pad ⑧ **Qp** **Qh** ♿   A
IOM: 100-02, 15, 120; 100-03, 4, 280.11;
100-03, 4, 280.12; 100-04, 4, 240

⊛ **L8330** Truss, addition to standard pad, scrotal
pad ⑧ **Qp** **Qh** ♂ ♿ A
IOM: 100-02, 15, 120; 100-03, 4, 280.11;
100-03, 4, 280.12; 100-04, 4, 240

Prosthetic Socks

⊛ **L8400** Prosthetic sheath, below knee,
each ⑧ **Qp** ♿   A
IOM: 100-02, 15, 200

⊛ **L8410** Prosthetic sheath, above knee,
each ⑧ **Qp** ♿   A
IOM: 100-02, 15, 200

⊛ **L8415** Prosthetic sheath, upper limb,
each ⑧ **Qp** ♿   A
IOM: 100-02, 15, 200

✳ **L8417** Prosthetic sheath/sock, including a gel
cushion layer, below knee or above
knee, each ⑧ **Qp** ♿   A

⊛ **L8420** Prosthetic sock, multiple ply, below
knee, each ⑧ **Qp** ♿   A
IOM: 100-02, 15, 200

⊛ **L8430** Prosthetic sock, multiple ply, above
knee, each ⑧ **Qp** ♿   A
IOM: 100-02, 15, 200

⊛ **L8435** Prosthetic sock, multiple ply, upper
limb, each ⑧ **Qp** ♿   A
IOM: 100-02, 15, 200

⊛ **L8440** Prosthetic shrinker, below knee,
each ⑧ **Qp** ♿   A
IOM: 100-02, 15, 200

⊛ **L8460** Prosthetic shrinker, above knee,
each ⑧ **Qp** ♿   A
IOM: 100-02, 15, 200

⊛ **L8465** Prosthetic shrinker, upper limb,
each ⑧ **Qp** ♿   A
IOM: 100-02, 15, 200

⊛ **L8470** Prosthetic sock, single ply, fitting, below
knee, each ⑧ **Qp** ♿   A
IOM: 100-02, 15, 200

⊛ **L8480** Prosthetic sock, single ply, fitting, above
knee, each ⑧ **Qp** ♿   A
IOM: 100-02, 15, 200

⊛ **L8485** Prosthetic sock, single ply, fitting, upper
limb, each ⑧ **Qp** ♿   A
IOM: 100-02, 15, 200

✳ **L8499** Unlisted procedure for miscellaneous
prosthetic services ⑧   A

Bill local carrier (⑧) if repair of
implanted prosthetic device.

Prosthetic Implants

Larynx, Tracheoesophageal

⊛ **L8500** Artificial larynx, any type ⑧ **Qp** **Qh** ♿ A
IOM: 100-02, 15, 120; 100-03, 1, 50.2;
100-04, 4, 240

⊛ **L8501** Tracheostomy speaking
valve ⑧ **Qp** **Qh** ♿   A
IOM: 100-03, 1, 50.4

✳ **L8505** Artificial larynx replacement battery/
accessory, any type ⑧   A

✳ **L8507** Tracheo-esophageal voice prosthesis,
patient inserted, any type,
each ⑧ **Qp** **Qh** ♿   A

✳ **L8509** Tracheo-esophageal voice prosthesis,
inserted by a licensed health care
provider, any type ⑧ **Qp** **Qh** ♿ A

⊛ **L8510** Voice amplifier ⑧ **Qp** **Qh** ♿ A
IOM: 100-03, 1, 50.2

✳ **L8511** Insert for indwelling tracheoesophageal
prosthesis, with or without valve,
replacement only, each ⑧ **Qp** **Qh** ♿ A

✳ **L8512** Gelatin capsules or equivalent, for use
with tracheoesophageal voice prosthesis,
replacement only, per 10 ⑧ ♿   A

✳ **L8513** Cleaning device used with
tracheoesophageal voice prosthesis,
pipet, brush, or equal, replacement
only, each ⑧ ♿   A

✳ **L8514** Tracheoesophageal puncture dilator,
replacement only, each ⑧ **Qp** **Qh** ♿ A

✳ **L8515** Gelatin capsule, application device
for use with tracheoesophageal voice
prosthesis, each ⑧ **Qp** **Qh** ♿ A

▶ New   ⟲ Revised   ✔ Reinstated   ~~deleted~~ Deleted   ⊘ Not covered or valid by Medicare
⊛ Special coverage instructions   ✳ Carrier discretion   ⑧ Bill local carrier   ⑧ Bill DME MAC

Breast

⊕ **L8600** Implantable breast prosthesis, silicone or equal ⑧ **Qp** **Qh** ♀ ⛨   N

IOM: 100-02, 15, 120; 100-3, 2, 140.2

Urinary System

⊕ **L8603** Injectable bulking agent, collagen implant, urinary tract, 2.5 ml syringe, includes shipping and necessary supplies ⑧ ⛨   N

Bill on paper, acquisition cost invoice required

IOM: 100-03, 4, 280.1

✳ **L8604** Injectable bulking agent, dextranomer/ hyaluronic acid copolymer implant, urinary tract, 1 ml, includes shipping and necessary supplies ⑧ **Qp** **Qh**   N

✳ **L8605** Injectable bulking agent, dextranomer/ hyaluronic acid copolymer implant, anal canal, 1 ml, includes shipping and necessary supplies ⑧ **Qp** **Qh** ⛨   A

⊕ **L8606** Injectable bulking agent, synthetic implant, urinary tract, 1 ml syringe, includes shipping and necessary supplies ⑨ **Qp** **Qh** ⛨   N

Bill on paper, acquisition cost invoice required

IOM: 100-03, 4, 280.1

Head (Skull, Facial Bones, and Temporomandibular Joint)

✳ **L8609** Artificial cornea ⑧ **Qp** **Qh** ⛨   N
⊕ **L8610** Ocular implant ⑧ **Qp** **Qh** ⛨   N

IOM: 100-02, 15, 120

⊕ **L8612** Aqueous shunt ⑧ **Qp** **Qh** ⛨   N

IOM: 100-02, 15, 120

Cross Reference Q0074

⊕ **L8613** Ossicula implant ⑧ **Qp** **Qh** ⛨   N

IOM: 100-02, 15, 120

⊕ **L8614** Cochlear device, includes all internal and external components ⑧ **Qp** **Qh** ⛨ N

IOM: 100-02, 15, 120; 100-03, 1, 50.3

⊕ **L8615** Headset/headpiece for use with cochlear implant device, replacement ⑧ **Qp** **Qh** ⛨   A

IOM: 100-03, 1, 50.3

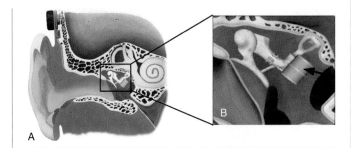

Figure 47   Cochlear device.

⊕ **L8616** Microphone for use with cochlear implant device, replacement ⑧ **Qp** **Qh** ⛨   A

IOM: 100-03, 1, 50.3

⊕ **L8617** Transmitting coil for use with cochlear implant device, replacement ⑨ **Qp** **Qh** ⛨   A

IOM: 100-03, 1, 50.3

⊕ **L8618** Transmitter cable for use with cochlear implant device, replacement ⑧ **Qp** **Qh** ⛨   A

IOM: 100-03, 1, 50.3

✳ **L8619** Cochlear implant, external speech processor and controller, integrated system, replacement ⑧ **Qp** **Qh** ⛨   A

IOM: 100-03, 1, 50.3

✳ **L8621** Zinc air battery for use with cochlear implant device, replacement, each ⑧ **Qp** **Qh** ⛨   A

✳ **L8622** Alkaline battery for use with cochlear implant device, any size, replacement, each ⑧ **Qp** **Qh** ⛨   A

✳ **L8623** Lithium ion battery for use with cochlear implant device speech processor, other than ear level, replacement, each ⑧ ⛨   A

✳ **L8624** Lithium ion battery for use with cochlear implant device speech processor, ear level, replacement, each ⑧ ⛨   A

⊕ **L8627** Cochlear implant, external speech processor, component, replacement ⑧ **Qp** **Qh** ⛨   A

IOM: 103-03, Part 1, 50.3

⊕ **L8628** Cochlear implant, external controller component, replacement ⑧ **Qp** **Qh** ⛨ A

IOM: 103-03, Part 1, 50.3

⊕ **L8629** Transmitting coil and cable, integrated, for use with cochlear implant device, replacement ⑧ **Qp** **Qh** ⛨   A

IOM: 103-03, Part 1, 50.3

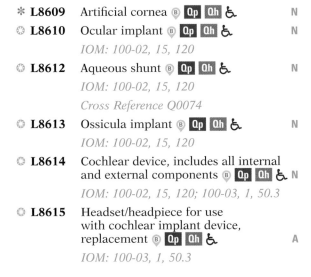

Ⓠ PQRS	**Qp** Quantity Physician Appendix A	**Qh** Quantity Hospital Appendix B	♀ Female only
♂ Male only	**A** Age	⛨ DMEPOS	A2-Z3 ASC Payment Indicator A-Y ASC Status Indicator *Coding Clinic*

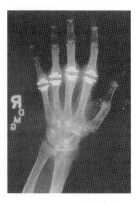

Figure 48 Metacarpophalangeal implant.

Upper Extremity

⊛ **L8630** Metacarpophalangeal joint implant ⑧ ⅋. N
IOM: 100-02, 15, 120

⊛ **L8631** Metacarpal phalangeal joint replacement, two or more pieces, metal (e.g., stainless steel or cobalt chrome), ceramic-like material (e.g., pyrocarbon), for surgical implantation (all sizes, includes entire system) ⑧ Qp Qh ⅋. N
IOM: 100-02, 15, 120

Lower Extremity (Joint: Knee, Ankle, Toe)

⊛ **L8641** Metatarsal joint implant ⑧ Qp Qh ⅋. N
IOM: 100-02, 15, 120

⊛ **L8642** Hallux implant ⑧ Qp Qh ⅋. N
May be billed by ambulatory surgical center or surgeon
IOM: 100-02, 15, 120
Cross Reference CPT Q0073

Miscellaneous Muscular-Skeletal

⊛ **L8658** Interphalangeal joint spacer, silicone or equal, each ⑧ Qp Qh ⅋. N
IOM: 100-02, 15, 120

⊛ **L8659** Interphalangeal finger joint replacement, 2 or more pieces, metal (e.g., stainless steel or cobalt chrome), ceramic-like material (e.g., pyrocarbon) for surgical implantation, any size ⑧ Qp Qh ⅋. N
IOM: 100-02, 15, 120

Cardiovascular System

⊛ **L8670** Vascular graft material, synthetic, implant ⑧ Qp Qh ⅋. N
IOM: 100-02, 15, 120

Neurostimulator

⊛ **L8679** Implantable neurostimulator, pulse generator, any type ⑧ Qp Qh N
IOM 100-03, 4, 280.4

⤺ ⊘ **L8680** Implantable neurostimulator electrode, each ⑧ E
Related CPT codes: 43647, 63650, 63655, 64553, 64555, 64560, 64561, 64565, 64573, 64575, 64577, 64580, 64581.

⊛ **L8681** Patient programmer (external) for use with implantable programmable neurostimulator pulse generator, replacement only ⑧ Qp Qh ⅋. A
IOM: 100-03, 4, 280.4

⊛ **L8682** Implantable neurostimulator radiofrequency receiver ⑧ Qp Qh N
IOM 100-03, 4, 280.4

⊛ **L8683** Radiofrequency transmitter (external) for use with implantable neurostimulator radiofrequency receiver ⑧ Qp Qh A
IOM 100-03, 4, 280.4

⊛ **L8684** Radiofrequency transmitter (external) for use with implantable sacral root neurostimulator receiver for bowel and bladder management, replacement ⑧ Qp Qh A
IOM 100-03, 4, 280.4

⊘ **L8685** Implantable neurostimulator pulse generator, single array, rechargeable, includes extension ⑧ Qp Qh E
Related CPT codes: 61885, 64590, 63685.

⊘ **L8686** Implantable neurostimulator pulse generator, single array, non-rechargeable, includes extension ⑧ Qp Qh E
Related CPT codes: 61885, 64590, 63685.

⊘ **L8687** Implantable neurostimulator pulse generator, dual array, rechargeable, includes extension ⑧ Qp Qh E
Related CPT codes: 64590, 63685, 61886.

▶ **New**   ⤺ **Revised**   ✔ **Reinstated**   ~~deleted~~ **Deleted**   ⊘ **Not covered or valid by Medicare**
⊛ **Special coverage instructions**   ✳ **Carrier discretion**   ⑧ **Bill local carrier**   ⑧ **Bill DME MAC**

⊘ **L8688** Implantable neurostimulator pulse generator, dual array, non-rechargeable, includes extension Ⓑ Qp Qh   E

Related CPT codes: 61885, 64590, 63685.

⊛ **L8689** External recharging system for battery (internal) for use with implantable neurostimulator, replacement only Ⓑ Qp Qh   A

IOM: 100-03, 4, 280.4

✱ **L8690** Auditory osseointegrated device, includes all internal and external components Ⓑ Qp Qh   N

Related CPT codes: 69714, 69715, 69717, 69718.

✱ **L8691** Auditory osseointegrated device, external sound processor, replacement Ⓑ Qp Qh   A

⊘ **L8692** Auditory osseointegrated device, external sound processor, used without osseointegration, body worn, includes headband or other means of external attachment Ⓑ Qp Qh   E

Medicare Statute 1862(a)(7)

✱ **L8693** Auditory osseointegrated device abutment, any length, replacement only Ⓑ Qp Qh   A

⊛ **L8695** External recharging system for battery (external) for use with implantable neurostimulator, replacement only Ⓑ Qp Qh   A

IOM: 100-03, 4, 280.4

▶ ⊛ **L8696** Antenna (external) for use with implantable diaphragmatic/phrenic nerve stimulation device, replacement, each   A

Unspecified

✱ **L8699** Prosthetic implant, not otherwise specified Ⓑ   N

✱ **L9900** Orthotic and prosthetic supply, accessory, and/or service component of another HCPCS "L" code Ⓑ   N

Bill local carrier (Ⓑ) if repair of implanted prosthetic device.

PQRS   Qp Quantity Physician Appendix A   Qh Quantity Hospital Appendix B   ♀ Female only   ♂ Male only   A Age   DMEPOS   A2-Z3 ASC Payment Indicator   A-Y ASC Status Indicator   Coding Clinic

PROSTHETICS L8688 – L9900

333

OTHER MEDICAL SERVICES (M0000-M0301)

~~M0064~~ ~~Brief office visit for the sole purpose~~ ✖
~~of monitoring or changing drug~~
~~prescriptions used in the treatment of~~
~~mental psychoneurotic and personality~~
~~disorders~~

⊘ **M0075** Cellular therapy ⓑ   E

⊘ **M0076** Prolotherapy ⓑ   E

Prolotherapy stimulates production of new ligament tissue. Not covered by Medicare

⊘ **M0100** Intragastric hypothermia using gastric freezing ⓑ   E

⊘ **M0300** IV chelation therapy (chemical endarterectomy) ⓑ   E

Non-covered by Medicare

⊘ **M0301** Fabric wrapping of abdominal aneurysm ⓑ   E

Treatment for abdominal aneurysms that involves wrapping aneurysms with cellophane or fascia lata. Fabric wrapping of abdominal aneurysms is not a covered Medicare procedure.

▶ **New**   ↻ **Revised**   ✔ **Reinstated**   ~~deleted~~ **Deleted**   ⊘ **Not covered or valid by Medicare**

✿ **Special coverage instructions**   ✳ **Carrier discretion**   ⓑ **Bill local carrier**   ⓑ **Bill DME MAC**

LABORATORY SERVICES (P0000-P9999)

Chemistry and Toxicology Tests

⊛ **P2028** Cephalin floculation, blood Ⓑ `Qp` `Qh` A

This code appears on a CMS list of codes that represent obsolete and unreliable tests and procedures. Verify before reporting.

IOM: 100-03, 4, 300.1

⊛ **P2029** Congo red, blood Ⓑ `Qp` `Qh` A

This code appears on a CMS list of codes that represent obsolete and unreliable tests and procedures. Verify before reporting.

IOM: 100-03, 4, 300.1

⊘ **P2031** Hair analysis (excluding arsenic) Ⓑ E

IOM: 100-03, 4, 300.1

⊛ **P2033** Thymol turbidity, blood Ⓑ `Qp` `Qh` A

This code appears on a CMS list of codes that represent obsolete and unreliable tests and procedures. Verify before reporting.

IOM: 100-03, 4, 300.1

⊛ **P2038** Mucoprotein, blood (seromucoid) (medical necessity procedure) Ⓑ `Qp` `Qh` A

This code appears on a CMS list of codes that represent obsolete and unreliable tests and procedures. Verify before reporting.

IOM: 100-03, 4, 300.1

Pathology Screening Tests

⊛ **P3000** Screening Papanicolaou smear, cervical or vaginal, up to three smears, by technician under physician supervision Ⓑ `Qp` `Qh` ♀ A

Co-insurance and deductible waived

Assign for Pap smear ordered for screening purposes only, conventional method, performed by technician

IOM: 100-03, 3, 190.2,

Laboratory Certification: Cytology

⊛ **P3001** Screening Papanicolaou smear, cervical or vaginal, up to three smears, requiring interpretation by physician Ⓑ `Qp` `Qh` ♀ B

Co-insurance and deductible waived

Report professional component for Pap smears requiring physician interpretation. There are CPT codes assigned for diagnostic Paps, such as, 88141; HCPCS are for screening Paps

IOM: 100-03, 3, 190.2

Laboratory Certification: Cytology

Microbiology Tests

⊘ **P7001** Culture, bacterial, urine; quantitative, sensitivity study Ⓑ E

Cross Reference CPT

Laboratory Certification: Bacteriology

Miscellaneous Pathology

⊛ **P9010** Blood (whole), for transfusion, per unit Ⓑ R

Blood furnished on an outpatient basis, subject to Medicare Part B blood deductible; applicable to first 3 pints of whole blood or equivalent units of packed red cells in calendar year

IOM: 100-01, 3, 20.5; 100-02, 1, 10

OPPS recognized blood/blood products

⊛ **P9011** Blood, split unit Ⓑ R

Reports all splitting activities of any blood component

IOM: 100-01, 3, 20.5; 100-02, 1, 10

OPPS recognized blood/blood products

⊛ **P9012** Cryoprecipitate, each unit Ⓑ R

IOM: 100-01, 3, 20.5; 100-02, 1, 10

OPPS recognized blood/blood products

⊛ **P9016** Red blood cells, leukocytes reduced, each unit Ⓑ R

IOM: 100-01, 3, 20.5; 100-02, 1, 10

OPPS recognized blood/blood products

⊛ **P9017** Fresh frozen plasma (single donor), frozen within 8 hours of collection, each unit Ⓑ R

IOM: 100-01, 3, 20.5; 100-02, 1, 10

OPPS recognized blood/blood products

⊛ **P9019** Platelets, each unit Ⓑ   R
IOM: 100-01, 3, 20.5; 100-02, 1, 10
OPPS recognized blood/blood products

⊛ **P9020** Platelet rich plasma, each unit Ⓑ   R
IOM: 100-01, 3, 20.5; 100-02, 1, 10
OPPS recognized blood/blood products

⊛ **P9021** Red blood cells, each unit Ⓑ   R
IOM: 100-01, 3, 20.5; 100-02, 1, 10
OPPS recognized blood/blood products

⊛ **P9022** Red blood cells, washed, each unit Ⓑ   R
IOM: 100-01, 3, 20.5; 100-02, 1, 10
OPPS recognized blood/blood products

⊛ **P9023** Plasma, pooled multiple donor, solvent/detergent treated, frozen, each unit Ⓑ   R
IOM: 100-01, 3, 20.5; 100-02, 1, 10
OPPS recognized blood/blood products

⊛ **P9031** Platelets, leukocytes reduced, each unit Ⓑ   R
IOM: 100-01, 3, 20.5; 100-02, 1, 10
OPPS recognized blood/blood products

⊛ **P9032** Platelets, irradiated, each unit Ⓑ   R
IOM: 100-01, 3, 20.5; 100-02, 1, 10
OPPS recognized blood/blood products

⊛ **P9033** Platelets, leukocytes reduced, irradiated, each unit Ⓑ   R
IOM: 100-01, 3, 20.5; 100-02, 1, 10
OPPS recognized blood/blood products

⊛ **P9034** Platelets, pheresis, each unit Ⓑ   R
IOM: 100-01, 3, 20.5; 100-02, 1, 10
OPPS recognized blood/blood products

⊛ **P9035** Platelets, pheresis, leukocytes reduced, each unit Ⓑ   R
IOM: 100-01, 3, 20.5; 100-02, 1, 10
OPPS recognized blood/blood products

⊛ **P9036** Platelets, pheresis, irradiated, each unit Ⓑ   R
IOM: 100-01, 3, 20.5; 100-02, 1, 10
OPPS recognized blood/blood products

⊛ **P9037** Platelets, pheresis, leukocytes reduced, irradiated, each unit Ⓑ   R
IOM: 100-01, 3, 20.5; 100-02, 1, 10
OPPS recognized blood/blood products

⊛ **P9038** Red blood cells, irradiated, each unit Ⓑ   R
IOM: 100-01, 3, 20.5; 100-02, 1, 10
OPPS recognized blood/blood products

⊛ **P9039** Red blood cells, deglycerolized, each unit Ⓑ   R
IOM: 100-01, 3, 20.5; 100-02, 1, 10
OPPS recognized blood/blood products

⊛ **P9040** Red blood cells, leukocytes reduced, irradiated, each unit Ⓑ   R
IOM: 100-01, 3, 20.5; 100-02, 1, 10
OPPS recognized blood/blood products

✳ **P9041** Infusion, albumin (human), 5%, 50 ml Ⓑ Qp Qh   K2 K

⊛ **P9043** Infusion, plasma protein fraction (human), 5%, 50 ml Ⓑ Qp Qh   R
IOM: 100-01, 3, 20.5; 100-02, 1, 10
OPPS recognized blood/blood products

⊛ **P9044** Plasma, cryoprecipitate reduced, each unit Ⓑ   R
IOM: 100-01, 3, 20.5; 100-02, 1, 10
OPPS recognized blood/blood products

✳ **P9045** Infusion, albumin (human), 5%, 250 ml Ⓑ Qp Qh   K2 K

✳ **P9046** Infusion, albumin (human), 25%, 20 ml Ⓑ Qp Qh   K2 K

✳ **P9047** Infusion, albumin (human), 25%, 50 ml Ⓑ Qp Qh   K2 K

✳ **P9048** Infusion, plasma protein fraction (human), 5%, 250 ml Ⓑ Qp Qh   R
OPPS recognized blood/blood products

✳ **P9050** Granulocytes, pheresis, each unit Ⓑ   R
OPPS recognized blood/blood products

⊛ **P9051** Whole blood or red blood cells, leukocytes reduced, CMV-negative, each unit Ⓑ   R
Medicare Statute 1833(t)
OPPS recognized blood/blood products

⊛ **P9052** Platelets, HLA-matched leukocytes reduced, apheresis/pheresis, each unit Ⓑ   R
Medicare Statute 1833(t)
OPPS recognized blood/blood products

▶ **New**   ↻ **Revised**   ✔ **Reinstated**   ~~deleted~~ **Deleted**   ⊘ **Not covered or valid by Medicare**
⊛ **Special coverage instructions**   ✳ **Carrier discretion**   Ⓑ **Bill local carrier**   Ⓑ **Bill DME MAC**

P9053 Platelets, pheresis, leukocytes reduced, CMV-negative, irradiated, each unit Ⓑ   R

Freezing and thawing are reported separately, see Transmittal 1487 (Hospital outpatient)

Medicare Statute 1833(t)

OPPS recognized blood/blood products

P9054 Whole blood or red blood cells, leukocytes reduced, frozen, deglycerol, washed, each unit Ⓑ   R

Medicare Statute 1833(t)

OPPS recognized blood/blood products

P9055 Platelets, leukocytes reduced, CMV-negative, apheresis/pheresis, each unit Ⓑ   R

Medicare Statute 1833(t)

OPPS recognized blood/blood products

P9056 Whole blood, leukocytes reduced, irradiated, each unit Ⓑ   R

Medicare Statute 1833(t)

OPPS recognized blood/blood products

P9057 Red blood cells, frozen/deglycerolized/washed, leukocytes reduced, irradiated, each unit Ⓑ   R

Medicare Statute 1833(t)

OPPS recognized blood/blood products

P9058 Red blood cells, leukocytes reduced, CMV-negative, irradiated, each unit Ⓑ   R

Medicare Statute 1833(t)

OPPS recognized blood/blood products

P9059 Fresh frozen plasma between 8-24 hours of collection, each unit Ⓑ   R

Medicare Statute 1833(t)

OPPS recognized blood/blood products

P9060 Fresh frozen plasma, donor retested, each unit Ⓑ   R

Medicare Statute 1833(t)

OPPS recognized blood/blood products

P9603 Travel allowance one way in connection with medically necessary laboratory specimen collection drawn from home bound or nursing home bound patient; prorated miles actually traveled Ⓑ   A

Fee for clinical laboratory travel (P9603) is $0.96 per mile for CY2011

IOM: 100-04, 16, 60

P9604 Travel allowance one way in connection with medically necessary laboratory specimen collection drawn from home bound or nursing home bound patient; prorated trip charge Ⓑ   A

For CY2010, the fee for clinical laboratory travel is $9.60 per flat rate trip for CY2011

IOM: 100-04, 16, 60

P9612 Catheterization for collection of specimen, single patient, all places of service Ⓑ Qp Qh   A

NCCI edits indicate that when 51701 is comprehensive or is a Column 1 code, P9612 cannot be reported. When the catheter insertion is a component of another procedure, do not report straight catheterization separately.

IOM: 100-04, 16, 60

Coding Clinic: 2007, Q3, P7

P9615 Catheterization for collection of specimen(s) (multiple patients) Ⓑ Qp Qh   N

IOM: 100-04, 16, 60

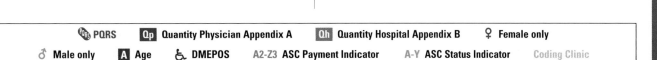

| ⓅPQRS PQRS | Qp Quantity Physician Appendix A | Qh Quantity Hospital Appendix B | ♀ Female only |
| ♂ Male only | A Age | & DMEPOS | A2-Z3 ASC Payment Indicator | A-Y ASC Status Indicator | Coding Clinic |

TEMPORARY CODES ASSIGNED BY CMS (Q0000-Q9999)

Cardiokymography

⚙ **Q0035** Cardiokymography ⑧ Qp Qh   S

Report modifier 26 if professional component only

IOM: 100-03, 1, 20.24

Chemotherapy

⚙ **Q0081** Infusion therapy, using other than chemotherapeutic drugs, per visit ⑧   B

IV piggyback only assigned one time per patient encounter per day. Report for hydration or the intravenous administration of antibiotics, anti-emetics, or analgesics. Bill on paper. Requires a report.

IOM: 100-03, 4, 280.14

Coding Clinic: 2004, Q2, P11; Q1, P5, 8; 2002, Q2, P10; Q1, P7

✳ **Q0083** Chemotherapy administration by other than infusion technique only (e.g., subcutaneous, intramuscular, push), per visit ⑧   B

Coding Clinic: 2002, Q1, P7

⚙ **Q0084** Chemotherapy administration by infusion technique only, per visit ⑧   B

IOM: 100-03, 4, 280.14

Coding Clinic: 2004, Q2, P11; 2002, Q1, P7

✳ **Q0085** Chemotherapy administration by both infusion technique and other technique(s) (e.g., subcutaneous, intramuscular, push), per visit ⑧ Qh   B

Coding Clinic: 2002, Q1, P7

Smear, Papanicolaou

⚙ **Q0091** Screening Papanicolaou smear; obtaining, preparing and conveyance of cervical or vaginal smear to laboratory ⑧ Qp Qh ♀   S

Medicare does not cover comprehensive preventive medicine services; however, services described by G0101 and Q0091 (only for Medicare patients) are covered. Includes the services necessary to procure and transport the specimen to the laboratory.

IOM: 100-03, 3, 190.2

Coding Clinic: 2002, Q4, P8

Equipment, X-Ray, Portable

⚙ **Q0092** Set-up portable x-ray equipment ⑧   N

IOM: 100-04, 13, 90

Laboratory

✳ **Q0111** Wet mounts, including preparations of vaginal, cervical or skin specimens ⑧ Qp Qh   A

Laboratory Certification: Bacteriology, Mycology, Parasitology

✳ **Q0112** All potassium hydroxide (KOH) preparations ⑧ Qp Qh   A

Laboratory Certification: Mycology

✳ **Q0113** Pinworm examinations ⑧ Qp Qh   A

Laboratory Certification: Parasitology

✳ **Q0114** Fern test ⑧ Qp Qh ♀   A

Laboratory certification: Routine chemistry

✳ **Q0115** Post-coital direct, qualitative examinations of vaginal or cervical mucous ⑧ Qp Qh ♀   A

Laboratory Certification: Hematology

Drugs

✳ **Q0138** Injection, ferumoxytol, for treatment of iron deficiency anemia, 1 mg (non-ESRD use)   K2 K

Feraheme is FDA approved for chronic kidney disease

NDC: Feraheme

✳ **Q0139** Injection, ferumoxytol, for treatment of iron deficiency anemia, 1 mg (for ESRD on dialysis)   K

NDC: Feraheme

⊘ **Q0144** Azithromycin dihydrate, oral, capsules/powder, 1 gm ⑧ Qp Qh   E

If incident to a physician's service, do not bill.

Other: Zithromax

✳ **Q0161** Chlorpromazine hydrochloride, 5 mg, oral, FDA approved prescription anti-emetic, for use as a complete therapeutic substitute for an IV anti-emetic at the time of chemotherapy treatment, not to exceed a 48 hour dosage regimen Qp Qh   N1 N

▶ **New**	↻ **Revised**	✔ **Reinstated**	~~deleted~~ **Deleted**	⊘ **Not covered or valid by Medicare**
⚙ **Special coverage instructions**		✳ **Carrier discretion**	⑧ **Bill local carrier**	⑧ **Bill DME MAC**

○ **Q0162** Ondansetron 1 mg, oral, FDA-approved prescription anti-emetic, for use as a complete therapeutic substitute for an iv anti-emetic at the time of chemotherapy treatment, not to exceed a 48 hour dosage regimen   N1   N

NDC: Zofran

Medicare Statute 4557

Coding Clinic: 2012, Q1, P9

○ **Q0163** Diphenhydramine hydrochloride, 50 mg, oral, FDA approved prescription anti-emetic, for use as a complete therapeutic substitute for an IV anti-emetic at time of chemotherapy treatment not to exceed a 48 hour dosage regimen Ⓑ   N1   N

Other: Alercap, Aler-Dryl, Allergy Children's, Allergy Relief Medicine, Allermax, Alertab, Anti-Hist, Antihistamine, Banophen, Complete Allergy Medication, Complete Allergy medicine, Diphedryl, Diphen, Diphenhist, Diphenyl, Dormin Sleep Aid, Geridryl, Good Sense Antihistamine Allergy Relief, Good Sense Nighttime Sleep Aid, Genahist, Hydramine, Medicine Shoppe Medi-Phedryl, Medicine Shoppe Nite Time Sleep, Mediphedryl, Night Time Sleep Aid, Nytol Quickcaps, Nytol Quickgels maximum strength, Q-Dryl, Quality Choice Sleep Aid, Quality Choice Rest Simply, Quenalin, Rite Aid Allergy, Serabrina La France, Siladryl Allergy, Silphen, Simply Sleep, Sleep Tabs, Sleep-ettes D, Sleepinal, Sominex, Twilite, Valu-Dryl Allergy

Medicare Statute 4557

Coding Clinic: 2012, Q2, P10

○ **Q0164** Prochlorperazine maleate, 5 mg, oral, FDA approved prescription anti-emetic, for use as a complete therapeutic substitute for an IV anti-emetic at the time of chemotherapy treatment, not to exceed a 48 hour dosage regimen Ⓑ   N1   N

Other: Compazine

Medicare Statute 4557

Coding Clinic: 2012, Q2, P10

○ **Q0166** Granisetron hydrochloride, 1 mg, oral, FDA approved prescription anti-emetic, for use as a complete therapeutic substitute for an IV anti-emetic at the time of chemotherapy treatment, not to exceed a 24 hour dosage regimen Ⓑ   N1   N

Other: Kytril

Medicare Statute 4557

Coding Clinic: 2012, Q2, P10

○ **Q0167** Dronabinol, 2.5 mg, oral, FDA approved prescription anti-emetic, for use as a complete therapeutic substitute for an IV anti-emetic at the time of chemotherapy treatment, not to exceed a 48 hour dosage regimen Ⓑ   N1   N

NDC: Marinol

Medicare Statute 4557

Coding Clinic: 2012, Q2, P10

○ **Q0169** Promethazine hydrochloride, 12.5 mg, oral, FDA approved prescription anti-emetic, for use as a complete therapeutic substitute for an IV anti-emetic at the time of chemotherapy treatment, not to exceed a 48 hour dosage regimen Ⓑ   N1   N

Other: Phenergan

Medicare Statute 4557

Coding Clinic: 2012, Q2, P10

○ **Q0173** Trimethobenzamide hydrochloride, 250 mg, oral, FDA approved prescription anti-emetic, for use as a complete therapeutic substitute for an IV anti-emetic at the time of chemotherapy treatment, not to exceed a 48 hour dosage regimen Ⓑ   N1   N

Other: Ticon, Tigan

Medicare Statute 4557

Coding Clinic: 2012, Q2, P10

○ **Q0174** Thiethylperazine maleate, 10 mg, oral, FDA approved prescription anti-emetic, for use as a complete therapeutic substitute for an IV anti-emetic at the time of chemotherapy treatment, not to exceed a 48 hour dosage regimen Ⓑ   E

Other: Torecan

Medicare Statute 4557

Coding Clinic: 2012, Q2, P10

ᴾᴼᴿₛ **PQRS**	**Qp** Quantity Physician Appendix A	**Qh** Quantity Hospital Appendix B	♀ **Female only**
♂ **Male only**	**A** Age	♿ **DMEPOS**	A2-Z3 **ASC Payment Indicator** A-Y **ASC Status Indicator** *Coding Clinic*

○ **Q0175** Perphenazine, 4 mg, oral, FDA approved prescription anti-emetic, for use as a complete therapeutic substitute for an IV anti-emetic at the time of chemotherapy treatment, not to exceed a 48 hour dosage regimen Ⓑ   **N1** **N**

Medicare Statute 4557

Coding Clinic: 2012, Q2, P10

○ **Q0177** Hydroxyzine pamoate, 25 mg, oral, FDA approved prescription anti-emetic, for use as a complete therapeutic substitute for an IV anti-emetic at the time of chemotherapy treatment, not to exceed a 48 hour dosage regimen Ⓑ   **N1** **N**

Other: Vistaril

Medicare Statute 4557

Coding Clinic: 2012, Q2, P10

○ **Q0180** Dolasetron mesylate, 100 mg, oral, FDA approved prescription anti-emetic, for use as a complete therapeutic substitute for an IV anti-emetic at the time of chemotherapy treatment, not to exceed a 24 hour dosage regimen Ⓑ   **N1** **N**

NDC: Anzemet

Medicare Statute 4557

Coding Clinic: 2012, Q2, P10

○ **Q0181** Unspecified oral dosage form, FDA approved prescription anti-emetic, for use as a complete therapeutic substitute for a IV anti-emetic at the time of chemotherapy treatment, not to exceed a 48 hour dosage regimen Ⓑ   **N**

Medicare Statute 4557

Coding Clinic: 2012, Q2, P10

Miscellaneous Devices

○ **Q0478** Power adapter for use with electric or electric/pneumatic ventricular assist device, vehicle type **Qp** **Qh** ♿   A

CMS has determined the reasonable useful lifetime is one year. Add modifier RA to claims to report when battery is replaced because it was lost, stolen, or irreparably damaged. (http://www.wpsmedicare.com/part_b/publications/communique/archived/_files/winter-2011-comm.pdf)

○ **Q0479** Power module for use with electric or electric/pneumatic ventricular assist device, replacement only **Qp** **Qh** ♿   A

CMS has determined the reasonable useful lifetime is one year. Add modifier RA in cases where the battery is being replaced because it was lost, stolen, or irreparably damaged. (http://www.wpsmedicare.com/part_b/publications/communique/archived/_files/winter-2011-comm.pdf)

○ **Q0480** Driver for use with pneumatic ventricular assist device, replacement only Ⓑ **Qp** **Qh** ♿   A

○ **Q0481** Microprocessor control unit for use with electric ventricular assist device, replacement only Ⓑ **Qp** **Qh** ♿   A

○ **Q0482** Microprocessor control unit for use with electric/pneumatic combination ventricular assist device, replacement only Ⓑ **Qp** **Qh** ♿   A

○ **Q0483** Monitor/display module for use with electric ventricular assist device, replacement only Ⓑ **Qp** **Qh** ♿   A

○ **Q0484** Monitor/display module for use with electric or electric/pneumatic ventricular assist device, replacement only Ⓑ **Qp** **Qh** ♿   A

○ **Q0485** Monitor control cable for use with electric ventricular assist device, replacement only Ⓑ **Qp** **Qh** ♿   A

○ **Q0486** Monitor control cable for use with electric/pneumatic ventricular assist device, replacement only Ⓑ **Qp** **Qh** ♿ A

○ **Q0487** Leads (pneumatic/electrical) for use with any type electric/pneumatic ventricular assist device, replacement only Ⓑ **Qp** **Qh** ♿   A

○ **Q0488** Power pack base for use with electric ventricular assist device, replacement only Ⓑ **Qp** **Qh**   A

○ **Q0489** Power pack base for use with electric/pneumatic ventricular assist device, replacement only Ⓑ **Qp** **Qh** ♿   A

○ **Q0490** Emergency power source for use with electric ventricular assist device, replacement only Ⓑ **Qp** **Qh** ♿   A

○ **Q0491** Emergency power source for use with electric/pneumatic ventricular assist device, replacement only Ⓑ **Qp** **Qh** ♿ A

○ **Q0492** Emergency power supply cable for use with electric ventricular assist device, replacement only Ⓑ **Qp** **Qh** ♿

▶ **New**   ↻ **Revised**   ✔ **Reinstated**   ~~deleted~~ **Deleted**   ⊘ **Not covered or valid by Medicare**

○ **Special coverage instructions**   ✱ **Carrier discretion**   Ⓑ **Bill local carrier**   Ⓑ **Bill DME MAC**

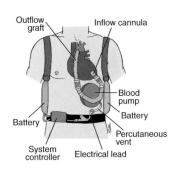

Figure 49 Ventricular assist device.

Labels: Outflow graft, Inflow cannula, Blood pump, Battery, Battery, Percutaneous vent, System controller, Electrical lead

○ **Q0493** Emergency power supply cable for use with electric/pneumatic ventricular assist device, replacement only ⓑ Qp Qh ㅤ A

○ **Q0494** Emergency hand pump for use with electric or electric/pneumatic ventricular assist device, replacement only ⓑ Qp Qh ㅤ A

○ **Q0495** Battery/power pack charger for use with electric or electric/pneumatic ventricular assist device, replacement only ⓑ Qp Qh ㅤ A

＊ **Q0496** Battery, other than lithium-ion, for use with electric or electric/pneumatic ventricular assist device, replacement only ⓑ ㅤ A

Reasonable useful lifetime is 6 months (CR3931).

○ **Q0497** Battery clips for use with electric or electric/pneumatic ventricular assist device, replacement only ⓑ Qp Qh ㅤ A

○ **Q0498** Holster for use with electric or electric/pneumatic ventricular assist device, replacement only ⓑ Qp Qh ㅤ A

○ **Q0499** Belt/vest/bag for use to carry external peripheral components of any type ventricular assist device, replacement only ⓑ Qp Qh ㅤ A

○ **Q0500** Filters for use with electric or electric/pneumatic ventricular assist device, replacement only ⓑ ㅤ A

○ **Q0501** Shower cover for use with electric or electric/pneumatic ventricular assist device, replacement only ⓑ Qp Qh ㅤ A

○ **Q0502** Mobility cart for pneumatic ventricular assist device, replacement only ⓑ Qp Qh ㅤ A

○ **Q0503** Battery for pneumatic ventricular assist device, replacement only, each ⓑ Qp Qh ㅤ A

Reasonable useful lifetime is 6 months (CR3931).

○ **Q0504** Power adapter for pneumatic ventricular assist device, replacement only, vehicle type ⓑ Qp Qh ㅤ A

○ **Q0506** Battery, lithium-ion, for use with electric or electric/pneumatic, ventricular assist device, replacement only ㅤ A

Reasonable useful lifetime is 12 months. Add -RA for replacement if lost, stolen, or irreparable damage.

○ **Q0507** Miscellaneous supply or accessory for use with an external ventricular assist device Qp Qh N1 N

○ **Q0508** Miscellaneous supply or accessory for use with an implanted ventricular assist device Qp Qh N1 N

○ **Q0509** Miscellaneous supply or accessory for use with any implanted ventricular assist device for which payment was not made under Medicare Part A Qp Qh N1 N

Fee, Pharmacy

○ **Q0510** Pharmacy supply fee for initial immunosuppressive drug(s), first month following transplant ⓑ Qp Qh B

○ **Q0511** Pharmacy supply fee for oral anti-cancer, oral anti-emetic or immunosuppressive drug(s); for the first prescription in a 30-day period ⓑ Qp Qh B

○ **Q0512** Pharmacy supply fee for oral anti-cancer, oral anti-emetic or immunosuppressive drug(s); for a subsequent prescription in a 30-day period ⓑ Qp Qh B

○ **Q0513** Pharmacy dispensing fee for inhalation drug(s); per 30 days ⓑ Qp Qh B

○ **Q0514** Pharmacy dispensing fee for inhalation drug(s); per 90 days ⓑ Qp Qh B

↻ ○ **Q0515** Injection, sermorelin acetate, 1 microgram ⓑ E

IOM: 100-02, 15, 50

Lens, Intraocular

○ **Q1004** New technology intraocular lens category 4 as defined in Federal Register notice ⓑ Qp Qh E

○ **Q1005** New technology intraocular lens category 5 as defined in Federal Register notice ⓑ Qp Qh E

Solutions and Drugs

⚙ **Q2004** Irrigation solution for treatment of bladder calculi, for example renacidin, per 500 ml Ⓑ `Qp` `Qh`   N

IOM: 100-02, 15, 50

Medicare Statute 1861S2B

✳ **Q2009** Injection, fosphenytoin, 50 mg phenytoin equivalent Ⓑ   N1 N

IOM: 100-02, 15, 50

Medicare Statute 1861S2B

⚙ **Q2017** Injection, teniposide, 50 mg Ⓑ   K2 K

IOM: 100-02, 15, 50

Medicare Statute 1861S2B

⚙ **Q2026** Injection, radiesse, 0.1 ml   B

Coding Clinic: 2010, Q3, P8

⚙ **Q2028** Injection, sculptra, 0.5 mg `Qp` `Qh`   B

⚙ **Q2034** Influenza virus vaccine, split virus, for intramuscular use (Agriflu) Sipuleucel-t, minimum of 50 million autologous CD54+ cells activated with PAP-GM-CSF, including leukapheresis and all other preparatory procedures, per infusion Ⓑ `Qp` `Qh`   L1

IOM 100-02, 15, 50

⚙ **Q2035** Influenza virus vaccine, split virus, when administered to individuals 3 years of age and older, for intramuscular use (Afluria) `Qp` `Qh` `A`   L1 L

Preventive service; no deductible

IOM: 100-02, 15, 50

Coding Clinic: 2011, Q1, P7; 2010, Q4, P8-9

⚙ **Q2036** Influenza virus vaccine, split virus, when administered to individuals 3 years of age and older, for intramuscular use (Flulaval) `Qp` `Qh` `A`   L1 L

Preventive service; no deductible

IOM: 100-02, 15, 50

Coding Clinic: 2011, Q1, P7; 2010, Q4, P8-9

⚙ **Q2037** Influenza virus vaccine, split virus, when administered to individuals 3 years of age and older, for intramuscular use (Fluvirin) `Qp` `Qh` `A`   L1 L

Preventive service; no deductible

IOM: 100-02, 15, 50

Coding Clinic: 2011, Q1, P7; 2010, Q4, P8-9

⚙ **Q2038** Influenza virus vaccine, split virus, when administered to individuals 3 years of age or older, for intramuscular use (Fluzone) `Qp` `Qh` `A`   L1 L

Preventive service; no deductible

IOM: 100-02, 15, 50

Coding Clinic: 2011, Q1, P7; 2010, Q4, P8-9

⚙ **Q2039** Influenza virus vaccine, split virus, when administered to individuals 3 years of age and older, for intramuscular use (not otherwise specified) `Qp` `Qh` `A`   L1 L

Preventive service; no deductible

IOM: 100-02, 15, 50

Coding Clinic: 2011, Q1, P7; 2010, Q4, P8-9

⚙ **Q2043** Sipuleucel-T, minimum of 50 million autologous CD54+ cells activated with PAP-GM-CSF, including leukapheresis and all other preparatory procedures, per infusion `Qp` `Qh`   K

Coding Clinic: 2012, Q2, P7; Q1, P7, 9; 2011, Q3, P9

✳ **Q2049** Injection, doxorubicin hydrochloride, liposomal, imported lipodox, 10 mg Ⓑ   K2

Bill local carrier (Ⓑ) if incident to a physician's service or used in an implanted infusion pump.

Coding Clinic: 2012, Q3, P10

⚙ **Q2050** Injection, doxorubicin hydrochloride, liposomal, not otherwise specified, 10 mg `Qp` `Qh`   K2 K

IOM 100-02, 15, 50

⚙ **Q2052** Services, supplies and accessories used in the home under the Medicare intravenous immune globulin (IVIG) demonstration `Qp` `Qh`   E

Coding Clinic: 2014, Q2, P6

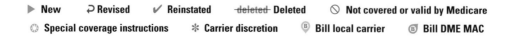

▶ **New**   ↻ **Revised**   ✔ **Reinstated**   ~~deleted~~ **Deleted**   ⊘ **Not covered or valid by Medicare**
⚙ **Special coverage instructions**   ✳ **Carrier discretion**   Ⓑ **Bill local carrier**   Ⓑ **Bill DME MAC**

Brachytherapy Radioelements

◎ **Q3001** Radioelements for brachytherapy, any type, each   B

IOM: 100-04, 12, 70; 100-04, 13, 20

Telehealth

＊ **Q3014** Telehealth originating site facility fee ⑧ Qp Qh   A

Effective January of each year, the fee for telehealth services is increased by the Medicare Economic Index (MEI). The telehealth originating facility site fee (HCPCS code Q3014) for 2011 was 80 percent of the lesser of the actual charge or $24.10.

Drugs

◎ **Q3027** Injection, interferon beta-1a, 1 mcg for intramuscular use ⑧ Qp Qh   K2   K

NDC: Avonex

IOM 100-02, 15, 50

⊘ **Q3028** Injection, interferon beta-1a, 1 mcg for subcutaneous use ⑧ Qp Qh   E

Test, Skin

◎ **Q3031** Collagen skin test ⑧ Qh   N1   N

IOM: 100-03, 4, 280.1

Supplies, Cast

Payment on a reasonable charge basis is required for splints, casts by regulations contained in 42 CFR 405.501.

↺＊ **Q4001** Casting supplies, body cast adult, with or without head, plaster ⑧ Qp Qh A ♿   B

↺＊ **Q4002** Cast supplies, body cast adult, with or without head, fiberglass ⑧ Qp Qh A ♿   B

↺＊ **Q4003** Cast supplies, shoulder cast, adult (11 years +), plaster ⑧ Qp Qh A ♿   B

↺＊ **Q4004** Cast supplies, shoulder cast, adult (11 years +), fiberglass ⑧ Qp Qh A ♿   B

↺＊ **Q4005** Cast supplies, long arm cast, adult (11 years +), plaster ⑧ A ♿   B

↺＊ **Q4006** Cast supplies, long arm cast, adult (11 years +), fiberglass ⑧ A ♿   B

↺＊ **Q4007** Cast supplies, long arm cast, pediatric (0-10 years), plaster ⑧ A ♿   B

↺＊ **Q4008** Cast supplies, long arm cast, pediatric (0-10 years), fiberglass ⑧ A ♿   B

↺＊ **Q4009** Cast supplies, short arm cast, adult (11 years +), plaster ⑧ A ♿   B

↺＊ **Q4010** Cast supplies, short arm cast, adult (11 years +), fiberglass ⑧ A ♿   B

↺＊ **Q4011** Cast supplies, short arm cast, pediatric (0-10 years), plaster ⑧ A ♿   B

↺＊ **Q4012** Cast supplies, short arm cast, pediatric (0-10 years), fiberglass ⑧ A ♿   B

↺＊ **Q4013** Cast supplies, gauntlet cast (includes lower forearm and hand), adult (11 years +), plaster ⑧ A ♿   B

↺＊ **Q4014** Cast supplies, gauntlet cast (includes lower forearm and hand), adult (11 years +), fiberglass ⑧ A ♿   B

↺＊ **Q4015** Cast supplies, gauntlet cast (includes lower forearm and hand), pediatric (0-10 years), plaster ⑧ A ♿   B

↺＊ **Q4016** Cast supplies, gauntlet cast (includes lower forearm and hand), pediatric (0-10 years), fiberglass A ♿   B

↺＊ **Q4017** Cast supplies, long arm splint, adult (11 years +), plaster ⑧ A ♿   B

↺＊ **Q4018** Cast supplies, long arm splint, adult (11 years +), fiberglass ⑧ A ♿   B

↺＊ **Q4019** Cast supplies, long arm splint, pediatric (0-10 years), plaster ⑧ A ♿   B

↺＊ **Q4020** Cast supplies, long arm splint, pediatric (0-10 years), fiberglass ⑧ A ♿   B

↺＊ **Q4021** Cast supplies, short arm splint, adult (11 years +), plaster ⑧ A ♿   B

↺＊ **Q4022** Cast supplies, short arm splint, adult (11 years +), fiberglass ⑧ A ♿   B

↺＊ **Q4023** Cast supplies, short arm splint, pediatric (0-10 years), plaster ⑧ A ♿   B

↺＊ **Q4024** Cast supplies, short arm splint, pediatric (0-10 years), fiberglass ⑧ A ♿   B

↺＊ **Q4025** Cast supplies, hip spica (one or both legs), adult (11 years +), plaster ⑧ Qp Qh A ♿   B

↺＊ **Q4026** Cast supplies, hip spica (one or both legs), adult (11 years +), fiberglass ⑧ Qp Qh A ♿   B

↺＊ **Q4027** Cast supplies, hip spica (one or both legs), pediatric (0-10 years), plaster ⑧ Qp Qh A ♿   B

↺＊ **Q4028** Cast supplies, hip spica (one or both legs), pediatric (0-10 years), fiberglass ⑧ Qp Qh A ♿   B

| 🅟 PQRS | Qp Quantity Physician Appendix A | Qh Quantity Hospital Appendix B | ♀ Female only |
| ♂ Male only | A Age | ♿ DMEPOS | A2-Z3 ASC Payment Indicator | A-Y ASC Status Indicator | Coding Clinic |

TEMPORARY CODES ASSIGNED BY CMS   Q3001 — Q4028

343

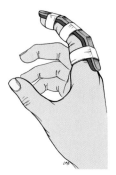

Figure 50 Finger splint.

○* **Q4029** Cast supplies, long leg cast, adult (11 years +), plaster ⓑ 🅐 ♿   B

○* **Q4030** Cast supplies, long leg cast, adult (11 years +), fiberglass ⓑ 🅐 ♿   B

○* **Q4031** Cast supplies, long leg cast, pediatric (0-10 years), plaster ⓑ 🅐 ♿   B

○* **Q4032** Cast supplies, long leg cast, pediatric (0-10 years), fiberglass ⓑ 🅐 ♿   B

○* **Q4033** Cast supplies, long leg cylinder cast, adult (11 years +), plaster ⓑ 🅐 ♿   B

○* **Q4034** Cast supplies, long leg cylinder cast, adult (11 years +), fiberglass ⓑ 🅐 ♿   B

○* **Q4035** Cast supplies, long leg cylinder cast, pediatric (0-10 years), plaster ⓑ 🅐 ♿   B

○* **Q4036** Cast supplies, long leg cylinder cast, pediatric (0-10 years), fiberglass ⓑ 🅐 ♿   B

○* **Q4037** Cast supplies, short leg cast, adult (11 years +), plaster ⓑ 🅐 ♿   B

○* **Q4038** Cast supplies, short leg cast, adult (11 years +), fiberglass ⓑ 🅐 ♿   B

○* **Q4039** Cast supplies, short leg cast, pediatric (0-10 years), plaster ⓑ 🅐 ♿   B

○* **Q4040** Cast supplies, short leg cast, pediatric (0-10 years), fiberglass ⓑ 🅐 ♿   B

○* **Q4041** Cast supplies, long leg splint, adult (11 years +), plaster ⓑ 🅐 ♿   B

○* **Q4042** Cast supplies, long leg splint, adult (11 years +), fiberglass ⓑ 🅐 ♿   B

○* **Q4043** Cast supplies, long leg splint, pediatric (0-10 years), plaster ⓑ 🅐 ♿   B

○* **Q4044** Cast supplies, long leg splint, pediatric (0-10 years), fiberglass ⓑ 🅐 ♿   B

○* **Q4045** Cast supplies, short leg splint, adult (11 years +), plaster ⓑ 🅐 ♿   B

○* **Q4046** Cast supplies, short leg splint, adult (11 years +), fiberglass ⓑ 🅐 ♿   B

○* **Q4047** Cast supplies, short leg splint, pediatric (0-10 years), plaster ⓑ 🅐 ♿   B

○* **Q4048** Cast supplies, short leg splint, pediatric (0-10 years), fiberglass ⓑ 🅐 ♿   B

○* **Q4049** Finger splint, static ⓑ ♿   B

* **Q4050** Cast supplies, for unlisted types and materials of casts ⓑ   B

* **Q4051** Splint supplies, miscellaneous (includes thermoplastics, strapping, fasteners, padding and other supplies) ⓑ   B

Drugs

* **Q4074** Iloprost, inhalation solution, FDA-approved final product, non-compounded, administered through DME, unit dose form, up to 20 micrograms 🆀🅿 🆀🅷   Y

NDC: Ventavis

◎ **Q4081** Injection, epoetin alfa, 100 units (for ESRD on dialysis) ⓑ   N

Bill local carrier (ⓑ) for method II home dialysis.

NDC: Epogen, Procrit

* **Q4082** Drug or biological, not otherwise classified, Part B drug competitive acquisition program (CAP) ⓑ   B

Skin Substitutes

* **Q4100** Skin substitute, not otherwise specified ⓑ   N1 N

Other: Orcel, Surgimend collagen matrix

Coding Clinic: 2012, Q2, P7

* **Q4101** Apligraf, per square centimeter ⓑ 🆀🅿 🆀🅷   N1 N

Coding Clinic: 2012, Q2, P7; 2011, Q1, P9

* **Q4102** Oasis Wound Matrix, per square centimeter ⓑ 🆀🅿 🆀🅷   N1 N

Coding Clinic: 2012, Q3, P8; Q2, P7; 2011, Q1, P9

* **Q4103** Oasis Burn Matrix, per square centimeter ⓑ 🆀🅿 🆀🅷   N1 N

Coding Clinic: 2012, Q2, P7; 2011, Q1, P9

* **Q4104** Integra Bilayer Matrix Wound Dressing (BMWD), per square centimeter ⓑ 🆀🅿 🆀🅷   N1 N

Coding Clinic: 2012, Q2, P7; 2011, Q1, P9; 2010, Q2, P8

* **Q4105** Integra Dermal Regeneration Template (DRT), per square centimeter ⓑ 🆀🅿 🆀🅷   N1 N

Coding Clinic: 2012, Q2, P7; 2011, Q1, P9; 2010, Q2, P8

* **Q4106** Dermagraft, per square centimeter ⓑ 🆀🅿 🆀🅷   N1 N

Coding Clinic: 2012, Q2, P7; 2011, Q1, P9

▶ **New**   ↺ **Revised**   ✔ **Reinstated**   ~~deleted~~ **Deleted**   ⊘ **Not covered or valid by Medicare**

◎ **Special coverage instructions**   * **Carrier discretion**   ⓑ **Bill local carrier**   ◎ **Bill DME MAC**

* **Q4107** Graftjacket, per square centimeter ⑬ **Qp** **Qh**   N1   N

NDC: Graftjacket Maxstrip, Graftjacket Small Ligament Repair Matrix, Graftjacket STD, Handjacket Scaffold Thin, Maxforce Thick, Ulcerjacket Scaffold, Ultra Maxforce

Coding Clinic: 2012, Q2, P7; 2011, Q1, P9

* **Q4108** Integra Matrix, per square centimeter ⑬ **Qp** **Qh**   N1   N

Coding Clinic: 2012, Q2, P7; 2011, Q1, P9; 2010, Q2, P8

* **Q4110** Primatrix, per square centimeter ⑬ **Qp** **Qh**   N1   N

Coding Clinic: 2012, Q2, P7; 2011, Q1, P9

* **Q4111** GammaGraft, per square centimeter ⑬ **Qp** **Qh**   N1   N

Coding Clinic: 2012, Q2, P7; 2011, Q1, P9

* **Q4112** Cymetra, injectable, 1cc **Qp** **Qh**   N1   N

Coding Clinic: 2012, Q2, P7; 2011, Q1, P9

* **Q4113** GraftJacket Xpress, injectable, 1cc ⑬ **Qp** **Qh**   N1   N

Coding Clinic: 2012, Q2, P7; 2011, Q1, P9

* **Q4114** Integra Flowable Wound Matrix, injectable, 1cc ⑬ **Qp** **Qh**   N1   N

Coding Clinic: 2012, Q2, P7; 2010, Q2, P8

* **Q4115** Alloskin, per square centimeter ⑬ **Qp** **Qh**   N1   N

Coding Clinic: 2012, Q2, P7; 2011, Q1, P9

* **Q4116** Alloderm, per square centimeter ⑬ **Qp** **Qh**   N1   N

Coding Clinic: 2012, Q2, P7; 2011, Q1, P9

* **Q4117** Hyalomatrix, per square centimeter **Qp** **Qh**   N

IOM: 100-02, 15, 50

* **Q4118** Matristem micromatrix, 1 mg **Qp** **Qh**   N1   N

Coding Clinic: 2013, Q4, P2; 2012, Q2, P7; 2011, Q1, P6

↺* **Q4119** Matristem wound matrix, per square centimeter **Qp** **Qh**   N1   N

Coding Clinic: 2012, Q2, P7; 2011, Q1, P6

* **Q4120** Matristem burn matrix, per square centimeter **Qp** **Qh**   N

↺* **Q4121** Theraskin, per square centimeter **Qp** **Qh**   K2   G

Coding Clinic: 2012, Q2, P7; 2011, Q1, P6

* **Q4122** Dermacell, per square centimeter **Qp** **Qh**   K2   G

Coding Clinic: 2012, Q2, P7; Q1, P8

* **Q4123** AlloSkin RT, per square centimeter **Qp** **Qh**   N1   N

* **Q4124** Oasis Ultra Tri-layer Wound Matrix, per square centimeter **Qp** **Qh**   N1   N

Coding Clinic: 2012, Q2, P7; Q1, P9

* **Q4125** Arthroflex, per square centimeter **Qp** **Qh**   N1   N

* **Q4126** Memoderm, dermaspan, tranzgraft or integuply, per square centimeter **Qp** **Qh**   N

* **Q4127** Talymed, per square centimeter **Qp** **Qh**   K2   G

* **Q4128** FlexHD, Allopatch HD, or Matrix HD, per square centimeter **Qp** **Qh**   N1   N

* **Q4129** Unite Biomatrix, per square centimeter **Qp** **Qh**   N

* **Q4130** Strattice TM, per square centimeter **Qp** **Qh**   N1   N

Coding Clinic: 2012, Q2, P7

↺* **Q4131** Epifix, per square centimeter ⑬ **Qp** **Qh**   N1   N

↺* **Q4132** Grafix core, per square centimeter ⑬ **Qp** **Qh**   N1   N

↺* **Q4133** Grafix prime, per square centimeter ⑬ **Qp** **Qh**   N1   N

* **Q4134** Hmatrix, per square centimeter ⑬ **Qp** **Qh**   N

* **Q4135** Mediskin, per square centimeter ⑬ **Qp** **Qh**   N

* **Q4136** Ez-derm, per square centimeter ⑬ **Qp** **Qh**   N

* **Q4137** Amnioexcel or biodexcel, per square centimeter   N1   N

* **Q4138** Biodfence dryflex, per square centimeter   N1   N

* **Q4139** Amniomatrix or biodmatrix, injectable, 1 cc   N1   N

* **Q4140** Biodfence, per square centimeter   N1   N

* **Q4141** Alloskin ac, per square centimeter   N1   N

* **Q4142** XCM biologic tissue matrix, per square centimeter   N1   N

* **Q4143** Repriza, per square centimeter   N1   N

* **Q4145** Epifix, injectable, 1 mg   N1   N

* **Q4146** Tensix, per square centimeter   N1   N

↺* **Q4147** Architect, architect PX, or architect FX, extracellular matrix, per square centimeter   N1   N

* **Q4148** Neox 1k, per square centimeter   N1   N

* **Q4149** Excellagen, 0.1 cc   N1   N

▶* **Q4150** AlloWrap DS or dry, per square centimeter   N1   N

PQRS PQRS	**Qp** Quantity Physician Appendix A	**Qh** Quantity Hospital Appendix B	♀ Female only
♂ **Male only**	**A** Age ♿ **DMEPOS**	A2-Z3 **ASC Payment Indicator**	A-Y **ASC Status Indicator** Coding Clinic

▶ ✳ **Q4151** Amnioband or guardian, per square centimeter N1 N

▶ ✳ **Q4152** DermaPure, per square centimeter N1 N

▶ ✳ **Q4153** Dermavest, per square centimeter N1 N

▶ ✳ **Q4154** Biovance, per square centimeter N1 N

▶ ✳ **Q4155** Neoxflo or clarixflo, 1 mg N1 N

▶ ✳ **Q4156** Neox 100, per square centimeter N1 N

▶ ✳ **Q4157** Revitalon, per square centimeter N1 N

▶ ✳ **Q4158** Marigen, per square centimeter N1 N

▶ ✳ **Q4159** Affinity, per square centimeter N1 N

▶ ✳ **Q4160** Nushield, per square centimeter N1 N

Hospice Care

⊘ **Q5001** Hospice or home health care provided in patient's home/residence ⑱ B

⊘ **Q5002** Hospice or home health care provided in assisted living facility ⑱ B

⊘ **Q5003** Hospice care provided in nursing long term care facility (LTC) or non-skilled nursing facility (NF) ⑱ B

⊘ **Q5004** Hospice care provided in skilled nursing facility (SNF) ⑱ B

⊘ **Q5005** Hospice care provided in inpatient hospital ⑱ B

⊘ **Q5006** Hospice care provided in inpatient hospice facility ⑱ B

Hospice care provided in an inpatient hospice facility. These are residential facilities, which are places for patients to live while receiving routine home care or continuous home care. These hospice residential facilities are not certified by Medicare or Medicaid for provision of General Inpatient (GIP) or respite care, and regulations at 42 CFR 418.202(e) do not allow provision of GIP or respite care at hospice residential facilities. (http://www.palmettogba.com/Palmetto/Providers.Nsf/files/Hospice_Coalition_QAs_03-2011.pdf/$File/Hospice_Coalition_QAs_03-2011.pdf)

⊘ **Q5007** Hospice care provided in long term care facility ⑱ B

⊘ **Q5008** Hospice care provided in inpatient psychiatric facility ⑱ B

⊘ **Q5009** Hospice or home health care provided in place not otherwise specified (NOS) ⑱ B

⊘ **Q5010** Hospice home care provided in a hospice facility B

Contrast

⊘ **Q9951** Low osmolar contrast material, 400 or greater mg/ml iodine concentration, per ml ⑱ N1 N

IOM: 100-04, 12, 70; 100-04, 13, 20; 100-04, 13, 90

Coding Clinic: 2012, Q3, P8

⊘ **Q9953** Injection, iron-based magnetic resonance contrast agent, per ml ⑱ N1 N

IOM: 100-04, 12, 70; 100-04, 13, 20; 100-04, 13, 90

Coding Clinic: 2012, Q3, P8

⊘ **Q9954** Oral magnetic resonance contrast agent, per 100 ml ⑱ N1 N

IOM: 100-04, 12, 70; 100-04, 13, 20; 100-04, 13, 90

Coding Clinic: 2012, Q3, P8

✳ **Q9955** Injection, perflexane lipid microspheres, per ml ⑱ **Qp** **Qh** N1 N

Coding Clinic: 2012, Q3, P8

✳ **Q9956** Injection, octafluoropropane microspheres, per ml ⑱ N1 N

NDC: Optison

Coding Clinic: 2012, Q3, P8

✳ **Q9957** Injection, perflutren lipid microspheres, per ml ⑱ N1 N

NDC: Definity

Coding Clinic: 2012, Q3, P8

⊘ **Q9958** High osmolar contrast material, up to 149 mg/ml iodine concentration, per ml ⑱ N1 N

NDC: Conray 30, Cysto-Conray II, Cystografin, Cystografin-Dilute, Reno-Dip

IOM: 100-04, 12, 70; 100-04, 13, 20; 100-04, 13, 90

Coding Clinic: 2012, Q3, P8; 2007, Q1, P6

⊘ **Q9959** High osmolar contrast material, 150-199 mg/ml iodine concentration, per ml ⑱ N1 N

IOM: 100-04, 12, 70; 100-04, 13, 20; 100-04, 13, 90

Coding Clinic: 2012, Q3, P8; 2007, Q1, P6

▶ **New**   ↻ **Revised**   ✔ **Reinstated**   ~~deleted~~ **Deleted**   ⊘ **Not covered or valid by Medicare**
⊘ **Special coverage instructions**   ✳ **Carrier discretion**   ⑱ **Bill local carrier**   ⑱ **Bill DME MAC**

⊙ **Q9960** High osmolar contrast material, 200-249 mg/ml iodine concentration, per ml Ⓑ   N1 N

NDC: Conray 43

IOM: 100-04, 12, 70; 100-04, 13, 20; 100-04, 13, 90

Coding Clinic: 2012, Q3, P8; 2007, Q1, P6

⊙ **Q9961** High osmolar contrast material, 250-299 mg/ml iodine concentration, per ml Ⓑ   N1 N

NDC: Conray, Cholografin Meglumine

IOM: 100-04, 12, 70; 100-04, 13, 20; 100-04, 13, 90

Coding Clinic: 2012, Q3, P8; 2007, Q1, P6

⊙ **Q9962** High osmolar contrast material, 300-349 mg/ml iodine concentration, per ml Ⓑ   N1 N

IOM: 100-04, 12, 70; 100-04, 13, 20; 100-04, 13, 90

Coding Clinic: 2012, Q3, P8; 2007, Q1, P6

⊙ **Q9963** High osmolar contrast material, 350-399 mg/ml iodine concentration, per ml Ⓑ   N1 N

NDC: Gastrografin, Md-76R, Md Gastroview, Sinografin

IOM: 100-04, 12, 70; 100-04, 13, 20; 100-04, 13, 90

Coding Clinic: 2012, Q3, P8; 2007, Q1, P6

⊙ **Q9964** High osmolar contrast material, 400 or greater mg/ml iodine concentration, per ml Ⓑ   N1 N

IOM: 100-04, 12, 70; 100-04, 13, 20; 100-04, 13, 90

Coding Clinic: 2012, Q3, P8; 2007, Q1, P6

⊙ **Q9965** Low osmolar contrast material, 100-199 mg/ml iodine concentration, per ml Ⓑ   N1 N

NDC: Omnipaque, Ultravist 150

IOM: 100-04, 12, 70; 100-04, 13, 20; 100-04, 13, 90

Coding Clinic: 2012, Q3, P8

⊙ **Q9966** Low osmolar contrast material, 200-299 mg/ml iodine concentration, per ml Ⓑ   N1 N

NDC: Isovue, Omnipaque, Optiray, Ultravist 240, Visipaque

IOM: 100-04, 12, 70; 100-04, 13, 20; 100-04, 13, 90

Coding Clinic: 2012, Q3, P8

⊙ **Q9967** Low osmolar contrast material, 300-399 mg/ml iodine concentration, per ml Ⓑ   N1 N

NDC: Hexabrix 320, Isovue-300, Isovue-370, Omnipaque 300, Omnipaque 350, Optiray, Oxilan, Ultravist 300, Ultravist 370, Vispaque

IOM: 100-04, 12, 70; 100-04, 13, 20; 100-04, 13, 90

Coding Clinic: 2012, Q3, P8

↻✳ **Q9968** Injection, non-radioactive, non-contrast, visualization adjunct (e.g., Methylene Blue, Isosulfan Blue), 1 mg   K2 K

✳ **Q9969** Tc-99m from non-highly enriched uranium source, full cost recovery add-on, per study dose Ⓑ   K

~~Q9970~~ ~~Injection, ferric carboxymaltose, 1 mg~~ ✖

~~Q9972~~ ~~Injection, epoetin beta, 1 microgram, (for ESRD on dialysis)~~ ✖

Cross Reference J0887

~~Q9973~~ ~~Injection, epoetin beta, 1 microgram, (non-ESRD use)~~ ✖

Cross Reference J0888

~~Q9974~~ ~~Injection, morphine sulfate, preservative-free for epidural or intrathecal use, 10 mg~~ ✖

Cross Reference J2274

ᴾᴼᴿˢ **PQRS**   **Qp** Quantity Physician Appendix A   **Qh** Quantity Hospital Appendix B   ♀ **Female only**

♂ **Male only**   **A** Age   ♿ **DMEPOS**   A2-Z3 **ASC Payment Indicator**   A-Y **ASC Status Indicator**   Coding Clinic

DIAGNOSTIC RADIOLOGY SERVICES (R0000-R9999)

Transportation/Setup of Portable Equipment

⊛ **R0070** Transportation of portable x-ray equipment and personnel to home or nursing home, per trip to facility or location, one patient seen ⑧ **Qp** **Qh**   B

CMS Transmittal B03-049; specific instructions to contractors on pricing

IOM: 100-04, 13, 90; 100-04, 13, 90.3

⊛ **R0075** Transportation of portable x-ray equipment and personnel to home or nursing home, per trip to facility or location, more than one patient seen ⑧ **Qp** **Qh**   B

This code would not apply to the x-ray equipment if stored at the location where the x-ray was performed (e.g., a nursing home).

IOM: 100-04, 13, 90; 100-04, 13, 90.3

⊛ **R0076** Transportation of portable ECG to facility or location, per patient ⑧ **Qh**   B

EKG procedure code 93000 or 93005 must be submitted on same claim as transportation code. Bundled status on physician fee schedule

IOM: 100-01, 5, 90.2; 100-02, 15, 80; 100-03, 1, 20.15; 100-04, 13, 90; 100-04, 16, 10; 100-04, 16, 110.4

▶ **New**   ↻ **Revised**   ✔ **Reinstated**   ~~deleted~~ **Deleted**   ⊘ **Not covered or valid by Medicare**
⊛ **Special coverage instructions**   ✳ **Carrier discretion**   ⑧ **Bill local carrier**   ⑧ **Bill DME MAC**

TEMPORARY NATIONAL CODES ESTABLISHED BY PRIVATE PAYERS (S0000-S9999)

Medicare and other federal payers do not recognize "S" codes; however, S codes may be useful for claims to some private insurers.

- ⊘ **S0012** Butorphanol tartrate, nasal spray, **25 mg**
- ⊘ **S0014** Tacrine hydrochloride, **10 mg**
- ⊘ **S0017** Injection, aminocaproic acid, **5 grams**
- ⊘ **S0020** Injection, bupivacaine hydrochloride, **30 ml**
- ⊘ **S0021** Injection, cefoperazone sodium, **1 gram**
- ⊘ **S0023** Injection, cimetidine hydrochloride, **300 mg**
- ⊘ **S0028** Injection, famotidine, **20 mg**
- ⊘ **S0030** Injection, metronidazole, **500 mg**
- ⊘ **S0032** Injection, nafcillin sodium, **2 grams**
- ⊘ **S0034** Injection, ofloxacin, **400 mg**
- ⊘ **S0039** Injection, sulfamethoxazole and tri-methoprim, **10 ml**
- ⊘ **S0040** Injection, ticarcillin disodium and clavulanate potassium, **3.1 grams**
- ⊘ **S0073** Injection, aztreonam, **500 mg**
  Other: Cayston
- ⊘ **S0074** Injection, cefotetan disodium, **500 mg**
- ⊘ **S0077** Injection, clindamycin phosphate, **300 mg**
- ⊘ **S0078** Injection, fosphenytoin sodium, **750 mg**
- ⊘ **S0080** Injection, pentamidine isethionate, **300 mg**
- ⊘ **S0081** Injection, piperacillin sodium, **500 mg**
- ⊘ **S0088** Imatinib, **100 mg**
- ⊘ **S0090** Sildenafil citrate, **25 mg** **A**
- ⊘ **S0091** Granisetron hydrochloride, **1 mg** (for circumstances falling under the Medicare Statute, use Q0166)
- ⊘ **S0092** Injection, hydromorphone hydrochloride, **250 mg** (loading dose for infusion pump)
- ⊘ **S0093** Injection, morphine sulfate, **500 mg** (loading dose for infusion pump)
- ⊘ **S0104** Zidovudine, oral, **100 mg**
- ⊘ **S0106** Bupropion HCl sustained release tablet, **150 mg,** per bottle of 60 tablets
- ⊘ **S0108** Mercaptopurine, oral, **50 mg**
- ⊘ **S0109** Methadone, oral, **5 mg**
- ⊘ **S0117** Tretinoin, topical, **5 grams**

- ⊘ **S0119** Ondansetron, oral, 4 mg (for circumstances falling under the medicare statute, use HCPCS Q code)
- ⊘ **S0122** Injection, menotropins, **75 IU**
- ⊘ **S0126** Injection, follitropin alfa, **75 IU** ♀
- ⊘ **S0128** Injection, follitropin beta, **75 IU**
- ⊘ **S0132** Injection, ganirelix acetate, **250 mcg** ♀
- ⊘ **S0136** Clozapine, **25 mg**
- ⊘ **S0137** Didanosine (DDI), **25 mg**
- ⊘ **S0138** Finasteride, **5 mg** ♂
- ⊘ **S0139** Minoxidil, **10 mg**
- ⊘ **S0140** Saquinavir, **200 mg**
- ⊘ **S0142** Colistimethate sodium, inhalation solution administered through DME, concentrated form, **per mg**
- ~~S0144 Injection, propofol, 10 mg~~ ✖
  Cross Reference J2704
- ⊘ **S0145** Injection, pegylated interferon alfa-2a, **180 mcg per ml**
- ⊘ **S0148** Injection, pegylated interferon ALFA-2b, **10 mcg**
- ⊘ **S0155** Sterile dilutant for epoprostenol, **50 ml**
- ⊘ **S0156** Exemestane, **25 mg**
- ⊘ **S0157** Becaplermin gel 0.01%, **0.5 gm**
- ⊘ **S0160** Dextroamphetamine sulfate, **5 mg**
- ⊘ **S0164** Injection, pantoprazole sodium, **40 mg**
- ⊘ **S0166** Injection, olanzapine, **2.5 mg**
- ⊘ **S0169** Calcitrol, **0.25 microgram**
- ⊘ **S0170** Anastrozole, oral, **1mg**
- ⊘ **S0171** Injection, bumetanide, **0.5 mg**
- ⊘ **S0172** Chlorambucil, oral, **2 mg**
- ⊘ **S0174** Dolasetron mesylate, oral **50 mg** (for circumstances falling under the Medicare Statute, use Q0180)
- ⊘ **S0175** Flutamide, oral, **125 mg**
- ⊘ **S0176** Hydroxyurea, oral, **500 mg**
- ⊘ **S0177** Levamisole hydrochloride, oral, **50 mg**
- ⊘ **S0178** Lomustine, oral, **10 mg**
- ⊘ **S0179** Megestrol acetate, oral, **20 mg**
- ⊘ **S0182** Procarbazine hydrochloride, oral, **50 mg**
- ⊅ ⊘ **S0183** Prochlorperazine maleate, oral, **5 mg** (for circumstances falling under the Medicare Statute, use Q0164)
- ⊘ **S0187** Tamoxifen citrate, oral, **10 mg**
- ⊘ **S0189** Testosterone pellet, **75 mg**
- ⊘ **S0190** Mifepristone, oral, **200 mg** ♀

PQRS | Quantity Physician Appendix A | Quantity Hospital Appendix B | ♀ Female only | ♂ Male only | A Age | DMEPOS | A2-Z3 ASC Payment Indicator | A-Y ASC Status Indicator | Coding Clinic

⊘ **S0191** Misoprostol, oral **200 mcg**

⊘ **S0194** Dialysis/stress vitamin supplement, oral, **100 capsules**

⊘ **S0195** Pneumococcal conjugate vaccine, polyvalent, intramuscular, for children from five years to nine years of age who have not previously received the vaccine **A**

⊘ **S0197** Prenatal vitamins, 30-day supply ♀

⊘ **S0199** Medically induced abortion by oral ingestion of medication including all associated services and supplies (e.g., patient counseling, office visits, confirmation of pregnancy by HCG, ultrasound to confirm duration of pregnancy, ultrasound to confirm completion of abortion) except drugs ♀

⊘ **S0201** Partial hospitalization services, less than 24 hours, per diem

⊘ **S0207** Paramedic intercept, non-hospital-based ALS service (non-voluntary), non-transport

⊘ **S0208** Paramedic intercept, hospital-based ALS service (non-voluntary), non-transport

⊘ **S0209** Wheelchair van, mileage, per mile

⊘ **S0215** Non-emergency transportation; mileage per mile

⊘ **S0220** Medical conference by a physician with interdisciplinary team of health professionals or representatives of community agencies to coordinate activities of patient care (patient is present); approximately 30 minutes

⊘ **S0221** Medical conference by a physician with interdisciplinary team of health professionals or representatives of community agencies to coordinate activities of patient care (patient is present); approximately 60 minutes

⊘ **S0250** Comprehensive geriatric assessment and treatment planning performed by assessment team **A**

⊘ **S0255** Hospice referral visit (advising patient and family of care options) performed by nurse, social worker, or other designated staff

⊘ **S0257** Counseling and discussion regarding advance directives or end of life care planning and decisions, with patient and/or surrogate (list separately in addition to code for appropriate evaluation and management service)

⊘ **S0260** History and physical (outpatient or office) related to surgical procedure (list separately in addition to code for appropriate evaluation and management service)

⊘ **S0265** Genetic counseling, under physician supervision, each 15 minutes

⊘ **S0270** Physician management of patient home care, standard monthly case rate (per 30 days)

⊘ **S0271** Physician management of patient home care, hospice monthly case rate (per 30 days)

⊘ **S0272** Physician management of patient home care, episodic care monthly case rate (per 30 days)

⊘ **S0273** Physician visit at member's home, outside of a capitation arrangement

⊘ **S0274** Nurse practitioner visit at member's home, outside of a capitation arrangement

⊘ **S0280** Medical home program, comprehensive care coordination and planning, initial plan

⊘ **S0281** Medical home program, comprehensive care coordination and planning, maintenance of plan

⊘ **S0302** Completed Early Periodic Screening Diagnosis and Treatment (EPSDT) service (list in addition to code for appropriate evaluation and management service) **A**

⊘ **S0310** Hospitalist services (list separately in addition to code for appropriate evaluation and management service)

⊘ **S0315** Disease management program; initial assessment and initiation of the program

⊘ **S0316** Disease management program; follow-up/reassessment

⊘ **S0317** Disease management program; per diem

⊘ **S0320** Telephone calls by a registered nurse to a disease management program member for monitoring purposes; per month

⊘ **S0340** Lifestyle modification program for management of coronary artery disease, including all supportive services; first quarter/stage

⊘ **S0341** Lifestyle modification program for management of coronary artery disease, including all supportive services; second or third quarter/stage

---

▶ New	↻ Revised	✔ Reinstated	~~deleted~~ Deleted	⊘ Not covered or valid by Medicare
✪ Special coverage instructions	✳ Carrier discretion	Ⓑ Bill local carrier	Ⓑ Bill DME MAC

⊘ **S0342** Lifestyle modification program for management of coronary artery disease, including all supportive services; fourth quarter/stage

✳ **S0353** Treatment planning and care coordination management for cancer, initial treatment

✳ **S0354** Treatment planning and care coordination management for cancer, established patient with a change of regimen

⊘ **S0390** Routine foot care; removal and/or trimming of corns, calluses and/or nails and preventive maintenance in specific medical conditions (e.g. diabetes), per visit

⊘ **S0395** Impression casting of a foot performed by a practitioner other than the manufacturer of the orthotic

⊘ **S0400** Global fee for extracorporeal shock wave lithotripsy treatment of kidney stone(s)

⊘ **S0500** Disposable contact lens, per lens

⊘ **S0504** Single vision prescription lens (safety, athletic, or sunglass), per lens

⊘ **S0506** Bifocal vision prescription lens (safety, athletic, or sunglass), per lens

⊘ **S0508** Trifocal vision prescription lens (safety, athletic, or sunglass), per lens

⊘ **S0510** Non-prescription lens (safety, athletic, or sunglass), per lens

⊘ **S0512** Daily wear specialty contact lens, per lens

⊘ **S0514** Color contact lens, per lens

⊘ **S0515** Scleral lens, liquid bandage device, per lens

⊘ **S0516** Safety eyeglass frames

⊘ **S0518** Sunglasses frames

⊘ **S0580** Polycarbonate lens (list this code in addition to the basic code for the lens)

⊘ **S0581** Nonstandard lens (list this code in addition to the basic code for the lens)

⊘ **S0590** Integral lens service, miscellaneous services reported separately

⊘ **S0592** Comprehensive contact lens evaluation

⊘ **S0595** Dispensing new spectacle lenses for patient supplied frame

⊘ **S0596** Phakic intraocular lens for correction of refractive error

⊘ **S0601** Screening proctoscopy

⊘ **S0610** Annual gynecological examination, new patient ♀

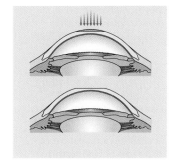

Figure 51
Phototherapeutic keratectomy (PRK).

⊘ **S0612** Annual gynecological examination, established patient ♀

⊘ **S0613** Annual gynecological examination; clinical breast examination without pelvic evaluation ♀

⊘ **S0618** Audiometry for hearing aid evaluation to determine the level and degree of hearing loss

⊘ **S0620** Routine ophthalmological examination including refraction; new patient

Many non-Medicare vision plans may require code for routine encounter, no complaints

⊘ **S0621** Routine ophthalmological examination including refraction; established patient

Many non-Medicare vision plans may require code for routine encounter, no complaints

⊘ **S0622** Physical exam for college, new or established patient (list separately) in addition to appropriate evaluation and management code **A**

⊘ **S0630** Removal of sutures; by a physician other than the physician who originally closed the wound

⊘ **S0800** Laser in situ keratomileusis (LASIK)

⊘ **S0810** Photorefractive keratectomy (PRK)

⊘ **S0812** Phototherapeutic keratectomy (PTK)

⊘ **S1001** Deluxe item, patient aware (list in addition to code for basic item)

⊘ **S1002** Customized item (list in addition to code for basic item)

⊘ **S1015** IV tubing extension set

⊘ **S1016** Non-PVC (polyvinyl chloride) intravenous administration set, for use with drugs that are not stable in PVC e.g. paclitaxel

---

PQRS PQRS   **Qp** Quantity Physician Appendix A   **Qh** Quantity Hospital Appendix B   ♀ Female only

♂ **Male only**   **A** Age   **Ⴑ DMEPOS**   A2-Z3 **ASC Payment Indicator**   A-Y **ASC Status Indicator**   Coding Clinic

⊘ **S1030** Continuous noninvasive glucose monitoring device, purchase (for physician interpretation of data, use CPT code)

⊘ **S1031** Continuous noninvasive glucose monitoring device, rental, including sensor, sensor replacement, and download to monitor (for physician interpretation of data, use CPT code)

▶ ⊘ **S1034** Artificial pancreas device system (eg., low glucose suspend (LGS) feature) including continuous glucose monitor, blood glucose device, insulin pump and computer algorithm that communicates with all of the devices

▶ ⊘ **S1035** Sensor; invasive (eg, subcutaneous), disposable, for use with artificial pancreas device system

▶ ⊘ **S1036** Transmitter; external, for use with artificial pancreas device system

▶ ⊘ **S1037** Receiver (monitor); external, for use with artificial pancreas device system

⊘ **S1040** Cranial remolding orthosis, pediatric, rigid, with soft interface material, custom fabricated, includes fitting and adjustment(s) **A**

⊘ **S1090** Mometasone furoate sinus implant, 370 micrograms

⊘ **S2053** Transplantation of small intestine and liver allografts

⊘ **S2054** Transplantation of multivisceral organs

⊘ **S2055** Harvesting of donor multivisceral organs, with preparation and maintenance of allografts; from cadaver donor

⊘ **S2060** Lobar lung transplantation

⊘ **S2061** Donor lobectomy (lung) for transplantation, living donor

⊘ **S2065** Simultaneous pancreas kidney transplantation

⊘ **S2066** Breast reconstruction with gluteal artery perforator (GAP) flap, including harvesting of the flap, microvascular transfer, closure of donor site and shaping the flap into a breast, unilateral ♀

⊘ **S2067** Breast reconstruction of a single breast with "stacked" deep inferior epigastric perforator (DIEP) flap(s) and/or gluteal artery perforator (GAP) flap(s), including harvesting of the flap(s), microvascular transfer, closure of donor site(s) and shaping the flap into a breast, unilateral ♀

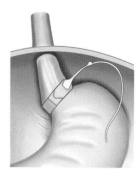

Figure 52 Gastric band.

⊘ **S2068** Breast reconstruction with deep inferior epigastric perforator (DIEP) flap, or superficial inferior epigastric artery (SIEA) flap, including harvesting of the flap, microvascular transfer, closure of donor site and shaping the flap into a breast, unilateral ♀

⊘ **S2070** Cystourethroscopy, with ureteroscopy and/or pyeloscopy; with endoscopic laser treatment of ureteral calculi (includes ureteral catheterization)

⊘ **S2079** Laparoscopic esophagomyotomy (Heller type)

⊘ **S2080** Laser-assisted uvulopalatoplasty (LAUP)

⊘ **S2083** Adjustment of gastric band diameter via subcutaneous port by injection or aspiration of saline

⊘ **S2095** Transcatheter occlusion or embolization for tumor destruction, percutaneous, any method, using yttrium-90 microspheres

⊘ **S2102** Islet cell tissue transplant from pancreas; allogeneic

⊘ **S2103** Adrenal tissue transplant to brain

⊘ **S2107** Adoptive immunotherapy i.e. development of specific anti-tumor reactivity (e.g. tumor-infiltrating lymphocyte therapy) per course of treatment

⊘ **S2112** Arthroscopy, knee, surgical for harvesting of cartilage (chondrocyte cells)

⊘ **S2115** Osteotomy, periacetabular, with internal fixation

⊘ **S2117** Arthroereisis, subtalar

⊘ **S2118** Metal-on-metal total hip resurfacing, including acetabular and femoral components

⊘ **S2120** Low density lipoprotein (LDL) apheresis using heparin-induced extracorporeal LDL precipitation

⊘ **S2140** Cord blood harvesting for transplantation, allogeneic

---

▶ New   ↻ Revised   ✔ Reinstated   ~~deleted~~ Deleted   ⊘ Not covered or valid by Medicare
⊛ Special coverage instructions   ✳ Carrier discretion   ⑧ Bill local carrier   ⑧ Bill DME MAC

⊘ **S2142** Cord blood-derived stem cell transplantation, allogeneic

⊘ **S2150** Bone marrow or blood-derived stem cells (peripheral or umbilical), allogeneic or autologous, harvesting, transplantation, and related complications; including: pheresis and cell preparation/storage; marrow ablative therapy; drugs, supplies, hospitalization with outpatient follow-up; medical/surgical, diagnostic, emergency, and rehabilitative services; and the number of days of pre- and post-transplant care in the global definition

⊘ **S2152** Solid organ(s), complete or segmental, single organ or combination of organs; deceased or living donor(s), procurement, transplantation, and related complications; including: drugs; supplies; hospitalization with outpatient follow-up; medical/surgical, diagnostic, emergency, and rehabilitative services, and the number of days of pre- and post-transplant care in the global definition

⊘ **S2202** Echosclerotherapy

⊘ **S2205** Minimally invasive direct coronary artery bypass surgery involving mini-thoracotomy or mini-sternotomy surgery, performed under direct vision; using arterial graft(s), single coronary arterial graft

⊘ **S2206** Minimally invasive direct coronary artery bypass surgery involving mini-thoracotomy or mini-sternotomy surgery, performed under direct vision; using arterial graft(s), two coronary arterial grafts

⊘ **S2207** Minimally invasive direct coronary artery bypass surgery involving mini-thoracotomy or mini-sternotomy surgery, performed under direct vision; using venous graft only, single coronary venous graft

⊘ **S2208** Minimally invasive direct coronary artery bypass surgery involving mini-thoracotomy or mini-sternotomy surgery, performed under direct vision; using single arterial and venous graft(s), single venous graft

⊘ **S2209** Minimally invasive direct coronary artery bypass surgery involving mini-thoracotomy or mini-sternotomy surgery, performed under direct vision; using two arterial grafts and single venous graft

⊘ **S2225** Myringotomy, laser-assisted

⊘ **S2230** Implantation of magnetic component of semi-implantable hearing device on ossicles in middle ear

⊘ **S2235** Implantation of auditory brain stem implant

⊘ **S2260** Induced abortion, 17 to 24 weeks ♀

⊘ **S2265** Induced abortion, 25 to 28 weeks ♀

⊘ **S2266** Induced abortion, 29 to 31 weeks ♀

⊘ **S2267** Induced abortion, 32 weeks or greater ♀

⊘ **S2300** Arthroscopy, shoulder, surgical; with thermally-induced capsulorrhaphy

⊘ **S2325** Hip core decompression

⊘ **S2340** Chemodenervation of abductor muscle(s) of vocal cord

⊘ **S2341** Chemodenervation of adductor muscle(s) of vocal cord

⊘ **S2342** Nasal endoscopy for post-operative debridement following functional endoscopic sinus surgery, nasal and/or sinus cavity(s), unilateral or bilateral

⊘ **S2348** Decompression procedure, percutaneous, of nucleus pulpous of intervertebral disc, using radiofrequency energy, single or multiple levels, lumbar

⊘ **S2350** Diskectomy, anterior, with decompression of spinal cord and/or nerve root(s), including osteophytectomy; lumbar, single interspace

⊘ **S2351** Diskectomy, anterior, with decompression of spinal cord and/or nerve root(s) including osteophytectomy; lumbar, each additional interspace (list separately in addition to code for primary procedure)

⊘ **S2360** Percutaneous vertebroplasty, one vertebral body, unilateral or bilateral injection; cervical

⊘ **S2361** Each additional cervical vertebral body (list separately in addition to code for primary procedure)

⊘ **S2400** Repair, congenital diaphragmatic hernia in the fetus using temporary tracheal occlusion, procedure performed in utero ♀ **A**

⊘ **S2401** Repair, urinary tract obstruction in the fetus, procedure performed in utero ♀ **A**

⊘ **S2402** Repair, congenital cystic adenomatoid malformation in the fetus, procedure performed in utero ♀ **A**

ⓟ PQRS	**Qp** Quantity Physician Appendix A	**Qh** Quantity Hospital Appendix B	♀ Female only	
♂ Male only	**A** Age	♿ DMEPOS	A2-Z3 ASC Payment Indicator	A-Y ASC Status Indicator	Coding Clinic

⊘ **S2403** Repair, extralobar pulmonary sequestration in the fetus, procedure performed in utero ♀ **A**

⊘ **S2404** Repair, myelomeningocele in the fetus, procedure performed in utero ♀ **A**

⊘ **S2405** Repair of sacrococcygeal teratoma in the fetus, procedure performed in utero ♀ **A**

⊘ **S2409** Repair, congenital malformation of fetus, procedure performed in utero, not otherwise classified ♀ **A**

⊘ **S2411** Fetoscopic laser therapy for treatment of twin-to-twin transfusion syndrome **A**

⊘ **S2900** Surgical techniques requiring use of robotic surgical system (list separately in addition to code for primary procedure)

Coding Clinic: 2010, Q2, P6

⊘ **S3000** Diabetic indicator; retinal eye exam, dilated, bilateral

⊘ **S3005** Performance measurement, evaluation of patient self assessment, depression

⊘ **S3600** STAT laboratory request (situations other than S3601)

⊘ **S3601** Emergency STAT laboratory charge for patient who is homebound or residing in a nursing facility

⊘ **S3620** Newborn metabolic screening panel, includes test kit, postage and the laboratory tests specified by the state for inclusion in this panel (e.g. galactose; hemoglobin, electrophoresis; hydroxyprogesterone, 17-D; phenylalanine (PKU); and thyroxine, total) **A**

⊘ **S3630** Eosinophil count, blood, direct

⊘ **S3645** HIV-1 antibody testing of oral mucosal transudate

⊘ **S3650** Saliva test, hormone level; during menopause ♀

⊘ **S3652** Saliva test, hormone level; to assess preterm labor risk ♀

⊘ **S3655** Antisperm antibodies test (immunobead) ♀

⊘ **S3708** Gastrointestinal fat absorption study

⊘ **S3721** Prostate cancer antigen 3 (PCA3) testing ♂

⊘ **S3722** Dose optimization by area under the curve (AUC) analysis, for infusional 5-fluorouracil

⊘ **S3800** Genetic testing for amyotrophic lateral sclerosis (ALS)

⊘ **S3840** DNA analysis for germline mutations of the RET proto-oncogene for susceptibility to multiple endocrine neoplasia type 2

⊘ **S3841** Genetic testing for retinoblastoma

⊘ **S3842** Genetic testing for von Hippel-Lindau disease

⊘ **S3844** DNA analysis of the connexin 26 gene (GJB2) for susceptibility to congenital, profound deafness

⊘ **S3845** Genetic testing for alpha-thalassemia

⊘ **S3846** Genetic testing for hemoglobin E beta-thalassemia

⊘ **S3849** Genetic testing for Niemann-Pick disease

⊘ **S3850** Genetic testing for sickle cell anemia

⊘ **S3852** DNA analysis for APOE epilson 4 allele for susceptibility to Alzheimer's disease

⊘ **S3853** Genetic testing for myotonic muscular dystrophy

⊘ **S3854** Gene expression profiling panel for use in the management of breast cancer treatment ♀

~~S3855~~ ~~Genetic testing for detection of mutations in the presenilin - 1 gene~~ ✖

⊘ **S3861** Genetic testing, sodium channel, voltage-gated, type V, alpha subunit (SCN5A) and variants for suspected Brugada syndrome

⊘ **S3865** Comprehensive gene sequence analysis for hypertrophic cardiomyopathy

⊘ **S3866** Genetic analysis for a specific gene mutation for hypertrophic cardiomyopathy (HCM) in an individual with a known HCM mutation in the family

⊘ **S3870** Comparative genomic hybridization (CGH) microarray testing for developmental delay, autism spectrum disorder and/or intellectual disability

⊘ **S3890** DNA analysis, fecal, for colorectal cancer screening

⊘ **S3900** Surface electromyography (EMG)

⊘ **S3902** Ballistrocardiogram

⊘ **S3904** Masters two step

Bill on paper. Requires a report.

⊘ **S4005** Interim labor facility global (labor occurring but not resulting in delivery) ♀

⊘ **S4011** In vitro fertilization; including but not limited to identification and incubation of mature oocytes, fertilization with sperm, incubation of embryo(s), and subsequent visualization for determination of development ♀

⊘ **S4013** Complete cycle, gamete intrafallopian transfer (GIFT), case rate ♀

⊘ **S4014** Complete cycle, zygote intrafallopian transfer (ZIFT), case rate ♀

⊘ **S4015** Complete in vitro fertilization cycle, not otherwise specified, case rate ♀

⊘ **S4016** Frozen in vitro fertilization cycle, case rate ♀

⊘ **S4017** Incomplete cycle, treatment cancelled prior to stimulation, case rate ♀

⊘ **S4018** Frozen embryo transfer procedure cancelled before transfer, case rate ♀

⊘ **S4020** In vitro fertilization procedure cancelled before aspiration, case rate ♀

⊘ **S4021** In vitro fertilization procedure cancelled after aspiration, case rate ♀

⊘ **S4022** Assisted oocyte fertilization, case rate ♀

⊘ **S4023** Donor egg cycle, incomplete, case rate ♀

⊘ **S4025** Donor services for in vitro fertilization (sperm or embryo), case rate

⊘ **S4026** Procurement of donor sperm from sperm bank ♂

⊘ **S4027** Storage of previously frozen embryos ♀

⊘ **S4028** Microsurgical epididymal sperm aspiration (MESA) ♂

⊘ **S4030** Sperm procurement and cryopreservation services; initial visit ♂

⊘ **S4031** Sperm procurement and cryopreservation services; subsequent visit ♂

⊘ **S4035** Stimulated intrauterine insemination (IUI), case rate ♀

⊘ **S4037** Cryopreserved embryo transfer, case rate ♀

⊘ **S4040** Monitoring and storage of cryopreserved embryos, per 30 days ♀

⊘ **S4042** Management of ovulation induction (interpretation of diagnostic tests and studies, non-face-to-face medical management of the patient), per cycle ♀

⊘ **S4981** Insertion of levonorgestrel-releasing intrauterine system ♀

⊘ **S4989** Contraceptive intrauterine device (e.g. Progestasert IUD), including implants and supplies ♀

⊘ **S4990** Nicotine patches, legend

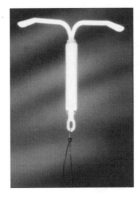

Figure 53 IUD.

⊘ **S4991** Nicotine patches, non-legend

⊘ **S4993** Contraceptive pills for birth control ♀

Only billed by Family Planning Clinics

⊘ **S4995** Smoking cessation gum

⊘ **S5000** Prescription drug, generic

⊘ **S5001** Prescription drug, brand name

⊘ **S5010** 5% dextrose and 0.45% normal saline, **1000 ml**

⊘ **S5011** 5% dextrose in lactated Ringer's, **1000 ml**

⊘ **S5012** 5% dextrose with potassium chloride, **1000 ml**

⊘ **S5013** 5% dextrose/0.45% normal saline with potassium chloride and magnesium sulfate, **1000 ml**

⊘ **S5014** 5% dextrose/0.45% normal saline with potassium chloride and magnesium sulfate, **1500 ml**

⊘ **S5035** Home infusion therapy, routine service of infusion device (e.g. pump maintenance)

⊘ **S5036** Home infusion therapy, repair of infusion device (e.g. pump repair)

⊘ **S5100** Day care services, adult; per 15 minutes **A**

⊘ **S5101** Day care services, adult; per half day **A**

⊘ **S5102** Day care services, adult; per diem **A**

⊘ **S5105** Day care services, center-based; services not included in program fee, per diem

⊘ **S5108** Home care training to home care client, per 15 minutes

⊘ **S5109** Home care training to home care client, per session

⊘ **S5110** Home care training, family; per 15 minutes

⊘ **S5111** Home care training, family; per session

⊘ **S5115** Home care training, non-family; per 15 minutes

PQRS PQRS	**Qp** Quantity Physician Appendix A	**Qh** Quantity Hospital Appendix B	♀ Female only
♂ Male only	**A** Age	DMEPOS	A2-Z3 ASC Payment Indicator	A-Y ASC Status Indicator	Coding Clinic

⊘ **S5116** Home care training, non-family; per session

⊘ **S5120** Chore services; per 15 minutes

⊘ **S5121** Chore services; per diem

⊘ **S5125** Attendant care services; per 15 minutes

⊘ **S5126** Attendant care services; per diem

⊘ **S5130** Homemaker service, NOS; per 15 minutes

⊘ **S5131** Homemaker service, NOS; per diem

⊘ **S5135** Companion care, adult (e.g. IADL/ADL); per 15 minutes **A**

⊘ **S5136** Companion care, adult (e.g. IADL/ADL); per diem **A**

⊘ **S5140** Foster care, adult; per diem **A**

⊘ **S5141** Foster care, adult; per month **A**

⊘ **S5145** Foster care, therapeutic, child; per diem **A**

⊘ **S5146** Foster care, therapeutic, child; per month **A**

⊘ **S5150** Unskilled respite care, not hospice; per 15 minutes

⊘ **S5151** Unskilled respite care, not hospice; per diem

⊘ **S5160** Emergency response system; installation and testing

⊘ **S5161** Emergency response system; service fee, per month (excludes installation and testing)

⊘ **S5162** Emergency response system; purchase only

⊘ **S5165** Home modifications; per service

⊘ **S5170** Home delivered meals, including preparation; per meal

⊘ **S5175** Laundry service, external, professional; per order

⊘ **S5180** Home health respiratory therapy, initial evaluation

⊘ **S5181** Home health respiratory therapy, NOS, per diem

⊘ **S5185** Medication reminder service, non-face-to-face; per month

⊘ **S5190** Wellness assessment, performed by non-physician

⊘ **S5199** Personal care item, NOS, each

⊘ **S5497** Home infusion therapy, catheter care/maintenance, not otherwise classified; includes administrative services, professional pharmacy services, care coordination, and all necessary supplies and equipment (drugs and nursing visits coded separately), per diem

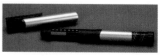

Figure 54 Nova Pen.

⊘ **S5498** Home infusion therapy, catheter care/maintenance, simple (single lumen), includes administrative services, professional pharmacy services, care coordination and all necessary supplies and equipment, (drugs and nursing visits coded separately), per diem

⊘ **S5501** Home infusion therapy, catheter care/maintenance, complex (more than one lumen), includes administrative services, professional pharmacy services, care coordination, and all necessary supplies and equipment (drugs and nursing visits coded separately), per diem

⊘ **S5502** Home infusion therapy, catheter care/maintenance, implanted access device, includes administrative services, professional pharmacy services, care coordination, and all necessary supplies and equipment, (drugs and nursing visits coded separately), per diem (use this code for interim maintenance of vascular access not currently in use)

⊘ **S5517** Home infusion therapy, all supplies necessary for restoration of catheter patency or declotting

⊘ **S5518** Home infusion therapy, all supplies necessary for catheter repair

⊘ **S5520** Home infusion therapy, all supplies (including catheter) necessary for a peripherally inserted central venous catheter (PICC) line insertion

Bill on paper. Requires a report.

⊘ **S5521** Home infusion therapy, all supplies (including catheter) necessary for a midline catheter insertion

⊘ **S5522** Home infusion therapy, insertion of peripherally inserted central venous catheter (PICC), nursing services only (no supplies or catheter included)

⊘ **S5523** Home infusion therapy, insertion of midline central venous catheter, nursing services only (no supplies or catheter included)

⊘ **S5550** Insulin, rapid onset, **5 units**

⊘ **S5551** Insulin, most rapid onset (Lispro or Aspart); **5 units**

⊘ **S5552** Insulin, intermediate acting (NPH or Lente); **5 units**

⊘ **S5553** Insulin, long acting; **5 units**

▶ **New**   ⟲ **Revised**   ✔ **Reinstated**   ~~deleted~~ **Deleted**   ⊘ **Not covered or valid by Medicare**

☼ **Special coverage instructions**   ✳ **Carrier discretion**   ⑧ **Bill local carrier**   ⑩ **Bill DME MAC**

⊘ **S5560** Insulin delivery device, reusable pen; **1.5 ml** size

⊘ **S5561** Insulin delivery device, reusable pen; **3 ml** size

⊘ **S5565** Insulin cartridge for use in insulin delivery device other than pump; **150 units**

⊘ **S5566** Insulin cartridge for use in insulin delivery device other than pump; **300 units**

⊘ **S5570** Insulin delivery device, disposable pen (including insulin); **1.5 ml** size

⊘ **S5571** Insulin delivery device, disposable pen (including insulin); **3 ml** size

⊘ **S8030** Scleral application of tantalum ring(s) for localization of lesions for proton beam therapy

▶ ⊘ **S8032** Low-dose computer tomography for lung cancer screening

⊘ **S8035** Magnetic source imaging

⊘ **S8037** Magnetic resonance cholangiopancreatography (MRCP)

⊘ **S8040** Topographic brain mapping

⊘ **S8042** Magnetic resonance imaging (MRI), low-field

⊘ **S8055** Ultrasound guidance for multifetal pregnancy reduction(s), technical component (only to be used when the physician doing the reduction procedure does not perform the ultrasound, guidance is included in the CPT code for multifetal pregnancy reduction - 59866) ♀

⊘ **S8080** Scintimammography (radioimmunoscintigraphy of the breast), unilateral, including supply of radiopharmaceutical ♀

⊘ **S8085** Fluorine-18 fluorodeoxyglucose (F-18 FDG) imaging using dual-head coincidence detection system (non-dedicated PET scan)

⊘ **S8092** Electron beam computed tomography (also known as ultrafast CT, cine CT)

⊘ **S8096** Portable peak flow meter

⊘ **S8097** Asthma kit (including but not limited to portable peak expiratory flow meter, instructional video, brochure, and/or spacer)

⊘ **S8100** Holding chamber or spacer for use with an inhaler or nebulizer; without mask

⊘ **S8101** Holding chamber or spacer for use with an inhaler or nebulizer; with mask

⊘ **S8110** Peak expiratory flow rate (physician services)

⊘ **S8120** Oxygen contents, gaseous, 1 unit equals 1 cubic foot

⊘ **S8121** Oxygen contents, liquid, 1 unit equals 1 pound

⊘ **S8130** Interferential current stimulator, 2 channel

⊘ **S8131** Interferential current stimulator, 4 channel

⊘ **S8185** Flutter device

⊘ **S8186** Swivel adaptor

⊘ **S8189** Tracheostomy supply, not otherwise classified

⊘ **S8210** Mucus trap

⊘ **S8262** Mandibular orthopedic repositioning device, each

⊘ **S8265** Haberman feeder for cleft lip/palate

⊘ **S8270** Enuresis alarm, using auditory buzzer and/or vibration device

⊘ **S8301** Infection control supplies, not otherwise specified

⊘ **S8415** Supplies for home delivery of infant **A**

⊘ **S8420** Gradient pressure aid (sleeve and glove combination), custom made

⊘ **S8421** Gradient pressure aid (sleeve and glove combination), ready made

⊘ **S8422** Gradient pressure aid (sleeve), custom made, medium weight

⊘ **S8423** Gradient pressure aid (sleeve), custom made, heavy weight

⊘ **S8424** Gradient pressure aid (sleeve), ready made

⊘ **S8425** Gradient pressure aid (glove), custom made, medium weight

⊘ **S8426** Gradient pressure aid (glove), custom made, heavy weight

⊘ **S8427** Gradient pressure aid (glove), ready made

⊘ **S8428** Gradient pressure aid (gauntlet), ready made

⊘ **S8429** Gradient pressure exterior wrap

⊘ **S8430** Padding for compression bandage, roll

⊘ **S8431** Compression bandage, roll

⊘ **S8450** Splint, prefabricated, digit (specify digit by use of modifier)

⊘ **S8451** Splint, prefabricated, wrist or ankle

⊘ **S8452** Splint, prefabricated, elbow

⊘ **S8460** Camisole, post-mastectomy

⊘ **S8490** Insulin syringes (100 syringes, any size)

⊘ **S8930** Electrical stimulation of auricular acupuncture points; each 15 minutes of personal one-on-one contact with the patient

---

⊘ **S8940**   Equestrian/Hippotherapy, per session

⊘ **S8948**   Application of a modality (requiring constant provider attendance) to one or more areas; low-level laser; each 15 minutes

⊘ **S8950**   Complex lymphedema therapy, each 15 minutes

⊘ **S8990**   Physical or manipulative therapy performed for maintenance rather than restoration

⊘ **S8999**   Resuscitation bag (for use by patient on artificial respiration during power failure or other catastrophic event)

⊘ **S9001**   Home uterine monitor with or without associated nursing services ♀

⊘ **S9007**   Ultrafiltration monitor

⊘ **S9015**   Automated EEG monitoring

⊘ **S9024**   Paranasal sinus ultrasound

⊘ **S9025**   Omnicardiogram/cardiointegram

⊘ **S9034**   Extracorporeal shockwave lithotripsy for gall stones (if performed with ERCP, use 43265)

⊘ **S9055**   Procuren or other growth factor preparation to promote wound healing

⊘ **S9056**   Coma stimulation per diem

⊘ **S9061**   Home administration of aerosolized drug therapy (e.g., pentamidine); administrative services, professional pharmacy services, care coordination, all necessary supplies and equipment (drugs and nursing visits coded separately), per diem

⊘ **S9083**   Global fee urgent care centers

⊘ **S9088**   Services provided in an urgent care center (list in addition to code for service)

⊘ **S9090**   Vertebral axial decompression, per session

⊘ **S9097**   Home visit for wound care

⊘ **S9098**   Home visit, phototherapy services (e.g. Bili-Lite), including equipment rental, nursing services, blood draw, supplies, and other services, per diem

⊘ **S9110**   Telemonitoring of patient in their home, including all necessary equipment; computer system, connections, and software; maintenance; patient education and support; per month

⊘ **S9117**   Back school, per visit

⊘ **S9122**   Home health aide or certified nurse assistant, providing care in the home; per hour

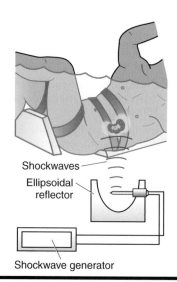

Shockwaves

Ellipsoidal reflector

Shockwave generator

Figure 55   Extracorporeal shockwave lithotripsy (ESWL).

⊘ **S9123**   Nursing care, in the home; by registered nurse, per hour (use for general nursing care only, not to be used when CPT codes 99500-99602 can be used)

⊘ **S9124**   Nursing care, in the home; by licensed practical nurse, per hour

⊘ **S9125**   Respite care, in the home, per diem

⊘ **S9126**   Hospice care, in the home, per diem

⊘ **S9127**   Social work visit, in the home, per diem

⊘ **S9128**   Speech therapy, in the home, per diem

⊘ **S9129**   Occupational therapy, in the home, per diem

⊘ **S9131**   Physical therapy; in the home, per diem

⊘ **S9140**   Diabetic management program, follow-up visit to non-MD provider

⊘ **S9141**   Diabetic management program, follow-up visit to MD provider

⊘ **S9145**   Insulin pump initiation, instruction in initial use of pump (pump not included)

⊘ **S9150**   Evaluation by ocularist

⊘ **S9152**   Speech therapy, re-evaluation

⊘ **S9208**   Home management of preterm labor, including administrative services, professional pharmacy services, care coordination, and all necessary supplies or equipment (drugs and nursing visits coded separately), per diem (do not use this code with any home infusion per diem code) ♀

▶ New	↻ Revised	✓ Reinstated	~~deleted~~ Deleted	⊘ Not covered or valid by Medicare
⊕ Special coverage instructions		✳ Carrier discretion	Ⓑ Bill local carrier	Ⓑ Bill DME MAC

⊘ **S9209** Home management of preterm premature rupture of membranes (PPROM), including administrative services, professional pharmacy services, care coordination, and all necessary supplies or equipment (drugs and nursing visits coded separately), per diem (do not use this code with any home infusion per diem code) ♀

⊘ **S9211** Home management of gestational hypertension, includes administrative services, professional pharmacy services, care coordination, and all necessary supplies and equipment (drugs and nursing visits coded separately); per diem (do not use this code with any home infusion per diem code) ♀

⊘ **S9212** Home management of postpartum hypertension, includes administrative services, professional pharmacy services, care coordination, and all necessary supplies and equipment (drugs and nursing visits coded separately); per diem (do not use this code with any home infusion per diem code) ♀

⊘ **S9213** Home management of preeclampsia, includes administrative services, professional pharmacy services, care coordination, and all necessary supplies and equipment (drugs and nursing services coded separately); per diem (do not use this code with any home infusion per diem code) ♀

⊘ **S9214** Home management of gestational diabetes, includes administrative services, professional pharmacy services, care coordination, and all necessary supplies and equipment (drugs and nursing visits coded separately); per diem (do not use this code with any home infusion per diem code) ♀

⊘ **S9325** Home infusion therapy, pain management infusion; administrative services, professional pharmacy services, care coordination, and all necessary supplies and equipment, (drugs and nursing visits coded separately), per diem (do not use this code with S9326, S9327 or S9328)

⊘ **S9326** Home infusion therapy, continuous (twenty-four hours or more) pain management infusion; administrative services, professional pharmacy services, care coordination, and all necessary supplies and equipment (drugs and nursing visits coded separately), per diem

⊘ **S9327** Home infusion therapy, intermittent (less than twenty-four hours) pain management infusion; administrative services, professional pharmacy services, care coordination, and all necessary supplies and equipment (drugs and nursing visits coded separately), per diem

⊘ **S9328** Home infusion therapy, implanted pump pain management infusion; administrative services, professional pharmacy services, care coordination, and all necessary supplies and equipment (drugs and nursing visits coded separately), per diem

⊘ **S9329** Home infusion therapy, chemotherapy infusion; administrative services, professional pharmacy services, care coordination, and all necessary supplies and equipment (drugs and nursing visits coded separately), per diem (do not use this code with S9330 or S9331)

⊘ **S9330** Home infusion therapy, continuous (twenty-four hours or more) chemotherapy infusion; administrative services, professional pharmacy services, care coordination, and all necessary supplies and equipment (drugs and nursing visits coded separately), per diem

⊘ **S9331** Home infusion therapy, intermittent (less than twenty-four hours) chemotherapy infusion; administrative services, professional pharmacy services, care coordination, and all necessary supplies and equipment (drugs and nursing visits coded separately), per diem

⊘ **S9335** Home therapy, hemodialysis; administrative services, professional pharmacy services, care coordination, and all necessary supplies and equipment (drugs and nursing services coded separately), per diem

⊘ **S9336** Home infusion therapy, continuous anticoagulant infusion therapy (e.g. heparin), administrative services, professional pharmacy services, care coordination, and all necessary supplies and equipment (drugs and nursing visits coded separately), per diem

⊘ **S9338** Home infusion therapy, immunotherapy, administrative services, professional pharmacy services, care coordination, and all necessary supplies and equipment (drug and nursing visits coded separately), per diem

🅟 PQRS	🆀p Quantity Physician Appendix A	🆀h Quantity Hospital Appendix B	♀ Female only
♂ Male only	🄰 Age	👤 DMEPOS	A2-Z3 ASC Payment Indicator	A-Y ASC Status Indicator	Coding Clinic

⊘ **S9339** Home therapy; peritoneal dialysis, administrative services, professional pharmacy services, care coordination and all necessary supplies and equipment (drugs and nursing visits coded separately), per diem

⊘ **S9340** Home therapy; enteral nutrition; administrative services, professional pharmacy services, care coordination, and all necessary supplies and equipment (enteral formula and nursing visits coded separately), per diem

⊘ **S9341** Home therapy; enteral nutrition via gravity; administrative services, professional pharmacy services, care coordination, and all necessary supplies and equipment (enteral formula and nursing visits coded separately), per diem

⊘ **S9342** Home therapy; enteral nutrition via pump; administrative services, professional pharmacy services, care coordination, and all necessary supplies and equipment (enteral formula and nursing visits coded separately), per diem

⊘ **S9343** Home therapy; enteral nutrition via bolus; administrative services, professional pharmacy services, care coordination, and all necessary supplies and equipment (enteral formula and nursing visits coded separately), per diem

⊘ **S9345** Home infusion therapy, anti-hemophilic agent infusion therapy (e.g. Factor VIII); administrative services, professional pharmacy services, care coordination, and all necessary supplies and equipment (drugs and nursing visits coded separately), per diem

⊘ **S9346** Home infusion therapy, alpha-1-proteinase inhibitor (e.g., Prolastin); administrative services, professional pharmacy services, care coordination, and all necessary supplies and equipment (drugs and nursing visits coded separately), per diem

⊘ **S9347** Home infusion therapy, uninterrupted, long-term, controlled rate intravenous or subcutaneous infusion therapy (e.g. Epoprostenol); administrative services, professional pharmacy services, care coordination, and all necessary supplies and equipment (drugs and nursing visits coded separately), per diem

⊘ **S9348** Home infusion therapy, sympathomimetic/inotropic agent infusion therapy (e.g., Dobutamine); administrative services, professional pharmacy services, care coordination, all necessary supplies and equipment (drugs and nursing visits coded separately), per diem

⊘ **S9349** Home infusion therapy, tocolytic infusion therapy; administrative services, professional pharmacy services, care coordination, and all necessary supplies and equipment (drugs and nursing visits coded separately), per diem

⊘ **S9351** Home infusion therapy, continuous or intermittent anti-emetic infusion therapy; administrative services, professional pharmacy services, care coordination, and all necessary supplies and equipment (drugs and visits coded separately), per diem

⊘ **S9353** Home infusion therapy, continuous insulin infusion therapy; administrative services, professional pharmacy services, care coordination, and all necessary supplies and equipment (drugs and nursing visits coded separately), per diem

⊘ **S9355** Home infusion therapy, chelation therapy; administrative services, professional pharmacy services, care coordination, and all necessary supplies and equipment (drugs and nursing visits coded separately), per diem

⊘ **S9357** Home infusion therapy, enzyme replacement intravenous therapy; (e.g. Imiglucerase); administrative services, professional pharmacy services, care coordination, and all necessary supplies and equipment (drugs and nursing visits coded separately), per diem

⊘ **S9359** Home infusion therapy, anti-tumor necrosis factor intravenous therapy; (e.g. Infliximab); administrative services, professional pharmacy services, care coordination, and all necessary supplies and equipment (drugs and nursing visits coded separately), per diem

⊘ **S9361** Home infusion therapy, diuretic intravenous therapy; administrative services, professional pharmacy services, care coordination, and all necessary supplies and equipment (drugs and nursing visits coded separately), per diem

---

▶ **New**　⟳ **Revised**　✔ **Reinstated**　~~deleted~~ **Deleted**　⊘ **Not covered or valid by Medicare**
⊛ **Special coverage instructions**　✳ **Carrier discretion**　Ⓑ **Bill local carrier**　Ⓓ **Bill DME MAC**

⊘ **S9363** Home infusion therapy, anti-spasmotic therapy; administrative services, professional pharmacy services, care coordination, and all necessary supplies and equipment (drugs and nursing visits coded separately), per diem

⊘ **S9364** Home infusion therapy, total parenteral nutrition (TPN); administrative services, professional pharmacy services, care coordination, and all necessary supplies and equipment including standard TPN formula (lipids, specialty amino acid formulas, drugs other than in standard formula, and nursing visits coded separately) per diem (do not use with home infusion codes S9365-S9368 using daily volume scales)

⊘ **S9365** Home infusion therapy, total parenteral nutrition (TPN); one liter per day, administrative services, professional pharmacy services, care coordination, and all necessary supplies and equipment including standard TPN formula (lipids, specialty amino acid formulas, drugs other than in standard formula and nursing visits coded separately), per diem

⊘ **S9366** Home infusion therapy, total parenteral nutrition (TPN); more than one liter but no more than two liters per day, administrative services, professional pharmacy services, care coordination, and all necessary supplies and equipment including standard TPN formula; (lipids, specialty amino acid formulas, drugs other than in standard formula and nursing visits coded separately), per diem

⊘ **S9367** Home infusion therapy, total parenteral nutrition (TPN); more than two liters but no more than three liters per day, administrative services, professional pharmacy services, care coordination, and all necessary supplies and equipment including standard TPN formula; (lipids, specialty amino acid formulas, drugs other than in standard formula and nursing visits coded separately), per diem

⊘ **S9368** Home infusion therapy, total parenteral nutrition (TPN); more than three liters per day, administrative services, professional pharmacy services, care coordination, and all necessary supplies and equipment (including standard TPN formula; lipids, specialty amino acid formulas, drugs other than in standard formula and nursing visits coded separately), per diem

⊘ **S9370** Home therapy, intermittent anti-emetic injection therapy; administrative services, professional pharmacy services, care coordination, and all necessary supplies and equipment (drugs and nursing visits coded separately), per diem

⊘ **S9372** Home therapy; intermittent anticoagulant injection therapy (e.g., heparin); administrative services, professional pharmacy services, care coordination, and all necessary supplies and equipment (drugs and nursing visits coded separately), per diem (do not use this code for flushing of infusion devices with heparin to maintain patency)

⊘ **S9373** Home infusion therapy, hydration therapy; administrative services, professional pharmacy services, care coordination, and all necessary supplies and equipment (drugs and nursing visits coded separately), per diem (do not use with hydration therapy codes S9374-S9377 using daily volume scales)

⊘ **S9374** Home infusion therapy, hydration therapy; one liter per day, administrative services, professional pharmacy services, care coordination, and all necessary supplies and equipment (drugs and nursing visits coded separately), per diem

⊘ **S9375** Home infusion therapy, hydration therapy; more than one liter but no more than two liters per day, administrative services, professional pharmacy services, care coordination, and all necessary supplies and equipment (drugs and nursing visits coded separately), per diem

⊘ **S9376** Home infusion therapy, hydration therapy; more than two liters but no more than three liters per day, administrative services, professional pharmacy services, care coordination, and all necessary supplies and equipment (drugs and nursing visits coded separately), per diem

⊘ **S9377** Home infusion therapy, hydration therapy; more than three liters per day, administrative services, professional pharmacy services, care coordination, and all necessary supplies (drugs and nursing visits coded separately), per diem

PQRS PQRS	**Qp** Quantity Physician Appendix A	**Qh** Quantity Hospital Appendix B	♀ Female only	
♂ Male only	**A** Age	♿ DMEPOS	A2-Z3 ASC Payment Indicator	A-Y ASC Status Indicator Coding Clinic

⊘ **S9379** Home infusion therapy, infusion therapy, not otherwise classified; administrative services, professional pharmacy services, care coordination, and all necessary supplies and equipment (drugs and nursing visits coded separately), per diem

⊘ **S9381** Delivery or service to high risk areas requiring escort or extra protection, per visit

⊘ **S9401** Anticoagulation clinic, inclusive of all services except laboratory tests, per session

⊘ **S9430** Pharmacy compounding and dispensing services

⊘ **S9433** Medical food nutritionally complete, administered orally, providing 100% of nutritional intake

⊘ **S9434** Modified solid food supplements for inborn errors of metabolism

⊘ **S9435** Medical foods for inborn errors of metabolism

⊘ **S9436** Childbirth preparation/Lamaze classes, non-physician provider, per session ♀

⊘ **S9437** Childbirth refresher classes, non-physician provider, per session ♀

⊘ **S9438** Cesarean birth classes, non-physician provider, per session ♀

⊘ **S9439** VBAC (vaginal birth after cesarean) classes, non-physician provider, per session ♀

⊘ **S9441** Asthma education, non-physician provider, per session

⊘ **S9442** Birthing classes, non-physician provider, per session ♀

⊘ **S9443** Lactation classes, non-physician provider, per session ♀

⊘ **S9444** Parenting classes, non-physician provider, per session

⊘ **S9445** Patient education, not otherwise classified, non-physician provider, individual, per session

⊘ **S9446** Patient education, not otherwise classified, non-physician provider, group, per session

⊘ **S9447** Infant safety (including CPR) classes, non-physician provider, per session

⊘ **S9449** Weight management classes, non-physician provider, per session

⊘ **S9451** Exercise classes, non-physician provider, per session

⊘ **S9452** Nutrition classes, non-physician provider, per session

⊘ **S9453** Smoking cessation classes, non-physician provider, per session

⊘ **S9454** Stress management classes, non-physician provider, per session

⊘ **S9455** Diabetic management program, group session

⊘ **S9460** Diabetic management program, nurse visit

⊘ **S9465** Diabetic management program, dietitian visit

⊘ **S9470** Nutritional counseling, dietitian visit

⊘ **S9472** Cardiac rehabilitation program, non-physician provider, per diem

⊘ **S9473** Pulmonary rehabilitation program, non-physician provider, per diem

⊘ **S9474** Enterostomal therapy by a registered nurse certified in enterostomal therapy, per diem

⊘ **S9475** Ambulatory setting substance abuse treatment or detoxification services, per diem

⊘ **S9476** Vestibular rehabilitation program, non-physician provider, per diem

⊘ **S9480** Intensive outpatient psychiatric services, per diem

⊘ **S9482** Family stabilization services, per 15 minutes

⊘ **S9484** Crisis intervention mental health services, per hour

⊘ **S9485** Crisis intervention mental health services, per diem

⊘ **S9490** Home infusion therapy, corticosteroid infusion; administrative services, professional pharmacy services, care coordination, and all necessary supplies and equipment (drugs and nursing visits coded separately), per diem

⊘ **S9494** Home infusion therapy, antibiotic, antiviral, or antifungal therapy; administrative services, professional pharmacy services, care coordination, and all necessary supplies and equipment (drugs and nursing visits coded separately) per diem, (do not use this code with home infusion codes for hourly dosing schedules S9497-S9504)

⊘ **S9497** Home infusion therapy, antibiotic, antiviral, or antifungal therapy; once every 3 hours; administrative services, professional pharmacy services, care coordination, and all necessary supplies and equipment (drugs and nursing visits coded separately), per diem

---

▶ **New**   ⟲ **Revised**   ✔ **Reinstated**   ~~deleted~~ **Deleted**   ⊘ **Not covered or valid by Medicare**

✪ **Special coverage instructions**   ✻ **Carrier discretion**   Ⓑ **Bill local carrier**   Ⓑ **Bill DME MAC**

⊘ **S9500** Home infusion therapy, antibiotic, antiviral, or antifungal therapy; once every 24 hours; administrative services, professional pharmacy services, care coordination, and all necessary supplies and equipment (drugs and nursing visits coded separately), per diem

⊘ **S9501** Home infusion therapy, antibiotic, antiviral, or antifungal therapy; once every 12 hours; administrative services, professional pharmacy services, care coordination, and all necessary supplies and equipment (drugs and nursing visits coded separately), per diem

⊘ **S9502** Home infusion therapy, antibiotic, antiviral, or antifungal therapy; once every 8 hours, administrative services, professional pharmacy services, care coordination, and all necessary supplies and equipment (drugs and nursing visits coded separately), per diem

⊘ **S9503** Home infusion therapy, antibiotic, antiviral, or antifungal; once every 6 hours; administrative services, professional pharmacy services, care coordination, and all necessary supplies and equipment (drugs and nursing visits coded separately), per diem

⊘ **S9504** Home infusion therapy, antibiotic, antiviral, or antifungal; once every 4 hours; administrative services, professional pharmacy services, care coordination, and all necessary supplies and equipment (drugs and nursing visits coded separately), per diem

⊘ **S9529** Routine venipuncture for collection of specimen(s), single home bound, nursing home, or skilled nursing facility patient

⊘ **S9537** Home therapy; hematopoietic hormone injection therapy (e.g. erythropoietin, G-CSF, GM-CSF); administrative services, professional pharmacy services, care coordination, and all necessary supplies and equipment (drugs and nursing visits coded separately), per diem

⊘ **S9538** Home transfusion of blood product(s); administrative services, professional pharmacy services, care coordination, and all necessary supplies and equipment (blood products, drugs, and nursing visits coded separately), per diem

⊘ **S9542** Home injectable therapy; not otherwise classified, including administrative services, professional pharmacy services, care coordination, and all necessary supplies and equipment (drugs and nursing visits coded separately), per diem

⊘ **S9558** Home injectable therapy; growth hormone, including administrative services, professional pharmacy services, care coordination, and all necessary supplies and equipment (drugs and nursing visits coded separately), per diem

⊘ **S9559** Home injectable therapy; interferon, including administrative services, professional pharmacy services, care coordination, and all necessary supplies and equipment (drugs and nursing visits coded separately), per diem

⊘ **S9560** Home injectable therapy; hormonal therapy (e.g., Leuprolide, Goserelin), including administrative services, professional pharmacy services, care coordination, and all necessary supplies and equipment (drugs and nursing visits coded separately), per diem

⊘ **S9562** Home injectable therapy, palivizumab, including administrative services, professional pharmacy services, care coordination, and all necessary supplies and equipment (drugs and nursing visits coded separately), per diem

⊘ **S9590** Home therapy, irrigation therapy (e.g. sterile irrigation of an organ or anatomical cavity); including administrative services, professional pharmacy services, care coordination, and all necessary supplies and equipment (drugs and nursing visits coded separately), per diem

⊘ **S9810** Home therapy; professional pharmacy services for provision of infusion, specialty drug administration, and/or disease state management, not otherwise classified, per hour (do not use this code with any per diem code)

⊘ **S9900** Services by journal-listed Christian Science Practitioner for the purpose of healing, per diem

▶ ⊘ **S9901** Services by a journal-listed Christian Science nurse, per hour

⊘ **S9960** Ambulance service, conventional air services, nonemergency transport, one way (fixed wing)

⊘ **S9961** Ambulance service, conventional air service, nonemergency transport, one way (rotary wing)

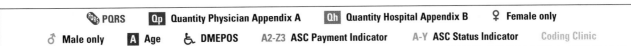

PQRS PQRS | Qp Quantity Physician Appendix A | Qh Quantity Hospital Appendix B | ♀ Female only

♂ Male only | A Age | ♿ DMEPOS | A2-Z3 ASC Payment Indicator | A-Y ASC Status Indicator | Coding Clinic

⊘ **S9970** Health club membership, annual

⊘ **S9975** Transplant related lodging, meals and transportation, per diem

⊘ **S9976** Lodging, per diem, not otherwise classified

⊘ **S9977** Meals, per diem, not otherwise specified

⊘ **S9981** Medical records copying fee, administrative

⊘ **S9982** Medical records copying fee, per page

⊘ **S9986** Not medically necessary service (patient is aware that service not medically necessary)

⊘ **S9988** Services provided as part of a Phase I clinical trial

⊘ **S9989** Services provided outside of the United States of America (list in addition to code(s) for services(s))

⊘ **S9990** Services provided as part of a Phase II clinical trial

⊘ **S9991** Services provided as part of a Phase III clinical trial

⊘ **S9992** Transportation costs to and from trial location and local transportation costs (e.g., fares for taxicab or bus) for clinical trial participant and one caregiver/companion

⊘ **S9994** Lodging costs (e.g., hotel charges) for clinical trial participant and one caregiver/companion

⊘ **S9996** Meals for clinical trial participant and one caregiver/companion

⊘ **S9999** Sales tax

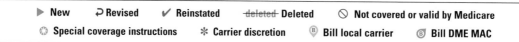

▶ New   ⟲ Revised   ✔ Reinstated   deleted Deleted   ⊘ Not covered or valid by Medicare

✿ Special coverage instructions   ✳ Carrier discretion   Ⓑ Bill local carrier   Ⓑ Bill DME MAC

TEMPORARY NATIONAL CODES ESTABLISHED BY MEDICAID (T1000-T9999)

Not Valid For Medicare

⊘ **T1000** Private duty/independent nursing service(s) - licensed, up to 15 minutes

⊘ **T1001** Nursing assessment/evaluation

⊘ **T1002** RN services, up to 15 minutes

⊘ **T1003** LPN/LVN services, up to 15 minutes

⊘ **T1004** Services of a qualified nursing aide, up to 15 minutes

⊘ **T1005** Respite care services, up to 15 minutes

⊘ **T1006** Alcohol and/or substance abuse services, family/couple counseling

⊘ **T1007** Alcohol and/or substance abuse services, treatment plan development and/or modification

⊘ **T1009** Child sitting services for children of the individual receiving alcohol and/or substance abuse services 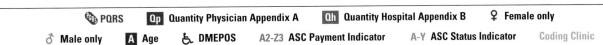 A

⊘ **T1010** Meals for individuals receiving alcohol and/or substance abuse services (when meals not included in the program)

⊘ **T1012** Alcohol and/or substance abuse services, skills development

⊘ **T1013** Sign language or oral interpretive services, per 15 minutes

⊘ **T1014** Telehealth transmission, per minute, professional services bill separately

⊘ **T1015** Clinic visit/encounter, all-inclusive

⊘ **T1016** Case Management, each 15 minutes

⊘ **T1017** Targeted Case Management, each 15 minutes

⊘ **T1018** School-based individualized education program (IEP) services, bundled

⊘ **T1019** Personal care services, per 15 minutes, not for an inpatient or resident of a hospital, nursing facility, ICF/MR or IMD, part of the individualized plan of treatment (code may not be used to identify services provided by home health aide or certified nurse assistant)

⊘ **T1020** Personal care services, per diem, not for an inpatient or resident of a hospital, nursing facility, ICF/MR or IMD, part of the individualized plan of treatment (code may not be used to identify services provided by home health aide or certified nurse assistant)

⊘ **T1021** Home health aide or certified nurse assistant, per visit

⊘ **T1022** Contracted home health agency services, all services provided under contract, per day

⊘ **T1023** Screening to determine the appropriateness of consideration of an individual for participation in a specified program, project or treatment protocol, per encounter

⊘ **T1024** Evaluation and treatment by an integrated, specialty team contracted to provide coordinated care to multiple or severely handicapped children, per encounter A

⊘ **T1025** Intensive, extended multidisciplinary services provided in a clinic setting to children with complex medical, physical, mental and psychosocial impairments, per diem A

⊘ **T1026** Intensive, extended multidisciplinary services provided in a clinic setting to children with complex medical, physical, medical and psychosocial impairments, per hour A

⊘ **T1027** Family training and counseling for child development, per 15 minutes A

⊘ **T1028** Assessment of home, physical and family environment, to determine suitability to meet patient's medical needs

⊘ **T1029** Comprehensive environmental lead investigation, not including laboratory analysis, per dwelling

⊘ **T1030** Nursing care, in the home, by registered nurse, per diem

⊘ **T1031** Nursing care, in the home, by licensed practical nurse, per diem

⊘ **T1502** Administration of oral, intramuscular and/or subcutaneous medication by health care agency/professional, per visit

⊘ **T1503** Administration of medication, other than oral and/or injectable, by a health care agency/professional, per visit

⊘ **T1505** Electronic medication compliance management device, includes all components and accessories, not otherwise classified

⊘ **T1999** Miscellaneous therapeutic items and supplies, retail purchases, not otherwise classified; identify product in "remarks"

⊘ **T2001** Non-emergency transportation; patient attendant/escort

⊘ **T2002** Non-emergency transportation; per diem

⊘ **T2003** Non-emergency transportation; encounter/trip

⊘ **T2004** Non-emergency transport; commercial carrier, multi-pass

⊘ **T2005** Non-emergency transportation: stretcher van

⊘ **T2007** Transportation waiting time, air ambulance and non-emergency vehicle, one-half (1/2) hour increments

⊘ **T2010** Preadmission screening and resident review (PASRR) level I identification screening, per screen

⊘ **T2011** Preadmission screening and resident review (PASRR) level II evaluation, per evaluation

⊘ **T2012** Habilitation, educational, waiver; per diem

⊘ **T2013** Habilitation, educational, waiver; per hour

⊘ **T2014** Habilitation, prevocational, waiver; per diem

⊘ **T2015** Habilitation, prevocational, waiver; per hour

⊘ **T2016** Habilitation, residential, waiver; per diem

⊘ **T2017** Habilitation, residential, waiver; 15 minutes

⊘ **T2018** Habilitation, supported employment, waiver; per diem

⊘ **T2019** Habilitation, supported employment, waiver; per 15 minutes

⊘ **T2020** Day habilitation, waiver; per diem

⊘ **T2021** Day habilitation, waiver; per 15 minutes

⊘ **T2022** Case management, per month

⊘ **T2023** Targeted case management; per month

⊘ **T2024** Service assessment/plan of care development, waiver

⊘ **T2025** Waiver services; not otherwise specified (NOS)

⊘ **T2026** Specialized childcare, waiver; per diem

⊘ **T2027** Specialized childcare, waiver; per 15 minutes

⊘ **T2028** Specialized supply, not otherwise specified, waiver

⊘ **T2029** Specialized medical equipment, not otherwise specified, waiver

⊘ **T2030** Assisted living, waiver; per month

⊘ **T2031** Assisted living; waiver, per diem

⊘ **T2032** Residential care, not otherwise specified (NOS), waiver; per month

⊘ **T2033** Residential care, not otherwise specified (NOS), waiver; per diem

⊘ **T2034** Crisis intervention, waiver; per diem

⊘ **T2035** Utility services to support medical equipment and assistive technology/ devices, waiver

⊘ **T2036** Therapeutic camping, overnight, waiver; each session

⊘ **T2037** Therapeutic camping, day, waiver; each session

⊘ **T2038** Community transition, waiver; per service

⊘ **T2039** Vehicle modifications, waiver; per service

⊘ **T2040** Financial management, self-directed, waiver; per 15 minutes

⊘ **T2041** Supports brokerage, self-directed, waiver; per 15 minutes

⊘ **T2042** Hospice routine home care; per diem

⊘ **T2043** Hospice continuous home care; per hour

⊘ **T2044** Hospice inpatient respite care; per diem

⊘ **T2045** Hospice general inpatient care; per diem

⊘ **T2046** Hospice long term care, room and board only; per diem

⊘ **T2048** Behavioral health; long-term care residential (non-acute care in a residential treatment program where stay is typically longer than 30 days), with room and board, per diem

⊘ **T2049** Non-emergency transportation; stretcher van, mileage; per mile

⊘ **T2101** Human breast milk processing, storage and distribution only ♀

⊘ **T4521** Adult sized disposable incontinence product, brief/diaper, small, each **A**
 IOM: 100-03, 4, 280.1

⊘ **T4522** Adult sized disposable incontinence product, brief/diaper, medium, each **A**
 IOM: 100-03, 4, 280.1

⊘ **T4523** Adult sized disposable incontinence product, brief/diaper, large, each **A**
 IOM: 100-03, 4, 280.1

⊘ **T4524** Adult sized disposable incontinence product, brief/diaper, extra large, each **A**
 IOM: 100-03, 4, 280.1

⊘ **T4525** Adult sized disposable incontinence product, protective underwear/pull-on, small size, each **A**
 IOM: 100-03, 4, 280.1

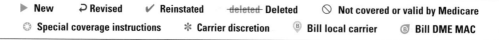

▶ **New**   ↻ **Revised**   ✔ **Reinstated**   ~~deleted~~ **Deleted**   ⊘ **Not covered or valid by Medicare**
✪ **Special coverage instructions**   ✳ **Carrier discretion**   ⑧ **Bill local carrier**   Ⓑ **Bill DME MAC**

⊘ **T4526**   Adult sized disposable incontinence product, protective underwear/pull-on, medium size, each **A**

IOM: 100-03, 4, 280.1

⊘ **T4527**   Adult sized disposable incontinence product, protective underwear/pull-on, large size, each **A**

IOM: 100-03, 4, 280.1

⊘ **T4528**   Adult sized disposable incontinence product, protective underwear/pull-on, extra large size, each **A**

IOM: 100-03, 4, 280.1

⊘ **T4529**   Pediatric sized disposable incontinence product, brief/diaper, small/medium size, each **A**

IOM: 100-03, 4, 280.1

⊘ **T4530**   Pediatric sized disposable incontinence product, brief/diaper, large size, each **A**

IOM: 100-03, 4, 280.1

⊘ **T4531**   Pediatric sized disposable incontinence product, protective underwear/pull-on, small/medium size, each **A**

IOM: 100-03, 4, 280.1

⊘ **T4532**   Pediatric sized disposable incontinence product, protective underwear/pull-on, large size, each **A**

IOM: 100-03, 4, 280.1

⊘ **T4533**   Youth sized disposable incontinence product, brief/diaper, each **A**

IOM: 100-03, 4, 280.1

⊘ **T4534**   Youth sized disposable incontinence product, protective underwear/pull-on, each **A**

IOM: 100-03, 4, 280.1

⊘ **T4535**   Disposable liner/shield/guard/pad/undergarment, for incontinence, each

IOM: 100-03, 4, 280.1

⊘ **T4536**   Incontinence product, protective underwear/pull-on, reusable, any size, each

IOM: 100-03, 4, 280.1

⊘ **T4537**   Incontinence product, protective underpad, reusable, bed size, each

IOM: 100-03, 4, 280.1

⊘ **T4538**   Diaper service, reusable diaper, each diaper

IOM: 100-03, 4, 280.1

⊘ **T4539**   Incontinence product, diaper/brief, reusable, any size, each

IOM: 100-03, 4, 280.1

⊘ **T4540**   Incontinence product, protective underpad, reusable, chair size, each

IOM: 100-03, 4, 280.1

⊘ **T4541**   Incontinence product, disposable underpad, large, each

⊘ **T4542**   Incontinence product, disposable underpad, small size, each

⊘ **T4543**   Adult sized disposable incontinence product, protective brief/diaper, above extra large, each **A**

IOM: 100-03, 4, 280.1

⊘ **T4544**   Adult sized disposable incontinence product, protective underwear/pull-on, above extra large, each **A**

IOM 100-03, 4, 280.1

⊘ **T5001**   Positioning seat for persons with special orthopedic needs, supply, not otherwise specified

⊘ **T5999**   Supply, not otherwise specified

PQRS   **Qp** Quantity Physician Appendix A   **Qh** Quantity Hospital Appendix B   ♀ **Female only**

♂ **Male only**   **A** Age   ⅙ **DMEPOS**   A2-Z3 **ASC Payment Indicator**   A-Y **ASC Status Indicator**   Coding Clinic

VISION SERVICES (V0000-V2999)

Frames

⊛ **V2020**   Frames, purchases Ⓑ Qp Qh ♿   A

Includes cost of frame/replacement and dispensing fee. One unit of service represents one pair of eyeglass frames.

IOM: 100-02, 15, 120

⊘ **V2025**   Deluxe frame Ⓑ   E

Not a benefit. Billing deluxe frames—submit V2020 on one line; V2025 on second line

IOM: 100-04, 1, 30.3.5

Spectacle Lenses

NOTE: If a CPT procedure code for supply of spectacles or a permanent prosthesis is reported, recode with the specific lens type listed below. For aphakic temporary spectacle correction, see CPT.

Single Vision, Glass or Plastic

✳ **V2100**   Sphere, single vision, plano to plus or minus 4.00, per lens Ⓑ Qp ♿   A

✳ **V2101**   Sphere, single vision, plus or minus 4.12 to plus or minus 7.00d, per lens Ⓑ Qp Qh ♿   A

✳ **V2102**   Sphere, single vision, plus or minus 7.12 to plus or minus 20.00d, per lens Ⓑ Qp Qh ♿   A

✳ **V2103**   Spherocylinder, single vision, plano to plus or minus 4.00d sphere, .12 to 2.00d cylinder, per lens Ⓑ Qp ♿   A

✳ **V2104**   Spherocylinder, single vision, plano to plus or minus 4.00d sphere, 2.12 to 4.00d cylinder, per lens Ⓑ Qp Qh ♿   A

✳ **V2105**   Spherocylinder, single vision, plano to plus or minus 4.00d sphere, 4.25 to 6.00d cylinder, per lens Ⓑ Qp Qh ♿   A

✳ **V2106**   Spherocylinder, single vision, plano to plus or minus 4.00d sphere, over 6.00d cylinder, per lens Ⓑ Qp Qh ♿   A

✳ **V2107**   Spherocylinder, single vision, plus or minus 4.25 to plus or minus 7.00 sphere, .12 to 2.00d cylinder, per lens Ⓑ Qp Qh ♿   A

✳ **V2108**   Spherocylinder, single vision, plus or minus 4.25d to plus or minus 7.00d sphere, 2.12 to 4.00d cylinder, per lens Ⓑ Qp Qh ♿   A

✳ **V2109**   Spherocylinder, single vision, plus or minus 4.25 to plus or minus 7.00d sphere, 4.25 to 6.00d cylinder, per lens Ⓑ Qp Qh ♿   A

✳ **V2110**   Sperocylinder, single vision, plus or minus 4.25 to 7.00d sphere, over 6.00d cylinder, per lens Ⓑ Qp Qh ♿   A

✳ **V2111**   Spherocylinder, single vision, plus or minus 7.25 to plus or minus 12.00d sphere, .25 to 2.25d cylinder, per lens Ⓑ Qp Qh ♿   A

✳ **V2112**   Spherocylinder, single vision, plus or minus 7.25 to plus or minus 12.00d sphere, 2.25d to 4.00d cylinder, per lens Ⓑ Qp Qh ♿   A

✳ **V2113**   Spherocylinder, single vision, plus or minus 7.25 to plus or minus 12.00d sphere, 4.25 to 6.00d cylinder, per lens Ⓑ Qp Qh ♿   A

✳ **V2114**   Spherocylinder, single vision, sphere over plus or minus 12.00d, per lens Ⓑ Qp Qh ♿   A

✳ **V2115**   Lenticular, (myodisc), per lens, single vision Ⓑ Qp Qh ♿   A

✳ **V2118**   Aniseikonic lens, single vision Ⓑ Qp Qh ♿   A

⊛ **V2121**   Lenticular lens, per lens, single Ⓑ Qp Qh ♿   A

IOM: 100-02, 15, 120; 100-04, 3, 10.4

✳ **V2199**   Not otherwise classified, single vision lens Ⓑ Qp Qh   A

Bill on paper. Requires report of type of single vision lens and optical lab invoice.

Bifocal, Glass or Plastic

✳ **V2200**   Sphere, bifocal, plano to plus or minus 4.00d, per lens Ⓑ Qp Qh ♿   A

✳ **V2201**   Sphere, bifocal, plus or minus 4.12 to plus or minus 7.00d, per lens Ⓑ Qp Qh ♿   A

✳ **V2202**   Sphere, bifocal, plus or minus 7.12 to plus or minus 20.00d, per lens Ⓑ Qp Qh ♿   A

✳ **V2203**   Spherocylinder, bifocal, plano to plus or minus 4.00d sphere, .12 to 2.00d cylinder, per lens Ⓑ Qp Qh ♿   A

✳ **V2204**   Spherocylinder, bifocal, plano to plus or minus 4.00d sphere, 2.12 to 4.00d cylinder, per lens Ⓑ Qp Qh ♿   A

✳ **V2205**   Spherocylinder, bifocal, plano to plus or minus 4.00d sphere, 4.25 to 6.00d cylinder, per lens Ⓑ Qp Qh ♿   A

▶ New   ↺ Revised   ✔ Reinstated   ~~deleted~~ Deleted   ⊘ Not covered or valid by Medicare
⊛ Special coverage instructions   ✳ Carrier discretion   Ⓟ Bill local carrier   Ⓑ Bill DME MAC

✳ **V2206** Spherocylinder, bifocal, plano to plus or minus 4.00d sphere, over 6.00d cylinder, per lens Ⓑ **Qp** **Qh** ♿ A

✳ **V2207** Spherocylinder, bifocal, plus or minus 4.25 to plus or minus 7.00d sphere, .12 to 2.00d cylinder, per lens Ⓑ **Qp** **Qh** ♿ A

✳ **V2208** Spherocylinder, bifocal, plus or minus 4.25 to plus or minus 7.00d sphere, 2.12 to 4.00d cylinder, per lens Ⓑ **Qp** **Qh** ♿ A

✳ **V2209** Spherocylinder, bifocal, plus or minus 4.25 to plus or minus 7.00d sphere, 4.25 to 6.00d cylinder, per lens Ⓑ **Qp** **Qh** ♿ A

✳ **V2210** Spherocylinder, bifocal, plus or minus 4.25 to plus or minus 7.00d sphere, over 6.00d cylinder, per lens Ⓑ **Qp** **Qh** ♿ A

✳ **V2211** Spherocylinder, bifocal, plus or minus 7.25 to plus or minus 12.00d sphere, .25 to 2.25d cylinder, per lens Ⓑ **Qp** **Qh** ♿ A

✳ **V2212** Spherocylinder, bifocal, plus or minus 7.25 to plus or minus 12.00d sphere, 2.25 to 4.00d cylinder, per lens Ⓑ **Qp** **Qh** ♿ A

✳ **V2213** Spherocylinder, bifocal, plus or minus 7.25 to plus or minus 12.00d sphere, 4.25 to 6.00d cylinder, per lens Ⓑ **Qp** **Qh** ♿ A

✳ **V2214** Spherocylinder, bifocal, sphere over plus or minus 12.00d, per lens Ⓑ **Qp** **Qh** ♿ A

✳ **V2215** Lenticular (myodisc), per lens, bifocal Ⓑ **Qp** **Qh** ♿ A

✳ **V2218** Aniseikonic, per lens, bifocal Ⓑ **Qp** **Qh** ♿ A

✳ **V2219** Bifocal seg width over 28mm Ⓑ **Qp** **Qh** ♿ A

✳ **V2220** Bifocal add over 3.25d Ⓑ **Qp** **Qh** ♿ A

◎ **V2221** Lenticular lens, per lens, bifocal Ⓑ **Qp** **Qh** ♿ A

IOM: 100-02, 15, 120; 100-04, 3, 10.4

✳ **V2299** Specialty bifocal (by report) Ⓑ **Qp** **Qh** A

Bill on paper. Requires report of type of specialty bifocal lens and optical lab invoice.

Trifocal, Glass or Plastic

✳ **V2300** Sphere, trifocal, plano to plus or minus 4.00d, per lens Ⓑ **Qp** **Qh** ♿ A

✳ **V2301** Sphere, trifocal, plus or minus 4.12 to plus or minus 7.00d per lens Ⓑ **Qp** **Qh** ♿ A

✳ **V2302** Sphere, trifocal, plus or minus 7.12 to plus or minus 20.00, per lens Ⓑ **Qp** **Qh** ♿ A

✳ **V2303** Spherocylinder, trifocal, plano to plus or minus 4.00d sphere, .12 to 2.00d cylinder, per lens Ⓑ **Qp** **Qh** A

✳ **V2304** Spherocylinder, trifocal, plano to plus or minus 4.00d sphere, 2.25-4.00d cylinder, per lens Ⓑ **Qp** **Qh** A

✳ **V2305** Spherocylinder, trifocal, plano to plus or minus 4.00d sphere, 4.25 to 6.00 cylinder, per lens Ⓑ **Qp** **Qh** ♿ A

✳ **V2306** Spherocylinder, trifocal, plano to plus or minus 4.00d sphere, over 6.00d cylinder, per lens Ⓑ **Qp** **Qh** ♿ A

✳ **V2307** Spherocylinder, trifocal, plus or minus 4.25 to plus or minus 7.00d sphere, .12 to 2.00d cylinder, per lens Ⓑ **Qp** **Qh** ♿ A

✳ **V2308** Spherocylinder, trifocal, plus or minus 4.25 to plus or minus 7.00d sphere, 2.12 to 4.00d cylinder, per lens Ⓑ **Qp** **Qh** ♿ A

✳ **V2309** Spherocylinder, trifocal, plus or minus 4.25 to plus or minus 7.00d sphere, 4.25 to 6.00d cylinder, per lens Ⓑ **Qp** **Qh** ♿ A

✳ **V2310** Spherocylinder, trifocal, plus or minus 4.25 to plus or minus 7.00d sphere, over 6.00d cylinder, per lens Ⓑ **Qp** **Qh** ♿ A

✳ **V2311** Spherocylinder, trifocal, plus or minus 7.25 to plus or minus 12.00d sphere, .25 to 2.25d cylinder, per lens Ⓑ **Qp** **Qh** ♿ A

✳ **V2312** Spherocylinder, trifocal, plus or minus 7.25 to plus or minus 12.00d sphere, 2.25 to 4.00d cylinder, per lens Ⓑ **Qp** **Qh** ♿ A

✳ **V2313** Spherocylinder, trifocal, plus or minus 7.25 to plus or minus 12.00d sphere, 4.25 to 6.00d cylinder, per lens Ⓑ **Qp** **Qh** ♿ A

✳ **V2314** Spherocylinder, trifocal, sphere over plus or minus 12.00d, per lens Ⓑ **Qp** **Qh** ♿ A

✳ **V2315** Lenticular, (myodisc), per lens, trifocal Ⓑ **Qp** **Qh** ♿ A

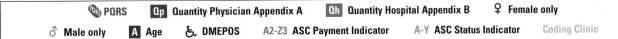

✳ **V2318**   Aniseikonic lens, trifocal Ⓑ Qp Qh ⚕   A

✳ **V2319**   Trifocal seg width over 28 mm Ⓑ Qp Qh ⚕   A

✳ **V2320**   Trifocal add over 3.25d Ⓑ Qp Qh ⚕   A

✿ **V2321**   Lenticular lens, per lens, trifocal Ⓑ Qp Qh ⚕   A

   IOM: 100-02, 15, 120; 100-04, 3, 10.4

✳ **V2399**   Specialty trifocal (by report) Ⓑ Qp Qh   A

   Bill on paper. Requires report of type of trifocal lens and optical lab invoice.

Variable Asphericity

✳ **V2410**   Variable asphericity lens, single vision, full field, glass or plastic, per lens Ⓑ Qp Qh ⚕   A

✳ **V2430**   Variable asphericity lens, bifocal, full field, glass or plastic, per lens Ⓑ Qp Qh ⚕   A

✳ **V2499**   Variable sphericity lens, other type Ⓑ Qp Qh   A

   Bill on paper. Requires report of other ptical lab invoice.

Contact Lenses

If a CPT procedure code for supply of contact lens is reported, recode with specific lens type listed below (per lens).

✳ **V2500**   Contact lens, PMMA, spherical, per lens Ⓑ Qp Qh ⚕   A

   Requires prior authorization for patients under age 21.

✳ **V2501**   Contact lens, PMMA, toric or prism ballast, per lens Ⓑ Qp Qh ⚕   A

   Requires prior authorization for clients under age 21.

✳ **V2502**   Contact lens PMMA, bifocal, per lens Ⓑ Qp Qh ⚕   A

   Requires prior authorization for clients under age 21. Bill on paper. Requires optical lab invoice.

✳ **V2503**   Contact lens PMMA, color vision deficiency, per lens Ⓑ Qp Qh ⚕   A

   Requires prior authorization for clients under age 21. Bill on paper. Requires optical lab invoice.

✳ **V2510**   Contact lens, gas permeable, spherical, per lens Ⓑ Qp Qh ⚕   A

   Requires prior authorization for clients under age 21.

✳ **V2511**   Contact lens, gas permeable, toric, prism ballast, per lens Ⓑ Qp Qh ⚕   A

   Requires prior authorization for clients under age 21.

✳ **V2512**   Contact lens, gas permeable, bifocal, per lens Ⓑ Qp Qh ⚕   A

   Requires prior authorization for clients under age 21.

✳ **V2513**   Contact lens, gas permeable, extended wear, per lens Ⓑ Qp Qh ⚕   A

   Requires prior authorization for clients under age 21.

✿ **V2520**   Contact lens, hydrophilic, spherical, per lens Ⓑ Qp Qh ⚕   A

   If "incident to" a physician's service, do not bill.

   Requires prior authorization for clients under age 21.

   IOM: 100-03, 1, 80.1; 100-03, 1, 80.4

✿ **V2521**   Contact lens, hydrophilic, toric, or prism ballast, per lens Ⓑ Qp Qh ⚕   A

   If "incident to" a physician's service, do not bill.

   Requires prior authorization for clients under age 21.

   IOM: 100-03, 1, 80.1; 100-03, 1, 80.4

✿ **V2522**   Contact lens, hydrophilic, bifocal, per lens Ⓑ Qp Qh ⚕   A

   If "incident to" a physician's service, do not bill.

   Requires prior authorization for clients under age 21.

   IOM: 100-03, 1, 80.1; 100-03, 1, 80.4

✿ **V2523**   Contact lens, hydrophilic, extended wear, per lens Ⓑ Qp Qh ⚕   A

   If "incident to" a physician's service, do not bill.

   Requires prior authorization for clients under age 21.

   IOM: 100-03, 1, 80.1; 100-03, 1, 80.4

✳ **V2530**   Contact lens, scleral, gas impermeable, per lens (for contact lens modification, see 92325) Ⓑ Qp Qh ⚕   A

   Requires prior authorization for clients under age 21.

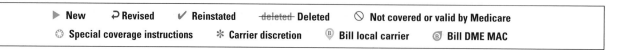

▶ **New**   ↻ **Revised**   ✔ **Reinstated**   ~~deleted~~ **Deleted**   ⊘ **Not covered or valid by Medicare**
✿ **Special coverage instructions**   ✳ **Carrier discretion**   Ⓑ **Bill local carrier**   Ⓑ **Bill DME MAC**

⊛ **V2531** Contact lens, scleral, gas permeable, per lens (for contact lens modification, see 92325) Ⓑ `Qp` `Qh` ♿   A

Requires prior authorization for clients under age 21. Bill on paper. Requires optical lab invoice.

IOM: 100-03, 1, 80.5

✳ **V2599** Contact lens, other type Ⓑ `Qp` `Qh`   A

If "incident to" a physician's service, do not bill.

Requires prior authorization for clients under age 21. Bill on paper. Requires report of other type of contact lens and optical invoice.

Low Vision Aids

If a CPT procedure code for supply of low vision aid is reported, recode with specific systems listed below.

✳ **V2600** Hand held low vision aids and other nonspectacle mounted aids Ⓑ `Qp` `Qh`   A

Requires prior authorization.

✳ **V2610** Single lens spectacle mounted low vision aids Ⓑ `Qp` `Qh`   A

Requires prior authorization.

✳ **V2615** Telescopic and other compound lens system, including distance vision telescopic, near vision telescopes and compound microscopic lens system Ⓑ `Qp` `Qh`   A

Requires prior authorization. Bill on paper. Requires optical lab invoice.

Prosthetic Eye

⊛ **V2623** Prosthetic eye, plastic, custom Ⓑ `Qp` `Qh` ♿   A

DME regional carrier. Requires prior authorization. Bill on paper. Requires optical lab invoice.

✳ **V2624** Polishing/resurfacing of ocular prosthesis Ⓑ `Qp` `Qh` ♿   A

Requires prior authorization. Bill on paper. Requires optical lab invoice.

✳ **V2625** Enlargement of ocular prosthesis Ⓑ `Qp` `Qh` ♿   A

Requires prior authorization. Bill on paper. Requires optical lab invoice.

✳ **V2626** Reduction of ocular prosthesis Ⓑ `Qp` `Qh` ♿   A

Requires prior authorization. Bill on paper. Requires optical lab invoice.

⊛ **V2627** Scleral cover shell Ⓑ `Qp` `Qh` ♿   A

DME regional carrier

Requires prior authorization. Bill on paper. Requires optical lab invoice.

IOM: 100-03, 4, 280.2

✳ **V2628** Fabrication and fitting of ocular conformer Ⓑ `Qp` `Qh` ♿   A

Requires prior authorization. Bill on paper. Requires optical lab invoice.

✳ **V2629** Prosthetic eye, other type Ⓑ `Qp` `Qh`   A

Requires prior authorization. Bill on paper. Requires optical lab invoice.

Intraocular Lenses

↺⊛ **V2630** Anterior chamber intraocular lens Ⓑ `Qp` `Qh` ♿   N1   N

IOM: 100-02, 15, 120

↺⊛ **V2631** Iris supported intraocular lens Ⓑ `Qp` `Qh` ♿   N1   N

IOM: 100-02, 15, 120

↺⊛ **V2632** Posterior chamber intraocular lens Ⓑ `Qp` `Qh` ♿   N1   N

IOM: 100-02, 15, 120

Miscellaneous

✳ **V2700** Balance lens, per lens Ⓑ `Qp` `Qh` ♿   A

⊘ **V2702** Deluxe lens feature Ⓑ   E

IOM: 100-02, 15, 120; 100-04, 3, 10.4

✳ **V2710** Slab off prism, glass or plastic, per lens Ⓑ `Qp` `Qh` ♿   A

✳ **V2715** Prism, per lens Ⓑ `Qp` ♿   A

✳ **V2718** Press-on lens, Fresnel prism, per lens Ⓑ `Qp` `Qh` ♿   A

✳ **V2730** Special base curve, glass or plastic, per lens Ⓑ `Qp` `Qh` ♿   A

⊛ **V2744** Tint, photochromatic, per lens Ⓑ `Qp` ♿   A

Requires prior authorization.

IOM: 100-02, 15, 120; 100-04, 3, 10.4

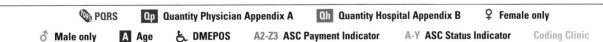

⒫ PQRS	`Qp` Quantity Physician Appendix A	`Qh` Quantity Hospital Appendix B	♀ Female only
♂ Male only **A** Age ♿ DMEPOS A2-Z3 ASC Payment Indicator A-Y ASC Status Indicator Coding Clinic			

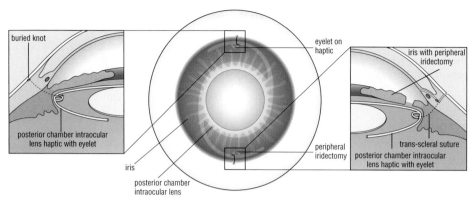

Figure 56 Posterior intraocular lens.

buried knot

posterior chamber intraocular lens haptic with eyelet

iris

posterior chamber intraocular lens

eyelet on haptic

peripheral iridectomy

iris with peripheral iridectomy

trans-scleral suture

posterior chamber intraocular lens haptic with eyelet

⊛ **V2745** Addition to lens, tint, any color, solid, gradient or equal, excludes photochroatic, any lens material, per lens Ⓑ **Qp** ♿   A

Includes photochromatic lenses (V2744) used as sunglasses, which are prescribed in addition to regular prosthetic lenses for aphakic patient will be denied as not medically necessary.

IOM: 100-02, 15, 120; 100-04, 3, 10.4

⊛ **V2750** Anti-reflective coating, per lens Ⓑ **Qp** ♿   A

Requires prior authorization.

IOM: 100-02, 15, 120; 100-04, 3, 10.4

⊛ **V2755** U-V lens, per lens Ⓑ **Qp** ♿   A

IOM: 100-02, 15, 120; 100-04, 3, 10.4

✳ **V2756** Eye glass case Ⓑ   E

✳ **V2760** Scratch resistant coating, per lens Ⓑ ♿   A

⊛ **V2761** Mirror coating, any type, solid, gradient or equal, any lens material, per lens Ⓑ **Qp** **Qh**   B

IOM: 100-02, 15, 120; 100-04, 3, 10.4

⊛ **V2762** Polarization, any lens material, per lens Ⓑ ♿   A

IOM: 100-02, 15, 120; 100-04, 3, 10.4

✳ **V2770** Occluder lens, per lens Ⓑ **Qp** **Qh** ♿   A

Requires prior authorization.

✳ **V2780** Oversize lens, per lens Ⓑ **Qp** **Qh** ♿   A

Requires prior authorization.

✳ **V2781** Progressive lens, per lens Ⓑ **Qp** **Qh**   B

Requires prior authorization.

⊛ **V2782** Lens, index 1.54 to 1.65 plastic or 1.60 to 1.79 glass, excludes polycarbonate, per lens Ⓑ **Qp** **Qh** ♿   A

Do not bill in addition to V2784

IOM: 100-02, 15, 120; 100-04, 3, 10.4

⊛ **V2783** Lens, index greater than or equal to 1.66 plastic or greater than or equal to 1.80 glass, excludes polycarbonate, per lens Ⓑ **Qp** **Qh** ♿   A

Do not bill in addition to V2784

IOM: 100-02, 15, 120; 100-04, 3, 10.4

⊛ **V2784** Lens, polycarbonate or equal, any index, per lens Ⓑ **Qp** ♿   A

Covered only for patients with functional vision in one eye—in this situation, an impact-resistant material is covered for both lenses if eyeglasses are covered. Claims with V2784 that do not meet this coverage criterion will be denied as not medically necessary.

IOM: 100-02, 15, 120; 100-04, 3, 10.4

✳ **V2785** Processing, preserving and transporting corneal tissue Ⓑ **Qp** **Qh**   F4 F

For ASC, bill on paper. Must attach eye bank invoice to claim.

For Hospitals, bill charges for corneal tissue to receive cost based reimbursement.

IOM: 100-4, 4, 200.1

⊛ **V2786** Specialty occupational multifocal lens, per lens Ⓑ ♿   A

IOM: 100-02, 15, 120; 100-04, 3, 10.4

⊘ **V2787** Astigmatism correcting function of intraocular lens Ⓑ   E

Medicare Statute 1862(a)(7)

⊘ **V2788** Presbyopia correcting function of intraocular lens Ⓑ   E

Medicare Statute 1862a7

▶ **New**	↻ **Revised**	✔ **Reinstated**	deleted **Deleted**	⊘ **Not covered or valid by Medicare**
⊛ **Special coverage instructions**		✳ **Carrier discretion**	⑧ **Bill local carrier**	Ⓑ **Bill DME MAC**

* **V2790** Amniotic membrane for surgical reconstruction, per procedure Ⓑ Qp Qh   N1 N

* **V2797** Vision supply, accessory and/or service component of another HCPCS vision code Ⓑ Qp Qh   A

↺* **V2799** Vision item or service, miscellaneous Ⓑ   A

Bill on paper. Requires report of miscellaneous service and optical lab invoice.

HEARING SERVICES (V5000-V5999)

NOTE: These codes are for non-physician services.

⊘ **V5008** Hearing screening Ⓑ Qp Qh   E
IOM: 100-02, 16, 90

⊘ **V5010** Assessment for hearing aid Ⓑ Qp Qh   E
Medicare Statute 1862a7

⊘ **V5011** Fitting/orientation/checking of hearing aid Ⓑ Qp Qh   E
Medicare Statute 1862a7

⊘ **V5014** Repair/modification of a hearing aid Ⓑ   E
Medicare Statute 1862a7

⊘ **V5020** Conformity evaluation Ⓑ   E
Medicare Statute 1862a7

⊘ **V5030** Hearing aid, monaural, body worn, air conduction Ⓑ   E
Medicare Statute 1862a7

⊘ **V5040** Hearing aid, monaural, body worn, bone conduction Ⓑ   E
Medicare Statute 1862a7

⊘ **V5050** Hearing aid, monaural, in the ear Ⓑ   E
Medicare Statute 1862a7

⊘ **V5060** Hearing aid, monaural, behind the ear Ⓑ   E
Medicare Statute 1862a7

⊘ **V5070** Glasses, air conduction Ⓑ   E
Medicare Statute 1862a7

⊘ **V5080** Glasses, bone conduction Ⓑ   E
Medicare Statute 1862a7

⊘ **V5090** Dispensing fee, unspecified hearing aid Ⓑ   E
Medicare Statute 1862a7

⊘ **V5095** Semi-implantable middle ear hearing prosthesis Ⓑ   E
Medicare Statute 1862a7

⊘ **V5100** Hearing aid, bilateral, body worn Ⓑ   E
Medicare Statute 1862a7

⊘ **V5110** Dispensing fee, bilateral Ⓑ   E
Medicare Statute 1862a7

⊘ **V5120** Binaural, body Ⓑ   E
Medicare Statute 1862a7

⊘ **V5130** Binaural, in the ear Ⓑ   E
Medicare Statute 1862a7

⊘ **V5140** Binaural, behind the ear Ⓑ   E
Medicare Statute 1862a7

⊘ **V5150** Binaural, glasses Ⓑ   E
Medicare Statute 1862a7

⊘ **V5160** Dispensing fee, binaural Ⓑ   E
Medicare Statute 1862a7

⊘ **V5170** Hearing aid, CROS, in the ear Ⓑ   E
Medicare Statute 1862a7

⊘ **V5180** Hearing aid, CROS, behind the ear Ⓑ   E
Medicare Statute 1862a7

⊘ **V5190** Hearing aid, CROS, glasses Ⓑ   E
Medicare Statute 1862a7

⊘ **V5200** Dispensing fee, CROS Ⓑ   E
Medicare Statute 1862a7

⊘ **V5210** Hearing aid, BICROS, in the ear Ⓑ   E
Medicare Statute 1862a7

⊘ **V5220** Hearing aid, BICROS, behind the ear Ⓑ   E
Medicare Statute 1862a7

⊘ **V5230** Hearing aid, BICROS, glasses Ⓑ   E
Medicare Statute 1862a7

⊘ **V5240** Dispensing fee, BICROS Ⓑ   E
Medicare Statute 1862a7

⊘ **V5241** Dispensing fee, monaural hearing aid, any type Ⓑ   E
Medicare Statute 1862a7

⊘ **V5242** Hearing aid, analog, monaural, CIC (completely in the ear canal) Ⓑ   E
Medicare Statute 1862a7

⊘ **V5243** Hearing aid, analog, monaural, ITC (in the canal) Ⓑ   E
Medicare Statute 1862a9

⊘ **V5244** Hearing aid, digitally programmable analog, monaural, CIC Ⓑ   E
Medicare Statute 1862a7

PQRS PQRS   **Qp** Quantity Physician Appendix A   **Qh** Quantity Hospital Appendix B   ♀ Female only
♂ Male only   **A** Age   ⅙ DMEPOS   A2-Z3 ASC Payment Indicator   A-Y ASC Status Indicator   Coding Clinic

373

⊘ **V5245** Hearing aid, digitally programmable, analog, monaural, ITC Ⓑ E

Medicare Statute 1862a7

⊘ **V5246** Hearing aid, digitally programmable analog, monaural, ITE (in the ear) Ⓑ E

Medicare Statute 1862a7

⊘ **V5247** Hearing aid, digitally programmable analog, monaural, BTE (behind the ear) Ⓑ E

Medicare Statute 1862a7

⊘ **V5248** Hearing aid, analog, binaural, CIC Ⓑ E

Medicare Statute 1862a7

⊘ **V5249** Hearing aid, analog, binaural, ITC Ⓑ E

Medicare Statute 1862a7

⊘ **V5250** Hearing aid, digitally programmable analog, binaural, CIC Ⓑ E

Medicare Statute 1862a7

⊘ **V5251** Hearing aid, digitally programmable analog, binaural, ITC Ⓑ E

Medicare Statute 1862a7

⊘ **V5252** Hearing aid, digitally programmable, binaural, ITE Ⓑ E

Medicare Statute 1862a7

⊘ **V5253** Hearing aid, digitally programmable, binaural, BTE Ⓑ E

Medicare Statute 1862a7

⊘ **V5254** Hearing aid, digital, monaural, CIC Ⓑ E

Medicare Statute 1862a7

⊘ **V5255** Hearing aid, digital, monaural, ITC Ⓑ E

Medicare Statute 1862a7

⊘ **V5256** Hearing aid, digital, monaural, ITE Ⓑ E

Medicare Statute 1862a7

⊘ **V5257** Hearing aid, digital, monaural, BTE Ⓑ E

Medicare Statute 1862a7

⊘ **V5258** Hearing aid, digital, binaural, CIC Ⓑ E

Medicare Statute 1862a7

⊘ **V5259** Hearing aid, digital, binaural, ITC Ⓑ E

Medicare Statute 1862a7

⊘ **V5260** Hearing aid, digital, binaural, ITE Ⓑ E

Medicare Statute 1862a7

⊘ **V5261** Hearing aid, digital, binaural, BTE Ⓑ E

Medicare Statute 1862a7

⊘ **V5262** Hearing aid, disposable, any type, monaural Ⓑ E

Medicare Statute 1862a7

⊘ **V5263** Hearing aid, disposable, any type, binaural Ⓑ E

Medicare Statute 1862a7

⊘ **V5264** Ear mold/insert, not disposable, any type Ⓑ E

Medicare Statute 1862a7

⊘ **V5265** Ear mold/insert, disposable, any type Ⓑ E

Medicare Statute 1862a7

⊘ **V5266** Battery for use in hearing device Ⓑ E

Medicare Statute 1862a7

⊘ **V5267** Hearing aid or assistive listening device/supplies/accessories, not otherwise specified Ⓑ E

Medicare Statute 1862a7

⊘ **V5268** Assistive listening device, telephone amplifier, any type Ⓑ E

Medicare Statute 1862a7

⊘ **V5269** Assistive listening device, alerting, any type Ⓑ E

Medicare Statute 1862a7

⊘ **V5270** Assistive listening device, television amplifier, any type Ⓑ E

Medicare Statute 1862a7

⊘ **V5271** Assistive listening device, television caption decoder Ⓑ E

Medicare Statute 1862a7

⊘ **V5272** Assistive listening device, TDD Ⓑ E

Medicare Statute 1862a7

⊘ **V5273** Assistive listening device, for use with cochlear implant Ⓑ E

Medicare Statute 1862a7

⊘ **V5274** Assistive listening device, not otherwise specified Ⓑ **Qp** **Qh** E

Medicare Statute 1862a7

⊘ **V5275** Ear impression, each Ⓑ E

Medicare Statute 1862a7

⊘ **V5281** Assistive listening device, personal FM/DM system, monaural, (1 receiver, transmitter, microphone), any type Ⓑ **Qp** **Qh** E

Medicare Statute 1862a7

▶ **New** ↻ **Revised** ✔ **Reinstated** ~~deleted~~ **Deleted** ⊘ **Not covered or valid by Medicare**
⟳ **Special coverage instructions** ✳ **Carrier discretion** Ⓑ **Bill local carrier** Ⓑ **Bill DME MAC**

⊘ **V5282** Assistive listening device, personal FM/DM system, binaural, (2 receivers, transmitter, microphone), any type Ⓑ `Qp` `Qh` E

Medicare Statute 1862a7

⊘ **V5283** Assistive listening device, personal FM/DM neck, loop induction receiver Ⓑ E

Medicare Statute 1862a7

⊘ **V5284** Assistive listening device, personal FM/DM, ear level receiver Ⓑ `Qp` `Qh` E

Medicare Statute 1862a7

⊘ **V5285** Assistive listening device, personal FM/DM, direct audio input receiver Ⓑ `Qp` `Qh` E

Medicare Statute 1862a7

⊘ **V5286** Assistive listening device, personal blue tooth FM/DM receiver Ⓑ `Qp` `Qh` E

Medicare Statute 1862a7

⊘ **V5287** Assistive listening device, personal FM/DM receiver, not otherwise specified Ⓑ `Qp` `Qh` E

Medicare Statute 1862a7

⊘ **V5288** Assistive listening device, personal FM/DM transmitter assistive listening device Ⓑ `Qp` `Qh` E

Medicare Statute 1862a7

⊘ **V5289** Assistive listening device, personal FM/DM adapter/boot coupling device for receiver, any type Ⓑ `Qp` `Qh` E

Medicare Statute 1862a7

⊘ **V5290** Assistive listening device, transmitter microphone, any type Ⓑ

Medicare Statute 1862a7

⊘ **V5298** Hearing aid, not otherwise classified Ⓑ E

Medicare Statute 1862a7

✪ **V5299** Hearing service, miscellaneous Ⓑ B

IOM: 100-02, 16, 90

Speech-Language Pathology Services

NOTE: These codes are for non-physician services.

⊘ **V5336** Repair/modification of augmentative communicative system or device (excludes adaptive hearing aid) Ⓑ E

Medicare Statute 1862a7

⊘ **V5362** Speech screening Ⓑ E

Medicare Statute 1862a7

⊘ **V5363** Language screening Ⓑ E

Medicare Statute 1862a7

⊘ **V5364** Dysphagia screening Ⓑ E

Medicare Statute 1862a7

⒫ **PQRS**	`Qp` **Quantity Physician Appendix A**	`Qh` **Quantity Hospital Appendix B**	♀ **Female only**
♂ **Male only**	**A Age**	♿ **DMEPOS**	A2-Z3 **ASC Payment Indicator** A-Y **ASC Status Indicator** *Coding Clinic*

APPENDIX A

GENERAL CORRECT CODING POLICIES FOR NATIONAL CORRECT CODING INITIATIVE POLICY MANUAL FOR MEDICARE SERVICES

Current Procedural Terminology © 2013 American Medical Association. All Rights Reserved.

Current Procedural Terminology (CPT) is copyright 2013 American Medical Association. All Rights Reserved. No fee schedules, basic units, relative values, or related listings are included in CPT. The AMA assumes no liability for the data contained herein. Applicable FARS/DFARS restrictions apply to government use.

CPT® is a trademark of the American Medical Association.

Chapter I

Revision Date 1/1/2014

GENERAL CORRECT CODING POLICIES

A. Introduction

Healthcare providers utilize HCPCS/CPT codes to report medical services performed on patients to Medicare Carriers (A/B MACs processing practitioner service claims) and Fiscal Intermediaries (FIs). HCPCS (Healthcare Common Procedure Coding System) consists of Level I CPT (Current Procedural Terminology) codes and Level II codes. CPT codes are defined in the American Medical Association's (AMA) *CPT Manual* which is updated and published annually. HCPCS Level II codes are defined by the Centers for Medicare and Medicaid Services (CMS) and are updated throughout the year as necessary. Changes in CPT codes are approved by the AMA CPT Editorial Panel which meets three times per year.

CPT and HCPCS Level II codes define medical and surgical procedures performed on patients. Some procedure codes are very specific defining a single service (e.g., CPT code 93000 (electrocardiogram)) while other codes define procedures consisting of many services (e.g., CPT code 58263 (vaginal hysterectomy with removal of tube(s) and ovary(s) and repair of enterocele)). Because many procedures can be performed by different approaches, different methods, or in combination with other procedures, there are often multiple HCPCS/CPT codes defining similar or related procedures.

CPT and HCPCS Level II code descriptors usually do not define all services included in a procedure. There are often services inherent in a procedure or group of procedures. For example, anesthesia services include certain preparation and monitoring services.

The CMS developed the NCCI to prevent inappropriate payment of services that should not be reported together. Prior to April 1, 2012, NCCI edits were placed into either the "Column One/Column Two Correct Coding Edit Table" or the "Mutually Exclusive Edit Table." However, on April 1, 2012, the edits in the "Mutually Exclusive Edit Table" were moved to the "Column One/Column Two Correct Coding Edit Table" so that all the NCCI edits are currently contained in this single table. Combining the two tables simplifies researching NCCI edits and online use of NCCI tables. Each edit table contains edits which are pairs of HCPCS/CPT codes that in general should not be reported together. Each edit has a column one and column two HCPCS/CPT code. If a provider reports the two codes of an edit pair, the column two code is denied, and

the column one code is eligible for payment. However, if it is clinically appropriate to utilize an NCCI-associated modifier, both the column one and column two codes are eligible for payment. (NCCI-associated modifiers and their appropriate use are discussed elsewhere in this chapter.)

When the NCCI was first established and during its early years, the "Column One/Column Two Correct Coding Edit Table" was termed the "Comprehensive/Component Edit Table." This latter terminology was a misnomer. Although the column two code is often a component of a more comprehensive column one code, this relationship is not true for many edits. In the latter type of edit the code pair edit simply represents two codes that should not be reported together. For example, a provider should not report a vaginal hysterectomy code and total abdominal hysterectomy code together.

In this chapter, Sections B–Q address various issues relating to NCCI edits.

Medically Unlikely Edits (MUEs) prevent payment for an inappropriate number/quantity of the same service on a single day. An MUE for a HCPCS/CPT code is the maximum number of units of service (UOS) under most circumstances reportable by the same provider for the same beneficiary on the same date of service. The ideal MUE value for a HCPCS/CPT code is one that allows the vast majority of appropriately coded claims to pass the MUE. More information concerning MUEs is discussed in Section V of this chapter.

In this Manual many policies are described utilizing the term "physician." Unless indicated differently the usage of this term does not restrict the policies to physicians only but applies to all practitioners, hospitals, providers, or suppliers eligible to bill the relevant HCPCS/CPT codes pursuant to applicable portions of the Social Security Act (SSA) of 1965, the Code of Federal Regulations (CFR), and Medicare rules. In some sections of this Manual, the term "physician" would not include some of these entities because specific rules do not apply to them. For example, Anesthesia Rules and Global Surgery Rules do not apply to hospitals.

Providers reporting services under Medicare's hospital outpatient prospective payment system (OPPS) should report all services in accordance with appropriate Medicare Internet Only Manual (IOM) instructions.

Physicians must report services correctly. This manual discusses general coding principles in Chapter I and principles more relevant to other specific groups of HCPCS/CPT codes in the other chapters. There are certain types of improper coding that physicians must avoid.

Procedures should be reported with the most comprehensive CPT code that describes the services performed. Physicians must not unbundle the services described by a HCPCS/CPT code. Some examples follow:

- A physician should not report multiple HCPCS/CPT codes when a single comprehensive HCPCS/CPT code describes these services. For example if a physician performs a vaginal hysterectomy on a uterus weighing less than 250 grams with bilateral salpingo-oophorectomy, the physician should report CPT code 58262 (Vaginal hysterectomy, for uterus 250 g or less; with removal of tube(s), and/or ovary(s)). The physician should not report CPT code 58260 (Vaginal hysterectomy, for uterus 250 g or less;) plus CPT code 58720 (Salpingo-oophorectomy, complete or partial, unilateral or bilateral (separate procedure)).
- A physician should not fragment a procedure into component parts. For example, if a physician performs an anal endoscopy with biopsy, the physician should report CPT code 46606 (Anoscopy; with biopsy, single or multiple). It is improper to unbundle this procedure and report CPT code 46600(Anoscopy; diagnostic,...) plus CPT code 45100 (Biopsy of anorectal wall, anal approach...). The latter code is not intended to be utilized with an endoscopic procedure code.
- A physician should not unbundle a bilateral procedure code into two unilateral procedure codes. For example if a physician performs bilateral mammography, the physician should report CPT code 77056 (Mammography; bilateral). The physician should not report CPT code 77055 (Mammography; unilateral) with two units of service or 77055LT plus 77055RT.
- A physician should not unbundle services that are integral to a more comprehensive procedure. For example, surgical access is integral to a surgical procedure. A physician should not report CPT code 49000 (Exploratory laparotomy,...) when performing an open abdominal procedure such as a total abdominal colectomy (e.g., CPT code 44150).

Physicians must avoid downcoding. If a HCPCS/CPT code exists that describes the services performed, the physician must report this code rather than report a less comprehensive code with other codes describing the services not included in the less comprehensive code. For example if a physician performs a unilateral partial mastectomy with axillary lymphadenectomy, the provider should report CPT code 19302 (Mastectomy, partial...; with axillary lymphadenectomy). A physician should not report CPT code 19301 (Mastectomy, partial...) plus CPT code 38745 (Axillary lymphadenectomy; complete).

Physicians must avoid upcoding. A HCPCS/CPT code may be reported only if all services described by that code have been performed. For example, if a physician performs a superficial axillary lymphadenectomy (CPT code 38740), the physician should not report CPT code 38745 (Axillary lymphadenectomy; complete).

Physicians must report units of service correctly. Each HCPCS/CPT code has a defined unit of service for reporting purposes. A physician should not report units of service for a HCPCS/CPT code using a criterion that differs from the code's defined unit of service. For example, some therapy codes are reported in fifteen minute increments (e.g., CPT codes 97110-97124). Others are reported per session (e.g., CPT codes 92507, 92508). A physician should not report a "per session" code using fifteen minute increments. CPT code 92507 or 92508 should be reported with one unit of service on a single date of service.

In 2010 the *CPT Manual* modified the numbering of codes so that the sequence of codes as they appear in the *CPT Manual* does not necessarily correspond to a sequential numbering of codes. In the *National Correct Coding Initiative Policy Manual for Medicare Services,* use of a numerical range of codes reflects all codes that numerically fall within the range regardless of their sequential order in the *CPT Manual.*

This chapter addresses general coding principles, issues, and policies. Many of these principles, issues, and policies are addressed further in subsequent chapters dealing with specific groups of HCPCS/CPT codes. In this chapter examples are often utilized to clarify principles, issues, or policies. The examples do not represent the only codes to which the principles, issues, or policies apply.

B. Coding Based on Standards of Medical/Surgical Practice

Most HCPCS/CPT code defined procedures include services that are integral to them. Some of these integral services have specific CPT codes for reporting the service when not performed as an integral part of another procedure. (For example, CPT code 36000 (introduction of needle or intracatheter into a vein) is integral to all nuclear medicine procedures requiring injection of a radiopharmaceutical into a vein. CPT code 36000 is not separately reportable with these types of nuclear medicine procedures. However, CPT code 36000 may be reported alone if the only service provided is the introduction of a needle into a vein. Other integral services do not have specific CPT codes. (For example, wound irrigation is integral to the treatment of all wounds and does not have a HCPCS/CPT code.) Services integral to HCPCS/CPT code defined procedures are included in those procedures based on the standards of medical/surgical practice. It is inappropriate to separately report services that are integral to another procedure with that procedure.

Many NCCI edits are based on the standards of medical/surgical practice. Services that are integral to another service are component parts of the more comprehensive service. When integral component services have their own HCPCS/CPT codes, NCCI edits place the comprehensive service in column one and the component service in column two. Since a component service integral to a comprehensive service is not separately reportable, the column two code is not separately reportable with the column one code.

Some services are integral to large numbers of procedures. Other services are integral to a more limited number of procedures. Examples of services integral to a large number of procedures include:

- Cleansing, shaving and prepping of skin
- Draping and positioning of patient
- Insertion of intravenous access for medication administration
- Insertion of urinary catheter
- Sedative administration by the physician performing a procedure (see Chapter II, Anesthesia Services)
- Local, topical or regional anesthesia administered by the physician performing the procedure
- Surgical approach including identification of anatomical landmarks, incision, evaluation of the surgical field, debridement of traumatized tissue, lysis of adhesions, and isolation of structures limiting access to the surgical field such as

bone, blood vessels, nerve, and muscles including stimulation for identification or monitoring

- Surgical cultures
- Wound irrigation
- Insertion and removal of drains, suction devices, and pumps into same site
- Surgical closure and dressings
- Application, management, and removal of postoperative dressings and analgesic devices (peri-incisional)
- Application of TENS unit
- Institution of Patient Controlled Anesthesia
- Preoperative, intraoperative and postoperative documentation, including photographs, drawings, dictation, or transcription as necessary to document the services provided
- Surgical supplies, except for specific situations where CMS policy permits separate payment

Although other chapters in this Manual further address issues related to the standards of medical/surgical practice for the procedures covered by that chapter, it is not possible because of space limitations to discuss all NCCI edits based on the principle of the standards of medical/surgical practice. However, there are several general principles that can be applied to the edits as follows:

1. The component service is an accepted standard of care when performing the comprehensive service.
2. The component service is usually necessary to complete the comprehensive service.
3. The component service is not a separately distinguishable procedure when performed with the comprehensive service.

Specific examples of services that are not separately reportable because they are components of more comprehensive services follow:

Medical:

1. Since interpretation of cardiac rhythm is an integral component of the interpretation of an electrocardiogram, a rhythm strip is not separately reportable.
2. Since determination of ankle/brachial indices requires both upper and lower extremity doppler studies, an upper extremity doppler study is not separately reportable.
3. Since a cardiac stress test includes multiple electrocardiograms, an electrocardiogram is not separately reportable.

Surgical:

1. Since a myringotomy requires access to the tympanic membrane through the external auditory canal, removal of impacted cerumen from the external auditory canal is not separately reportable.
2. A "scout" bronchoscopy to assess the surgical field, anatomic landmarks, extent of disease, etc., is not separately reportable with an open pulmonary procedure such as a pulmonary lobectomy. By contrast, an initial diagnostic bronchoscopy is separately reportable. If the diagnostic bronchoscopy is performed at the same patient encounter as the open pulmonary procedure and does not duplicate an earlier diagnostic bronchoscopy by the same or another physician, the diagnostic bronchoscopy may be reported with modifier –58 appended to the open pulmonary procedure code to indicate a staged procedure. A cursory examination of the upper airway during a bronchoscopy with the bronchoscope should not be reported separately as a laryngoscopy. However, separate en-

doscopies of anatomically distinct areas with different endoscopes may be reported separately (e.g., thoracoscopy and mediastinoscopy).
3. Since a colectomy requires exposure of the colon, the laparotomy and adhesiolysis to expose the colon are not separately reportable.

C. Medical/Surgical Package

Most medical and surgical procedures include pre-procedure, intra-procedure, and post-procedure work. When multiple procedures are performed at the same patient encounter, there is often overlap of the pre-procedure and post-procedure work. Payment methodologies for surgical procedures account for the overlap of the pre-procedure and post-procedure work.

The component elements of the pre-procedure and post-procedure work for each procedure are included component services of that procedure as a standard of medical/surgical practice. Some general guidelines follow:

1. Many invasive procedures require vascular and/or airway access. The work associated with obtaining the required access is included in the pre-procedure or intra-procedure work. The work associated with returning a patient to the appropriate post-procedure state is included in the post-procedure work.

Airway access is necessary for general anesthesia and is not separately reportable. There is no CPT code for elective endotracheal intubation. CPT code 31500 describes an emergency endotracheal intubation and should not be reported for elective endotracheal intubation. Visualization of the airway is a component part of an endotracheal intubation, and CPT codes describing procedures that visualize the airway (e.g., nasal endoscopy, laryngoscopy, bronchoscopy) should not be reported with an endotracheal intubation. These CPT codes describe diagnostic and therapeutic endoscopies, and it is a misuse of these codes to report visualization of the airway for endotracheal intubation.

Intravenous access (e.g., CPT codes 36000, 36400, 36410) is not separately reportable when performed with many types of procedures (e.g., surgical procedures, anesthesia procedures, radiological procedures requiring intravenous contrast, nuclear medicine procedures requiring intravenous radiopharmaceutical).

After vascular access is achieved, the access must be maintained by a slow infusion (e.g., saline) or injection of heparin or saline into a "lock". Since these services are necessary for maintenance of the vascular access, they are not separately reportable with the vascular access CPT codes or procedures requiring vascular access as a standard of medical/surgical practice. CPT codes 37211-37214 (Transcatheter therapy with infusion for thrombolysis) should not be reported for use of an anticoagulant to maintain vascular access.

The global surgical package includes the administration of fluids and drugs during the operative procedure. CPT codes 96360-96376 should not be reported separately. Under OPPS, the administration of fluids and drugs during or for an operative procedure are included services and are not separately reportable (e.g., CPT codes 96360-96376).

When a procedure requires more invasive vascular access services (e.g., central venous access, pulmonary artery access), the more invasive vascular service is separately reportable if it is not typical of the procedure and the work of the more invasive vascular service has not been included in the valuation of the procedure.

Insertion of a central venous access device (e.g., central venous catheter, pulmonary artery catheter) requires passage of a catheter through central venous vessels and, in the case of a pulmonary artery catheter, through the right atrium and ventricle. These services often require the use of fluoroscopic guidance. Separate reporting of CPT codes for right heart catheterization, selective venous catheterization, or pulmonary artery catheterization is not appropriate when reporting a CPT code for insertion of a central venous access device. Since CPT code 77001 describes fluoroscopic guidance for central venous access device procedures, CPT codes for more general fluoroscopy (e.g., 76000, 76001, 77002) should not be reported separately.

2. Medicare Anesthesia Rules prevent separate payment for anesthesia services by the same physician performing a surgical or medical procedure. The physician performing a surgical or medical procedure should not report CPT codes 96360-96376 for the administration of anesthetic agents during the procedure. If it is medically reasonable and necessary that a separate provider (anesthesia practitioner) perform anesthesia services (e.g., monitored anesthesia care) for a surgical or medical procedure, a separate anesthesia service may be reported by the second provider.

Under OPPS, anesthesia for a surgical procedure is an included service and is not separately reportable. For example, a provider should not report CPT codes 96360-96376 for anesthesia services.

When anesthesia services are not separately reportable, physicians and facilities should not unbundle components of anesthesia and report them in lieu of an anesthesia code.

3. Many procedures require cardiopulmonary monitoring either by the physician performing the procedure or an anesthesia practitioner. Since these services are integral to the procedure, they are not separately reportable. Examples of these services include cardiac monitoring, pulse oximetry, and ventilation management (e.g., 93000-93010, 93040-93042, 94760, 94761, 94770).

4. A biopsy performed at the time of another more extensive procedure (e.g., excision, destruction, removal) is separately reportable under specific circumstances.

If the biopsy is performed on a separate lesion, it is separately reportable. This situation may be reported with anatomic modifiers or modifier -59.

If the biopsy is performed on the same lesion on which a more extensive procedure is performed, it is separately reportable only if the biopsy is utilized for immediate pathologic diagnosis prior to the more extensive procedure, and the decision to proceed with the more extensive procedure is based on the diagnosis established by the pathologic examination. The biopsy is not separately reportable if the pathologic examination at the time of surgery is for the purpose of assessing margins of resection or verifying resectability. When separately reportable modifier -58 may be reported to indicate that the biopsy and the more extensive procedure were planned or staged procedures.

If a biopsy is performed and submitted for pathologic evaluation that will be completed after the more extensive procedure is performed, the biopsy is not separately reportable with the more extensive procedure.

If a single lesion is biopsied multiple times, only one biopsy code may be reported with a single unit of service. If multiple lesions are non-endoscopically biopsied, a biopsy code may be reported for each lesion appending a modifier indicating that each biopsy was performed on a separate lesion. For endoscopic biopsies, multiple biopsies of a single or multiple lesions are reported with one unit of service of the biopsy code. If it is medically reasonable and necessary to submit multiple biopsies of the same or different lesions for separate pathologic examination, the medical record must identify the precise location and separate nature of each biopsy.

5. Exposure and exploration of the surgical field is integral to an operative procedure and is not separately reportable. For example, an exploratory laparotomy (CPT code 49000) is not separately reportable with an intra-abdominal procedure. If exploration of the surgical field results in additional procedures other than the primary procedure, the additional procedures may generally be reported separately. However, a procedure designated by the CPT code descriptor as a "separate procedure" is not separately reportable if performed in a region anatomically related to the other procedure(s) through the same skin incision, orifice, or surgical approach.

6. If a definitive surgical procedure requires access through diseased tissue (e.g., necrotic skin, abscess, hematoma, seroma), a separate service for this access (e.g., debridement, incision and drainage) is not separately reportable. For example, debridement of skin to repair a fracture is not separately reportable.

7. If removal, destruction, or other form of elimination of a lesion requires coincidental elimination of other pathology, only the primary procedure may be reported. For example, if an area of pilonidal disease contains an abscess, incision and drainage of the abscess during the procedure to excise the area of pilonidal disease is not separately reportable.

8. An excision and removal (–ectomy) includes the incision and opening (–otomy) of the organ. A HCPCS/CPT code for an –otomy procedure should not be reported with an –ectomy code for the same organ.

9. Multiple approaches to the same procedure are mutually exclusive of one another and should not be reported separately.

For example, both a vaginal hysterectomy and abdominal hysterectomy should not be reported separately.

10. If a procedure utilizing one approach fails and is converted to a procedure utilizing a different approach, only the completed procedure may be reported. For example, if a laparoscopic hysterectomy is converted to an open hysterectomy, only the open hysterectomy procedure code may be reported.

11. If a laparoscopic procedure fails and is converted to an open procedure, the physician should not report a diagnostic laparoscopy in lieu of the failed laparoscopic procedure. For example, if a laparoscopic cholecystectomy is converted to an open cholecystectomy, the physician should not report the failed laparoscopic cholecystectomy nor a diagnostic laparoscopy.

12. If a diagnostic endoscopy is the basis for and precedes an open procedure, the diagnostic endoscopy may be reported with modifier -58 appended to the open procedure code. However, the medical record must document the

medical reasonableness and necessity for the diagnostic endoscopy. A scout endoscopy to assess anatomic landmarks and extent of disease is not separately reportable with an open procedure. When an endoscopic procedure fails and is converted to another surgical procedure, only the completed surgical procedure may be reported. The endoscopic procedure is not separately reportable with the completed surgical procedure.

13. Treatment of complications of primary surgical procedures is separately reportable with some limitations. The global surgical package for an operative procedure includes all intra-operative services that are normally a usual and necessary part of the procedure. Additionally the global surgical package includes all medical and surgical services required of the surgeon during the postoperative period of the surgery to treat complications that do not require return to the operating room. Thus, treatment of a complication of a primary surgical procedure is not separately reportable (1) if it represents usual and necessary care in the operating room during the procedure or (2) if it occurs postoperatively and does not require return to the operating room. For example, control of hemorrhage is a usual and necessary component of a surgical procedure in the operating room and is not separately reportable. Control of postoperative hemorrhage is also not separately reportable unless the patient must be returned to the operating room for treatment. In the latter case, the control of hemorrhage may be separately reportable with modifier -78.

D. Evaluation and Management (E&M) Services

Medicare Global Surgery Rules define the rules for reporting evaluation and management (E&M) services with procedures covered by these rules. This section summarizes some of the rules.

All procedures on the Medicare Physician Fee Schedule are assigned a Global period of 000, 010, 090, XXX, YYY, ZZZ, or MMM. The global concept does not apply to XXX procedures. The global period for YYY procedures is defined by the Carrier (A/B MAC processing practitioner service claims). All procedures with a global period of ZZZ are related to another procedure, and the applicable global period for the ZZZ code is determined by the related procedure. Procedures with a global period of MMM are maternity procedures.

Since NCCI edits are applied to same day services by the same provider to the same beneficiary, certain Global Surgery Rules are applicable to NCCI. An E&M service is separately reportable on the same date of service as a procedure with a global period of 000, 010, or 090 under limited circumstances.

If a procedure has a global period of 090 days, it is defined as a major surgical procedure. If an E&M is performed on the same date of service as a major surgical procedure for the purpose of deciding whether to perform this surgical procedure, the E&M service is separately reportable with modifier –57. Other preoperative E&M services on the same date of service as a major surgical procedure are included in the global payment for the procedure and are not separately reportable. NCCI does not contain edits based on this rule because Medicare Carriers (A/B MACs processing practitioner service claims) have separate edits.

If a procedure has a global period of 000 or 010 days, it is defined as a minor surgical procedure. *In general* E&M services on the same date of service as the minor surgical procedure are included in the payment for the procedure. The decision to perform a minor surgical procedure is included in the payment for the minor surgical procedure and should not be reported separately as an E&M service. However, a significant and separately identifiable E&M service unrelated to the decision to perform the minor surgical procedure is separately reportable with modifier -25. The E&M service and minor surgical procedure do not require different diagnoses. If a minor surgical procedure is performed on a new patient, the same rules for reporting E&M services apply. The fact that the patient is "new" to the provider is not sufficient alone to justify reporting an E&M service on the same date of service as a minor surgical procedure. NCCI contains *many, but not all, possible* edits based on these principles.

Example: If a physician determines that a new patient with head trauma requires sutures, confirms the allergy and immunization status, obtains informed consent, and performs the repair, an E&M service is not separately reportable. However, if the physician also performs a medically reasonable and necessary full neurological examination, an E&M service may be separately reportable.

For major and minor surgical procedures, postoperative E&M services related to recovery from the surgical procedure during the postoperative period are included in the global surgical package as are E&M services related to complications of the surgery. Postoperative visits unrelated to the diagnosis for which the surgical procedure was performed unless related to a complication of surgery may be reported separately on the same day as a surgical procedure with modifier 24 ("Unrelated Evaluation and Management Service by the Same Physician or Other Qualified Health Care Professional During a Postoperative Period").

Procedures with a global surgery indicator of "XXX" are not covered by these rules. Many of these "XXX" procedures are performed by physicians and have inherent pre-procedure, intra-procedure, and post-procedure work usually performed each time the procedure is completed. This work should never be reported as a separate E&M code. Other "XXX" procedures are not usually performed by a physician and have no physician work relative value units associated with them. A physician should never report a separate E&M code with these procedures for the supervision of others performing the procedure or for the interpretation of the procedure. With most "XXX" procedures, the physician may, however, perform a significant and separately identifiable E&M service on the same date of service which may be reported by appending modifier -25 to the E&M code. This E&M service may be related to the same diagnosis necessitating performance of the "XXX" procedure but cannot include any work inherent in the "XXX" procedure, supervision of others performing the "XXX" procedure, or time for interpreting the result of the "XXX" procedure. Appending modifier -25 to a significant, separately identifiable E&M service when performed on the same date of service as an "XXX" procedure is correct coding.

E. Modifiers and Modifier Indicators

1. The AMA *CPT Manual* and CMS define modifiers that may be appended to HCPCS/CPT codes to provide additional information about the services rendered. Modifiers consist of two alphanumeric characters.

Modifiers may be appended to HCPCS/CPT codes only if the clinical circumstances justify the use of the modifier. A modifier should not be appended to a HCPCS/CPT code solely to bypass an NCCI edit if the clinical circumstances do not justify its use. If the Medicare program imposes restrictions on the use of a modifier, the modifier may only be used to bypass an NCCI edit if the Medicare restrictions are fulfilled.

Modifiers that may be used under appropriate clinical circumstances to bypass an NCCI edit include:

Anatomic modifiers: E1-E4, FA, F1-F9, TA, T1-T9, LT, RT, LC, LD, RC, LM, RI
Global surgery modifiers: -24, -25, -57, -58, -78, -79
Other modifiers: -27,-59, -91

Modifiers 76 ("repeat procedure or service by same physician") and 77 ("repeat procedure by another physician") are not NCCI-associated modifiers. Use of either of these modifiers does not bypass an NCCI edit.

Each NCCI edit has an assigned modifier indicator. A modifier indicator of "0" indicates that NCCI-associated modifiers cannot be used to bypass the edit. A modifier indicator of "1" indicates that NCCI-associated modifiers may be used to bypass an edit under appropriate circumstances. A modifier indicator of "9" indicates that the edit has been deleted, and the modifier indicator is not relevant.

It is very important that NCCI-associated modifiers only be used when appropriate. In general these circumstances relate to separate patient encounters, separate anatomic sites or separate specimens. (See subsequent discussion of modifiers in this section.) Most edits involving paired organs or structures (e.g., eyes, ears, extremities, lungs, kidneys) have modifier indicators of "1" because the two codes of the code pair edit may be reported if performed on the contralateral organs or structures. Most of these code pairs should not be reported with NCCI-associated modifiers when performed on the ipsilateral organ or structure unless there is a specific coding rationale to bypass the edit. The existence of the NCCI edit indicates that the two codes generally cannot be reported together unless the two corresponding procedures are performed at two separate patient encounters or two separate anatomic locations. However, if the two corresponding procedures are performed at the same patient encounter and in contiguous structures, NCCI-associated modifiers generally should not be utilized.

The appropriate use of most of these modifiers is straight-forward. However, further explanation is provided about modifiers -25, -58, and -59. Although modifier -22 is not a modifier that bypasses an NCCI edit, its use is occasionally relevant to an NCCI edit and is discussed below.

a) **Modifier -22:** Modifier -22 is defined by the *CPT Manual* as "Increased Procedural Services." This modifier should not be reported routinely but only when the service(s) performed is(are) substantially more extensive than the usual service(s) included in the procedure described by the HCPCS/CPT code reported.

Occasionally a provider may perform two procedures that should not be reported together based on an NCCI edit. If the edit allows use of NCCI-associated modifiers to bypass it and the clinical circumstances justify use of one of these modifiers, both services may be reported with the NCCI-associated modifier. However, if the NCCI edit does not allow use of NCCI-associated modifiers to bypass it and the procedure qualifies as an unusual procedural service, the physician may report the column one HCPCS/CPT code of the NCCI edit with modifier

-22. The Carrier (A/B MAC processing practitioner service claims) may then evaluate the unusual procedural service to determine whether additional payment is justified.

For example, CMS limits payment for CPT code 69990 (microsurgical techniques, requiring use of operating microscope . . .) to procedures listed in the Internet-Only Manual (IOM) (*Claims Processing Manual*, Pub. 100-4, 12-§20.4.5). If a physician reports CPT code 69990 with two other CPT codes and one of the codes is not on this list, an NCCI edit with the code not on the list will prevent payment for CPT code 69990. Claims processing systems do not determine which procedure is linked with CPT code 69990. In situations such as this, the physician may submit his claim to the local carrier (A/B MAC processing practitioner service claims) for readjudication appending modifier 22 to the CPT code. Although the carrier (A/B MAC processing practitioner service claims) cannot override an NCCI edit that does not allow use of NCCI-associated modifiers, the carrier (A/B MAC processing practitioner service claims) has discretion to adjust payment to include use of the operating microscope based on modifier 22.

b) **Modifier -25:** The *CPT Manual* defines modifier -25 as a "significant, separately identifiable evaluation and management service by the same physician *or other qualified health care professional* on the same day of the procedure or other service." Modifier -25 may be appended to an evaluation and management (E&M) CPT code to indicate that the E&M service is significant and separately identifiable from other services reported on the same date of service. The E&M service may be related to the same or different diagnosis as the other procedure(s).

Modifier -25 may be appended to E&M services reported with minor surgical procedures (global period of 000 or 010 days) or procedures not covered by global surgery rules (global indicator of XXX). Since minor surgical procedures and XXX procedures include pre-procedure, intra-procedure, and post-procedure work inherent in the procedure, the provider should not report an E&M service for this work. Furthermore, Medicare Global Surgery rules prevent the reporting of a separate E&M service for the work associated with the decision to perform a minor surgical procedure whether the patient is a new or established patient.

c) **Modifier -58:** Modifier -58 is defined by the *CPT Manual* as a "staged or related procedure or service by the same physician *or other qualified health care professional* during the postoperative period." It may be used to indicate that a procedure was followed by a second procedure during the post-operative period of the first procedure. This situation may occur because the second procedure was planned prospectively, was more extensive than the first procedure, or was therapy after a diagnostic surgical service. Use of modifier -58 will bypass NCCI edits that allow use of NCCI-associated modifiers.

If a diagnostic endoscopic procedure results in the decision to perform an open procedure, both procedures may be reported with modifier -58 appended to the HCPCS/CPT code for the open procedure. However, if the endoscopic procedure preceding an open procedure is a "scout" procedure to assess anatomic landmarks and/or extent of disease, it is not separately reportable.

Diagnostic endoscopy is never separately reportable with another endoscopic procedure of the same organ(s) when performed at the same patient encounter. Similarly, diagnostic laparoscopy is never separately reportable with a surgical laparoscopic procedure of the same body cavity when performed at the same patient encounter.

If a planned laparoscopic procedure fails and is converted to an open procedure, only the open procedure may be reported. The failed laparoscopic procedure is not separately reportable. The NCCI contains many, but not all, edits bundling laparoscopic procedures into open procedures. Since the number of possible code combinations bundling a laparoscopic procedure into an open procedure is much greater than the number of such edits in NCCI, the principle stated in this paragraph is applicable regardless of whether the selected code pair combination is included in the NCCI tables. A provider should not select laparoscopic and open HCPCS/CPT codes to report because the combination is not included in the NCCI tables.

d) **Modifier -59:** Modifier -59 is an important NCCI-associated modifier that is often used incorrectly. For the NCCI its primary purpose is to indicate that two or more procedures are performed at different anatomic sites or different patient encounters. It should only be used if no other modifier more appropriately describes the relationships of the two or more procedure codes. The *CPT Manual* defines modifier -59 as follows:

Modifier -59:11 Distinct Procedural Service: Under certain circumstances, *it* may *be necessary* to indicate that a procedure or service was distinct or independent from other *non E/M* services performed on the same day. Modifier -59 is used to identify procedures/services *other than E/M services* that are not normally reported together, but are appropriate under the circumstances. *Documentation must support* a different session, different procedure or surgery, different site or organ system, separate incision/excision, separate lesion, or separate injury (or area of injury in extensive injuries) not ordinarily encountered or performed on the same day by the same *individual*. However, when another already established modifier is appropriate, it should be used rather than modifier -59. Only if no more descriptive modifier is available, and the use of modifier -59 best explains the circumstances, should modifier -59 be used. *Note: Modifier 59 should not be appended to an E/M service. To report a separate and distinct E/M service with a non-E/M service performed on the same date, see modifier 25.*

NCCI edits define when two procedure HCPCS/CPT codes may not be reported together except under special circumstances. If an edit allows use of NCCI-associated modifiers, the two procedure codes may be reported together when the two procedures are performed at different anatomic sites or different patient encounters. Carrier (A/B MAC processing practitioner service claims) processing systems utilize NCCI-associated modifiers to allow payment of both codes of an edit. Modifier -59 and other NCCI-associated modifiers should NOT be used to bypass an NCCI edit unless the proper criteria for use of the modifier are met. Documentation in the medical record must satisfy the criteria required by any NCCI-associated modifier used.

Some examples of the appropriate use of modifier -59 are contained in the individual chapter policies.

One of the common misuses of modifier -59 is related to the portion of the definition of modifier -59 allowing its use to describe "different procedure or surgery." The code descriptors of the two codes of a code pair edit consisting of two surgical procedures, *two non-surgical therapeutic procedures, and/or two diagnostic procedures* usually represent different procedures or surgeries. The edit indicates that the two procedures/surgeries cannot be reported together if performed at the same anatomic site and same patient encounter. The

provider cannot use modifier -59 for such an edit based on the two codes being different procedures/surgeries. However, if the two procedures/surgeries are performed at separate anatomic sites or at separate patient encounters on the same date of service, modifier -59 may be appended to indicate that they are different procedures/surgeries on that date of service.

There are several exceptions to this general principle about misuse of modifier -59 *that* apply *to some code pair edits for procedures performed at the same patient encounter.*

(1) If *a* diagnostic procedure precedes *a* surgical or *non-surgical therapeutic* procedure and is the basis on which the decision to perform the surgical *or non-surgical therapeutic* procedure is made, the two procedures may be reported with modifier -59 appended to the column two HCPCS/CPT code under appropriate circumstances. However, if the diagnostic procedure is an inherent component of the surgical *or non-surgical therapeutic* procedure, it cannot be reported separately.

(2) If *a* diagnostic procedure follows *a* surgical procedure *or non-surgical therapeutic procedure* at the same patient encounter *and the post-procedure diagnostic procedure is not an inherent component or otherwise included (or not separately payable) post-procedure service of the surgical procedure or non-surgical therapeutic procedure, the two procedures may be reported with* modifier 59 if appropriate.

Use of modifier -59 to indicate different procedures/surgeries does not require a different diagnosis for each HCPCS/CPT coded procedure/surgery. Additionally, different diagnoses are not adequate criteria for use of modifier -59. The HCPCS/CPT codes remain bundled unless the procedures/surgeries are performed at different anatomic sites or separate patient encounters.

From an NCCI perspective, the definition of different anatomic sites includes different organs or different lesions in the same organ. However, it does not include treatment of contiguous structures of the same organ. For example, treatment of the nail, nail bed, and adjacent soft tissue constitutes treatment of a single anatomic site. Treatment of posterior segment structures in the ipsilateral eye constitutes treatment of a single anatomic site. Arthroscopic treatment of a shoulder injury in adjoining areas of the ipsilateral shoulder constitutes treatment of a single anatomic site.

If the same procedure is performed at different anatomic sites, it does not necessarily imply that a HCPCS/CPT code may be reported with more than one unit of service (UOS) for the procedure. Determining whether additional UOS may be reported depends upon the HCPCS/CPT code descriptor and the code's UOS.

Example: The column one/column two code edit with column one CPT code 38221 (bone marrow biopsy) and column two CPT code 38220 (bone marrow, aspiration only) includes two distinct procedures when performed at separate anatomic sites or separate patient encounters. In these circumstances, it would be acceptable to use modifier -59. However, if both 38221 and 38220 are performed through the same skin incision at the same patient encounter which is the usual practice, modifier -59 should NOT be used. Although CMS does not allow separate payment for CPT code 38220 with CPT code 38221 when bone marrow aspiration and biopsy are performed through the same skin incision at a single patient encounter, CMS does allow separate payment for HCPCS level II code G0364 (bone marrow aspiration performed with bone marrow biopsy through same incision on the same date of service) with CPT code 38221 under these circumstances.

F. Standard Preparation/Monitoring Services for Anesthesia

With few exceptions anesthesia HCPCS/CPT codes do not specify the mode of anesthesia for a particular procedure. Regardless of the mode of anesthesia, preparation and monitoring services are not separately reportable with anesthesia service HCPCS/CPT codes when performed in association with the anesthesia service. However, if the provider of the anesthesia service performs one or more of these services prior to and unrelated to the anticipated anesthesia service or after the patient is released from the anesthesia practitioner's postoperative care, the service may be separately reportable with modifier -59.

G. Anesthesia Service Included in the Surgical Procedure

Under the CMS Anesthesia Rules, with limited exceptions, Medicare does not allow separate payment for anesthesia services performed by the physician who also furnishes the medical or surgical service. In this case, payment for the anesthesia service is included in the payment for the medical or surgical procedure. For example, separate payment is not allowed for the physician's performance of local, regional, or most other anesthesia including nerve blocks if the physician also performs the medical or surgical procedure. However, Medicare allows separate reporting for moderate conscious sedation services (CPT codes 99143-99145) when provided by same physician performing a medical or surgical procedure except for those procedures listed in Appendix G of the *CPT Manual*.

CPT codes describing anesthesia services (00100-01999) or services that are bundled into anesthesia should not be reported in addition to the surgical or medical procedure requiring the anesthesia services if performed by the same physician. Examples of improperly reported services that are bundled into the anesthesia service when anesthesia is provided by the physician performing the medical or surgical procedure include introduction of needle or intracatheter into a vein (CPT code 36000), venipuncture (CPT code 36410), intravenous infusion/injection (CPT codes 96360-96368, 96374-96376) or cardiac assessment (e.g., CPT codes 93000-93010, 93040-93042). However, if these services are not related to the delivery of an anesthetic agent, or are not an inherent component of the procedure or global service, they may be reported separately.

The physician performing a surgical or medical procedure should not report an epidural/subarachnoid injection (CPT codes 62310-62319) or nerve block (CPT codes 64400-64530) for anesthesia for that procedure.

H. HCPCS/CPT Procedure Code Definition

The HCPCS/CPT code descriptors of two codes are often the basis of an NCCI edit. If two HCPCS/CPT codes describe redundant services, they should not be reported separately. Several general principles follow:

1. A family of CPT codes may include a CPT code followed by one or more indented CPT codes. The first CPT code descriptor includes a semicolon. The portion of the descriptor of the first code in the family preceding the semicolon is a common part of the descriptor for each subsequent code of the family. For example,

CPT code 70120   Radiologic examination, mastoids; less than three views per side
CPT code 70130   Complete, minimum of three views per side

The portion of the descriptor preceding the semicolon ("Radiologic examination, mastoids") is common to both CPT codes 70120 and 70130. The difference between the two codes is the portion of the descriptors following the semicolon. Often as in this case, two codes from a family may not be reported separately. A physician cannot report CPT codes 70120 and 70130 for a procedure performed on ipsilateral mastoids at the same patient encounter. It is important to recognize, however, that there are numerous circumstances when it may be appropriate to report more than one code from a family of codes. For example, CPT codes 70120 and 70130 may be reported separately if the two procedures are performed on contralateral mastoids or at two separate patient encounters on the same date of service.

2. If a HCPCS/CPT code is reported, it includes all components of the procedure defined by the descriptor. For example, CPT code 58291 includes a vaginal hysterectomy with "removal of tube(s) and/or ovary(s)." A physician cannot report a salpingo-oophorectomy (CPT code 58720) separately with CPT code 58291.

3. CPT code descriptors often define correct coding relationships where two codes may not be reported separately with one another at the same anatomic site and/or same patient encounter. A few examples follow:
   a) A "partial" procedure is not separately reportable with a "complete" procedure.
   b) A "partial" procedure is not separately reportable with a "total" procedure.
   c) A "unilateral" procedure is not separately reportable with a "bilateral" procedure.
   d) A "single" procedure is not separately reportable with a "multiple" procedure.
   e) A "with" procedure is not separately reportable with a "without" procedure.
   f) An "initial" procedure is not separately reportable with a "subsequent" procedure.

I. *CPT Manual* and CMS Coding Manual Instructions

CMS often publishes coding instructions in its rules, manuals, and notices. Physicians must utilize these instructions when reporting services rendered to Medicare patients.

The *CPT Manual* also includes coding instructions which may be found in the "Introduction", individual chapters, and appendices. In individual chapters the instructions may appear at the beginning of a chapter, at the beginning of a subsection of the chapter, or after specific CPT codes. Physicians should follow *CPT Manual* instructions unless CMS has provided different coding or reporting instructions.

The American Medical Association publishes *CPT Assistant* which contains coding guidelines. CMS does not review nor approve the information in this publication. In the development of NCCI edits, CMS occasionally disagrees with the information in this publication. If a physician utilizes information from *CPT Assistant* to report services rendered to Medicare patients, it is possible that Medicare Carriers (A/B MACs processing practitioner service claims) and Fiscal Intermediaries may utilize different criteria to process claims.

J. CPT "Separate Procedure" Definition

If a CPT code descriptor includes the term "separate procedure", the CPT code may not be reported separately with a related procedure. CMS interprets this designation to prohibit the separate reporting of a "separate procedure" when performed with another procedure in an anatomically related region often through the same skin incision, orifice, or surgical approach.

A CPT code with the "separate procedure" designation may be reported with another procedure if it is performed at a separate patient encounter on the same date of service or at the same patient encounter in an anatomically unrelated area often through a separate skin incision, orifice, or surgical approach. Modifier -59 or a more specific modifier (e.g., anatomic modifier) may be appended to the "separate procedure" CPT code to indicate that it qualifies as a separately reportable service.

K. Family of Codes

The *CPT Manual* often contains a group of codes that describe related procedures that may be performed in various combinations. Some codes describe limited component services, and other codes describe various combinations of component services. Physicians must utilize several principles in selecting the correct code to report:

1. A HCPCS/CPT code may be reported if and only if all services described by the code are performed.
2. The HCPCS/CPT code describing the services performed should be reported. A physician should not report multiple codes corresponding to component services if a single comprehensive code describes the services performed. There are limited exceptions to this rule which are specifically identified in this Manual.
3. HCPCS/CPT code(s) corresponding to component service(s) of other more comprehensive HCPCS/CPT code(s) should not be reported separately with the more comprehensive HCPCS/CPT code(s) that include the component service(s).
4. If the HCPCS/CPT codes do not correctly describe the procedure(s) performed, the physician should report a "not otherwise specified" CPT code rather than a HCPCS/CPT code that most closely describes the procedure(s) performed.

L. More Extensive Procedure

The *CPT Manual* often describes groups of similar codes differing in the complexity of the service. Unless services are performed at separate patient encounters or at separate anatomic sites, the less complex service is included in the more complex service and is not separately reportable. Several examples of this principle follow:

1. If two procedures only differ in that one is described as a "simple" procedure and the other as a "complex" procedure, the "simple" procedure is included in the "complex" procedure and is not separately reportable unless the two proce-

dures are performed at separate patient encounters or at separate anatomic sites.
2. If two procedures only differ in that one is described as a "simple" procedure and the other as a "complicated" procedure, the "simple" procedure is included in the "complicated" procedure and is not separately reportable unless the two procedures are performed at separate patient encounters or at separate anatomic sites.
3. If two procedures only differ in that one is described as a "limited" procedure and the other as a "complete" procedure, the "limited" procedure is included in the "complete" procedure and is not separately reportable unless the two procedures are performed at separate patient encounters or at separate anatomic sites.
4. If two procedures only differ in that one is described as an "intermediate" procedure and the other as a "comprehensive" procedure, the "intermediate" procedure is included in the "comprehensive" procedure and is not separately reportable unless the two procedures are performed at separate patient encounters or at separate anatomic sites.
5. If two procedures only differ in that one is described as a "superficial" procedure and the other as a "deep" procedure, the "superficial" procedure is included in the "deep" procedure and is not separately reportable unless the two procedures are performed at separate patient encounters or at separate anatomic sites.
6. If two procedures only differ in that one is described as an "incomplete" procedure and the other as a "complete" procedure, the "incomplete" procedure is included in the "complete" procedure and is not separately reportable unless the two procedures are performed at separate patient encounters or at separate anatomic sites.
7. If two procedures only differ in that one is described as an "external" procedure and the other as an "internal" procedure, the "external" procedure is included in the "internal" procedure and is not separately reportable unless the two procedures are performed at separate patient encounters or at separate anatomic sites.

M. Sequential Procedure

Some surgical procedures may be performed by different surgical approaches. If an initial surgical approach to a procedure fails and a second surgical approach is utilized at the same patient encounter, only the HCPCS/CPT code corresponding to the second surgical approach may be reported. If there are different HCPCS/CPT codes for the two different surgical approaches, the two procedures are considered "sequential", and only the HCPCS/CPT code corresponding to the second surgical approach may be reported. For example, a physician may begin a cholecystectomy procedure utilizing a laparoscopic approach and have to convert the procedure to an open abdominal approach. Only the CPT code for the open cholecystectomy may be reported. The CPT code for the failed laparoscopic cholecystectomy is not separately reportable.

N. Laboratory Panel

The *CPT Manual* defines organ and disease specific panels of laboratory tests. If a laboratory performs all tests included in one of these panels, the laboratory may report the CPT code for the panel or the CPT codes for the individual tests. If the laboratory repeats one of these component tests as a medically reasonable and necessary service on the same date of service, the CPT code corresponding to the repeat laboratory test may be reported with modifier -91 appended.

O. Misuse of Column Two Code with Column One Code

CMS manuals and instructions often describe groups of HCPCS/CPT codes that should not be reported together for the Medicare program. Edits based on these instructions are often included as misuse of column two code with column one code.

A HCPCS/CPT code descriptor does not include exhaustive information about the code. Physicians who are not familiar with a HCPCS/CPT code may incorrectly report the code in a context different than intended. The NCCI has identified HCPCS/CPT codes that are incorrectly reported with other HCPCS/CPT codes as a result of the misuse of the column two code with the column one code. If these edits allow use of NCCI-associated modifiers (modifier indicator of "1"), there are limited circumstances when the column two code may be reported on the same date of service as the column one code. Two examples follow:

1. Three or more HCPCS/CPT codes may be reported on the same date of service. Although the column two code is misused if reported as a service associated with the column one code, the column two code may be appropriately reported with a third HCPCS/CPT code reported on the same date of service. For example, CMS limits separate payment for use of the operating microscope for microsurgical techniques (CPT code 69990) to a group of procedures listed in the online *Claims Processing Manual* (Chapter 12, Section 20.4.5 (Allowable Adjustments)). The NCCI has edits with column one codes of surgical procedures not listed in this section of the manual and column two CPT code of 69990. Some of these edits allow use of NCCI-associated modifiers because the two services listed in the edit may be performed at the same patient encounter as a third procedure for which CPT code 69990 is separately reportable.
2. There may be limited circumstances when the column two code is separately reportable with the column one code. For example, the NCCI has an edit with column one CPT code of 80061 (lipid profile) and column two CPT code of 83721 (LDL cholesterol by direct measurement). If the triglyceride level is less than 400 mg/dl, the LDL is a calculated value utilizing the results from the lipid profile for the calculation, and CPT code 83721 is not separately reportable. However, if the triglyceride level is greater than 400 mg/dl, the LDL may be measured directly and may be separately reportable with CPT code 83721 utilizing an NCCI-associated modifier to bypass the edit.

P. Mutually Exclusive Procedures

Many procedure codes cannot be reported together because they are mutually exclusive of each other. Mutually exclusive procedures cannot reasonably be performed at the same anatomic site or same patient encounter. An example of a mutually exclusive situation is the repair of an organ that can be performed by two different methods. Only one method can be chosen to repair the organ. A second example is a service

that can be reported as an "initial" service or a "subsequent" service. With the exception of drug administration services, the initial service and subsequent service cannot be reported at the same patient encounter.

Q. Gender-Specific Procedures (formerly Designation of Sex)

The descriptor of some HCPCS/CPT codes includes a gender-specific restriction on the use of the code. HCPCS/CPT codes specific for one gender should not be reported with HCPCS/CPT codes for the opposite gender. For example, CPT code 53210 describes a total urethrectomy including cystostomy in a female, and CPT code 53215 describes the same procedure in a male. Since the patient cannot have both the male and female procedures performed, the two CPT codes cannot be reported together.

R. Add-on Codes

Some codes in the *CPT Manual* are identified as "add-on" codes which describe a service that can only be reported in addition to a primary procedure. *CPT Manual* instructions specify the primary procedure code(s) for most add-on codes. For other add-on codes, the primary procedure code(s) is(are) not specified. When the *CPT Manual* identifies specific primary codes, the add-on code should not be reported as a supplemental service for other HCPCS/CPT codes not listed as a primary code.

Add-on codes permit the reporting of significant supplemental services commonly performed in addition to the primary procedure. By contrast, incidental services that are necessary to accomplish the primary procedure (e.g., lysis of adhesions in the course of an open cholecystectomy) are not separately reportable with an add-on code. Similarly, complications inherent in an invasive procedure occurring during the procedure are not separately reportable. For example, control of bleeding during an invasive procedure is considered part of the procedure and is not separately reportable.

In general, NCCI procedure to procedure edits do not include edits with most add-on codes because edits related to the primary procedure(s) are adequate to prevent inappropriate payment for an add-on coded procedure. (I.e., if an edit prevents payment of the primary procedure code, the add-on code should not be paid.) However, NCCI does include edits for some add-on codes when coding edits related to the primary procedures must be supplemented. Examples include edits with add-on *HCPCS/CPT* codes 69990 (microsurgical techniques requiring use of operating microscope) and 95940/95941/ *G0453* (intraoperative neurophysiology testing).

HCPCS/CPT codes that are not designated as add-on codes should not be misused as an add-on code to report a supplemental service. A HCPCS/CPT code may be reported if and only if all services described by the CPT code are performed. A HCPCS/CPT code should not be reported with another service because a portion of the service described by the HCPCS/CPT code was performed with the other procedure. For example: If an ejection fraction is estimated from an echocardiogram study, it would be inappropriate to additionally report CPT code 78472 (cardiac blood pool imaging with ejection fraction) with the echocardiography (CPT code 93307). Although the procedure described by CPT code 78472 includes an ejection fraction, it is measured by gated equilibrium with a radionuclide which is not utilized in echocardiography.

S. Excluded Service

The NCCI does not address issues related to HCPCS/CPT codes describing services that are excluded from Medicare coverage or are not otherwise recognized for payment under the Medicare program.

T. Unlisted Procedure Codes

The *CPT Manual* includes codes to identify services or procedures not described by other HCPCS/CPT codes. These unlisted procedure codes are generally identified as XXX99 or XXXX9 codes and are located at the end of each section or subsection of the manual. If a physician provides a service that is not accurately described by other HCPCS/CPT codes, the service should be reported utilizing an unlisted procedure code. A physician should not report a CPT code for a specific procedure if it does not accurately describe the service performed. It is inappropriate to report the best fit HCPCS/CPT code unless it accurately describes the service performed, and all components of the HCPCS/CPT code were performed. Since unlisted procedure codes may be reported for a very diverse group of services, the NCCI generally does not include edits with these codes.

U. Modified, Deleted, and Added Code Pairs/Edits

Information moved to Introduction chapter, Section (Purpose), Page Intro-5 of this Manual.

V. Medically Unlikely Edits (MUEs)

To lower the Medicare Fee-For-Service Paid Claims Error Rate, CMS has established units of service edits referred to as Medically Unlikely Edit(s) (MUEs).

An MUE for a HCPCS/CPT code is the maximum number of units of service (UOS) under most circumstances allowable by the same provider for the same beneficiary on the same date of service. The ideal MUE value for a HCPCS/CPT code is the unit of service that allows the vast majority of appropriately coded claims to pass the MUE.

All practitioner claims submitted to Carriers (A/B MACs processing practitioner service claims), outpatient facility services claims (Type of Bill 13X, 14X, 85X) submitted to Fiscal Intermediaries (A/B MACs processing facility claims), and supplier claims submitted to Durable Medical Equipment (DME) MACs are tested against MUEs.

*Prior to April 1, 2013, e*ach line of a claim *was* adjudicated separately against the MUE value for the HCPCS/CPT code

reported on that *claim* line. If the unit*s* of service on that claim line exceed*ed* the MUE value, the entire *claim* line *was* denied.

In the April 1, 2013 version of MUE, CMS began introducing date of service (DOS) MUEs. Over time CMS will convert many, but not all, MUEs to DOS MUEs. Since April 1, 2013, MUEs are adjudicated either as claim line edits or DOS edits. If the MUE is adjudicated as a claim line edit, the units of service (UOS) on each claim line are compared to the MUE value for the HCPCS/ CPT code on that claim line. If the UOS exceed the MUE value, all UOS on that claim line are denied. If the MUE is adjudicated as a DOS MUE, all UOS on each claim line for the same date of service for the same HCPCS/CPT code are summed, and the sum is compared to the MUE value. If the summed UOS exceed the MUE value, all UOS for the HCPCS/CPT code for that date of service are denied. Denials due to claim line MUEs or DOS MUEs may be appealed to the local claims processing contractor. DOS MUEs are utilized for HCPCS/CPT codes where it would be extremely unlikely that more UOS than the MUE value would ever be performed on the same date of service for the same patient.

If a *HCPCS/CPT code has an MUE that is adjudicated as a claim line edit,* appropriate use of CPT modifiers (e.g., -59, -76, -77, -91, anatomic) *may be used to the* same HCPCS/CPT code on separate lines of a claim. *E*ach line *of the claim with that HCPCS/ CPT code will be* separately adjudicated against the MUE value for that HCPCS/CPT code. Claims processing contractors have rules limiting use of these modifiers with some HCPCS/CPT codes.

UOS denied based on an MUE may be appealed.

The MUE value for each HCPCS/CPT code is based on one or more of the following considerations:

(1) Anatomic considerations may limit units of service based on anatomic structures. For example, the MUE value for an appendectomy is 1 since there is only one appendix.
(2) CPT code descriptors/CPT coding instructions in the *CPT Manual* may limit units of service. For example, a procedure described as the "initial 30 minutes" would have an MUE value of 1 because of the use of the term "initial".
(3) Edits based on established CMS policies may limit units of service. For example,the bilateral surgery indicator on the Medicare Physician Fee Schedule Database(MPFSDB) may limit reporting of bilateral procedures.
(4) The nature of an analyte may limit units of service and is in general determined by one of three considerations:
    a) The nature of the specimen may limit the units of service as for a test requiring a 24 hour urine specimen.
    b) The nature of the test may limit the units of service as for a test that requires 24 hours to perform.
    c) The physiology, pathophysiology, or clinical application of the analyte is such that a maximum unit of service for a single date of service can be determined. For example, the MUE for RBC folic acid level is one since the test would only be necessary once on a single date of service.
(5) The nature of a procedure/service may limit units of service and is in general determined by the amount of time required to perform a procedure/service (e.g., overnight sleep studies) or clinical application of a procedure/service (e.g., motion analysis tests).
(6) The nature of equipment may limit units of service and is in general determined by the number of items of equipment that would be utilized (e.g., cochlear implant or wheelchair).

(7) Clinical judgment considerations are based on input from numerous physicians and certified coders.

(8) Submitted claims data (100%) from a six month period is utilized.

HCPCS J code and drug related C and Q code MUEs are based on prescribing information and 100% claims data for a six month period of time. Utilizing the prescribing information the highest total daily dose for each drug was determined. This dose and its corresponding units of service were evaluated against paid and submitted claims data. Some of the guiding principles utilized in developing these edits are as follows:

(1) If the prescribing information defined a maximum daily dose, this value was used to determine the MUE value. For some drugs there is an absolute maximum daily dose. For others there is a maximum "recommended" or "usual" dose. In the latter of the two cases, the daily dose calculation was evaluated against claims data.

(2) If the maximum daily dose calculation is based on actual body weight, a dose based on a weight range of 110-150 kg was evaluated against the claims data. If the maximum daily dose calculation is based on ideal body weight, a dose based on a weight range of 90-110 kg was evaluated against claims data. If the maximum daily dose calculation is based on body surface area (BSA), a dose based on a BSA range of 2.4-3.0 square meters was evaluated against claims data.

(3) For "as needed" (PRN) drugs and drugs where maximum daily dose is based on patient response, prescribing information and claims data were utilized to establish MUE values.

(4) Published off label usage of a drug was considered for the maximum daily dose calculation.

(5) The MUE values for some drug codes are set to 0. The rationale for such values include but are not limited to: discontinued manufacture of drug, non-FDA approved compounded drug, practitioner MUE values for oral anti-neoplastic, oral anti-emetic, and oral immune suppressive drugs which should be billed to the DME MACs, and outpatient hospital MUE values for inhalation drugs which should be billed to the DME MACs.

The first MUEs were implemented January 1, 2007. Additional MUEs are added on a quarterly basis on the same schedule as NCCI updates. Prior to implementation proposed MUEs are sent to numerous national healthcare organizations for a sixty day review and comment period.

Many surgical procedures may be performed bilaterally. Instructions in the CMS *Internet Only Manual* (Publication 100-04 *Medicare Claims Processing Manual,* Chapter 12 (Physicians/Nonphysician Practitioners), Section 40.7.B. and Chapter 4 (Part B Hospital (Including Inpatient Hospital Part B and OPPS)), Section 20.6.2 require that bilateral surgical procedures be reported using modifier 50 with one unit of service. If a bilateral surgical procedure is performed at different sites bilaterally (e.g.,transforaminal epidural injections (CPT codes 64480, 64484)), one unit of service may be reported for each site. That is, the HCPCS/CPT code may be reported with modifier 50 and one unit of service for each site at which it was performed bilaterally.

Some A/B MACs allow providers to report repetitive services performed over a range of dates on a single line of a claim with multiple units of service. If a provider reports services in this fashion, the provider should report the "from date" and "to date" on the claim line. Contractors are instructed to divide the units of service reported on the claim line by the number of days in the date span and round to the nearest whole number. This number is compared to the MUE value for the code on the claim line.

Suppliers billing services to the DME MACs typically report some HCPCS codes for supply items for a period exceeding a single day. The DME MACs have billing rules for these codes. For some codes the DME MACs require that the "from date" and "to date" be reported. The MUEs for these codes are based on the maximum number of units of service that may be reported for a single date of service. For other codes the DME MACs permit multiple days' supply items to be reported on a single claim line where the "from date" and "to date" are the same. The DME MACs have rules allowing supply items for a maximum number of days to be reported at one time for each of these types of codes. The MUE values for these codes are based on the maximum number of days that may be reported at one time. As with all MUEs, the MUE value does not represent a utilization guideline. Suppliers should not assume that they may report units of service up to the MUE value on each date of service. Suppliers may only report supply items that are medically reasonable and necessary.

A denial of services due to an MUE is a coding denial, not a medical necessity denial. A provider/supplier may not issue an Advanced Beneficiary Notice of Noncoverage (ABN) in connection with services denied due to an MUE and cannot bill the beneficiary for units of service denied based on an MUE.

Most MUE values are set so that a provider or supplier would only very occasionally have a claim line denied. If a provider encounters a code with frequent denials due to the MUE, or frequent use of a CPT modifier to bypass the MUE, the provider or supplier should consider the following: (1) Is the HCPCS/CPT code being used correctly? (2) Is the unit of service being counted correctly? (3) Are all reported services medically reasonable and necessary? and (4) Why does the provider's or supplier's practice differ from national patterns? A provider or supplier may choose to discuss these questions with the local Medicare contractor or a national healthcare organization whose members frequently perform the procedure.

Most MUE values are published on the CMS MUE webpage (http://www.cms.gov/medicare/coding/NationalCorrectCodInitEd/MUE.html). However, some MUE values are not published and are confidential. These values should not be published in oral or written form by any party that acquires one or more of them.

MUEs are not utilization edits. Although the MUE value for some codes may represent the commonly reported units of service (e.g., MUE of "1" for appendectomy), the usual units of service for many HCPCS/CPT codes is less than the MUE value. Claims reporting units of service less than the MUE value may be subject to review by claims processing contractors, Program Safeguard Contractors (PSCs), Zoned Program Integrity Contractors (ZPICs), Recovery Audit Contractors (RACs), and Department of Justice (DOJ).

Since MUEs are coding edits rather than medical necessity edits, claims processing contractors may have units of service edits that are more restrictive than MUEs. In such cases, the more restrictive claims processing contractor edit would be applied to the claim. Similarly, if the MUE is more restrictive than a claims processing contractor edit, the more restrictive MUE would apply.

A provider, supplier, healthcare organization, or other interested party may request reconsideration of an MUE value for a HCPCS/CPT code. A written request proposing an alternative MUE with rationale may be sent to:

National Correct Coding Initiative
Correct Coding Solutions, LLC
P.O. Box 907
Carmel, IN 46082-0907
Fax: 317-571-1745

W. Add-on Code Edit Tables

Add-on codes are discussed in Chapter I, Section R (Add-on Codes). *CMS publishes a list of add-on codes and their primary codes annually prior to January 1. The list is updated quarterly based on the AMA's "CPT Errata" documents or implementation of new HCPCS/CPT add-on codes. CMS identifies add-on codes and their primary codes based on CPT Manual instructions, CMS interpretation of HCPCS/CPT codes, and CMS coding instructions.*

The NCCI program includes three Add-on Code Edit Tables, one table for each of three "Types" of add-on codes. Each table lists the add-on code with its primary codes. An add-on code, with one exception, is eligible for payment if and only if one of its primary codes is also eligible for payment.

The "Type I Add-on Code Edit Table" lists add-on codes for which the CPT Manual or HCPCS tables define all acceptable primary codes. Claims processing contractors should not allow other primary codes with Type I add-on codes. CPT code 99292 (Critical care, evaluation and management of the critically ill or critically injured patient; each additional 30 minutes (List separately in addition to code for primary service)) is included as a Type I add-on code since its only primary code is CPT code 99291 (Critical care, evaluation and management of the critically ill or critically injured patient; first 30-74 minutes). For Medicare purposes, CPT code 99292 may be eligible for payment to a physician without CPT code 99291 if another physician of the same specialty and physician group reports and is paid for CPT code 99291.

The "Type II Add-on Code Edit Table" lists add-on codes for which the CPT Manual and HCPCS tables do not define any primary codes. Claims processing contractors should develop their own lists of acceptable primary codes.

The "Type III Add-on Code Edit Table" lists add-on codes for which the CPT Manual or HCPCS tables define some, but not all, acceptable primary codes. Claims processing contractors should allow the listed primary codes for these add-on codes but may develop their own lists of additional acceptable primary codes.

Although the add-on code and primary code are normally reported for the same date of service, there are unusual circumstances where the two services may be reported for different dates of service (e.g., CPT codes 99291 and 99292).

The first Add-On Code edit tables were implemented April 1, 2013. For subsequent years, new Add-On Code edit tables will be published to be effective for January 1 of the new year based on changes in the new year's CPT Manual. CMS also issues quarterly updates to the Add-On Code edit tables if required due to publication of new HCPCS/CPT codes or changes in add-on codes or their primary codes. The changes in the quarterly update files (April 1, July 1, or October 1) are retroactive to the implementation date of that year's annual Add-On Code edit files unless the files specify a different effective date for a change. Since the first Add-On Code edit files were implemented on April 1, 2013, changes in the July 1 and October 1 quarterly updates for 2013 were retroactive to April 1, 2013 unless the files specified a different effective date for a change.

FIGURE CREDITS

1. From Little J et al: *Dental management of the medically compromised patient*, ed 7, St. Louis, 2008, Mosby. *(Courtesy Medtronic, Minneapolis)*
2. From Roberts J, Hedges J: *Clinical procedures in emergency medicine*, ed 4, Philadelphia, 2004, Saunders.
3. Modified from Grosfeld J et al: *Pediatric surgery*, ed 6, Philadelphia, 2006, Mosby.
4. Modified from Hsu J, Michael J, Fisk J: *AAOS atlas of orthoses and assistive devices*, ed 4, Philadelphia, 2008, Mosby.
5. From Dionne R, Phero J, Becker D: *Management of pain and anxiety in the dental office*, ed 1, St. Louis, 2002, Saunders.
6. Modified from Roberts J, Hedges J: *Clinical procedures in emergency medicine*, ed 4, St. Louis, 2004, Saunders.
7. From Auerbach P: *Wilderness medicine*, ed 5, Philadelphia, 2007, Mosby. (Courtesy Black Diamond Equipment, Ltd.)
8. *(Original to book).*
9. Modified from Abeloff M et al: *Clinical oncology*, ed 3, Philadelphia, 2004, Churchill Livingstone.
10. *(Original to book).*
11. Modified from Duthie E, Katz P, Malone M: *Practice of geriatrics*, ed 4, Philadelphia, 2007, Saunders.
12. Modified from Roberts J, Hedges J: *Clinical procedures in emergency medicine*, ed 4, St. Louis, 2004, Saunders.
13. From Albert R, Spiro S, Jett J: *Clinical respiratory medicine*, ed 2, Philadelphia, 2004, Mosby.
14. From Young A, Proctor D: *Kinn's the medical assistant*, ed 9, St. Louis, 2003, Saunders.
15. From Bonewit-West K: *Clinical procedures for medical assistants*, ed 5, Philadelphia, 2000, WB Saunders.
16. From Roberts J, Hedges J: *Clinical procedures in emergency medicine*, ed 4, St. Louis, 2004, Saunders.
17. From Yeo: *Shackelford's surgery of the alimentary tract*, ed 6, Philadelphia, 2007, Saunders.
18. Redrawn from Bragg D, Rubin P, Hricak H: *Oncologic imaging*, ed 2, 2002, Saunders.
19. From Lewis S, Bain B, Bates I: *Dacie and Lewis practical haematology*, ed 10, Philadelphia, 2006, Churchill Livingstone.
20. From Roberts J, Hedges J: *Clinical procedures in emergency medicine*, ed 4, St. Louis, 2004, Saunders. *(Courtesy Atrium Medical Corp., Hudson, NH 03051)*
21. **A** From Auerbach P: *Wilderness medicine*, ed 5, Philadelphia, 2007, Mosby. **B** Modified from Hsu J, Michael J, Fisk J: *AAOS atlas of orthoses and assistive devices*, ed 4, Philadelphia, 2008, Mosby.
22. Modified from Lusardi M, Nielsen C: *Orthotics and prosthetics in rehabilitation*, ed 2, St. Louis, 2006, Butterworth-Heinemann.
23. Modified from Lusardi M, Nielsen C: *Orthotics and prosthetics in rehabilitation*, ed 2, St. Louis, 2006, Butterworth-Heinemann.
24. Modified from Lusardi M, Nielsen C: *Orthotics and prosthetics in rehabilitation*, ed 2, St. Louis, 2006, Butterworth-Heinemann.
25. From Buck C: *The next step, advanced medical coding 2009 edition*, St. Louis, 2008, Saunders.
26. From Lusardi M, Nielsen C: *Orthotics and prosthetics in rehabilitation*, ed 2, St. Louis, 2006, Butterworth-Heinemann.
27. From Hsu J, Michael J, Fisk J: *AAOS atlas of orthoses and assistive devices*, ed 4, Philadelphia, 2008, Mosby.
28. Modified from Hsu J, Michael J, Fisk J: *AAOS atlas of orthoses and assistive devices*, ed 4, Philadelphia, 2008, Mosby.
29. Modified from Hsu J, Michael J, Fisk J: *AAOS atlas of orthoses and assistive devices*, ed 4, Philadelphia, 2008, Mosby.
30. From Hsu J, Michael J, Fisk J: *AAOS atlas of orthoses and assistive devices*, ed 4, Philadelphia, 2008, Mosby.
31. From Lusardi M, Nielsen C: *Orthotics and prosthetics in rehabilitation*, ed 2, St. Louis, 2006, Butterworth-Heinemann.
32. From Lusardi M, Nielsen C: *Orthotics and prosthetics in rehabilitation*, ed 2, St. Louis, 2006, Butterworth-Heinemann.
33. Modified from Lusardi M, Nielsen C: *Orthotics and prosthetics in rehabilitation*, ed 2, St. Louis, 2006, Butterworth-Heinemann.
34. From Hsu J, Michael J, Fisk J: *AAOS atlas of orthoses and assistive devices*, ed 4, Philadelphia, 2008, Mosby.
35. *(Original to book.)*
36. From Lusardi M, Nielsen C: *Orthotics and prosthetics in rehabilitation*, ed 2, St. Louis, 2006, Butterworth-Heinemann.
37. Modified from Hsu J, Michael J, Fisk J: *AAOS atlas of orthoses and assistive devices*, ed 4, Philadelphia, 2008, Mosby.
38. From Canale S: *Campbell's operative orthopaedics*, ed 10, St. Louis, 2003, Mosby.
39. Modified from Canale S: *Campbell's operative orthopaedics*, ed 10, St. Louis, 2003, Mosby.
40. From Canale S: *Campbell's operative orthopaedics*, ed 10, St. Louis, 2003, Mosby.
41. From Lusardi M, Nielsen C: *Orthotics and prosthetics in rehabilitation*, ed 2, St. Louis, 2006, Butterworth-Heinemann.
42. Modified from Lusardi M, Nielsen C: *Orthotics and prosthetics in rehabilitation*, ed 2, St. Louis, 2006, Butterworth-Heinemann.
43. From Lusardi M, Nielsen C: *Orthotics and prosthetics in rehabilitation*, ed 2, St. Louis, 2006, Butterworth-Heinemann. *(Courtesy Michael Curtain)*
44. Modified from Lusardi M, Nielsen C: *Orthotics and prosthetics in rehabilitation*, ed 2, St. Louis, 2006, Butterworth-Heinemann.
45. Modified from Bland K, Copeland E: *The breast: comprehensive management of benign and malignant disorders*, ed 3, St. Louis, 2004, Saunders.
46. From Cummings C et al: *Cummings otolaryngology: head and neck surgery*, ed 4, Philadelphia, 2005, Mosby.
47. Modified from Cummings C et al: *Cummings otolaryngology: head and neck surgery*, ed 4, Philadelphia, 2005, Mosby.
48. From Weinzweig J: *Plastic surgery secrets*, ed 1, Philadelphia, 1999, Hanley & Belfus, p 543.
49. Modified from Mann D: *Heart failure: a companion to Braunwald's heart disease*, ed 1, Philadelphia, 2004, Saunders.
50. Modified from Roberts J, Hedges J: *Clinical procedures in emergency medicine*, ed 4, Philadelphia, 2004, Saunders.
51. From Yanoff M, Duker J: *Ophthalmology*, ed 2, St. Louis, 2004, Mosby.
52. From Feldman M, Friedman L, Brandt L: *Sleisenger and Fordtran's gastrointestinal and liver disease*, ed 8, Philadelphia, 2006, Saunders.
53. From Katz V et al: *Comprehensive gynecology*, ed 5, Philadelphia, 2007, Mosby.
54. From Young A, Proctor D: *Kinn's the medical assistant*, ed 10, St. Louis, 2007, Saunders.
55. Modified from National Kidney and Urologic Diseases Information Clearinghouse: (http://kidney.niddk.nih.gov/kudiseases/pubs/stonesadults/index.htm)
56. From Yanoff M, Duker J: *Ophthalmology*, ed 2, St. Louis, 2004, Mosby.

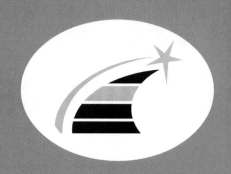
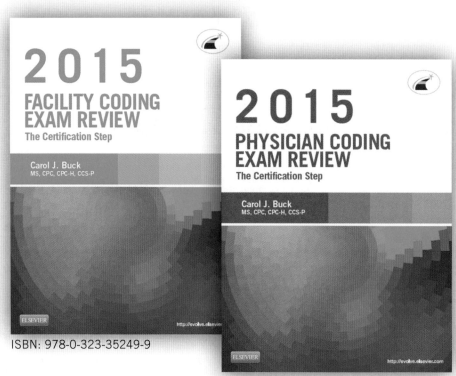
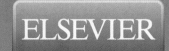

Trust Elsevier.
We've got you covered.

When it comes to preparing for ICD-10,

we've got you covered.

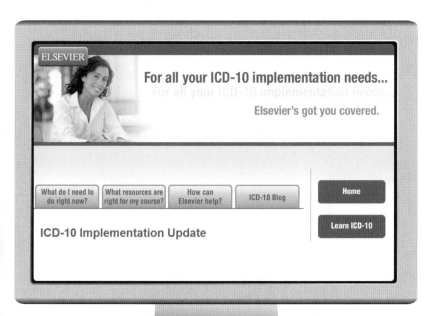

- Learn how to transition from ICD-9-CM to ICD-10-CM/PCS.

- Develop your plan to teach ICD-10-CM/PCS to students.

- Articles, updates, and webinars provide guidance for integrating ICD-10 into your program.

Count on the leader in coding education for everything you need to train your staff, teach your students, and transition your program.

Learn more at www.icd10educators.com!

ELSEVIER

Content

Simulations

Courses

Study Tools

Educator Support

Trust Elsevier
to provide your complete curriculum solution!

Content

978-0-323-27981-9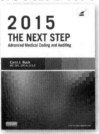

2015
STEP-BY-STEP
Medical Coding

Carol J. Buck

978-0-323-27983-3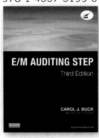

2015
THE NEXT STEP
Advanced Medical Coding and Auditing

Carol J. Buck

978-1-4557-5199-0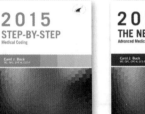

E/M AUDITING STEP
Third Edition

CAROL J. BUCK

Study Tools

978-0-323-27980-2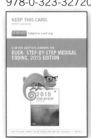

WORKBOOK

2015
STEP-BY-STEP
Medical Coding

Carol J. Buck

978-0-323-32720-6

KEEP THIS CARD.

ELSEVIER Adaptive Learning

ELSEVIER ADAPTIVE LEARNING FOR
BUCK: STEP-BY-STEP MEDICAL
CODING, 2015 EDITION

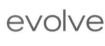

evolve

Simulations

978-0-323-23937-0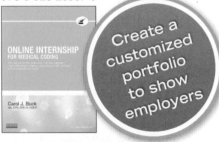

ONLINE INTERNSHIP
FOR MEDICAL CODING

Carol J. Buck

 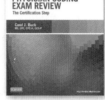

Create a customized portfolio to show employers

978-0-323-35248-2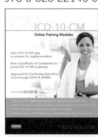

2015
PHYSICIAN CODING
EXAM REVIEW
The Certification Step

Carol J. Buck

978-0-323-35249-9

2015
FACILITY CODING
EXAM REVIEW
The Certification Step

Carol J. Buck

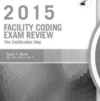

More study tools available

Courses

978-0-323-31994-2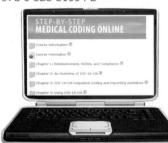

STEP-BY-STEP
MEDICAL CODING ONLINE

Course Information
Course Orientation
Chapter 1: Reimbursement, HIPAA, and Compliance
Chapter 2: An Overview of ICD-10-CM
Chapter 3: ICD-10-CM Outpatient Coding and Reporting Guidelines
Chapter 4: Using ICD-10-CM

Educator Support

978-0-323-22145-0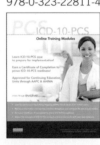

ICD-10-CM
Online Training Modules

978-0-323-22811-4

ICD-10-PCS
Online Training Modules

evolve

Learn more at Elsevieradvantage.com!